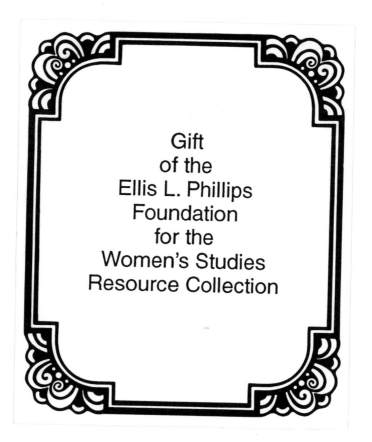

NURSE-MIDWIFERY

Second Edition

NURSE-MIDWIFERY

Second Edition

Helen Varney, C.N.M., M.S.N.

Professor and Chairperson
Maternal-Newborn Nursing/Nurse-Midwifery Program
Yale University School of Nursing
New Haven, Connecticut

BLACKWELL SCIENTIFIC PUBLICATIONS

BOSTON OXFORD LONDON EDINBURGH PALO ALTO MELBOURNE

Blackwell Scientific Publications, Inc.
© 1980, 1987 by Blackwell Scientific Publications, Inc.
Printed in the United States of America
5

Library of Congress Cataloging-in-Publication Data

Varney, Helen.
    Nurse-midwifery.

    Includes bibliographies and index.
    1. Obstetrical nursing.   2. Obstetrics.
3. Midwives.   I. Title.
RG951.V35   1987   618.2   86-34340
ISBN 0-86542-027-0

Blackwell Scientific Publications
Editorial Offices:
    52 Beacon Street, Boston, Massachusetts 02108, USA
    Osney Mead, Oxford OX2 0EL, England
    8 John Street, London, WC1N 2ES, England
    23 Ainslie Place, Edinburgh, EH3 6AJ, Scotland
    107 Barry Street, Carlton, Victoria 3053, Australia
    667 Lytton Avenue, Palo Alto, California 94301, USA

Distributors:
USA
    Blackwell Mosby Book Distributors
    11830 Westline Industrial Drive
    St. Louis, MO 63146
Canada
    The C.V. Mosby Company
    5240 Finch Avenue East
    Scarborough, Ontario
Australia
    Blackwell Scientific Publications, Pty., Ltd.
    107 Barry Street
    Carlton, Victoria, 3053
Outside North American and Australia
    Blackwell Scientific Publications, Ltd.
    Osney Mead
    Oxford OX2 0EL
    England

Typeset by Setrite Typesetters Ltd.
Printed and bound by the Maple Vail Book
    Manufacturing Group
Cover by BEC Design

*In tribute to Therese Dondero and all other
Certified Nurse-Midwives whose masterly
contributions to our profession were tragically
curtailed because of untimely death.*

Dedication to the first edition

*For my students, peers, and colleagues; the
profession of nurse-midwifery; and the women,
mothers, babies, and families who receive health
care from those who study this book*

Contents

VII. Skills (Continued)

Preface

The First Edition of this book reflected the basic practice of nurse-midwifery in the United States. The Second Edition addresses the full scope of nurse-midwifery practice in the United States thereby adding the two ends of a continuum that extends from home birth to collaborative management of high-risk patients with physicians in tertiary medical centers.

The process of addressing the full scope of nurse-midwifery practice entailed a rethinking of the philosophy and definition of nurse-midwifery. A commonly held viewpoint is that nurse-midwifery is the management of the health care of *only* normal, or essentially normal, women. A review of our history is instructive because it is quickly obvious that nurse-midwifery was never limited to "normal" or "low-risk" childbearing women. The women in the remote areas of the Kentucky mountains in 1925, or in the Madera County, California project, or in Mississippi, or in the city hospitals of New York City, or any of the number of other underserved areas where nurse-midwives have reduced perinatal and infant mortality and prematurity rates and increased birth weights, were high-risk, or at-risk, and rarely low-risk. The education of

nurse-midwives has always emphasized screening for the earliest possible signs and symptoms of an existing or developing complication. The profession has unshakably believed that nurse-midwives must work in a health care system that provides for physician consultation, collaboration, and referral. Such emphasis on screening and relationships with physicians clearly reflects concerns emanating from working with at-risk or high-risk populations from the beginning of our profession in the United States.

In the days when nurse-midwives worked only with underserved, and therefore at-risk or high-risk, populations, it was assumed that the nurse-midwife managed the care of the woman as long as she was essentially normal, consulted when there was any evidence of complications, and continued to care for the woman in a collaborative relationship with the physician. It was always entirely possible that if a woman remained essentially healthy that she would never see a physician. This did not deny, however, the role of the nurse-midwife in contributing to the collaborative management of at-risk or high-risk patients if they developed complications nor the focus of the nurse-midwife upon those aspects of childbearing which are normal in any woman, regardless of how complex her obstetric care becomes.

It was not until nurse-midwifery included the private patient sector in the early 1970's that nurse-midwives began taking care of women from an essentially healthy, largely normal or low-risk population. Many of these women were seeking health care that involved them and their families in knowledgeable participatory decision making and which supported natural, normal processes. They found this in the care given by nurse-midwives. Some of them were disenchanted with technology and displeased with routine hospital maternity care. Nurse-midwives responded by being advocates for the women (both normal and complicated) who remained within the hospital health care system and by providing care to carefully screened, normal childbearing women in out-of-hospital settings.

Being able to work with a variety of populations has meant that some nurse-midwives focus on one or another of these populations and thus apply the basic practice of nurse-midwifery to either end of the continuum. Those who work solely with a middle/upper class, educated, healthy population in an out-of-hospital setting have a different world view of the practice of nurse-midwifery than those nurse-midwives who work solely with a lower socio-economic, complicated population in a tertiary medical center. This has led at times to a sense of dichotomy or of nurse-midwives on either end of the continuum being out of harmony with either accepted practice or with our basic definition. Not true. Our history encompasses the care of women in all settings. Our focus on normal does not define or limit our patient populations; it simply defines our area of expertise regardless of the population.

This edition of *Nurse-Midwifery*, thus adds the two ends of the continuum. Chapter 20 is a new chapter which focuses on out-of-hospital birth and the responsibilities of both the consumer and the nurse-midwife in that setting.

At the other end of the continuum Chapters 9 and 14 on antepartal and intrapartal complications have been completely rewritten and expanded to reflect the contribution the nurse-midwife makes to the collaborative management of complicated patients. These two chapters also add topics not included in the First Edition such as size/dates discrepancy, small-for-dates, large-for-dates, postdates, oligohydramnios, preterm labor, etc. Chapters 57 and 58 on manual removal of the placenta and intrauterine exploration were added because of recognition that these are essential skills for a nurse-midwife to know in any setting in the event of an emergency. This led to changes in Chapters 17 and 19 on the management of third and fourth stage hemorrhage.

All chapters and bibliographies have been critically scrutinized, updated, and content expanded, added or deleted as indicated. I made a deliberate last minute decision to retain the chapter on intrauterine contraceptive devices (Chapter 31) after they were removed from the market because 1) some women we care for still have them, 2) some Certified Nurse-Midwives practice in other countries where they are still available, and 3) I believe they someday once again will be available in the United States and we need to have that knowledge. The removal of Nisentil from the market did not happen until too late to make changes in Chapter 12. The dedication, preface, and acknowledgments to the First Edition were retained for historical purposes and because the purpose of this book and the educational principles used in its writing have not changed and are articulated in the preface to the First Edition.

Once again I welcome comments from readers including suggestions "which will enable me to ever better meet the needs of our students, our colleagues, and ourselves in this book."

Helen Varney Burst
New Haven, Connecticut

Preface to the First Edition

This book was written because it needed to be written. As a nurse-midwifery educator I quickly became aware of my students' frustration in trying to piece together what the practice of nurse-midwifery is from a conglomeration of American nursing and medical literature and English midwifery texts. The former was either too superficial or too much in depth with too little detail, while the latter were not always applicable to the practice of nurse-midwifery in the United States. This affected, in part, the content of this book. For example, the section on skills (Part VII) was written because the medical texts are woefully inadequate in explaining to non-physicians how to perform traditionally medical procedures. Consequently faculty in the different nurse-midwifery programs have written their own procedures or borrowed from other programs. Nurse-midwifery educators are characterized by their willingness to help each other and to share their materials with their peers. This has resulted in a sizable body of unpublished literature. What a student in any given program might actually get, however, varies considerably from program to program. The rest has been taught in the oral tradition from teacher to student, from demonstration to demonstration, from generation to generation. All have learned, and learned well, but at the price of frustration for the student and endless repetition for the teacher.

Several educational principles have guided the writing of this book. A primary one has been that learning takes place best when used. For this reason the anatomical, physiological, and psychological bases for what is being observed and the rationale for action are given together rather than in separate and discrete chapters. This has been reinforced by my belief that the nurse-midwifery management process is the core of any nurse-midwifery curriculum. I first articulated the rudiments of this process in Mississippi based in part on my observations and analyses of my own and others' thought processes when managing the care of patients. Others have since added their own interpretations. The one presented in this book is a composite drawn from many minds. Learning the nurse-midwifery management process is facilitated by basic educational principles of application and reinforcement. In turn, the design of the process is such as to foster the utilization of these basic educational principles in teaching.

This book has a definite hospital orientation, in part because this is what I know, and in part because this is where the basic education of students usually takes place. This orientation is not meant to imply any questioning of the value of out-of-hospital birth settings nor to reflect any personal reservations on my part in relation to them. Future editions of NURSE-MIDWIFERY will include expanded coverage of nurse-midwifery practice in out-of-hospital birth settings, additional aspects of care during the interconceptional period, and comprehensive care of the pregnant adolescent as a specialty area.

Finally, I have designed this book so that it will be of value as a permanent reference not only to nurse-midwifery students but to all those who are involved in the care of women and of the childbearing family. I welcome comments from readers including suggestions which will enable me to ever better meet the needs of our students, our colleagues, and ourselves in this book.

Helen Varney Burst
New Haven, Connecticut

Acknowledgments

Writing a new edition is quite different from writing the original text. The original text was based on what I knew, had practiced and taught for a number of years. I wanted, however, in the Second Edition to include some aspects of practice with which I was not as well versed. Since I refuse to write what I do not know and have not done myself, writing the Second Edition required some preparation and expansion of my own scope of practice.

I owe a debt of gratitude to four very special C.N.M. friends who generously gave of themselves and allowed me to practice with them in their settings. With three of them I had the greatest joy and fulfillment a teacher can have: that of working with former students who now were teaching me.

My odyssey for the Second Edition began with Judy Edwards, C.N.M., M.S. with whom I began the transition away from 20 years experience in delivery rooms in tertiary medical centers. The patients in the obstetrical practice Judy is in deliver in a Level I New Hampshire community hospital which has a nursing staff supportive of all possible alternatives and delivery positions. Judy's experienced, laid-back and honest approach provided a safe setting for me to accept the welcome challenge of learning what for me were new methods of delivery.

My education in this vein culminated with Judy Kier, C.N.M., M.S.N. in her combination birth center and home birth practice, Women's Health Care Associates in Houston, Texas. Under Judy's thoughtful, analytical, and articulate toutelage I expanded my mind in the realm of alternative modalities. I also learned the basics of out-of-hospital practice. This learning is reflected in Chapter 20. A special thank you goes to Cheryl, Tom, and Ashley Marie Linn who shared their life and home birth with me and to Susan Melnikow, C.N.M. who completely integrated me into the experience.

Susan Wente, C.N.M., M.P.H., Director of Midwifery at Baylor Medical College/Jefferson Davis Hospital in Houston, Texas spent precious time with me as I learned the procedures of manual removal of the placenta and intrauterine exploration (Chapters 57 and 58). What Susan has accomplished in a health care and hospital system that has the largest number of deliveries in the country is a pre-eminent model which served to remind me of the immense impact public health oriented nurse-midwifery can have.

Therese Dondero, C.N.M., B.S.N., Director

of Midwifery, North Central Bronx Hospital, New York, not only shared her unique setting with me but challenged me to remember my own early teachings and to rethink, again, the philosophy, definition, and scope of practice of nurse-midwifery. She entered this soul-searching thought process with me and then joined with me in the outcome of this process by co-authoring the total rewrite and expansion of Chapters 9 and 14. She also was influential in the review and discussion of parts of Chapters 3, 15, 17, 19, 20, 57, and 58. A year and a half of driving down and up the Merritt Parkway to accomplish this not only reinforced my enjoyment of that drive but also built a fund of shared time and thoughts with Therese which I treasure.

Kate McHugh, C.N.M., M.S.N. accepted the job of reviewing, updating, and rewriting the section on the Neonate (Chapters 21, 22, and 23). Kate is a former neonatal intensive care nurse specialist and a former Yale nurse-midwifery faculty member who taught the Neonatal Module. It was good to once again work and enjoy lively and purposeful discussion with her.

I said in the preface to the first edition that I would welcome comments and suggestions. A few wrote thoughtful and specifically detailed letters: Doris Abbott, C.N.M., M.P.H., Patricia Deibel, C.N.M., B.S.N., Helen Gabel, C.N.M., M.S.N., Mary Alice Johnson, C.N.M., M.S.N., and Phyllis Long, C.N.M., M.S.N. Into this category must also go the helpful book review written by Mary Widhalm, C.N.M., M.S. Many other C.N.M.'s wrote or spoke to me with useful tidbits which ranged from clinical observations to missing categories in the index. Elisabeth Genley, C.N.M., M.S.N. felt so strongly about the deficits of the index while a student that she became the indexer for this edition. In addition, Rochelle Kanell, C.N.M., M.S. undertook the initial critical review of Section VI (Chapters 26, 27, 28, 29, 30, and 31) to identify content that needed to be updated and added.

Samuel G. Oberlander, M.D., FACOG, Assistant Clinical Professor, Department of Obstetrics-Gynecology, Albert Einstein College of Medicine, Bronx, New York, graciously reviewed the new and updated material in Chapters 9, 14, 17, 19, 57, and 58 for obstetric theoretical accuracy. Ellen Harrison, M.D., Associate Director of Medicine, Montefiore-North Central Bronx Hospital Affiliation and Assistant Clinical Professor, Department of Medicine, Albert Einstein College of Medicine, Bronx, New York was critically helpful in her review of the segments on hepatitis and tuberculosis. I retain, however, full responsibility for any inaccuracies and the determination of clinical judgement presented in this book.

Friends and family again played a critical role in the writing of the book. Margaret-Ann Corbett, C.N.M., J.D., Anne Malley-Corrinet, C.N.M., M.S., and Jerrilyn Meyer, C.N.M., M.S. took primary care of me as a person. My parents, Theodore R. and Helene Hahn Varney, sacrificed precious time for us to be together and were unfailingly interested and encouraging.

Finally, I wish to acknowledge the editorial help of Richard Zorab, Editor in Chief, and of Elizabeth McGuire, Production Manager, at Blackwell Scientific Publications; and of Patricia Sheehan. Richard was especially supportive and facilitative when contracted copyediting proved problematic and delayed the publication of this edition by several months.

A heartfelt thank you to all.

Acknowledgments to the First Edition

This book would not exist were it not for a number of helping and helpful people, some whose contributions have been highly visible and others who have been supportive in various indirect ways. There have been the many who posed for pictures, took pictures, sent pictures, sent professional literature and materials, typed, photocopied and, most of all, patiently waited. And there have been the many who have touched and shaped my life and beliefs in nurse-midwifery: from Ernestine Wiedenbach, C.N.M., M.A., my teacher and mentor from the beginning; through nurse-midwifery faculty and staff in the institutions where I have studied; to the nurse-midwifery faculty, staff, and students at the University of Mississippi Medical Center (1969–1974); the faculty, staff and students at the Medical University of South Carolina (1974–1979); the faculty in the nurse-midwifery education programs I have served as a consultant; the Certified Nurse-Midwives who have shared so much with me during my terms of office as President of the American College of Nurse-Midwives; and now the faculty and students at Yale University.

There has been one person who has lived the book with me. To my friend, Margaret-Ann Corbett, C.N.M., M.S., goes the most special acknowledgment and thank you for her never-failing encouragement, wise counsel, performance of innumerable detailed tasks, and provision of a sane counterbalance to the demands of the book.

A special acknowledgment and thank you also goes to Sally Ann Yeomans, C.N.M., M.S.N., who has given much personally and professionally out of her conviction that the book should be written. This included her assuming the Chairpersonship of the Division of Examiners of the American College of Nurse-Midwives which I held, so I would have the time to write.

A very special thank you must be said to Joy M. Brands, C.N.M., M.P.H., who rescued me and the book at one low point by volunteering to write the Neonatal Section. She enlisted the aid of Mary J. Banigan, R.N., Ph.D. in that project and the results are Chapters 20, 21, and 22. They were assisted in their endeavors by Sally Ann Yeomans.

A number of professionals reviewed parts of the book. Foremost among these is Henry A. Thiede, M.D., FACOG, Professor and Chairman, Department of Obstetrics-Gynecology, The University of Rochester School of Medicine and Dentistry and Strong Memorial Hospital. He reviewed the entire book for medical accuracy — always with ready willingness and a prompt response. Alfred W. Brann, Jr., M.D., FAAP and Linda Book, M.D., FAAP, reviewed the section on the Management of the Newborn. Agnes Higgins, C.M., B.Sc., P.Dt., F.R.S.H., LL.D., Executive Director of the Montreal Diet Dispensary, reviewed Chapter 8. Helen E. Browne, C.N.M., Sc.D. (Hon.), C.B.E., Aileen Hogan, C.N.M., M.A., Ruth Lubic, C.N.M., Ph.D., Agnes Reinders, C.N.M., M.S. in N.Ed., and Ernestine Wiedenbach, C.N.M., M.A., reviewed parts of the first two chapters. Margaret-Ann Corbett, C.N.M., M.S., and Linda Wheeler, C.N.M., Ed.D. reviewed other chapters throughout the book. All reviewers undertook this work at my request as personal favors and I whole-heartedly thank them all, while assuming full responsibility for any inaccuracies which may exist.

I learned a great deal about the arts from Betty Goodwin, Chief, Section of Illustration and Design, Division of Audiovisual Production, Medical University of South Carolina, who drew the original illustrations in this book, and from John Watts Clark, A.R.P.S., Supervisor of Photograph Department, Medical University of South Carolina, the photographer who took most of the original photographs in this book. Their helpfulness and pleasant ways made my learning what is entailed in their respective fields a most enjoyable experience.

I have known several editors throughout the process of writing this book. A special thank you goes to Christopher Campbell and Martha White Tenney of Blackwell Scientific Publications, Inc., and to Eleanor Mora. Without Chris and Marty urging and helping me through the last stages of production, the book would have stopped at the point of an edited manuscript. Special thanks must be given to Donna Diers, R.N., M.S.N., F.A.A.N., Dean and Professor of Yale University School of Nursing, for instigating and encouraging the contacts between Christopher Campbell and myself that led to the finalization and realization of the book.

In the end it was my local friends who enabled the book to be finished. The bulk of the six hundred pages of galleys were divided up and proofread by Joy Ruth Cohen, C.N.M., M.S.N., Margaret-Ann Corbett, C.N.M., M.S., Anne Malley-Corrinet, C.N.M., M.S., Donna Diers, R.N., M.S.N., F.A.A.N., Charlotte (Pixie) Elsberry, C.N.M., M.S.N., Elizabeth Grob, C.N.M., B.S.N., and Elizabeth Cole Rogers, C.N.M., M.N.

Finally, not least but most, I acknowledge and thank my parents, Theodore R. and Helene Hahn Varney, who have provided both personal encouragement and financial support through the years it has taken to write this book, and in whose honor I have decided to publish this book under my maiden name.

I Nurse-Midwifery

1

The Profession of Nurse-Midwifery

And it came to pass, when she was in hard labour, that the midwife said unto her, Fear not ...

Genesis 35:17

Midwifery is as old as the history of Homo sapiens. Reference is made to midwives at the beginning of biblical history (in the book of Genesis); these Hebrew midwives are the first midwives found in literature. Beginning in simplicity, midwifery has survived through the centuries, fulfilling its meaning of "with woman" as birth, the renewal of life, continues through the ages.

DEFINITION AND PRACTICE

A Certified Nurse-Midwife (CNM) is an individual educated in the two disciplines of nursing and midwifery, who possesses evidence of certification according to the requirements of the American College of Nurse-Midwives [1].

Nurse-midwifery practice is the independent management of care of essentially normal newborns and women, antepartally, intrapartally, postpartally, and/or gynecologically, occurring within a health care system which provides for medical consultation, collaborative management, or referral and is in accord with the Qualifications, Standards, and Functions for the Practice of Nurse-Midwifery as defined by the American College of Nurse-Midwives [2].

Analysis of these definitions reveals key philosophical stances and practical considerations pertaining to the preparation and functioning of a nurse-midwife. They are as follows.

1. "A certified nurse-midwife is ... educated in the two disciplines of nursing and midwifery." This phrase reflects the unique nature of nurse-midwifery as it encompasses two professional disciplines. This nature can be illustrated as in Figure 1-1.

The *nurse* part of the term nurse-midwifery acknowledges that being a registered nurse is prerequisite to being a certified nurse-midwife. It also emphasizes the primary focus of the professional nurse on the experiencing individual patient as well as on patient education, counseling, and supportive care.

Midwifery is an internationally recognized

3

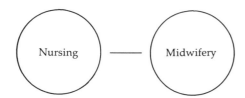

FIGURE 1-1. Graphic representation of the principle that Certified Nurse-Midwives are educated in the two disciplines of nursing and midwifery.

profession with practitioners throughout the world. The international definition of a midwife and her sphere of practice has been accepted by the International Confederation of Midwives, the Federation of International Gynecologists and Obstetricians, the World Health Organization, and others. It is as follows:

A Midwife is a person who, having been regularly admitted to a midwifery educational program fully recognized in the country in which it is located, has successfully completed the prescribed course of studies in midwifery and has acquired the requisite qualifications to be registered and/or legally licensed to practice midwifery.

She must be able to give the necessary supervision, care and advice to women during pregnancy, labor and postpartum period, to conduct deliveries on her own responsibility, and to care for the newborn and the infant. This care includes preventive measures, the detection of abnormal condition in mother and child, the procurement of medical assistance, and the execution of emergency measures in the absence of medical help.

She has an important task in counseling and education — not only for patients, but also within the family and community. The work should involve antenatal education and preparation for parenthood and extends to certain areas of gynecology, family planning, and child care.

She may practice in hospitals, clinics, health units, domiciliary conditions or any other service [3].

In the United States, nurse-midwifery education goes beyond the scope of practice

defined as midwifery in this international definition to include preventive gynecologic health care for all women. Nurse-midwives in the United States are taught normal obstetrics, gynecology, and neonatal pediatrics and its medical management; beliefs, knowledge, skills, and judgment for the facilitation of natural processes and nonintervention in these normal processes unless indicated; beliefs in continuity of care; beliefs and knowledge in the promotion and implementation of family-centered maternity care; beliefs in consumer rights; and beliefs, knowledge, and skills in educating patients for knowledgeable participation and decision making in their health care and for experiencing of their bodily processes. Midwifery also encompasses the primary focus of medicine on the diagnosis and treatment of a condition as it pertains to the essentially normal woman and neonate.

Nurse-midwifery thus is comprised of education in two disciplines that also incorporate components of a third discipline — medicine, specifically normal obstetrics, gynecology, and neonatal medicine. In practice, nurse-midwifery encompasses all of midwifery plus components from both nursing and medicine. Thus, nurse-midwifery is not totally nursing, not totally midwifery, and not totally medicine; it is a unique profession in its own right.

2. A certified nurse-midwife "... possesses evidence of certification according to the requirements of the American College of Nurse-Midwives." Nurse-midwifery certification is conferred upon an individual who has met eligibility requirements for and successfully passed the national certification examination of the American College of Nurse-Midwives (ACNM). Certification gives official recognition to an individual who has met professional standards for safe practice. This both protects the public and differentiates the well-educated and highly prepared certified nurse-midwife from a nurse who is functioning as a birth attendant or lay midwife, from the poorly

educated "granny" midwife, and from the lay or empirical midwife who may or may not be well educated in midwifery.

3. "Nurse-midwifery practice is the independent management of care ... occurring within a health care system which provides for medical consultation, collaborative management, or referral." *Independent management* refers to the fact that a patient may never see a physician if her course is essentially normal and her care is managed by a nurse-midwife. Thus, the practice of nurse-midwifery *within* the protocols for practice, which define the practice and provide for medical consultation and referral, is independent. This independence differentiates the nurse-midwife from those nonphysician practitioners who use the term management to mean fundamentally gathering a data base for the physician to use in decision making and action. Such "management" carries neither the responsibilities nor the accountability inherent in the functioning of a nurse-midwife, for whom management involves decision making and action as well.

In addition, independent management is clearly not the same as independent practice, which differentiates the nurse-midwife from nurses in independent practice. *Independent practice* means providing patient care without a professional practice agreement with a physician which provides for medical protocols and physician backup. A certified nurse-midwife always functions within a health care system in a team relationship with a physician and is never independent of physician backup for consultation, collaborative management, or referral (Fig. 1-2).

Professional practice agreements, however, are not the same as business practice agreements. Nurse-midwives across the country have a variety of business practice arrangements. These include being the employee of a physician, being the employee of a health care institution, and being self-employed in their own practice while employing the consulting physician. This latter business arrangement is

often referred to as "independent practice," meaning that the certified nurse-midwife has established her own independent business.

The critical delineation to be made in discussing independent practice is whether one means a business relationship or a professional relationship. Independent practice for certified nurse-midwives is the establishment and direction of their own business. Setting up an independent practice includes negotiating a written professional practice agreement with a physician for consultation, collaborative management, and referral. This professional practice agreement provides for independent management but not for independent practice.

Management of care indicates not only the medical practice aspects of nurse-midwifery but also the responsibilities and accountability the nurse-midwife assumes in accepting management of medical care functions and the mandatory relationship this requires with a physician. A nurse-midwife functions as an inherent member of the obstetrical team, working always in conjunction with a physician whom she consults if a patient exhibits any signs or symptoms of complications. To this end a nurse-midwife always functions within a circumscribed scope of practice as defined by medical protocols and standing orders developed and accepted by both the physicians and the nurse-midwives involved in any particular practice setting.

In joint statements made in 1971 and 1975, the American College of Obstetricians and Gynecologists, the Nurses Association of the American College of Obstetricians and Gynecologists, and the American College of Nurse-Midwives endorsed the concept of obstetric health care teams and recognized the contribution that each category of health personnel makes to this team effort based on a common goal of providing health services for maternity care. In 1982, these statements were superseded by a new joint statement made by the American College of Nurse-Midwives and the American College of Obstetricians and Gynecologists.

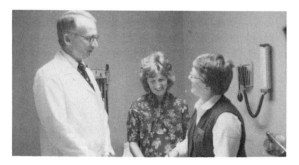

FIGURE 1-2.   A nurse-midwife and patient consulting with a physician.

The 1982 statement, entitled Joint Statement of Practice Relationships Between Obstetrician/Gynecologists and Certified Nurse-Midwives, appears in Appendix I, at the end of this chapter.

4. "Nurse-midwifery practice is the . . . care of essentially normal newborns and women, antepartally, intrapartally, postpartally, and/or gynecologically." This phrase states that the practice of nurse-midwifery, insofar as assumption of responsibility for the total management of care is concerned, is limited to the essentially normal child-bearing woman and neonate. This does not mean, however, that if a patient develops complications that the nurse-midwife no longer makes a contribution to the management of care. Rather, depending on the severity of the complication and on the setting, the nurse-midwife either consults and collaborates with the physician in the management of the care or refers the patient to the physician but may continue to see the patient in order to provide continuity of care.

Essentially normal also reflects again the team relationship with the physician, because *normal*, and therefore the circumscribed scope of nurse-midwifery practice in the "gray zone" of normality, is defined by the nurse-midwives and physicians in a particular practice setting. The limits of this gray zone vary from practice setting to practice setting and are reflected in the use of the word *essentially*.

Use of the term *normal* also reflects a philosophic view of childbearing and childbirth as a natural, normal process. Words such as uncomplicated or low risk neither connote the same meaning nor give the same sense of expectation of outcome.

5. *Newborn* means the baby during the neonatal period and reflects care during fetal life. *Women* reflects that nurse-midwives manage the care of nonpregnant women, who may or may not be mothers, with interconceptional, family planning, and well-woman gynecology health care needs. The term *women* also includes those who are pregnant and in the process of becoming, or who already are, a mother.

6. The phrase *antepartally, intrapartally, postpartally, and/or gynecologically* reflects a key belief in the practice of nurse-midwifery. Continuity of care is an inherent component of nurse-midwifery practice and a philosophic denial of nurse-midwives to subspecialize or fragment the childbearing cycle. Nurse-midwifery thus functions as an interdisciplinary bridge not only between nursing and medicine as it pertains to the health care of childbearing women and neonates but also between the fields of obstetrics, gynecology, and pediatrics (specifically neonatology) as the nurse-midwife provides continuity of care throughout the childbearing cycle and early family relationships.

The *and/or* in this phrase recognizes the role of the nurse-midwife in well-woman gynecology either as a continuation of the childbearing cycle or separate from maternity.

7. "Nurse-midwifery practice is . . . in accord with the Qualifications, Standards, and Functions for the Practice of Nurse-Midwifery as defined by the American College of Nurse-Midwives." The *ACNM Statement of Functions, Standards, and Qualifications* (see Appendix II at the end of this chapter) reflects the philosophy of the American College of Nurse-Midwives,

dictates activities of the professional organization, and more explicitly defines the practice of nurse-midwifery. It does not specifically list detailed functions because doing so would restrict its serving as a guide for current and developing practice. Such detailing of functions is developed as appropriate to individual practice settings and outlined in the protocols and standing orders for each site.

Other Beliefs Characterizing Nurse-Midwifery

The foregoing definitions do not reflect all the beliefs that are central to nurse-midwifery practice and characterize the patient care given by nurse-midwives. These include family-centered maternity care, promotion and facilitation of the natural and normal processes of childbearing, and consumer orientation and advocacy. Nurse-midwives were in the forefront of the early movements in the 1940s in the United States relative to family-centered maternity care, including preparation for childbirth and parenthood, inclusion of fathers or significant others in the labor and delivery rooms, and rooming-in.

Specialization in management of essentially normal childbearing women means that nurse-midwives have perfected skills which promote and facilitate the natural, normal processes of childbearing as well as skills which may be obstetrically indicated. A nurse-midwife has the knowledge, judgment, and skill to perform pudendal blocks, deliver in lithotomy position, and cut and repair episiotomies. A nurse-midwife can also provide the alternative of delivering over an intact perineum in left lateral position with no analgesia or anesthesia while coaching the patient in her breathing. These choices and others may be combined in various ways; the decisions are made in conjunction with the patient and within the obstetrical limits of safety as dictated by the patient's condition.

Currently, nurse-midwives are again listening to consumer concerns and desires and are in the forefront of developing alternatives to the all too frequently sterile, pathologically-oriented obstetrical units in hospitals. Alternatives are being sought which will provide all the safety features and emergency equipment for both mother and baby if needed and which will utilize the advantages, while modifying or avoiding the disadvantages, of the present in-hospital health care system. Such alternatives include promoting obstetrical team (physician/nurse-midwife) efforts geared toward deliveries in the labor room, or in specially designed family-oriented birthing rooms, and early discharge from the hospital; family-oriented childbirth centers with emergency equipment and arrangements with nearby hospitals; and carefully selected home deliveries with arrangements for transportation and a back-up hospital.

The philosophy of the American College of Nurse-Midwives states beliefs which are supportive of and provide a base for the characteristics of patient care given by nurse-midwives as described previously. These beliefs are:

Every individual has the right to safe, satisfying health care with respect for human dignity and cultural variations. The individual has the right to self-determination, to adequate information, and to active participation in all aspects of care.

Nurse-midwifery's primary focus is on women of childbearing age, and its practice may be extended to preventive health care of all women. This comprehensive health maintenance is most effectively and efficiently delivered by interdependent health disciplines.

Nurse-midwifery, as a discipline, focuses on the individual's and family's needs for physical care, emotional and social support, and health education.

The profession of nurse-midwifery assumes the responsibility for ensuring that Certified Nurse-Midwives are provided with excellence in educational preparation and that they demonstrate professional standards of practice in keeping with these stated beliefs [4].

THE AMERICAN COLLEGE OF NURSE-MIDWIVES

The American College of Nurse-Midwives (ACNM) is the professional organization for nurse-midwives. Incorporated in 1955, it was founded as the outgrowth of a series of circumstances which rendered its creation necessary.

During the mid-1940s the National Organization of Public Health Nurses (NOPHN) established a section for nurse-midwives. In 1949 the nurse midwifery section of this organization published the first national descriptive data gathered about nurse-midwives [5]. A few years later, when there was a general reorganization of the national nursing organizations, the NOPHN was absorbed into the American Nurses' Association (ANA) and the National League for Nursing (NLN) and there was no provision within these organizations for a recognizable entity of nurse-midwives. Instead, the nurse-midwives had been assigned to belong to the Maternal and Child Health — National League for Nursing Interdivisional Council, which encompassed the areas of obstetrics, pediatrics, orthopedics, crippled children, and school nursing. The membership and concerns of this Council were simply too broad to serve as a forum or voice for nurse-midwifery. Ironically, even though nurse-midwives were in positions of leadership in maternal-child nursing in educational, professional, and federal organizations pertaining to health care, they were usually not thought of as being nurse-midwives.

The Committee on Organization

Since the identity of nurse-midwives could not be maintained within the existing situation, the nurse-midwives present at an ANA convention in the spring of 1954 agreed to establish The Committee on Organization. This committee was formed with Sister M. Theophane Shoemaker, the director of the then existing Catholic Maternity Center in Santa Fe, New Mexico, as chair.

The Committee on Organization, while professing its progress as being slow and tedious, had within 2 months identified reasons for organizing; discussed ways in which organization could be accomplished; written a definition of a nurse-midwife, functions of a new organization if one was to be established, and educational standards for nurse-midwifery schools including a statement of purpose and basic admission requirements; designed and mailed a questionnaire to locate nurse-midwives and ascertain their desire to organize; written and mailed two of the eventual six Organization Bulletins of The Committee on Organization; and organized a meeting of nurse-midwives for December 1954.

Forty-six nurse-midwives attended the meeting in December, reviewed the work done thusfar and the results of the questionnaire (to which 147 nurse-midwives had replied), and approved the definition of a nurse-midwife and a statement of purposes of a nurse-midwifery organization. The major issue, however, was how organization could be accomplished. Possible options had been identified as follows:

1. Organization within the American Nurses' Association (ANA) as a conference group
2. Organization within the National League for Nursing (NLN) as a council
3. Reorganization of the American Association of Nurse-Midwives (AANM) into a national organization
4. Formation of an entirely new organization of nurse-midwives to be known as the American College of Nurse-Midwifery

The American Association of Nurse-Midwives had been started in 1928 as the Kentucky State Association of Midwives, incorporated by nurse-midwives working with the Frontier Nursing Service. Mary Breckinridge, then director of the Frontier Nursing Service, was president of AANM during her lifetime. Its function, which was akin to that of an alumnae association although not limited to alumnae, and its organization were such that it could not serve the purposes of this national movement of nurse-midwives. AANM, therefore, was eliminated as a possible option because of its own self-analysis and statement of preference not to be considered.

The remaining options, thus, were either to organize within one of the national nursing organizations or to create a new organization. It was decided to defer this decision until letters requesting a conference group and a council, respectively, were submitted to, and replies received from, ANA and NLN. The letters were approved during the meeting.

The reply from NLN expressed interest and concern but pointed out that its bylaws for organization of a council were not facilitative to the needs of the nurse-midwives. The reply from ANA was not encouraging. ANA was interested in a plan to establish an interdisciplinary committee of ANA and NLN, with additional representatives from the public, to study the improvement of the care of mothers and children. Nurse-midwifery could be a part of this committee.

This information was published in the fourth Organization Bulletin along with the plans for the next meeting of The Committee on Organization and a request for any comments regarding what the obvious direction for organization had to be. At this meeting in May 1955, The Committee on Organization voted unanimously to proceed with the formation of the American College of Nurse-Midwifery. They based their action on the fact that all the other options had essentially been ruled out, the fact that 133 of the 147 nurse-midwives answering the questionnaire had responded positively to the idea of belonging to a new organization of nurse-midwives, the obvious conclusion that formation of a separate organization seemed to be the only way that nurse-midwives could work together and accomplish anything constructive as had been delineated in the statement of purposes, and the fact that only one response had been received from the request in the Organization Bulletin for comments regarding this direction. The Committee on Organization had done such a splendid job of keeping all the nurse-midwives informed and involved that there was nothing further to be said.

The Committee on Organization then instituted work on developing what needed to be done to actually incorporate and establish the new organization. The result was the incorporation of the American College of Nurse-Midwifery, November 7, 1955, in the state of New Mexico. New Mexico was chosen because it was one of the few states in which nurse-midwives were practicing and it involved the least amount of red tape, time, and expense.

ACNM as an Organization

The first annual meeting of the American College of Nurse-Midwifery was held November 12 and 13, 1955, in Kansas City, Missouri. Hattie Hemschemeyer, then director of Maternity Center Association School of Nurse-Midwifery, was elected the first president of the American College of Nurse-Midwifery. In her first message to members in the *Bulletin of the American College of Nurse-Midwifery* she wrote about the driving force and movement of nurse-midwifery in terms equally applicable to today:

The College must select carefully the work it undertakes and then do well the work it has undertaken. We need to work with dedication and conviction. We are beginning at a time when education has concentrated too heavily on techniques and too little on the human factors involved. It is essential that education relate in a responsible and practical way with the problems and moral issues of our times.

We nurse-midwives are a specialized group and our education, experience, and service have led us to the considered conclusion that in our present society it is neither desirable nor necessary to eliminate specialization. We believe that creative imagination, plus the ability to utilize ideas, is one of the most powerful influences in the world today...

The nurse-midwives have not substituted rationalization nor routines for reason; they have not been helpless when it comes to effecting mass movements for the care of human beings where helplessness, faith in reason, responsibility, and the dignity of the individual were concerned. They know the difference between supplying verbal allegiance and action ...

We have a pioneer job to do, and if we work as well and as constructively in a group as we have in the past as individuals, we can help to improve professional competence, provide better service and educational programs, and make fuller use of resources. The future looks bright [6].

At another time she stated, "Our identity as a College gives us fundamental rights and grave responsibilities" [7].

The objectives of the American College of Nurse-Midwives as found in the Articles of Incorporation, Revised, 1975, reflect both nurse-midwifery's concern for quality maternity care and the assumption of the "grave responsibilities" alluded to by Hattie Hemschemeyer:

That the objectives of said corporation shall be:
a. To study, develop and evaluate standards for nurse-midwifery care of women and infants;
b. To study, develop and evaluate standards for nurse-midwifery education;
c. To support and assist in the development of nurse-midwifery services and educational programs, in association with allied professional groups;
d. To evaluate and approve nurse-midwifery services and educational programs;
e. To determine the eligibility of individuals to practice as Certified Nurse-Midwives, and to assume responsibility for National Nurse-Midwifery Certification;
f. To facilitate and coordinate the efforts of nurse-midwives who in the public interest provide quality services to individuals and childbearing families;
g. To establish channels for communication and cooperation with other professional and non-professional groups who in the public interest

share the objectives of ensuring sufficient quality services to individuals and childbearing families;
h. To establish channels for interpretation of nurse-midwifery to allied professional and non-professional groups on a regional, national and international basis;
i. To promote research and the development of literature in the field of nurse-midwifery [8].

In 1956 both the American College of Nurse-Midwifery and the American Association of Nurse-Midwives were accepted in the International Confederation of Midwives (ICM) upon the recommendation of England and Scotland and the unanimous vote of the executive council of the ICM. In 1968 the American Association of Nurse-Midwives (AANM) merged with the American College of Nurse-Midwifery (ACNM) to form the American College of Nurse-Midwives (ACNM). The American College of Nurse-Midwives is now the United States member organization in the ICM and in October 1972 hosted the triennial congress of the ICM in Washington, D.C., when Lucille Woodville, then nursing consultant to the Bureau of Indian Health Affairs and past president of the ACNM (1969–1971), was president of the ICM (1969–1972).

The seal of the ACNM (Fig. 1-3) reflects basic philosophical beliefs of nurse-midwifery. Rita Kroska, who designed the seal in 1955, interprets its symbols as follows:

The large shield is comprised of four symbols: a small shield of stars and stripes exemplify the United States of America; three intertwined circles exemplify the family with the lower circle containing crosshatching to illustrate the crib containing the child; a tripod with flames rising exemplifies continuance and warmth in dedication to the American family; and, lastly, the large shield contains an undulating band above the tripod but beneath the smaller shield and circles. The undulation portrays movement, persistence, steadiness, and steadfastness to the word written within. That word is VIVANT, an expletive in French which means Let Them Live! It is there to fill out the sentence of the symbols, to give emphasis short of exclamatory

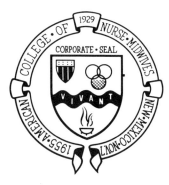

FIGURE 1-3. The seal of the American College of Nurse-Midwives.

oath, that of unremitting dedication to safeguarding and promoting the health and wellbeing of family life, particularly the mother and infant.

The large shield is encircled by a ribboned band containing the inscription, "AMERICAN COLLEGE OF NURSE-MIDWIVES, NEW MEXICO, Nov. 7, 1955." Originally, between 1955 and 1969, the word "nurse-midwives" was "nurse-midwifery," and without the year 1929 included within the inscription. The two changes took place in 1969 when the American Association of Nurse-Midwives with headquarters at the Frontier Nursing Service in Wendover, Kentucky, and the American College of Nurse-Midwifery joined and became the American College of Nurse-Midwives. The year 1929 was the founding of the American Association of Nurse-Midwives [9].

Activities of the ACNM

The membership of the American College of Nurse-Midwives has been characterized from the beginning by its dedication, commitment, hard work, articulateness, personal sacrifice, vision, and pioneering spirit. The annals of the ACNM's brief history are peopled with creative giants who were also willing to do the necessary detail work while dipping into their own pocketbooks to finance it. Starting with a charter membership of 124, the ACNM had grown to a membership of 860 by its twentieth anniversary in 1975. By 1980 the membership, now including students, had increased to over

1500 and by 1984 numbered 2534. This figure reflects the fact that approximately 87 percent of the total number of certified nurse-midwives belong to the ACNM (10). Seventeen nurse-midwives attended the first annual meeting in Kansas City in 1955; 291 members were in attendance at the twentieth annual meeting in Jackson, Mississippi, in 1975. Convention attendance first passed the 1000 mark with 863 members and 138 guests in Philadelphia in 1984.

The rapid expansion of nurse-midwifery and proliferation of nurse-midwives placed stress on the professional organization. It was faced with having to change from a small, intimate group of hard-working, dedicated nurse-midwives with an organizational structure for the same to an organizational structure and management style that could cope with both a rapid increase in membership (the total number of nurse-midwives had tripled in less than 10 years) and the continuation of its dedication and ideals. This was done. The productivity of the American College of Nurse-Midwives since its founding in 1955 is inspirational in showing what a small group can do. Against what appeared to be insurmountable odds this small membership accomplished major tasks in minimal time, to the astonishment of larger organizations struggling with the same tasks. A review of the first 20 years of ACNM shows the following (subsequent updates are also given where applicable):

Three education workshops (1958, 1967, and 1973 [combined with service]); there are now annual meetings of the directors of nurse-midwifery education programs and of the directors of nurse-midwifery services

Trebling of the number of educational programs

Massive proliferation of nurse-midwifery services in all types of health care systems

A comprehensive and continuing survey of legislation (first survey done in 1970–1971; latest published survey done in 1983)

Writing and acceptance of nurse-midwifery definition (1955, 1962, 1978); philosophy (1963, 1972, 1983); and functions, standards, and qualifications (1966, 1975, 1983)

Publication of "Descriptive Data, Nurse-Midwives — U.S.A." (1963, 1968, 1971, 1976—1977, 1982)

Writing and acceptance of articles of incorporation and bylaws (1955, revised 1974—1975 in accord with organizational restructuring)

Initiation, implementation (1962), and evaluation of accreditation of nurse-midwifery educational programs

Initiation, implementation (1971), and evaluation of a national certification examination and ACNM certification process

Formulation and approval of guidelines for establishing nurse-midwifery services (1971—1972)

Formulation and approval of guidelines for establishing new basic educational programs in nurse-midwifery (1973)

Formulation and implementation of a consultation service (1974—1975)

Publication of a professional journal (*Journal of Nurse-Midwifery*, formerly *Bulletin of the American College of Nurse-Midwifery*, started in 1955)

Formation of the A.C.N.M. Foundation (1967)

Formation of ACNM local chapters (1962)

Service as host for the sixteenth triennial congress of the International Confederation of Midwives (1972)

Establishment of a national headquarters office (1959, moved in 1974, 1978, and 1981)

Establishment of ACNM archives (1972)

Appendix III (see end of this chapter) lists what could be called the essential documents of the ACNM. These essential documents are the product of the above enumerated and other subsequent activities and affect the direction of nurse-midwifery and the practice of each individual nurse-midwife.

ACNM has also been active in both national and international interorganizational activities with official representation to, and membership in, The Federation of Specialty Nursing Organizations and the ANA, the International Confederation of Midwives, The Interorganizational Committee on Obstetric-Gynecologic Health Personnel, The Interprofessional Task Force on Health Care of Women and Children, the National Perinatal Association, and the National Commission for Health Certifying Agencies. In addition, there have been and are innumerable occasions of official representation at specific organizational and interorganizational meetings. This emphasizes the fact that, while the ACNM is an autonomous professional organization, nurse-midwifery collaborates with all other professional groups that share its primary concern of quality maternal-infant health care for all women and babies.

REFERENCES

1. Definition accepted by the American College of Nurse-Midwives, 1978.
2. Definition accepted by the American College of Nurse-Midwives, 1978.
3. Definition accepted by the International Confederation of Midwives, the Federation of International Gynecologists and Obstetricians, and the World Health Organization, Rev., 1972.
4. Philosophy adopted by the American College of Nurse Midwives, revised, 1983.
5. Nurse midwifery today. *Public Health Nursing* (May) 1949.
6. Hemschemeyer, H. Sends message to members. *Bull. Am. Coll. Nurse-Midwifery* 1:5, 1956.
7. Hemschemeyer, H. Report of the first president of the American College of Nurse-Midwifery. *Bull. Am. Coll. Nurse-Midwifery* 10:8, 1965. (Anniversary issue)
8. Articles of Incorporation, Revised. American College of Nurse-Midwives, 1975.
9. Kroska, R. The emblem of the American College of Nurse-Midwives. *J. Nurse-Midwifery* 18:23, 1973.

10. *Nurse-Midwifery in the United States: 1982.* American College of Nurse-Midwives, Washington, D.C. 1984, p. 18.

APPENDIX I

JOINT STATEMENT OF PRACTICE RELATIONSHIPS BETWEEN OBSTETRICIAN/GYNECOLOGISTS AND CERTIFIED NURSE-MIDWIVES*

It is critical that obstetrician/gynecologists and certified nurse-midwives have a clear understanding of their individual, collaborative and interdependent responsibilities. As agreed upon in previous Joint Statements by the American College of Nurse-Midwives, the American College of Obstetricians and Gynecologists, and the Nurses Association of the American College of Obstetricians and Gynecologists, the maternity care team should be directed by a qualified obstetrician/gynecologist. The American College of Obstetricians and Gynecologists and the American College of Nurse-Midwives believe that the appropriate practice of the certified nurse-midwife includes the participation and involvement of the obstetrician/gynecologist as mutually agreed upon in written medical guideline/protocols. The American College of Obstetricians and Gynecologists and the American College of Nurse-Midwives also believe that the obstetrician/gynecologist should be responsive to the desire of certified nurse-midwives for the participation and involvement of the obstetrician/gynecologist. The following principles represent a

---

* This statement supersedes previous Joint Statements of Maternity Care by the American College of Obstetricians and Gynecologists, the American College of Nurse-Midwives, and the Nurses Association of the American College of Obstetricians and Gynecologists dated 1971 and 1975.

November 1, 1982

joint statement of the American College of Obstetricians and Gynecologists and the American College of Nurse-Midwives and are recommended for consideration in all practice relationships and agreements.

1. Clinical practice relationship between the obstetrician/gynecologist and the certified nurse-midwife should provide for:
   a. mutually agreed upon written medical guidelines/protocols for clinical practice which define the individual and shared responsibilities of the certified nurse-midwife and the obstetrician/gynecologist in the delivery of health care services;
   b. mutually agreed upon written medical guidelines/protocols for ongoing communication which provide for and define appropriate consultation between the obstetrician/gynecologist and the certified nurse-midwife;
   c. informed consent about the involvement of the obstetrician/gynecologist, certified nurse-midwife, and other health care providers in the services offered;
   d. periodic and joint evaluation of services rendered, e.g., chart review, case review, patient evaluation, review of outcome statistics; and
   e. periodic and joint review and updating of the written medical guidelines/protocols.

2. Quality of care is enhanced by the interdependent practice of the obstetrician/gynecologist and the certified nurse-midwife working in a relationship of mutual respect, trust and professional responsibility. This does not necessarily imply the physical presence of the physician when care is being given by the certified nurse-midwife.

3. Administrative relationships, including employment agreements, reimbursement mechanisms, and corporate structures, should be mutually agreed upon by the participating parties.

4. Access to practice within the hospital setting for the obstetrician/gynecologist and

the certified nurse-midwife who have a practice relationship in concurrence with these principles is strongly urged by the respective professional organizations.

The American College of Obstetricians and Gynecologists and the American College of Nurse-Midwives strongly urge the implementation of these principles in all practice relationships between obstetrician/gynecologists and certified nurse-midwives, and consider the preceding an ideal model of practice.

APPENDIX II

ACNM STATEMENT OF FUNCTIONS, STANDARDS, AND QUALIFICATIONS

Functions for the Practice of Nurse-Midwifery

The nurse-midwife:
1. Assumes the responsibility for management of care of the essentially healthy woman and newborn throughout the childbearing process.
2. Assumes responsibility for the management of care of the essentially healthy woman as related to her gynecologic and interconceptional needs.
3. Develops with the woman a plan of care appropriate for her total health care needs, recognizing the unique role of the family in this process.
4. Provides to clients individual and/or group counseling and teaching appropriate to their needs.
5. Collaborates with the physician in the management of care of medically complicated women.
6. Collaborates with other health professionals in the delivery and evaluation of health care.
7. Conducts an ongoing assessment of own professional abilities and functions.
8. Assumes responsibility for maintaining currency and safety in professional practice.

9. Utilizes Guidelines for Evaluation of Nurse-Midwifery Procedural Functions in development and evaluation of practice [Addendum 1].
10. Promotes and assists the education of nurse-midwifery students.
11. Assists with the education of other health care personnel.
12. Practices according to the philosophy and offical policies of the American College of Nurse-Midwives.

Standards for the Practice of Nurse-Midwifery

Nurse-midwifery practice:
1. Fosters the delivery of safe and satisfying care to women.
2. Upholds the right to self-determination of consumers within the boundaries of safe care.
3. Endeavors to provide comprehensive health care to women including continuity of care, emotional and social support, and health education.
4. Encompasses the provision of care during the childbearing years recognizing that this is a family experience and encourages the active involvement of family members in this care.
5. Stimulates community awareness of and responsiveness to the need for quality family-centered care, recognizing variations in family patterns.
6. Includes the provision of interconceptional and gynecological services to women who request preventive health care.
7. Recognizes the client's health and growth as developmental processes occurring throughout the life cycle.
8. Occurs interdependently within a health care delivery system.
9. Demonstrates a safe mechanism for physician consultation, collaboration and referral within an alliance agreement which includes mutually approved protocols.

10. Requires continuing professional growth and development which includes an on-going process of evaluation as defined by the American College of Nurse-Midwives.

Qualifications for the Practice of
Nurse-Midwifery

1. Certification by the American College of Nurse-Midwives.
2. Compliance with legal requirements of the jurisdiction in which nurse-midwifery practice will occur.

Revised and approved April 1983

ADDENDUM 1

GUIDELINES FOR EVALUATION OF
NURSE-MIDWIFERY PROCEDURAL
FUNCTIONS

The following guidelines were adopted by the Executive Board of the American College of Nurse-Midwives as a way of approaching the clinical practice of the nurse-midwife. Practice is continually evolving and it varies depending upon the institution and the demands for service within each setting. Because of this, the nurse-midwife may frequently be in a position of having to evaluate a new function for possible inclusion into her practice. This need for evaluation may be stimulated by the obstetrician, the demands of the patient or community, pressure from other groups, or desires of the nurse-midwife herself. In any case, the answer as to the worth and safety of a new procedure for inclusion into nurse-midwifery may not be clear.

No one of these guidelines can stand alone. It is only by employing each of them and then surveying the whole that an accurate feeling for the safety and suitability of the procedure for nurse-midwifery practice can be obtained.

Guidelines help to direct but they do not necessarily guarantee that the direction will be completely clear. Systematic review of new procedures will help to assure that the statements on qualifications, standards and functions are up to date.

1. The procedure assists the nurse-midwife in managing the care of the normal child-bearing woman and infant.
   a. It does not conflict with the basic philosophy of nurse-midwifery as outlined by the ACNM and with that outlined by the nurse-midwifery service.
   b. The procedure can be done competently by the nurse-midwife, i.e., the practitioner has obtained sound theory and supervised clinical experience from qualified faculty.
   c. The nurse-midwife is prepared to handle possible complications from the procedure until help arrives.
2. The procedure is within accepted obstetrical practice within the institution.
   a. It is presently an established procedure.
   b. It is a new procedure that is being instituted by the obstetric service.
3. The procedure fills a demonstrated need.
   a. There is consumer demand.
   b. Within the obstetric team it is appropriate that the nurse-midwife carry out the procedure.
   c. The nurse-midwife feels the procedure will contribute to the provision of optimal care.
4. The procedure is evaluated in the literature and/or in practice.
   a. The literature has been reviewed with both indications and contraindications identified.
   b. There is consideration of what other institutions and other nurse-midwives are doing.
5. The procedure is within legal limits.
6. There is an on-going plan for the evaluation of the procedure.
   a. The plan is filed with the Clinical Practice

Committee at the time of initiation of the procedure.

  b. Progress reports are periodically submitted to the Clinical Practice Committee.

The Committee requests that if a nurse-midwifery service or a nurse-midwife intends to initiate a new procedure, the Clinical Practice Committee be notified. This will enable the Committee to record changes in practice throughout the United States and will also facilitate the dissemination of information of nurse-midwifery practice. It is hoped that periodic reports to the Committee will be made which are evaluative and in summary form. The collection of this type of data is important to the development of nurse-midwifery and will provide a resource for other services which may be considering the initiation of the same procedures.

Accepted January 27, 1972

APPENDIX III

ESSENTIAL DOCUMENTS OF THE
AMERICAN COLLEGE OF
NURSE-MIDWIVES*

1. *Definition of a Certified Nurse-Midwife* (1978)
2. *Definition of Nurse-Midwifery Practice* (1978)
3. *Philosophy* (1983)
4. *Functions, Standards, and Qualifications for the Practice of Nurse-Midwifery* (1983) and Addendum 1, *Guidelines for Evaluation of*

Nurse-Midwifery Procedural Functions (1972); reproduced as Appendix II of the present text
5. *Articles of Incorporation and Bylaws*
6. *Standing Rules of Procedure*
7. *Procedure for Initiation of New ACNM Chapters*
8. *Working Document of ACNM* (1974)
9. *Joint Statement of Practice Relationships between Obstetrician/Gynecologists and Certified Nurse-Midwives* (1982); reproduced as Appendix I of the present text
10. *Position Statement on Nurse-Midwifery Legislation* (1974) with *Sample Law: Statute and Rules and Regulations* (1978)
11. Special legislative issue, *Journal of Nurse-Midwifery*, vol. 29, no. 2, March/April, 1984.
12. *A Framework for Establishing a Nurse-Midwifery Practice in a Variety of Settings*
13. *Guidelines for Establishing a Nurse-Midwifery Service* (1972)
14. *Guidelines (legislative) for Establishing a Nurse-Midwifery Practice*
15. *Community Orientation Package*
16. *Statement on Practice Settings* (1980)
17. *Guidelines for Establishing a Hospital Birth Room* (1979)
18. *Guidelines for Establishing an Alternative Birth Center* (1979)
19. *Guidelines for Establishing a Home Birth Service* (1979)
20. *Guide to Quality Assurance/Peer Review* (1984)
21. *Statement on Abortion* (1971)
22. *Grievance Procedure*
23. *Nurse-Midwifery in the United States: 1982* (1984)
24. *Guidelines for Establishing New Basic Educational Programs for Nurse-Midwifery*
25. *ACNM Core Competencies in Nurse-Midwifery* (1985). Reproduced as Appendix V in the present text, at the end of Chapter 2
26. *Policies and Procedure Manual for Accreditation of Basic Certificate, Basic Graduate,*

---

* This listing was assembled by the author in 1984. The author also considers *The International (ICM/FIGO/WHO) Definition of a Midwife* an essential document. In addition, two informational pamphlets, *What Is A Nurse-Midwife?* and *The A.C.N.M. Foundation*, may be obtained upon request from the American College of Nurse-Midwives, 1522 K Street, N.W., Suite 1120, Washington, D.C., 20005

2

History of Nurse-Midwifery in the United States

The history of nurse-midwifery in the United States must be prefaced by midwifery history from the time of the arrival of colonists in the New World. There were midwives among the first women to settle the colonies. Modern nurse-midwifery still feels the effects of this pre-nurse-midwifery history.

EARLY HISTORY

Midwives were considered vital to colonial community life and were treated with dignity. Special courtesies were extended and arrangements made for housing, land, food, and salary as payment for their services. This information is noted in town records and charters of the mid-1600s.

During the 1800s pioneer women crossed the plains in covered wagons, settled the Wild West, and bore children with the aid of midwives who were a part of the westward movement. Mormon history documents the honorable role and heroic functioning of midwives during their trek from Illinois to Utah in the period of 1846 to 1847.

Despite the initial honor afforded midwives in the colonies and their importance to other segments of the population through the years, a series of factors reduced midwifery from a status of respect to one of disrepute by the early 1900s. These factors include religious attitudes, economic demands, replacement by physicians, inadequate education, lack of organization, influx of immigrants, and the status of women.

Factors Leading to Disrepute

Religious factors plagued midwives from the beginning. Most of the early midwives came from England, where at that time license to practice midwifery was under the auspices of the Church of England. Criteria were moralistically judgmental; they emphasized good character and granted the ability to denounce sins and to baptize. The midwives' oath included pressuring the mother into naming the true father. The results of such actions were not always appreciated. On the other hand, in the Puritan communities midwives were often suspected of witchcraft, especially if a malformed baby was born.

By the early 1700s compensation was not always adequate for the midwife; her services were no longer economically feasible. This was especially true in the rapidly growing towns and cities. There was no organization or authority to establish guidelines for fees.

European society in the late 1700s made it fashionable to have male midwives (physicians) for lying-in. This trend soon crossed the ocean and was capitalized on by physicians. Fox, in her analysis of historical roots of antipathy towards the midwife, states

As the practice of medicine became highly competitive, physicians and medical students were advised that their presence at a delivery would insure the entire family as grateful patients thereafter. For example, the outspoken and highly influential Dr. Walter Channing, of Harvard, objected strongly to the practice of midwifery by women in his "Remarks on the Employment of Females as Practitioners in Midwifery", (1820) and pointed out that:

"... Women seldom forget a practitioner who has conducted them tenderly and safely through parturition — they feel a familiarity with him, a confidence and reliance upon him which is of the most essential mutual advantage ... It is principally on this account that the practice of midwifery becomes desirable to physicians. It is this which ensures to them the permanency and security of all their other business." [1]

Male physicians thus replaced the female midwife.

The 1700s and 1800s mark a time of rapid development in medical and nursing science and of discoveries and teaching pertinent to obstetric practice. These developments include the end of the Chamberlen family secret of forceps and the refinement of these instruments, technical advances which decreased the risks involved in cesarean section, pioneering efforts in obstetric anesthesia, conquest of puerperal fever, emergence of modern nursing in the 1860s, and inclusion of obstetrics in medical practice. The observations and teachings of William Smellie (1697–1763), who developed teaching manikins and kept meticulous records of his patients, identified the mechanisms of labor and refuted any number of myths and misconceptions.

The anatomical studies of William Hunter (1718–1783) included discoveries pertaining to the lymphatic system, placental circulation, and pregnant uterus. William Shippen, Jr. (1736–1808), the first lecturer on obstetrics, and Samuel Bard (1742–1821), author of the first American textbook on obstetrics, are attributed with promoting obstetrical teaching in the United States. All made measurable contributions to the science and art of obstetrics.

None of these developments, new knowledge, and teachings were accessible to the midwife because there was neither a legal or professional organization of, nor any educational programs for, midwives. Any one of these structures would have provided a channel for learning. Without them the knowledge and practice of the midwife became sadly out-of-date while medicine advanced and modern nursing began.

An influx of immigrants from a number of European countries formed pockets of cultural communities within cities, each such community having its own midwives who came from the "old country." These untrained urban midwives, like their counterparts in the rural South, frequently passed the practice of midwifery from mother to daughter, learned through experience, and relied heavily on patience, home remedies, and prayer since these were the only resources available to the midwives and the women they served. Lack of licensure, organization, and supervision prevented these midwives from being a part of the official health care system.

The low status of women in general at the turn of the twentieth century affected the work of midwives. Norma Swenson, in her analysis of social factors affecting the history of midwifery in the United States, makes the following comments:

But the final and I think more significant point was that the status of women at the turn of the century was at a particularly low ebb. At that point in time women were regarded as economically exploitable but at the same time socially and politically incompetent, in the sense that they were perceived as being unfit to exercise good judgment concerning their own affairs or the affairs of others, and in fact were legally prevented from doing so. Paternal domination of home and society was at an all-time high.

It was then in this kind of atmosphere that midwives were outlawed and women were, therefore, in effect blamed for the appalling conditions under which mothers and babies died at that time, when in fact women were powerless to control social conditions, and coped as midwives as well as they could with circumstances which were largely the product of a man-made industrial and social revolution [2].

These events and social factors combined by the end of the 1800s to render a system of health care education and service to which the descendants of the midwives in the colonies, the urban ethnic immigrant midwives, their rural midwife counterparts in the South, and the native American midwives could not have access.

THE EARLY 1900s

The first 2 decades of the twentieth century are notable for the recognition of woefully inadequate maternity care and subsequent actions taken to improve this care; and for the establishment of two organizations, the Children's Bureau in Washington, D.C., and Maternity Center Association in New York City, both of which have had an immense influence on the development of maternal-infant health care and of nurse-midwifery.

In 1906 a study was made of maternal and infant mortality in New York City. The study, attributed to the New York City Health Department, stated that over 40 percent of deliveries were attended by approximately 3000 incompetent and ignorant midwives. While these midwives were not solely responsible for the high maternal and infant mortality rates at that time, they received the brunt of the blame. Other factors of obstetrical care contributing to maternal and infant mortality at that time included the following:

1. The hospital was not viewed as a setting for obstetrical care, so there was a lack of hospital resources for treatment of emergencies or complications arising during childbirth in the home (where the vast majority of deliveries were taking place).
2. The study of obstetrics was not an identified essential component of medical education except in isolated teaching institutions.
3. The practice of obstetrics was virtually limited to the intrapartal and postpartal periods.
4. There were few state laws and regulations for the licensure and supervision of midwives.
5. There was no organized system of education for midwives.

Progress in improving care was slow. In 1915 the registration of births occurred in only ten states, and it was not until 1935 that the registration of births was mandatory in every state.

The Children's Bureau

In 1903 Lillian Wald, a nurse, suggested a federal children's bureau. President Theodore Roosevelt recommended a bill to establish such a bureau in 1909, but it was 1912 before the Congress of the United States passed a bill, which President Taft signed, establishing the Children's Bureau.

The first act of the Children's Bureau was to conduct a study of infant deaths, which, according to available statistics, produced an infant mortality rate of approximately 124 per 1000 live births. It is to the Children's Bureau's credit that in analyzing the data from their first study they identified the inescapable link between infant health and maternal health during the maternity cycle. The Children's Bureau then conducted studies of maternal mortality and conclusively established the importance of early and continuous prenatal care in reducing both maternal and infant mortality. With this information the idea of prenatal care gained respectability and the concept of health care throughout the intraconceptional period began to grow.

The Maternity Center Association in New York City

In 1915 the New York City health commissioner made another study of maternal and infant mortality. The findings of this study, which again demonstrated the connection between mortality and lack of prenatal care, yielded a plan in which the city was zoned and a maternity center established in each zone. The first such maternity center opened in 1917. The need for central organization became quickly evident and the Maternity Center Association (MCA) was established in 1918. By 1920, MCA had 30 maternity centers in New York City. From this grew MCA's first endeavors in developing teaching materials and educational exhibits for use by individuals and agencies. In 1921 the association decided to concentrate efforts on a demonstration of providing complete maternity care in one district and to cease the scattered effort in the multitudinous centers, although some of the other clinics were still maintained for a while

longer. This decision was based on the belief that most nursing agencies and hospitals caring for families were now giving sufficient emphasis to prenatal care in their health care services.

In the meantime MCA and the Henry Street Visiting Nurse Association collaborated in the conduct of a study which illustrated the value of specialized maternity care within a generalized public health nursing program. Subsequently MCA embarked upon an intensive educational program in maternity care for both the public and professional health personnel, especially physicians and public health nurses.

MCA expanded its efforts beyond New York City; it endeavored to supply information about the need for maternity care to expectant parents throughout the United States. Mother's Day was dedicated to this endeavor for several years with an emphasis on saving mothers' lives. The mayors of cities made Mothers' Day proclamations regarding saving mothers' lives and ministers preached their Mother's Day sermons on the subject, using packets of educational materials sent by MCA.

On the basis of their demonstration of providing complete maternity care, their collaboration with the Henry Street Visiting Nurse Association, and a study of maternity care in other countries, MCA concluded that the need existed to prepare nurses to do normal obstetrics and discussed opening a school of nurse-midwifery. This idea was temporarily thwarted in the early 1920s by bitter opposition from both medicine and nursing and by a lack of cooperation from city officials.

The "Midwife Problem"

In the early 1900s a debate over what was known as "the midwife problem" took place. The factors mentioned earlier as contributing to the disrepute of midwifery converged around 1912 to 1914 to make a heated issue of the licensing and practice of the midwife.

During this time medical schools began to include obstetrics in their curricula, and obstetrics became an established medical specially by 1930. Obstetric care began a mass movement out of the home into the hospital, and laws were passed to regulate the practice of the indigenous midwives. The heated debate ensued.

On the one side of the debate were a majority who believed that all midwifery should be abolished; on the other side were those who believed midwives could perform a valuable function. The former feared the status legality would give the midwives as they believed improving the practice of midwives was an impossible task. Those in favor felt midwifery was practical with proper training, licensing, and supervision.

Two significant events took place while the debate raged. The first event grew out of realities. Some states had already passed laws granting legal recognition to midwives and including requirements and specifications aimed at control of their practice. These laws were passed in an effort to reduce the high mortality rates since it was evident that the medical profession could not assume the entire task of obstetric care.

Several schools were established as a result of the laws to regulate midwifery practice. Two of these schools, designed to instruct the indigenous midwives in meeting requirements for practice, are best known: The Bellevue School of Midwifery in New York City and the Preston Retreat Hospital in Philadelphia. The Preston Retreat Hospital opened in 1923 but dwindled in enrollment after 1930. The Bellevue School of Midwifery existed from 1911 until 1935, when it was closed by order of the New York City commissioner of hospitals, a physician. In his opinion, changing social and medical standards rendered the school superfluous and an unnecessary expense to the city. He cited a decrease in the number of midwives as deliveries within hospitals had increased to 81 percent in New York City (3).

The laws and schools to upgrade midwifery had served their purpose, and obstetric care for a large number of mothers and infants was improved. In addition, Congress passed the Sheppard-Towner Act in 1921; this legislation assigned money, administered through the Children's Bureau, for providing better maternal-infant care. Included in this Act was the specification that public health nurses should be employed for the instruction of untrained midwives.

The second significant event was the introduction of nurse-midwives from Europe. Nurse-midwives had proven their effectiveness in European countries where they were an established part of the health care system.

The Frontier Nursing Service

The first nurse-midwives to practice in the United States were British-trained nurse-midwives brought to this country in 1925 by Mary Breckinridge as part of her plan to provide health care for the remote rural people in the Kentucky mountains. This endeavor was organized as the Kentucky Committee for Mothers and Babies in May 1925; through a change in its articles of incorporation it became the Frontier Nursing Service (FNS) in 1928.

Breckinridge was admirably suited for the task she initiated and undertook. Her qualifications included a family background and upbringing which gave her a wealth of influential contacts, professional preparation as a registered nurse in the United States and as a state certified midwife in England, personal and professional life experiences, and a carefully self-designed program of observation and study of the Highlands and Islands Medical and Nursing Service in Scotland, concentrating on the Outer Hebrides with further study in England. From this background she crystallized a plan involving outpost nursing centers staffed by nurse-midwives and backed by a medical director located at a small, local, rural hospital. Breckinridge's program was to be administered by a director overseen by an executive com-

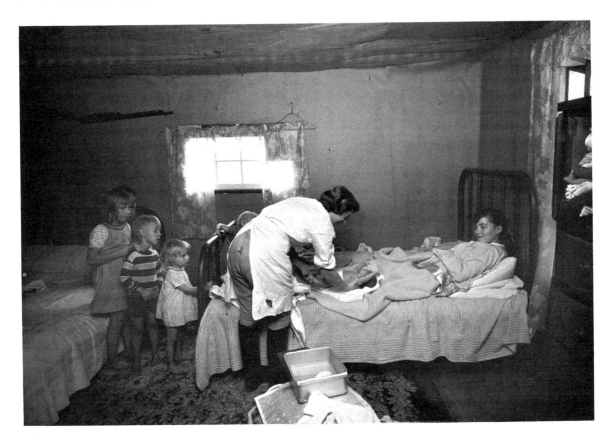

FIGURE 2-1. A nurse-mildwife of the Frontier Nursing Service in a home in Kentucky, circa 1950. (Reproduced by permission from Frontier Nursing Service, Hyden, Kentucky.)

mittee and board of trustees, and supported by local committees throughout the United States. Before the work began, a survey of births and deaths in the region was conducted to provide baseline data for subsequent statistics and research. In her book *Wide Neighborhoods* [4], Breckinridge writes in fascinating detail of the myriad activities, people, concerns, and problems involved in bringing her plan to fruition.

The work and record of the Frontier Nursing Service (Fig. 2-1) is legendary. The records kept during the earlier years were in accord with a statistical system set up by the Carnegie Corporation and tabulated by statisticians from the Metropolitan Life Insurance Com-

pany. In 1951 the Frontier Nursing Service statistics showed that 8596 registered nurse-midwifery patients had been delivered since 1925, 6533 of which were delivered in mostly primitive homes, with a gross maternal death rate of 1.2 per thousand for the 25 years studied. This was in contrast to a national maternal mortality rate of 6.73 per thousand in 1931; 3.76 per thousand in 1940; and 0.83 per thousand in 1950, or an average of 3.4 per thousand for the same overall period of time. In addition, a comprehensive scope of health care services had been brought to the people including general dental, pediatric, medical, and surgical services; general eye, tonsil, and worm treatment services; special tuberculosis and trachoma services; and social services supported by Alpha Omicron Pi, national sorority of social workers, as its national philanthropic project.

World War II had a great effect on the Frontier Nursing Service both in manpower and in the direction it mandated for nurse-midwifery education at FNS. Great Britain had been both the source of British nurse-midwives working in the Frontier Nursing Service and also the provider of midwifery education for United States registered nurses, who were sent to Great Britain for their education and returned to work at the FNS. With the advent of war the British nurse-midwives wanted to return to their homeland to be of service to their country. It became evident that a long-deferred plan for an educational program in nurse-midwifery had to be instituted immediately. The Frontier Graduate School of Midwifery started with a class of two students in November 1939. By the summer of 1976, 460 nurse-midwives had graduated from the school of the Frontier Nursing Service. In 1970 it changed its name to the Frontier School of Midwifery and Family Nursing. It was not, however, the first nurse-midwifery education program in the United States.

The First Nurse-Midwifery Education Program

The School of the Association for the Promotion and Standardization of Midwifery, more commonly known as the Lobenstine Midwifery School, was the first nurse-midwifery education program in the United States. Actually, the Association for the Promotion and Stand-ardization of Midwifery was the creation of the Maternity Center Association in New York City. MCA was convinced of the need for nurse-midwives whose education would combine United States education in obstetric nursing with the education received by the professional European mid-wife. Much had happened to create a more favorable atmosphere since the abortive attempt by MCA in the early 1920s to establish a nurse-midwifery education program. There was growing recognition of the poor obstetric conditions in the United States as contrasted to other countries with much lower mortality rates but a well organized system of educated and supervised midwives. Publicity spread about the conclusive proof by the Frontier Nursing Service of the value of a system utilizing nurse-midwives, the work of Maternity Center Association in parent education, and their demonstration with the Henry Street Visiting Nurse Association illustrating the value of specialized maternity nursing care.

The Association for the Promotion and Standardization of Midwifery was incorporated in early 1931 by three members of the medical board of the Maternity Center Association and its general director, Hazel Corbin, R.N. Ralph Waldo Lobenstine, M.D., chairman of the medical board of MCA since 1918, was one of the charter members, as was Mary Breckinridge, director of the Frontier Nursing Service. Lobenstine worked tirelessly until his death in 1931 to bring about the establishment of nurse-midwifery services and education. The determination of the members of the Association for the Promotion and Standardization of Midwifery and the financial support of a group of 60 former patients and friends of Lobenstine led to the establishment of the Lobenstine Midwifery Clinic, Inc., in November 1931.

Organization and administrative details of the clinic were worked out and a curriculum was designed for the school, the latter guided by British curricula and modified to meet the needs, cultural patterns, and health care systems in the United States. Hattie Hemschemeyer, a public health nurse educator, was named director of the Lobenstine Midwifery Clinic and School. Rose McNaught, a public health nurse who had obtained her midwifery preparation in London and then returned to work at the Frontier Nursing Service, was loaned by

FNS to help develop the program and joined the Lobenstein staff as clinician and faculty. The school opened in September 1932 and had six graduates in 1933, including Hattie Hemschemeyer. The memorial funds which had been pledged to establish and maintain the school and clinic for 3 years were exhausted in 1934. Therefore, in 1935, Maternity Center Association and the Lobenstine Midwifery Clinic consolidated under the name and auspices of Maternity Center Association, which also assumed administrative and financial responsibility for the School of the Association for the Promotion and Standardization of Midwifery.

The nurse-midwifery services through the clinic consisted of providing antepartal care and patient education at the clinic, intrapartal and postpartal care in the patient's home except when hospitalization was required for medical reasons, and postpartum checkups at 14 days and 6 weeks in the clinic. Four attending obstetricians provided medical clinics and round-the-clock consultation and, if necessary, were present in the patient's home for delivery. During the 26 years this service was provided (1932–1958), a total of 7099 deliveries were attended, of which 6116 took place in the patient's home. The maternal mortality rate of the clinic was 0.9 per thousand live births as contrasted to a maternal death rate of 10.4 per thousand live births for the same geographic district as a whole and 1.2 per thousand live births for a leading hospital in New York City.

The Maternity Center Association School of Nurse-Midwifery (Fig. 2-2) graduated 320 students from 1933 to 1959, utilizing the services provided by the clinic for educational purposes. In 1958 the Maternity Center Association School of Nurse-Midwifery moved inside a major medical and educational institution and was established in the Downstate Medical Center, State University of New York in Brooklyn, New York, utilizing Kings County Hospital for clinical experience. This move was facilitated by Hazel Corbin, R.N., executive director of

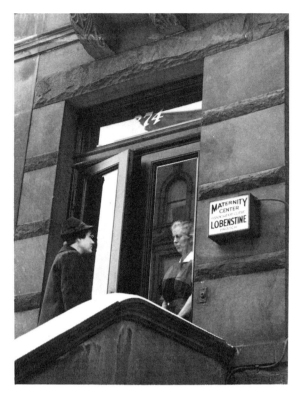

FIGURE 2-2. A new nurse-midwifery student (Margaret Thomas) in the 1930s being greeted by Rose McNaught, first nurse-midwifery educator in the United States, at the Maternity Center Association Lobenstine Clinic and School. (Reproduced by permission from Maternity Center Association, New York, New York.)

MCA, Marion Strachan, C.N.M., director of the nurse-midwifery program, and Louis Hellman, M.D., chairman and professor of obstetrics and gynecology at Downstate Medical Center and Kings County Hospital.

Subsequent Programs of Education

All of nurse-midwifery education today can trace its beginnings to the Maternity Center Association's School of Nurse-Midwifery because all schools, with the exception of the program at the Frontier Nursing Service, have been started by either graduates or students of graduates of the MCA program. By 1965 there were nine nurse-midwifery education programs. They are listed here with their starting dates and locations:

1932 School of the Association for the Promotion and Standardization of Midwifery. (Became the Maternity Center Association School of Nurse-Midwifery in 1934. Affiliated with Downstate Medical Center, State University of New York and Kings County Hospital, Brooklyn, New York, in 1958.)
1939 Frontier Graduate School of Midwifery of the Frontier Nursing Service, Hyden, Kentucky.
1945 Catholic Maternity Institute School of Nurse-Midwifery, Santa Fe, New Mexico.
1947 Catholic University of America, Washington, D.C. (Affiliated with Catholic Maternity Institute.)
1955 Columbia University Graduate Program in Maternity Nursing, New York City, New York.
1956 The Johns Hopkins University Nurse-Midwifery Program, Baltimore, Maryland.
1956 Yale University Graduate Maternal and Newborn Health Nursing Program, New Haven, Connecticut.
1963 New York Medical College Graduate School of Nursing Nurse-Midwifery Program, New York City, New York.
1965 University of Utah Graduate Maternal-Infant Nursing Program, Salt Lake City, Utah.

Four of these programs subsequently closed — Catholic Maternity Institute (1968); Catholic University of America (1968), which had the distinction of being the first nurse-midwifery education program to be part of a master's degree program; New York Medical College (1972); and The Johns Hopkins University Nurse-Midwifery Program (1981). In addition, three other schools opened and closed during the 1930s and 1940s:

1933–1942 The Preston Retreat School of Nurse Midwifery in Philadelphia. Originally designed to aid indigenous midwives meet requirements for practice; changed to educating nurses as nurse-midwives. Graduated six students.
1941–1946 The Tuskegee School of Nurse-Midwifery in Tuskegee, Alabama. Joint project of the Tuskegee Institute and the Alabama State Department of Health. Graduated 25 students.
1942–1943 The Flint Goodridge School of Nurse-Midwifery in New Orleans, Louisiana. In connection with Flint Goodridge Hospital and Dillard University. Graduated two students.

THE 1940s AND 1950s

The early graduates from MCA went into a variety of positions, the only common denominator being that of improving maternity care. The majority of graduates either practiced clinical nurse-midwifery in the MCA or FNS programs or became involved with various aspects of public health. A number of nurse-midwives in public health went into positions in state health departments designed for the supervision, teaching, and control of indigenous midwives. This was in keeping with the original thought in the Sheppard-Towner Act that public health nurses be employed for the instruction of untrained midwives. Since many of the early MCA graduates were also public health nurses, they were ideally prepared for working in rural maternity care, where the majority of indigenous midwives were.

Other graduates held positions as maternal-child health consultants for the state boards of health. Still other graduates became involved in projects which became Tuskegee Institute's program in Alabama and the Flint Goodrich program in Louisiana.

In 1944 members of the Medical Mission Sisters, a Roman Catholic order, who were graduates of the MCA program, started the Catholic Maternity Institute (CMI) in Santa Fe. CMI long stood as an outstanding example of what could be accomplished through inter-agency cooperation and commitment to patient care.

In the middle and late 1940s, graduates of MCA at Yale University were central in deve-loping the concept and practice of rooming-in and in studying the effects of natural (prepared) childbirth on a woman's antepartal, intrapartal, and postpartal experience. From this work evolved the concept of family-centered maternity care.

The 1950s saw the development of three more educational programs by MCA graduates at Columbia University, The Johns Hopkins University, and Yale University. Maternity Center Association was directly involved in initiating two of these programs by sending nurse-midwives to start them (Columbia and Johns Hopkins).

In the 1940s and 1950s there was consider-able demand for nurse-midwives as nursing educators in maternity nursing; for nursing service staff, supervisory, and consultant positions in hospital obstetrics departments; and as consultants in federal and international health organizations. These employment possibilities, combined with a lack of oppor-tunities for clinical nurse-midwifery practice, created the situation in which a large per-centage of the early graduate nurse-midwives did not actually practice clinical nurse-midwifery.

THE 1960s

A nurse-midwife graduating in the early 1960s was severely limited in opportunities to prac-tice clinical nurse-midwifery. Only three legal jurisdictions provided for the practice of nurse-midwifery at that time: New Mexico, Kentucky, and New York City. Another legal jurisdiction,

Maryland, had nurse-midwives practicing under an old granny midwife law.

In brief, a graduate could join the faculty of one of the six existing nurse-midwifery schools; practice at Catholic Maternity Institute in Santa Fe, Frontier Nursing Service in Kentucky, Baltimore City Hospital and Johns Hopkins University in Baltimore, or Kings County Hospital or Cumberland Hospital in New York City; or go to an overseas mission field. A few other isolated service positions or projects existed but generally were not known or were, as in the case of the Madera County project in California, known to be limited for long-term employment by virtue of being a demonstration project. Therefore, the majority of graduates of that era went into teaching, supervisory, ad-ministrative, or consultative positions in related fields. This situation led to the need for re-fresher programs for nurse-midwives wanting to return to the practice of clinical nurse-midwifery when, less than a decade later, there was a rapid expansion in service sites in which to practice.

In the late 1950s and during the 1960s nurse-midwives made a deliberate and concerted effort to get into hospitals because this was where the majority of births (approximately 70 percent at that time) were taking place. The movement of nurse-midwives into hospitals brought concepts of family-centered maternity care and a consumer advocate to childbearing women who delivered in hospitals. Nurse-midwives were now working in both in-hospital and out-of-hospital settings.

By 1967 approximately 23 percent of 468 employed nurse-midwives responding to a questionnaire [5] were actually practicing clinical nurse-midwifery. This was an increase from 11 percent in 1963. Of the 468 employed nurse-midwives in 1967, 103 (22 percent) were in foreign countries, mostly through church missions or international health organizations. Fifty-six percent of the employed nurse-midwives in 1967 were in service areas related to nurse-midwifery but not actually practicing nurse-midwifery (e.g., working in obstetrics, pediatrics, maternal-child health programs, and public health departments as supervisors, administrators, staff nurses, head nurses, consultants, educators, and researchers); 75 percent held positions above the staff level. Of the 23 percent practicing nurse-midwifery, 35 percent were also on faculties of schools of nurse-midwifery; 53 percent were giving nurse-midwifery services throughout the maternity cycle; and the remaining 12 percent were functioning as nurse-midwives in one or more, but not all, of the phases of the maternity cycle.

Development of opportunities to practice clinical nurse-midwifery was slow into the late 1960s with a few isolated areas utilizing practicing nurse-midwives and the remaining nurse-midwives contributing to maternal-infant health care in related fields. A number of obstacles contributed to this situation. Paramount among these were misconceptions and stereotypes regarding nurse-midwives. These mistaken ideas led to outright hostility by some professionals at the same time still other professionals came to believe in and support the development of nurse-midwifery. Hostility and support have emanated from both professional groups of colleagues with whom nurse-midwives work — physicians and nurses.

The misconceptions and stereotypes which hindered the development of nurse-midwifery in the 1960s and the factual rebuttal to them at that time included the following:

Stereotype: "Midwives" are all alike. Frequently, when only the *midwife* part of *nurse-midwife* is used or heard, a negative image is conjured up. This image is of the good-hearted, loving, but untrained midwife either of past history or in rural areas of the South today, or functioning as a birth attendant for those disenchanted with the present health care system. It leads to the irrational conclusion that nurse-midwives

are an uneducated menace representing a backwards step into illiteracy in the provision of maternal-infant health care.

Fact: The name *nurse-midwife* actually specifies exactly who and what a nurse-midwife is. Either part of the name alone does not fully describe the unique profession of the nurse-midwife in the United States.

The *nurse* part recognizes the prerequisite education in nursing, differentiates the nurse-midwife from the lay midwife of both history and today, and assures a continuing emphasis on patient education, support, and counseling. All certified nurse-midwives are registered nurses. Two-thirds of the nurse-midwifery education programs are in schools granting the master's degree.

The *midwife* part of the name recognizes the additional specialized preparation and functioning of the nurse-midwife, tempers the medical focus in normal obstetrics, and identifies the nurse-midwife with professional midwife counterparts the world over.

Misconception: Nurse-midwives are trying to be "little doctors." Thus some physicians think that nurse-midwives don't know "their place," while some nurses think that nurse-midwives have "sold out" to the physicians and are, therefore, traitors to nursing.

Fact: Nurse-midwifery is a clearly defined profession. Nurse-midwives believe fervently in who they are, what they have to offer, and what they can do. In fact, lack of acceptance for years by both medicine and nursing meant that the profession of nurse-midwifery attracted only those individuals who were highly dedicated and committed to contributing to the improvement and provision of maternal-infant health care in this capacity.

Nurse-midwives are experts in the normal childbearing cycle. They wish to be precisely who they are and to be doing precisely what they do — encouraging and facilitating natural, normal childbearing processes with a minimum of interference; educating, supporting, and instigating personal and family growth; fostering self-confidence and independence; dispelling fear and providing an atmosphere of love and joy (not possible when there are life-threatening complications requiring necessary machines and medical or surgical intervention).

Nurse-midwives have the best of two worlds — nursing and medicine. Nurse-midwives are neither sell-outs nor traitors to either. Instead, they realistically recognize the need for the support of both the nursing and medical professions in order for real growth in nurse-midwifery to take place. For the benefit of mothers and babies, nurse-midwives continue to seek accord with both.

THE 1970s

It was in the late 1960s and early 1970s that it all changed. Suddenly nurse-midwifery was not only acceptable but inundated with requests for practitioners and berated for the lack of nurse-midwives to meet the demand. The late 1960s and early 1970s were a time of rapid development in nurse-midwifery, with widespread proliferation of nurse-midwifery services and educational programs. A number of factors contributed to this growth:

1. Official recognition by organized obstetrics. A joint statement in 1971 from the American College of Obstetricians and Gynecologists, the Nurses Association of the American College of Obstetricians and Gynecologists, and the American College of Nurse-Midwives recognized and supported the development and utilization of nurse-midwives.
2. Increased visibility and involvement of the women's movement and feminism, which increased feelings of self-worth and self-confidence in all women. This led to

a natural alliance between women who wanted to participate in and be responsible for their childbearing experience and nurse-midwives, who facilitate the natural and normal processes, provide family-centered care, and promote parental self-determination.

3. Recognition by the consumer. An increasing number of articles about the "new midwife" were published in major lay magazines, Sunday newsmagazines, and newspapers, such as *Redbook, Newsweek, Life, McCall's, The New York Times, The Wall Street Journal.* Consumer awareness and satisfaction of those experiencing nurse-midwifery care and writing about it led to consumer demand for nurse-midwifery services.
4. Utilization of nurse-midwives in federally funded projects such as Maternal-Infant Care (MIC), Family Planning Monies (314E), Agency for International Development (AID), and demonstration projects geared towards improving maternal-infant health care and providing family planning services. Through these projects more professionals became familiar with nurse-midwifery. This familiarity dispelled misconceptions, and many physicians and nurses subsequently became ardent supporters of nurse-midwifery.
5. The children of the post-World War II baby boom were having babies during the mid-1960s and 1970s. This population peak led to the thought that there was not, and was not going to be, a sufficient supply of obstetricians to care for all of the childbearing women in the country. This, combined with the small number of general practitioners doing obstetrics, made a lack of manpower during this period of time obvious. This shortage led to scrutiny about how to utilize the optimal capabilities of each health care worker and promoted commitment to the obstetric team concept.
6. Demonstration of the efficacy of the obstetric team concept. The effectiveness of

nurse-midwives has been statistically proven again and again since the first studies at the Frontier Nursing Service, reproven again in the Madera County Demonstration Program in California, shown in every service where nurse-midwives have worked, and again dramatically shown in the team concept which decreased by half the infant mortality in Holmes County, Mississippi, in 1971.

7. The involvement of nurse-midwives in interconceptional health care, i.e., family planning, human sexuality, and gynecological screening, and in neonatal care including promotion of parenting. This involvement fully rounds out nurse-midwifery management throughout the childbearing cycle, thereby providing continuity of care to the developing family.

The first private practice with nurse-midwives was in the early 1970s. With the consumer "discovery" of the nurse-midwife there was a burgeoning of private practice nurse-midwives and another inhibiting misconception was laid to rest:

Misconception: Nurse-midwifery is second-class care for second-class citizens. Therefore it follows that nurse-midwives can be utilized only for care of the indigent and will never be accepted by middle- and upper-class patients.

Fact: By the mid-1970s nurse-midwives were in practice with physicians all over the country taking care of middle- and upper-class patients. According to the 1976–1977 survey [6], approximately 26 percent of all nurse-midwives practicing nurse-midwifery were in some form of private practice arrangement. Nurse-midwives are well accepted by these patients, who often prefer to be seen in the office and to be delivered by the nurse-midwife as long as their condition does not require the physician member of the team. This preference is largely a result of the time the nurse-midwife spends in explanations and teaching during the office visits, the commitment of the nurse-midwife to the patient throughout labor, and the practical application of the beliefs of the nurse-midwife in promoting a family-centered, normal childbearing experience. This places the obstetrician in the difficult position of feeling displaced at the same time the obstetrician is initially introducing the nurse-midwife into his or her private practice and is creating the environment for acceptance of the nurse-midwife until the nurse-midwife earns this acceptance from the patients by virtue of the care she or he gives them. Mutual professional understanding and patience are required in order for the patient to obtain the maximum benefit and advantages of the physician/nurse-midwife team approach.

The misconception came from the fact that nurse-midwifery practice for years was mainly in large medical centers and city hospitals serving the medically indigent or in remote rural areas where physicians were few. This initial concentration of nurse-midwives in lower socioeconomic patient care settings occurred because the professional services a nurse-midwife can give was welcomed first in areas where help was most desperately needed.

Nurse-midwifery had become not only acceptable but also desirable and demanded. Now the problem was that, after years during which nurse-midwives struggled for existence, there was nowhere near the supply to meet the demand. Varney discussed the conflicting pressure on nurse-midwives in the 1970s in her 1980 edition of this book as follows:

On the one hand is the need for providing quantity services sufficient to warrant the expense of utilizing nurse-midwives by the established health care system and the need for nurse-midwives to be able to function within this system to benefit mothers and babies either desiring or needing care in the system. On the other hand, there is a small but growing number of consumers who are dissatisfied with the health care provided by the system, who desire care outside of the system, and who look to nurse-midwives for support and services. Lack of response with childbirth alternatives (e.g., hospital birthing rooms, childbirth centers, or carefully selected home births) further disenchants the consumer with professional health care and fosters the development of often untrained lay midwives or birth attendants, and a do-it-yourself movement. Affecting this conflict is the issue of nurse-midwives being able to collect third party payment for services. The resolution of this conflict has far-reaching implications and ramifications and constitutes the challenge nurse-midwifery has had in the latter half of the 1970s (7).

THE EARLY 1980s

Nurse-midwives were now practicing in the full range of possible practice arenas: from clinics and federally funded programs to hospital delivery services, from in-hospital delivery services to out-of-hospital delivery services or a mix of both, from being employed by physicians to employing the physicians. By the 1980s, nurse-midwives were perceived to be competitors for the obstetric health care dollar. While supportive physicians continued to enable nurse-midwifery practice to exist by providing necessary physician consultation, collaboration, and referral systems, opposing physicians tried to restrict the growth of nurse-midwifery through state legislative battles over statutory recognition of nurse-midwives, denial of hospital practice privileges, attempts to keep nurse-midwives from getting direct third party reimbursement, and pressure on supportive physicians vis-a-vis their malpractice insurance.

An investigative congressional hearing into the problems nurse-midwives were having was held in 1980 and the Federal Trade Commission became actively concerned with possible and real restraint of trade issues. At the same time health care costs had become unacceptably high and some services run by nurse-midwives were demonstrating that they were cost effective.

The entire situation was exacerbated by the fact that there was an overabundance of physi-

cians and would continue to be an excess for the foreseeable future. In the viewpoint of many physicians, nurse-midwives were no longer needed.

The late 1970s and early 1980s also saw the rapid development of out-of-hospital childbirth centers, with Maternity Center Association again leading the way as it spearheaded this movement. The history of out-of-hospital childbirth centers is detailed in Chapter 20.

Educational Programs

Between 1969 and January 1979, nurse-midwifery education proliferated to a total of 21 basic educational programs, thereby more than doubling in 10 years the number of programs developed during the preceding 37 years. By the end of 1985 there were 26 basic educational programs. A listing of all the basic educational programs accredited by the American College of Nurse-Midwives in 1985 is presented in Appendix IV, at the end of this chapter. Four educational programs opened and closed between 1969 and 1985:

1969–1985 University of Mississippi Medical Center Nurse-Midwifery Program
1971–1974 Loma Linda University Nurse-Midwifery Program
1973–1984 St. Louis University Graduate Program in Nurse-Midwifery
1977–1985 University of Arizona Nurse-Midwifery Program.

Nurse-midwives have cooperated with each other in the provision of clinical facilities and clinical faculty for educational purposes. This has meant sacrifice on the part of many, for the joy and motivation of the practicing nurse-midwife is to be directly providing services to women, their babies, and their families.

There are two types of basic nurse-midwifery education programs which prepare nurse-midwives for practice and for taking the national certification examination of the American

College of Nurse-Midwives (ACNM). These are certificate programs and higher degree programs. A little over half of the nurse-midwifery programs are included in the requirements leading to a master's degree. The master's degree programs are 18 months to 2 years in length. The certificate programs are for those registered nurses who either do not have the academic credentials to be accepted in a graduate program (i.e., diploma and associate degree nurses) or already have a master's or doctoral degree and simply want to obtain the clinical expertise and practice of a nurse-midwife. Most certificate programs are 9 to 12 months in length. One basic nurse-midwifery education program is included in the requirements leading to a doctor in nursing science.

The actual nurse-midwifery clinical component curriculum in all basic educational programs takes from 9 to 12 months, although it may spread out over a longer period of time in the degree programs. This curriculum is essentially the same in all the programs and includes preparation for the core competencies in nurse-midwifery which have been identified by the American College of Nurse-Midwives as expected outcomes of nurse-midwifery education. Appendix V at the end of this chapter presents the ACNM document on core competencies.

All basic nurse-midwifery education programs have to be within or affiliated with institutions of higher learning as a prerequisite for obtaining program accreditation from the American College of Nurse-Midwives. The majority of nurse-midwifery education programs are administratively located in university schools or colleges of nursing. A few are in schools of medicine (department of obstetrics and gynecology), allied health, or public health.

In order for graduates of a nurse-midwifery education program to be eligible to sit for the national certification examination of the American College of Nurse-Midwives, the program must be accredited by the American College of Nurse-Midwives. The accreditation process is similar to that of the National League for Nursing (NLN) in their accreditation of schools of nursing. At times joint NLN and ACNM accreditation site visits have been arranged.

There are refresher programs for nurse-midwives who have been out of practice for a period of time and for foreign-trained nurse-midwives preparatory for taking the ACNM certification examination. The refresher programs vary in length in accord with individual need but generally take 4 months. Some basic nurse-midwifery education programs which have mastery learning curricula and utilize modules thereby allowing for student self-pacing accept refresher students with the expectation that they will finish the program in much less time than a basic student.

The Practice of Nurse-Midwifery

A survey made of nurse-midwives in 1971 showed that 37 percent of the respondents were in the direct practice of nurse-midwifery as opposed to 23 percent in 1967 and 18 percent of those nurse-midwives practicing in the United States in 1963. By 1976–1977, 51 percent of 1218 respondents living in the United States and replying to a questionnaire [6] were actually practicing nurse-midwifery. Within 15 years active nurse-midwifery services increased in number from 6 services in 3 states and New York City to multiple services in 35 states, with more in planning stages. By 1982, 67 percent of 1584 survey participants living in the United States stated they were practicing nurse-midwifery [8]. In 1984 nurse-midwives were practicing in all 50 states.

The legal practice of nurse-midwifery had gone from 3 states and New York City in 1963, with the possible legal status in the other states largely unknown, to a very clear understanding of the legal status in all 50 states and 4 jurisdictions (District of Columbia, Guam, Puerto Rico, Virgin Islands) as a result of extensive and intensive work by the legislation committee of the American College of Nurse-

Midwives. In 1984, only one state had an unclear legal basis for nurse-midwifery practice (North Dakota — CNMs, however, do practice at the U.S. Air Force base in North Dakota; Nebraska passed nurse-midwifery legislation in 1984) [9]. From practicing almost exclusively in large medical centers, city hospitals, and remote rural areas in the early 1960s, nurse-midwives were practicing in every possible type of setting by the late 1970s and early 1980s. Because continuity of care is an essential component of nurse-midwifery care, a nurse-midwife may utilize more than one practice setting.

REFERENCES

1. Fox, C.G. Toward a sound historical basis for nurse-midwifery. *Bull. Am. Col. Nurse-Midwifery* 14:77, 1969.
2. Swenson, N. The role of the nurse-midwife on the health team as viewed by the family. *Bull. Am. Coll. Nurse-Midwifery* 13:128, 1968.
3. Newspaper article, 1934.
4. Breckinridge, M. *Wide Neighborhoods: A story of the Frontier Nursing Service.* New York: Harper & Brothers, 1952.
5. American College of Nurse-Midwifery. *Descriptive Data, Nurse-Midwives — U.S.A., 1968.*
6. American College of Nurse-Midwives. *Nurse-Midwifery in the United States: 1976—1977,* 1978.
7. Varney, H. *Nurse-Midwifery.* Boston: Blackwell Scientific Publishing, 1980, p. 26.
8. American College of Nurse-Midwives. *Nurse-Midwifery in the United States: 1982,* Washington, D.C., 1984.
9. Cohn, S., Cuddihy, N., Kraus, N., and Tom, S. Legislation and nurse-midwifery practice in the USA. (Special legislative issue.) *J. Nurse-Midwifery* 29(2) (March/April) 1984.

BIBLIOGRAPHY

American College of Nurse-Midwifery. *Descriptive Data, Nurse-Midwives — U.S.A., 1963.* New York, 1963.

American College of Nurse-Midwifery. *Descriptive Data, Nurse-Midwives — U.S.A., 1968.* New York, 1968.

American College of Nurse-Midwives. *Descriptive Data, Nurse-Midwives — U.S.A., 1971.* New York, 1971.

American College of Nurse-Midwives. *Nurse-Midwifery in the United States: 1976—1977.* Washington, D.C., 1978.

American College of Nurse-Midwives. *Nurse-Midwifery in the United States: 1982.* Washington, D.C., 1984.

American College of Nurse-Midwives. *What is a Nurse-Midwife?* Washington, D.C., 1978.

Breckinridge, M. *Wide Neighborhoods: A Story of the Frontier Nursing Service.* New York: Harper and Brothers, 1952.

Browne, H.E. and Isaacs, G. The Frontier Nursing Service. *Am. J. Obstet. Gynecol.* 124:16, 1976.

Burnett, J.E., Jr. A physician-sponsored community nurse-midwife program. *Obstet. Gynecol.* 40:719, 1972.

Burst, H.V. Harmonious unity. *J. Nurse-Midwifery* 22:10, 1977.

Burst, H.V. Our three-ring circus. *J. Nurse-Midwifery* 23:11, 1978.

Burst, H.V. The American College of Nurse-Midwives: A professional organization. *J. Nurse-Midwifery* 25(1):4—6 (January/February) 1980.

Burst, H.V. The influence of consumers on the birthing movement. In J. Strawn (Ed.). *Topics in Clinical Nursing: Rehumanizing the Acute Care Setting* 5(3):42—54 (October) 1983.

Cameron, J. The history and development of midwifery in the United States. *Can Maternity Nursing Meet Today's Challenge?* Columbus, Ohio: Ross Laboratories, 1967.

Chaney, J.A. Birthing in early America. *J. Nurse-Midwifery* 25(2):5—13 (March/April) 1980.

Cherry, J., and Foster, J.C. Comparison of hospital charges generated by certified nurse-midwives' and physicians' clients. *J. Nurse-Midwifery* 27(1):7—11 (January/February) 1982.

Cohn, S., Cuddihy, N., Kraus, N., and Tom, S. Legislation and nurse-midwifery practice in the USA. (Special legislative issue.) *J. Nurse-Midwifery* 29(2) (March/April) 1984.

Corbin, H. *Forty-Fifth Annual Report.* New York: Maternity Center Association, 1963.

Corbin, H. Historical development of nurse-midwifery in this country and present trends.

Bull. Am. Coll. Nurse-Midwifery 4:13, 1959.

Crowe-Carraco, C. Mary Breckinridge and the Frontier Nursing Service. *The Register of the Kentucky Historical Society* July, 1978.

Diers, D., and Burst, H.V. Effectiveness of policy related research: nurse-midwifery as case study. *Image* 15(3):68–74 (Summer) 1983.

Ernst, E.K.M., and Gordon, K.A. Fifty-three years of home birth experience at the Frontier Nursing Service, Kentucky: 1925–1978. In L. Stewart and D. Stewart (Eds.). *Compulsory Hospitalization: Freedom of Choice in Childbirth? Vol. 2.* Marble Hill, Missouri: NAPSAC Publications, 1979.

Forman, A.M., and Cooper, E.M. Legislation and nurse-midwifery practice in the USA: Report on a survey conducted by the legislation committee of the American College of Nurse-Midwives. *J. Nurse-Midwifery* 21:1, 1976.

Fox, C.G. Toward a sound historical basis for nurse-midwifery, *Bull. Am. Coll. Nurse-Midwives* 14:76, 1969.

Gatewood, T.S., and Stewart, R.B. Obstetricians and nurse-midwives: The team approach in private practice. *Am. J. Obstet. Gynecol.* 123:35, 1975.

Harris, D. The development of nurse-midwifery in New York City. *Bull. Am. Coll. Nurse-Midwifery* 14:4, 1969.

Hellman, L.M., and O'Brien, F.B. Nurse-midwifery: an experiment in maternity care. *Obstet. Gynecol.* 24:343–349, 1964.

Hellman, L.M. Nurse-midwifery in the United States. *Obstet. Gynecol.* 30:883, 1967.

Hemschemeyer, H. Report of the first president of the American College of Nurse-Midwifery. *Bull. Am. Coll. Nurse-Midwifery* 10:8, 1965.

Hemschemeyer, H. Sends message to members. *Bull. Am. Coll. Nurse-Midwifery* 1:5, 1956.

Hogan, A. A tribute to the pioneers. *J. Nurse-Midwifery* 20:6, 1975.

Hosford, E. Alternative patterns of nurse-midwifery care: III. The home birth movement. *J. Nurse-Midwifery* 21:27, 1976.

Kroska, R. The emblem of the American College of Nurse-Midwives, *J. Nurse-Midwifery* 28: 23, 1973.

Lang, D.M. Providing maternity care through a nurse-midwifery service program, *Nurs. Clin. North Am.* 4:509, 1969.

Lazarus, W., Levine, E.S., and Lewin, L.S. *Competition among Health Practitioners: The Influence of the Medical Profession on the Health Manpower Market. Vol. 1: Executive Summary and Final Report; Vol. 2: The Childbearing Center Case Study.* Washington, D.C.: Federal Trade Commission, February, 1981.

Levy, B.S., Wilkinson, F.S., and Marine, W.M. Reducing neonatal mortality rate with nurse-midwives. *Am. J. Obstet. Gynecol.* 109:50, 1971.

Litoff, J.B. *American Midwives: 1860 to the Present.* Westport, Ct.: Greenwood Press, 1978.

Litoff, J.B. The midwife throughout history. *J. Nurse-Midwifery* 27(6):3–11 (November/December) 1982.

Lubic, R.W. Evaluation of an out-of-hospital maternity center for low risk patients. In L.H. Aiken (Ed.), *Hospital Policy and Nursing Practice.* New York: McGraw-Hill, 1980.

Lubic, R.W. The nurse-midwife joins the obstetrical team. *Bull. Am. Coll. Nurse-Midwives* 27:73, 1972.

Lubic, R.W., and Ernst, E.K.M. The childbearing center: An alternative to conventional care. *Nurs. Outlook* 26:754, 1978.

Maternity Center Association. *Maternity Center Association, 1918–1943.* New York: Maternity Center Association, 1943.

Maternity Center Association. *Twenty Years of Nurse-Midwifery, 1933–1953.* New York: Maternity Center Association, 1955.

Meglen, M.C. Nurse-midwife program in the southeast cuts mortality rates. *Contemporary OB/GYN* 8:79, 1976.

Meglen, M.C., and Burst, H.V. Nurse-midwives make a difference. *Nurs. Outlook* 22:382, 1974.

Metropolitan Life Insurance Company. Summary of the ten thousand confinement records of the Frontier Nursing Service. *Frontier Nursing Service Quart. Bull.* 1958, 33. Reprinted in *Bull. Am. Coll. Nurse-Midwives* 5:1–9, 1960.

Nurse-midwifery today. *Public Health Nursing* (May) 1949.

Perry, D.S. The early midwives of Missouri. *J. Nurse-Midwifery* 28(6):15–22 (November/December) 1983.

Robinson, S. A historical development of midwifery in the black community: 1600–1940. *J. Nurse-Midwifery* 29(4):247–250 (July/August) 1984.

Rooks, J.B. American nurse-midwifery: Are we making an impact? *J. Nurse-Midwifery* 23:15, 1978.

Roush, R.E. The development of midwifery — Male and female, yesterday and today. *J. Nurse-Midwifery* 24(3):27–37 (May/June) 1979.

Shoemaker, Sister M. (idem: Agnes Reinders). *History of Nurse-Midwifery in the United States*. Washington, D.C.: The Catholic University of America Press, 1947.

Swenson, N. The role of the nurse-midwife on the health team as viewed by the family. *Bull. Am. Coll. Nurse-Midwifery* 13:125, 1968.

The Committee on Organization. *Organization Bulletin*. Vol. 1: No. 1, 2, and 3, 1954 and Vol. 2: No. 1, 2, and 3, 1955.

Thiede, H.A. A presumptuous experiment in rural maternal-child health care. *Am. J. Obstet. Gynecol.* 111:736, 1971.

Thiede, H.A. Interdisciplinary MCH teams can function within the system with proper planning. *Am. J. Dis. Child.* 127:633, 1974.

Thomas, M.W. *The Practice of Nurse-Midwifery in the United States*. Washington, D.C.: Children's Bureau, U.S. Department of Health, Education and Welfare, 1965.

Thoms, H. *Our Obstetrical Heritage: The Story of Safe Childbirth*. Hamden, Connecticut: The Shoe String Press, 1960.

Tom, S.A. The evolution of nurse-midwifery: 1900–1960, *J. Nurse-Midwifery* 27(4):4–13 (July/August) 1982.

Transcript of the Testimony Given to the Subcommittee on Oversight and Investigation, Interstate and Foreign Commerce Committee, U.S. House of Representatives. Washington, D.C., December 18, 1980.

Varney, H. *Nurse-Midwifery*. Boston: Blackwell Scientific Publishing, 1980.

Wertz, R.W., and Wertz, D.C. *Lying-In, A History of Childbirth in America*. New York: The Free Press, 1977.

Wiedenbach, E. Nurse-midwifery . . . purpose, practice, and opportunity. *Nurs. Outlook* 8:256, 1960.

Williams, H.V. (idem: Burst). Nursing, nurse-midwifery, and the history of nurse-midwifery in the United States. Unpublished paper, 1969.

APPENDIX IV

NURSE-MIDWIFERY BASIC EDUCATION PROGRAMS THAT ARE ACCREDITED OR HAVE PREACCREDITATION STATUS, 1985

Baylor Medical College Nurse-Midwifery Program	CB
Case Western Reserve Frances Payne Bolton School of Nursing	MB
Columbia University Graduate Program in Maternity Nursing and Nurse Midwifery	MB
Emory University Nell Hodgson Woodruff School of Nursing	MB
Frontier School of Midwifery and Family Nursing Frontier Nursing Service	CB
Georgetown University School of Nursing Graduate Program in Nurse-Midwifery	MB
Medical University of South Carolina Nurse-Midwifery Program, College of Nursing	CB
Meharry Medical College Nurse-Midwifery Program, Dept. of Nursing Education	CB
Oregon Health Sciences University School of Nursing, Dept. of Family Nursing Nurse-Midwifery Program	MB
Rush-Presbyterian-St. Luke's Medical Center	DNSc
Stanford University Woman's Health Care Training Project Primary Care Project	CB
State University of New York Downstate Medical Center College of Health Related Professions Nurse-Midwifery Program	CB

United States Air Force (USAF)   CB
Nurse-Midwifery Program

University of California at San Diego   MB
UCSF/UCSD Intercampus Graduate
  Studies
Family Nurse Practice
Nurse-Midwifery

University of California at San   CB
  Francisco
San Francisco General Hospital

University of Colorado Health   MB
  Sciences Center
School of Nursing Graduate Program
Nurse-Midwifery Tract

University of Florida at Gainesville   MB
J. Hillis Miller Health Center
College of Nursing

University of Illinois at the Medical   MB
  Center
College of Nursing
Department of Maternal-Child
  Nursing
Nurse-Midwifery Program

University of Kentucky   MB
College of Nursing

University of Miami   MB
School of Nursing

University of Minnesota   MB
School of Nursing

University of Medicine and   CB
  Dentistry of New Jersey
School of Allied Health Professions
Nurse-Midwifery Program

University of Pennsylvania   MB
School of Nursing

University of Southern California   CB
Nurse-Midwifery Program

University of Utah   MB
College of Nursing
Graduate Specialty in
  Nurse-Midwifery

Yale University   MB, CM
School of Nursing
Maternal Newborn
  Nursing/Nurse-Midwifery Program

Key: CB: Certificate basic program
        MB: Master's degree basic program
        CM: Combined RN and master's degree
          program
        DNSc: Doctoral degree basic program
Note: Complete addresses of, and up-to-date
information on, the nurse-midwifery
education programs can be obtained upon
request from the American College of Nurse-
Midwives, 1522 K Street, N.W., Suite 1120,
Washington, D.C., 20005.

APPENDIX V

ACNM CORE COMPETENCIES IN NURSE-
MIDWIFERY

Nurse-midwifery education is based upon
theoretical preparation in the sciences and
clinical preparation for the judgment and skills
necessary for management and care of essentially normal women and newborns. The care
as defined by the American College of Nurse-
Midwives includes antepartum, intrapartum,
postpartum, and family planning/ gynecology,
and occurs within a health care system which
provides for medical consultation, collaborative
management, or referral. Nurse-midwifery
practice is based upon a management process
that is used in all aspects of care. It includes
knowledge and skills for competent practice
and incorporates the Functions, Standards and
Qualifications of the American College of
Nurse-Midwives.

Core competencies are the fundamental
knowledge, skills and behaviors expected of a
new graduate. This statement identifies the

core of knowledge and skills basic to preparation for nurse-midwifery practice. Because we recognize that nurse-midwifery practice continues to be a dynamic and changing discipline, these core competencies are presented as a guideline only for educators, physicians and other professionals, consumers and employers of nurse-midwives. They will continue to evolve with the practice of nurse-midwifery. The concepts and skills identified below and the aspects of the nurse-midwifery management process outlined in the following section apply to all components of nurse-midwifery care. This document must therefore be used in its entirety.

Because creativity, individuality and experimentation in nurse-midwifery education are essential to the vitality of the profession, educational programs are encouraged to be innovative. Each program will develop its own characteristics and may extend into other areas of health care. (It is the responsibility of each graduate to adapt practice to be consistent with state laws and institutional protocols.) Core competencies remain, however, as the basic requisites for the graduate of any educational program.

Certain concepts and skills from the behavioral sciences, communication, and public health permeate all aspects of nurse-midwifery practice. The following have been identified:

1. Family-centered approach to client care.
2. Constructive use of communication and of guidance and counseling skills.
3. Communication and collaboration with other members of the health team.
4. Client education.
5. Continuity of care.
6. Use of appropriate community resources.
7. Health promotion and disease prevention.
8. Pregnancy as a normal physiologic process.
9. Informed client choice and decision making.
10. Bioethical considerations related to reproductive health.

NURSE-MIDWIFERY MANAGEMENT

The nurse-midwifery management process has three aspects: primary management, collaborative management, and referral as well as medical consultation. Implicit in the management process is the documentation of all its aspects.

I. Primary Management

A. Systematically obtains or updates a complete and relevant data base for assessment of the client's health status.
B. Accurately identifies problems/diagnoses based upon correct interpretation of the data base.
C. Formulates and communicates a complete needs/problems list with corroboration from the client.
D. Identifies need for consultation/collaboration/referral with appropriate members of the health care team.
E. Provides information to enable clients to make appropriate decisions and to assume appropriate responsibility for their own health.
F. Assumes direct responsibility for the development, with the client, of a comprehensive plan of care based upon supportive rationale.
G. Assumes direct responsibility for implementing the plan of care.
H. Initiates emergency management of specific complications/deviations.
I. Evaluates, with corroboration from the client, the achievement of health care goals and modifies the plan of care appropriately.

II. Collaborative Management

Collaborative management builds upon the steps of primary management; additionally the nurse-midwife:

A. Anticipates and identifies problems and related complications.
B. Plans and implements physician consultation and nurse-midwifery/physician management.
C. Carries out the plan of care as appropriate.
D. Continues nurse-midwifery care, including teaching, counseling, support, and advocacy.

III. Referral

A. Identifies the need for management and/or care outside the scope of nurse-midwifery practice.
B. Selects an appropriate source of care in collaboration with the client.
C. Transfers the care of the client to medical management as appropriate.

COMPONENTS OF NURSE-MIDWIFERY CARE

Implicit in a nurse-midwifery knowledge base is the ability to perform skills pertinent to each of the outlined areas of practice.

I. Antepartum Care

A. Assumes responsibility for management of the care of the pregnant woman, using the nurse-midwifery management process.
B. Uses a foundation for nurse-midwifery practice that includes but is not limited to the knowledge of:
   1. Female anatomy and physiology.
   2. Anatomy and physiology of conception and pregnancy.
   3. Anatomy of the female bony pelvis.
   4. Preconceptional factors likely to influence pregnancy outcome.
   5. Clinical application of genetics, embryology, and fetal development.

6. Effects of pregnancy on the woman.
7. The etiology and management of common discomforts of pregnancy.
8. Parameters and methods for assessing the progress of pregnancy.
9. Parameters and methods for assessing fetal well-being.
10. Nutritional assessment of the maternal-fetal unit.
11. Environmental influences on the maternal-fetal unit.
12. Psychosocial/emotional/sexual changes during pregnancy.
13. Common screening/diagnostic tests used during pregnancy.
14. Pharmacology of medications commonly used during pregnancy.
15. Indicators of risk in pregnancy and appropriate intervention.
16. Assessment of relevant historical data regarding the client and her family.
17. Assessment of physical status.
18. Assessment of the soft and bony structures of the pelvis.
19. Assessment of the emotional status of the client and the dynamics in her support system.
20. Diagnosis of pregnancy.
21. Nutritional counseling.
22. Counseling in the physical and emotional changes of pregnancy and preparation for birth, parenthood, and change in the family constellation.
23. Prescription of medications.
24. Planning for individual/family birth experiences.
25. Planning and implementation of individual and/or group education.

II. Intrapartum Care

A. Assumes responsibility for management of the care of the client and neonate during the intrapartum period.
B. Uses a foundation for nurse-midwifery

practice that includes but is not limited to the knowledge of:

1. Normal labor process, including the mechanisms of labor and delivery.
2. Pelvic anatomy and physiology.
3. Anatomy of the fetal skull and its critical landmarks.
4. Parameters and methods for assessing progress of labor and delivery.
5. Parameters and methods for assessing maternal and fetal status.
6. Common screening/diagnostic tests used during labor.
7. Emotional changes during labor and delivery.
8. Pharmacology of medications commonly used during labor and birth, including effects on mother and fetus.
9. Comfort and support measures used during labor and birth.
10. Anatomy, physiology, and indicators of normal adaptation of newborn to extrauterine life.
11. Methods to facilitate newborn's adaptation to extrauterine life.
12. Indicators of deviations from normal and appropriate interventions.
13. Assessment of relevant historical data about clients.
14. Assessment of general physical and emotional status of clients.
15. Diagnosis and assessment of labor and its progress through the four stages.
16. Prescription or administration of appropriate medications/solutions during labor and birth.
17. Techniques for spontaneous vaginal delivery.
18. Techniques for placental expulsion.
19. Techniques for repair of episiotomy and episiotomy/laceration.
20. Techniques for administration of local and pudendal anesthesia.
21. Establishment of maternal/infant/family bonds.

III. Postpartum Care

A. Assumes responsibility for management of the care of the client and neonate during the postpartum period, using the nurse-midwifery management process.
B. Uses a foundation for nurse-midwifery practice that includes but is not limited to the knowledge of:

1. Anatomy and physiology of the puerperium, including the involutional process.
2. Anatomy and physiology of lactation and methods for its facilitation or suppression.
3. Parameters and methods for assessing the puerperium.
4. Etiology and methods for managing discomforts of the puerperium.
5. Emotional/psychosocial/sexual changes of the puerperium.
6. Establishment of maternal/infant/family bonds.
7. Pharmacology of medications commonly used during the puerperium, including effects on lactation and the infant.
8. Prescription or administration of appropriate medications and solutions.
9. Common screening/diagnostic tests used during the puerperium.
10. Assessment of relevant historical data about the client.
11. Assessment of client's general physical and emotional status.
12. Nutritional needs during the puerperium.
13. Indicators of deviations from normal and appropriate interventions.
14. Appropriate anticipatory guidance regarding self-care, infant care, family planning, and family relationships.

IV. Neonatal Care

A. Assumes responsibility for management

of the care of the neonate using the nurse-midwifery management process.

B. Uses a foundation for nurse-midwifery practice that includes but is not limited to the knowledge of:
  1. Anatomy and physiology of continuing adaptation to extrauterine life and stabilization of the neonate.
  2. Parameters and methods for assessing neonatal status.
  3. Parameters and methods for assessing gestational age of the neonate.
  4. Nutritional needs of the neonate.
  5. Establishment of maternal/infant/family bonds.
  6. Pharmacology of medications commonly used for the neonate.
  7. Screening/diagnostic tests performed on the neonate.
  8. Assessment of relevant historical data about maternal and neonatal course.
  9. Indicators of deviations from normal and appropriate intervention.
  10. Resuscitation and emergency care of the newborn.

V. Family Planning/Gynecological Care

A. Assumes responsibility for management of the care of women seeking family planning and/or gynecological services, using the nurse-midwifery management process.
B. Uses a foundation for nurse-midwifery practice that includes but is not limited to the knowledge of:
  1. Anatomy and physiology of the reproductive systems through the life cycle.
  2. Anatomy and physiology of the female breast.
  3. Anatomy, physiology, and psychosocial components of human sexuality.
  4. Factors relating to steroid, mechanical, chemical, physiological, and surgical conception control methods, including:

  (a) Rationale for use.
  (b) Contraindications to use.
  (c) Effectiveness rates.
  (d) Mechanisms of action.
  (e) Advantages/disadvantages.
  (f) Side effects/complications.
  (g) Cost.
  (h) Client instructions/counseling.
  (i) Psychosocial factors.
  (j) Provision of appropriate method, including but not limited to, oral contraception, vaginal diaphragms, and IUDs.
  (k) Discontinuation or change of method.
  5. Indicators of common problems of sexuality and methods for counseling.
  6. Factors involved in decision making regarding unplanned and/or undesirable pregnancies and resources for counseling and referral.
  7. Indicators of deviations from normal and appropriate interventions including but not limited to:
  (a) Vaginal/pelvic infections.
  (b) Sexually transmitted diseases.
  (c) Pelvic and breast masses.
  (d) Abnormal Pap smears.
  (e) Problems related to menstrual cycle.
  (f) Pelvic relaxation.
  (g) Urinary tract infections.
  (h) Infertility.
  8. Assessment of relevant historical data about client/partner.
  9. Assessment of general physical and emotional status of client.
  10. Common screening and diagnostic tests.

VI. Complications

As members of the health care team, nurse-midwives might manage some deviations in collaboration with a physician, or they might refer clients to a physician with or without continued nurse-midwifery support and teaching. Basic knowledge of the more common complications is essential to preparation for nurse-midwifery practice. The depth of knowledge needed will vary with the frequency of the complication and the role of the nurse-midwife. This basic knowledge generally includes:

A. Causative and risk factors and preventive measures.
B. Anatomical and/or physiological deviations from normal.
C. Effect of these changes on the health of the woman.
D. Effects of these changes on the health of the fetus or infant.
E. Signs and symptoms for screening and detecting existing abnormality.
F. Adjunctive laboratory data.

PROFESSIONAL ASPECT

Assumes the role and professional responsibilities of nurse-midwifery practice. As a leader or change agent, the nurse-midwife demonstrates:

1. Knowledge of the historical development of nurse-midwifery in the U.S., structure and function of the American College of Nurse-Midwives, and the legal base for nurse-midwifery practice.
2. Knowledge of contemporary issues and trends in maternal-child health care nationally and internationally.
3. Knowledge of standards for quality maternal and child health services.
4. Knowledge of current and pending health legislation.
5. Knowledge of the role and responsibilities of the nurse-midwife in supporting legislative contributions to high-quality maternal and child health services.
6. Knowledge of the various nurse-midwifery practice options and the resources available for their development and evaluation.
7. The ability to carry out the philosophy of the American College of Nurse-Midwives.
8. Respect for the dignity and rights of health care providers and clients.
9. Responsibility and accountability for:
   a. Personal management decisions made in caring for clients.
   b. Periodic self-evaluation and peer review.
   c. Administration and delivery of services to families in collaboration with other health care providers.
10. The ability to use and collaborate in research.
11. Awareness of the responsibility of the professional to participate in the education of nurse midwives.

Approved, 1985.

3   Management

THE MANAGEMENT PROCESS

The management process is a problem-solving process. It provides a method of organizing thoughts and actions in a logical sequence for the benefit of both the patient and the examiner. It is written in terms of expected behaviors of the examiner. These clearly state not only the thought and action process involved but also the behavioral level at which each step is to be achieved in order to provide safe, comprehensive patient care. Since the management process follows a logical sequence, it is also most useful to students in learning the management of care of patients because it provides a means of putting together isolated fragments of knowledge, findings, skills, and judgments into a meaningful whole and focuses upon the transition into the role of patient management.

The management process comprises seven sequential steps [1, 2]. It starts with the collection of a data base and ends with evaluation. The seven steps compose an overall format which is a framework applicable in all situa-

tions. Each step, however, may be broken down into finite tasks, and these vary in accord with whatever the patient's condition is. The seven steps follow:

1. Investigate by obtaining all necessary data for complete evaluation of the patient.
2. Make an accurate identification of problems or diagnoses based on correct interpretation of the data.
3. Anticipate other potential problems or diagnoses that might be expected because of the identified problems or diagnoses.
4. Evaluate patient need for immediate nurse-midwife intervention and/or for physician consultation and collaborative management and/or physician referral when there is a deviation from normal.
5. Develop a comprehensive plan of care which is supported by explanations of valid rationale underlying the decisions made and is based on the preceding steps.
6. Direct or implement the plan of care efficiently and safely.
7. Evaluate the effectiveness of the care given,

recycling appropriately through the management process for any aspect of care which has been ineffective.

The steps of the management process are essentially self-explanatory. However, a brief discussion and examples of what may be included in the tasks of each of these steps may clarify the thought process involved in this action-oriented clinical process.

The first step is the gathering of a complete data base for evaluation of the patient. This data base includes history, physical and pelvic examination as indicated, review of current chart or old hospital records, review of laboratory data, and, in short, collection of all pertinent information from all sources that have a bearing on the patient's condition. The nurse-midwife gathers a complete initial data base even if the patient has a complication that will need to be presented to a physician for consultation, collaboration, or referral. At times, thus, step 1 may overlap with steps 5 and 6 (or be part of a continuing sequence) in the process of obtaining necessary data from laboratory tests or other diagnostic studies. Sometimes the nurse-midwife will need to make an initial pass through step 4 in order to acquire the complete initial data base for presentation to a physician. This juncture should be specified in the medical management protocols agreed upon by each nurse-midwife and physician consultant.

From the data base the second step evolves: the interpretation of the data into specifically identified problems or diagnoses. The words *problems* and *diagnoses* are both used as some problems cannot necessarily be defined as diagnoses but do need to be considered in developing a comprehensive plan of care for the patient. Problems are frequently related to how the patient is experiencing the fact of her diagnosis and are often identified by the nurse-midwife's focus on the experiencing individual patient. For example, the diagnosis might

be that the patient is pregnant, and a related problem might be that the patient does not want the pregnancy. Another example is a patient in her third trimester who is frightened by her impending labor and delivery. Being frightened does not fit a category of standard diagnostic nomenclature but certainly creates a problem which needs to be explored and for which a plan needs to be developed for reducing this fear.

The third step — identifying other potential problems or diagnoses based on the current set of problems and diagnoses — is a matter of anticipation, prevention when possible, watchful waiting, and preparation for possible eventuality. This step is vital to safe care. Take, for example, a patient with an overdistended uterus for whatever reason (diagnosis), e.g., polyhydramnios, large-for-dates baby, diabetic mother, or multiple gestation. One should anticipate, take precautionary measures in relationship to, and be prepared for the possibility of an immediate postpartum hemorrhage as a result of uterine atony from the overdistention. In the event of a single large baby one should also anticipate and be prepared for the possibility of shoulder dystocia and the need for infant resuscitation. Another example is the patient with sickle cell trait. One should be alert to the possibility of this patient's developing a urinary tract infection, which in turn increases the possibility of either premature labor or a small-for-dates baby. Simple preventive measures, pertinent history taking at each prenatal visit, laboratory tests for asymptomatic bacteriuria, and immediate therapeutic treatment if a urinary tract infection does develop are indicated.

The fourth step reflects the continual and ongoing nature of the management process not only during periodic prenatal visits but during the time when one is constantly with the patient, such as in labor. New data are constantly obtained and evaluated. Some data indicate emergency situations in which the nurse-midwife must act immediately in the interest of the life of the mother or baby, e.g., third stage or immediate postpartal hemorrhage, shoulder dystocia, or a low Apgar score. Some data indicate immediate action while awaiting the physician for referral of the patient, such as a prolapsed cord. Other situations are not emergencies but may require physician consultation or referral. Early signs of preeclampsia, for example, require physician consultation. On the other hand, an initial history and physical and pelvic examination that yield the findings of heart disease, diabetes, or any major medical problem require collaboration with, or referral of the patient to, a physician. The nurse-midwife must evaluate each patient situation for management of the patient's care by the most appropriate health team member.

The fifth step — developing a comprehensive plan of care — is determined by the preceding steps, is an outgrowth of the identified current and anticipated problems and diagnoses, and also involves obtaining any missing or necessary additional pieces of information for the data base. A comprehensive plan of care includes not only what is indicated by the patient's condition and any related problems but also anticipatory guidance for the patient as to what to expect next, patient teaching and counseling, and any necessary referrals for social, economic, religious, family, cultural, or psychological problems. In other words, anything that pertains to any aspect of her health care is included. A plan of care must be mutually agreed upon by the examiner and the patient in order for it to be effective, because it is the patient, especially while an outpatient, who will or will not implement the plan. Therefore, tasks in this step include formulation and discussion of the plan with the patient as well as confirmation of agreement.

All decisions made in developing a comprehensive plan of care must reflect valid rationale based on pertinent, appropriate, and up-to-date theoretical knowledge and validated assumptions about what the patient will or will not do. Rationale based on unvalidated assumptions of patient behavior, erroneous or deficient theoretical knowledge, or an incomplete data base is not valid and yields patient care which is incomplete and may be unsafe.

The sixth step is implementation of the comprehensive plan of care. This may be done in part or in whole by the nurse-midwife or in part by the patient, nurse-midwife, and other health team members. If the nurse-midwife is not doing it herself, she assumes the responsibility for directing its implementation, i.e., seeing that it is indeed done. In settings where the nurse-midwife collaborates with a physician and contributes to the management of care of patients with complications, the nurse-midwife also may assume responsibility for the implementation of the collaborative comprehensive plan of care. Efficient implementation cuts time and cost and enhances the quality of patient care.

The final step — evaluation — is really one of checking whether the plan of care, which involves meeting needs-for-help, did indeed meet the needs-for-help identified in the problems and diagnoses. The plan is deemed effective if it did, ineffective if it did not. It is possible for parts of the plan to have been effective while other parts have been ineffective. Again, perceiving the management process as a continuum, it is necessary to recycle any ineffective care back through the management process to identify why it was ineffective and to adjust the plan of care accordingly.

Since this book is clinically oriented, a modified version of the first five steps of this management process is used in presenting the content in the management sections. The steps are modified for the purpose of adding relevant theoretical knowledge necessary as background information in the pursuit of clinical management of the patient. Because the management process is a process that takes place in the clinical setting and the last two steps are dependent on the patient and the clinical situation, it is not possible to include them in a textbook.

SCREENING FOR ABNORMALITY AND DIFFERENTIAL DIAGNOSIS

Screening for abnormality and differential diagnosis are vital, and unfortunately sometimes misunderstood, functions of the nurse-midwife. Differential diagnosis is considered the purview of the physician. However, within certain limits, the nurse-midwife does make differential diagnoses and at all times identifies and does the initial workup of the complicated patient for evaluation by the physician. Clarity as to what is being talked about is of utmost importance.

The primary diagnosis the nurse-midwife makes is one of normality. To this end the nurse-midwife must differentiate, for example, between the normality of the minor discomforts of pregnancy and the complications of pregnancy. The minor discomfort of nausea and vomiting of the first trimester is not the same as hyperemesis gravidarum nor is it a sign of hydatidiform mole. Likewise, right-sided round ligament pain must be differentiated from appendicitis, false labor differentiated from true labor or a urinary tract infection, bloody show differentiated from frank bleeding, and so forth.

To make these differential diagnoses the nurse-midwife must know, in depth and in detail, normal obstetrics and normal findings of the history, physical assessment, and pelvic examination in order to detect when there is deviation from normal. Aiding in the recognition of deviation from normal is a thorough knowledge of the signs and symptoms of complications known to affect pregnancy. Similarly, a thorough knowledge of how pregnancy affects pre-existing medical conditions

is also required. The purpose is to screen the patient for abnormality and to differentiate normal from abnormal.

Differential diagnosis by a nurse-midwife does not mean pretending to be a diagnostician of medical complications. If the nurse-midwife finds a medical abnormality she or he consults with the physician for diagnosis, disposition, or possible referral of the patient to a specialist.

On the other hand, the nurse-midwife is expected to begin the process of making a differential diagnosis. It is not enough for a nurse-midwife to report to a physician that a patient's labor is failing to progress normally. The report needs to include specific patient data indicating differentiation between hypertonic and hypotonic uterine dysfunction and, further, differentiation as to possible causes, such as cephalopelvic disproportion, by stating clinical evaluation of the pelvis and station; poorly-timed administration of analgesia; or malposition or malpresentation of the fetus.

Further, since normality is often poorly defined, there are a number of "gray zone" complications which the nurse-midwife diagnoses and treats. These commonly include urinary tract infections, vaginitis, borderline anemia, need for RhoGam, spotting with an intrauterine contraceptive device, breakthrough bleeding with oral contraceptives, condylomata accuminata (nonpregnant patient), and uncomplicated gonorrhea and syphilis (nonpregnant patients). This type of listing, however, may vary considerably from practice setting to practice setting.

For other complications the nurse-midwife is expected to go beyond the initial signs and symptoms indicating a complication, and order laboratory or other adjunctive tests for confirmation of the diagnosis and presentation to the physician for evaluation and treatment. Complications in this category include suspected diabetes, unresponding anemia, small-for-dates and large-for-dates fetuses, endometritis, and postmaturity.

Nurse-midwifery comprises the management of care of the essentially normal childbearing patient. Therefore the nurse-midwife must be astutely alert to that which is abnormal and to complications which may develop in the course of childbearing, both generally and in relation to a specific patient situation.

The definition of normality, however, is not always clearly defined and varies from practice setting to practice setting, thereby creating a gray zone area of what the nurse-midwife is managing. Limits of practice are established by definitions; by functions, standards, and qualifications as stated by the American College of Nurse-Midwives; by local standing orders and policies; and by the nurse-midwife's own limitations of knowledge and capabilities. Thus there are four different types of limits — professional, local, personal, and legal [3] — and they have certain elastic qualities. For this reason "collaboration with the physician" and "contribution of the nurse-midwife to management" rather than "consultation and referral to the physician" is stressed in the management of patients with complications, as will be illustrated in later chapters. In many practice settings nurse-midwives see all of the patients, managing the normal and collaborating with the physician in the management of the patients with complications.

There is a precise thought process involved in making differential diagnoses. This process must be followed in sequence to assure not missing the diagnosis. The thought process starts with the recognition of a sign or symptom either indicative of abnormality or needing to be processed to determine if normal or not. The next step is to list all the possible conditions or complications of which the sign or symptom could be indicative. The third step is to go methodically through each possible condition or complication listed, obtaining additional pertinent data (history, physical, pelvic, laboratory, or other adjunctive studies) that will either confirm or rule out each complication

on the list. All such findings are documented and, unless the condition or complication can be managed by the nurse-midwife, presented to the physician for evaluation. If the complications are within the purview of the nurse-midwife, the findings are documented on the patient's chart.

Differential diagnosis as done by a nurse-midwife, therefore, is primarily differentiation of normal from abnormal, since the role of the nurse-midwife includes continually screening the patient for deviation from normal. "Gray zone" areas of differential diagnosis of actual obstetric or gynecologic complications are defined in each individual practice setting and establish the limits of the nurse-midwife's practice in that setting. Close collaboration with the physician throughout is the essential element in this aspect of the practice of a nurse-midwife.

PHYSICAL EXAMINATION FOR A DATA BASE

The following presentation on history and physical and pelvic examination is not meant to be a definitive work on the subject of physical assessment. Several excellent textbooks detailing the content, procedures, and skills used in physical diagnosis are listed in the bibliography. What is presented here, rather, is an outline of what is included in a history, physical examination, and pelvic examination that will screen a woman of childbearing age for abnormality and determine normality. Assessment of the neonate is included in Chapter 22, Evaluation and Management of the Neonate.

Before 1970, physical assessment by nurse-midwives consisted primarily of thorough examination of the breasts and the pelvis and limited examination of the mouth, throat, thyroid gland, abdomen, and extremities. Early in the 1970s, however, nurse-midwives were adding interconceptional care to the totality of their care by virtue of their involvement in family planning and in accord with their philosophy of providing continuity of care. It was then realized that the only physical examination many women received from year to year was the one the nurse-midwives were doing when the patient returned for her annual or semiannual family planning visit. Obviously the physical examination being done was inadequate for purposes of detecting medical problems not related to contraceptive methods. The solution was for nurse-midwives to learn the content, procedures, and skills of a total history and physical examination. This was added to the curriculum in nurse-midwifery education programs while in-service education was held for staff nurse-midwives. By 1974 physical assessment was an accepted part of nurse-midwifery practice. However, a problem was identified in the form of a question — how much needs to be included in the physical assessment for the singular purpose of screening for abnormality?

The following outline of a history and physical is one attempt to include only what is needed for screening purposes. A screening examination is for recognition of relatively gross evidence of abnormalities and disease for the purpose of referral to a physician for diagnosis and treatment. It does not go into the detail necessary for diagnosis of an abnormality; this is the responsibility of the physician. For example, it is the role of the nurse-midwife to detect an abnormality while listening to the heart. If the nurse-midwife hears a murmur, that patient needs to have the murmur evaluated by a physician. It is not the role of the nurse-midwife to diagnose the heart problem or even the type or grade of the murmur. The nurse-midwife does have the responsibility of obtaining a relevant history in relation to any abnormality detected for presentation to the physician. Such a history includes the following:

Is the patient aware of the abnormality?
What brought the abnormality to her attention

(e.g., has pain; was told during previous physical)?
Length of time abnormality has been present and its course since discovery?
Has the patient ever been seen and treated for the abnormality?
    By whom?
    When?
    Diagnosis as patient understands it?
    Treated with what?
    Effectiveness of the treatment?
    Continuing care?

On the other hand, nurse-midwives go into greater detail in taking a history and doing a physical and pelvic examination in those areas germane to childbearing, pregnancy, simple gynecology (e.g., vaginal infections, pelvic relaxations), and family planning than is usual for a patient admitted to a medical unit for a diagnostic workup. This is not surprising, because it is for conditions relevant to the reproductive tract that a woman is seen by a nurse-midwife. Therefore the screening physical is for the body systems other than the reproductive system.

For this reason the following outline of a history and physical and pelvic examination lacks detail for some body systems and is in considerable detail for aspects related to obstetrics and gynecology. It also includes specific skills, detailed in Part VII, that are not strictly related to the reproductive system but are frequently used in identifying complications related to pregnancy. Examples include checking for costovertebral angle (CVA) tenderness, since urinary tract infections are a common complication of pregnancy, and checking deep tendon reflexes, essential in evaluating the possible severity of preeclampsia.

History

Principles of History Taking (Fig. 3–1):
1.   Observe all rules of interviewing:
     a. use open-ended, not closed-ended, questions

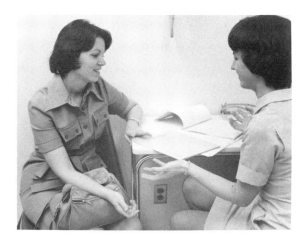

FIGURE 3-1. A nurse-midwife taking a woman's history.

    b. avoid putting answers in the woman's mouth

    c. clarify what the woman's behavior means to her

    d. use level of terminology understood by the woman

2. Introduce yourself and state what you are going to do and your purpose for doing it.

3. Be tactful and respectful of the woman's right to privacy about her person and personal life at all times.

4. Be responsive to what the woman is saying. For example, if she is talking about a past difficult time in her life a response denoting sympathetic understanding is appropriate.

5. Be precise, thorough, and accurate in obtaining all essential information.

6. By the same token, screen out, stop, and delete from recording all irrelevant material.

7. Allow the woman time to answer. Don't interrupt unless she starts to ramble or clarification is needed.

8. Listen to the woman with interest and concern.

9. Listen to the woman — she may in one answer be giving you the answer to a later question as well. Don't repeat the later question.

10. Listen to the woman — don't have her repeat what she just said because you weren't paying attention.

11. Be sure you understand what the woman is saying. Such things as accents and expressions vary from one part of the country to the next. Don't hesitate to ask the woman to spell or explain words she is using.

12. Do not be judgmental by facial expression, body language, or tonal inflection.

13. Provide as much privacy from being overheard as possible.

14. Speak in well-modulated, soothing, calming tones.

15. Maintain eye contact — don't always be reading from the history form, writing responses, and charting.

Identifying Information

1. Name	6. Address
2. Age	7. Religion
3. Race	8. Marital status
4. Sex	9. Occupation
5. Gravida and para	10. Date of interview

Chief Complaint (CC)
The reason why the woman is in the clinic, office, or hospital as stated in her own words.

History of Present Illness (HPI): relates to the chief complaint or problem

1. Date and time of onset
2. Mode of onset
3. Precipitating or predisposing factors related to onset
4. Course since onset — including duration and recurrence
5. Specific location
6. Type of pain or discomfort and severity or intensity
7. Other associated symptoms
8. Relationship to bodily functions and activities

9. Factors influencing the problem, either aggravating or relieving
10. Previous medical help (and from whom) for this problem; diagnosis and treatment
11. Effectiveness of any treatments or medications used (self- or medically initiated)

Past Medical History
1. Childhood diseases, e.g., measles (type), mumps, chickenpox
2. Major illnesses, e.g., pneumonia, hepatitis, diphtheria, polio
3. Hospitalizations
4. Surgery
5. Accidents — fractures? injuries? unconsciousness?
6. Blood transfusions — reaction?
7. Allergies, e.g., food, hay fever, environmental (dust), asthma
8. Drug allergies
9. Alcohol abuse/alcoholism
10. Drug abuse/addiction
11. Habits
    a. smoking
    b. alcohol
    c. coffee, tea
    d. "recreational" drugs
12. Specific diseases:
    a. diabetes
    b. kidney/urinary tract infections (UTI)
    c. heart disease, including rheumatic fever
    d. varicosities/thrombophlebitis
    e. tuberculosis
    f. glandular/endocrine
    g. cancer
    h. liver
    i. hypertension
    j. mental illness
    k. epilepsy
    l. blood dyscrasias, e.g., anemia (type: iron deficiency, sickle cell)
13. Medications
    a. prescription
    b. nonprescription

Family History (pertains to mother, father, siblings, grandparents, aunts, and uncles)
1. Mother, father, siblings — age? living and well? if deceased, what was the cause of death?
2. Cancer
3. Heart disease
4. Hypertension
5. Diabetes
6. Kidney disease
7. Mental illness
8. Congenital anomalies
9. Multiple pregnancies
10. Tuberculosis
11. Epilepsy
12. Blood dyscrasias, e.g., anemia (type)
13. Allergies

Menstrual History
1. Age at menarche
2. Frequency — range if irregular
3. Duration
4. Amount of flow
5. Characteristics of flow, e.g., clots
6. Last menstrual period (LMP) — normal duration and amount?
7. Dysmenorrhea
8. Dysfunctional uterine bleeding (i.e., intermenstrual spotting or bleeding, menorrhagia, metrorrhagia)
9. Toxic shock syndrome
10. Premenstrual symptoms/premenstrual syndrome (PMS)
11. Perimenopausal symptoms

Obstetric History
1. Gravida/para (four digit system)
2. Rh and ABO blood type
3. For each pregnancy:
    a. date of termination
    b. weeks gestation
    c. where delivered, i.e., hospital (name), childbirth center (name), or home
    d. length of labor
    e. type of delivery, i.e., spontaneous, C-section, forceps

f. RhoGam received
g. any obstetric, medical problems during:
   (1) pregnancy, e.g., preeclampsia, UTI
   (2) labor and delivery, e.g., malpresentation, malposition, preeclampsia, eclampsia, pitocin induction, or pitocin stimulation
   (3) postpartum period, e.g., UTI, hemorrhage, uterine infection
h. weight of baby at birth
i. sex of baby
j. any congenital anomalies or neonatal complications, e.g., jaundice, respiratory problems
k. status of infant at birth, i.e., alive or dead
l. present status of infant, e.g., living and well, problems, or cause of death

Gynecologic History
1. Infertility
2. Diethylstilbestrol (DES) exposure
3. Vaginal infections, i.e., monilia, trichomonas, gardnerella
4. Condylomata acuminata
5. Sexually transmitted diseases (STD), i.e., chlamydia, syphillis, gonorrhea, herpes, acquired immune deficiency syndrome (AIDS)
6. Chronic cervicitis
7. Endometritis
8. Pelvic inflammatory disease (PID)
9. Cysts (Bartholin, ovarian)
10. Endometriosis
11. Myomas
12. Pelvic relaxations (cystocele, rectocele)
13. Polyps
14. Breast masses
15. Abnormal Pap smears
16. Biopsies (cervical, endometrical, breast)
17. Gynecologic cancer
18. Gynecologic surgery
19. Rape and/or battering

Sexual, Contraceptive, and Douching History
1. Sexual history

a. nature of sexual relationship
b. frequency of sexual relations
c. satisfaction with sexual frequency
d. satisfaction with sexual relationship
e. problems
   (1) insufficient foreplay
   (2) insufficient lubrication
   (3) lack of personal consideration
   (4) pain
   (5) fear of becoming pregnant
   (6) fear of hurting the fetus, if pregnant
   (7) problems of partner, e.g., impotence, premature ejaculation
   (8) postcoital bleeding
2. Contraceptive history
a. present contraceptive method:
   (1) type
   (2) satisfaction
   (3) side effects
   (4) consistency of use
   (5) length of time using this method
b. previous contraceptive methods:
   (1) types
   (2) duration of use for each
   (3) side effects of each
   (4) reasons for discontinuing each
3. Douching history
a. frequency
b. method (how)
c. solution used
d. reasons for douching
e. length of time woman has been douching
f. last time douched

Personal History

This area includes social, occupational, economic, educational, and housing information and history. Much of the information which can be sought and obtained in these areas is not always necessary information to have. Neither is it desirable to obtain it without a purpose, since questions may be interpreted by the woman as prying into her personal life. She may then rightfully respond with hostility which affects her ability to carry out instructions pertinent to her condition.

A good rule of thumb is to ask yourself if the information is essential either for assisting in making a diagnosis or for formulating a plan of care which the woman can implement. The most appropriate time for asking these questions is at the time one needs the information. Examples follow.

1. Knowing a woman's occupation and household responsibilities is important during pregnancy for planning rest periods with her feet elevated. This information is not routinely necessary for the family planning patient.
2. Before talking about taking showers or soaking in a tub of warm/hot water it is useful to know what bathing facilities a woman has.
3. Before talking about diet and meal preparation with a woman one should know if she actually does the grocery shopping and meal preparation. One needs to talk to the person who does — who may not be the patient.

Review of Systems

The review of systems (ROS) is a structured inquiry about past or current symptoms or complaints related to each body system. Because some examiners prefer to do the review of systems during the physical examination, usually in the interest of saving time, and because it makes sense to ask questions about specific systems, organs, or body parts while they are being examined, the ROS is included in the following outline of the physical examination and designated as such. Combining the ROS with the examination has caused information about some systems (lymphatic and hematopoietic systems, central nervous system, and endocrine system) to be split up

in order to tie them to specific body structures. The history and physical examination outline presented in this book includes all information pertaining to these systems. One should review the symptoms pertaining to each of these body systems, using any physical diagnosis book, in order to identify the system involved if any symptoms are reported. The advantage of proceding this way is that it eliminates repetition.

Physical Examination

Principles of Doing a Physical Examination (Fig. 3–2):
1. Wash your hands immediately before doing the examination.
2. Be sure that your fingernails are clean and cut at a length that will not hurt the woman.
3. Warm your hands prior to touching the woman by using warm water to wash them, or by rubbing them together, or by holding them under a lamp.
4. Tell the woman what you will be doing in general. During the examination itself tell the woman more specifically what you will be doing just before doing it. *Specifically* means letting her know where you will be touching her, what you want her to do, and whether or not this portion of the examination will be uncomfortable.
5. Utilize a gentle approach to the woman, yet make your touch firm enough not to tickle her and as firm as needed to elicit accurate information.
6. Let your approach and touch bespeak respect for her body as well as respect for her right to modesty and privacy.
7. Drape the woman in such a way that only the area being examined at any one point during the examination is exposed.
8. Organize your examination so that:
   a. it progresses naturally from head to toe
   b. it minimizes movement of the woman;

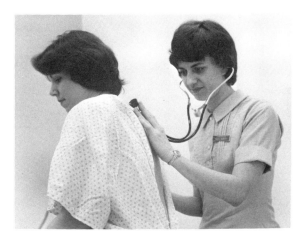

FIGURE 3-2. A nurse-midwife doing a physical examination of a woman.

e.g., while having her sit up for inspection of her breasts also listen to her lungs from the back, observe and palpate for spinal deformities, and check for CVA tenderness rather than having her return to this position several times during the examination

c. you do not touch parts of the body that will necessitate rewashing your hands if you have to return to other parts of the body; e.g., the bottom of her feet, until the end of the examination

d. the progression of your examination is the same for every woman; this aids you in remembering everything

9. Share your findings with the woman. If she is anxious about something that you find normal, immediately tell her your findings. If you find something of concern to you as a possible deviation from normal, tell her that you are not sure of what you have found and want a physician to check it. Remember, it is the woman's body and she has a right to know everything about it. Be honest and truthful with her.

Physical Measurements

1. Temperature   4. Blood pressure
2. Pulse   5. Height
3. Respirations   6. Weight

General
ROS:
1. Woman's evaluation of own health status
2. Woman's evaluation of own dietary patterns
3. Unusual weight changes
4. Weakness
5. Fatigue
6. Malaise
7. Fever, chills, sweating
8. Woman's evaluation of own emotional status
9. Ability to carry out daily living activities

Observations:
1. Appropriateness of appearance for age
2. General nutritional status
3. Apparent state of health
4. General personal appearance
5. General mental and emotional state: speech; appropriateness of mood or affect; general mood (e.g., anxiety, depression); orientation to time, place, person; memory; logic and coherence of thought processes; general behavior (e.g., hostile, friendly, cooperative, confused)
6. Striking obvious findings (e.g., pallor, cyanosis, respiratory distress, persistent cough, voice or speech abnormality, facial asymmetry, orthopedic abnormalities)
7. General posture, gait, body movements

Skin and Hair
ROS:
1. Skin
   a. pruritus
   b. rashes
   c. moles — any change noted
   d. lesions
   e. tendency to bruise
   f. general character (i.e., dry, oily)
   g. hirsutism
2. Hair and scalp
   a. general character (i.e., dry, oily)

b. loss of hair
c. wearing wig or not, and, if so, why
d. scalp infections, dandruff, lice

Observations and examination:
1. Skin
   a. temperature
   b. color (e.g., pigmentation, pallor, cyanosis, jaundice)
   c. moisture
   d. scars
   e. moles
   f. rashes, lesions, bruises
   g. tumors
   h. turgor
2. Hair and scalp
   a. hair pattern
   b. scalp infections, dandruff, lice, lesions
   c. bald spots (alopecia)
   d. general character (i.e., dry, oily)
   e. lumps

Head
ROS:
1. Headaches — location, duration, time of day when they occur, frequency, type of pain, severity, relief measures and their effectiveness, any known causative factors, associated symptoms (e.g., nausea and vomiting, dizziness)
2. Dizziness
3. Syncope (fainting)
4. Sinusitis

Observation and examination:
1. Size, shape, contour, symmetry
2. Facial symmetry
3. Location of facial structures
4. Involuntary movements
5. Tenderness over frontal and maxillary sinuses

Eyes
ROS:
1. Blurring of vision
2. Scotomata (blind spots in vision)

3. Diplopia (double vision)
4. Spots before eyes
5. Flashing lights
6. Pressure or pain symptoms
7. Photophobia (sensitivity to light)
8. Lacrimation (excessive tearing)
9. Discharge, redness, burning
10. Woman's evaluation of own visual acuity and any recent changes
11. Glasses or contact lenses — for what, last time eyes examined, last time prescription changed
12. Injuries
13. Diseases or conditions

Observations and examination:
1. Eyelids — closure, edema, signs of infection, blinking, squinting, masses, lesions, ptosis (drooping eyelid)
2. Eyelashes — matting from discharge, absence
3. Lacrimal ducts — signs of infection, tenderness
4. Involuntary eye movements
5. Color of lower conjunctival sac
6. Color of sclera
7. Abrasions or opacities of lens and cornea
8. Strabismus (cross-eyes)
9. Size, shape, and equality of pupils
10. Parallel movement of eyes and gross visual fields
11. Pupillary reaction to light and accommodation
12. Protrusion of eyeball and intraocular pressure as determined by finger tension
13. Ophthalmoscopic examination
    a. presence of red reflex
    b. color and outline of optic disc
    c. color, size, and shape of retinal vessels
    d. hemorrhagic areas
    e. color and shape of macula and fovea
    f. papilledema

Ears
ROS:
1. Woman's evaluation of own hearing acuity

and any recent changes
2. Earaches
3. Discharge
4. Tinnitus (ringing in the ears)
5. Vertigo (lack of balance)
6. Infections, injuries
7. Pain

Observation and examination:
1. Enlargement or tenderness of mastoid
2. General hearing acuity
3. Placement of ears on head
4. Shape, growths, lesions, and discharge noted in auricles and outlet of external ear canal
5. Color, obstruction, lesions, edema, discharge, foreign objects in external auditory canal
6. Otoscopic examination of tympanic membrane
   a. color
   b. bulging or retraction
   c. bony landmarks
   d. cone of light — presence or absence
   e. scars, perforations

Nose
ROS:
1. Nasal obstruction (difficulty with nasal breathing)
2. Epistaxis (nosebleeds)
3. Discharge — nasal and postnasal
4. Woman's evaluation of own sense of smell
5. Injuries
6. Frequency of colds

Observation and examination:
1. Flaring of nares
2. Deformity or septal deviation
3. Symmetry, size, placement — including symmetry of nasolabial fold
4. Patency of nostrils
5. Perforation of nasal septum
6. Nasal speculum examination
   a. size, signs of infection, edema of turbinates

b. polyps, growths, obstructions
c. ulcerations, lesions, bleeding points
d. discharge
e. color of mucosa

Mouth and Throat
ROS:
1. Toothaches
2. Bleeding, lesions, pain, or edema of gums
3. Extractions and dentures
4. Any difficulty with eating — chewing or swallowing
5. Pain, lesions, bleeding, or edema of lips
6. Pain, lesions, tumors, or bleeding of mouth
7. Pain, lesions, color, texture, tumors, bleeding, edema of tongue
8: Frequency of sore throats
9. Number of cigarettes per day
10. Surgery (e.g., tonsillectomy)
11. Woman's evaluation of own sense of taste
12. Hoarseness or voice change
13. Any difficulty with talking or speech
14. Dental care

Observation and examination
1. Odor of breath
2. Lips — symmetry, color, lesions, edema, tumors, fissures
3. Mouth and mucosa — lesions, tumors, plaques, intactness of palate, color, vascular spots
4. Teeth — state of repair, missing teeth, caries
5. Gums — bleeding, lesions, edema, tumors, color, retraction, pus/exudate
6. Tongue — symmetry, position, texture, color, lesions, tumors, moistness, coating, mobility, deviation
7. Uvula — deviation, size, enlargement
8. Oropharynx — signs of infection in posterior pharynx, tonsillar fossae, and tonsillar pillars; inflammation, edema, bleeding, exudate, pus patches, color, lesions, tumors, size, symmetry, and enlargement of tonsils

Neck

ROS:

1. Pain or stiffness
2. Limitation of motion
3. Node enlargement or tenderness
4. Thyroid enlargement — history of goiter
5. Injuries, deformities
6. Thyroid (endocrine system)
   a. sensitivity to environmental temperature and weather changes
   b. amount of sweating — excessive
   c. changes in scalp and hair, breasts, skin, genitalia, neck, secondary sex characteristics
   d. changes in emotional lability
   e. changes in heart rate, tremors, nervousness
   f. change in body weight in relationship to appetite
   g. change in energy levels and activity pattern
   h. results of previous BMR (basal metabolism rate) and thyroid function tests
   i. known history of thyroid disease and medications

Observation and examination:

1. Enlargement or tenderness of the salivary, submaxillary, anterior, posterior, and deep cervical, preauricular and postauricular, and supraclavicular lymph nodes and glands; note size, shape, consistency, and mobility of any palpable nodes and glands
2. Carotid pulse
3. Abnormal pulsations
4. Vein distention
5. Range of motion
6. Enlargement or tumor of parotid gland
7. Enlargement, tumor, symmetry, size, shape, tenderness, or nodules of thyroid gland
8. Symmetry and deviation (position) of trachea

Cardiorespiratory

ROS:

1. Dyspnea (shortness of breath)
2. Orthopnea
3. Tachypnea
4. Wheezing
5. Cough
6. Pleurisy
7. Sputum production — color, consistency, amount
8. Hemoptysis
9. Chest pain
10. Stridor ("crowing" inspiratory sounds)
11. History of bronchitis, pneumonia, asthma
12. Any contact with tuberculosis
13. Date of last chest x-ray film and result
14. Night sweats
15. Palpitations
16. Cyanosis
17. Dependent edema
18. Any known abnormalities of heart rate or rhythm
19. History of rheumatic heart disease, anemia, hypertension, coronary artery disease

Observation and examination:

1. Chest and lungs
   a. configuration, deformities, symmetry, shape, masses, lesions, scars of chest structure and walls
   b. intercostal and/or subclavicular retractions or bulging
   c. equilateral respiratory excursion and symmetry with respiratory movement
   d. rate, depth, rhythm, and type (chest, abdominal) or respirations
   e. tactile fremitus
   f. auscultation of lungs
      (1) normal breath sounds
      (2) rales
      (3) rhonchi
      (4) wheezes
      (5) friction rub
      (6) adventitious sounds
2. Heart
   a. size
   b. location of point of maximum impulse (PMI)

c. Palpable thrills, rubs, impulses, shocks
d. Observable bulgings, heavings, pulsations
e. auscultation of heart
    (1) rate, rhythm, and quality of heart sounds at the four valvular areas
    (2) extra sounds, murmurs, splitting, rubs, thrills

Breasts
ROS:
1. Pain
2. Nipple discharge
3. Lumps, biopsies
4. Whether or not woman does self-breast examination (see Chapter 40 for more complete history related to the breasts)

Observation and Examination:
See Chapter 40 for observations, examination, and significance of findings.

Abdomen (Gastrointestinal System)
ROS:
1. Appetite, anorexia (lack of appetite)
2. Nausea or vomiting
3. Heartburn
4. Eructation (belching)
5. Hematemesis
6. Pain
7. Flatulence
8. Color of stools
9. Character of stools (soft, diarrhea, constipation)
10. Any recent change in bowel habits or stools.
11. Jaundice
12. Rectal itching, pain, bleeding, hemorrhoids, sphincter control
13. Known history of gallbladder disease, liver disease (hepatitis), appendicitis, colitis, ulcers, pancreatitis, parasites, hernia
14. Food allergies and idiosyncrasies
15. Any gastrointestinal x-ray examinations; date and results
16. Use of cathartics, laxatives, antacids, and

17. Pancreas (endocrine system) antiemetics
   a. polyruia, polydipsia, polyphagia in relation to food ingestion
   b. hypoglycemia symptoms (weakness, nervousness, sweating, tachycardia, hunger) in relation to food ingestion
   c. known history of diabetes

Observation and examination (Fig. 3–3):
1. Symmetry, shape, contour, scars, distention, striae, lesions, pigmentation, bruises, abnormal pulsations
2. Masses, tenderness, organomegaly, rigidity, guarding, distention, peristaltic activity
3. Femoral pulses
4. Umbilical, inguinal, or femoral hernias
5. Diastasis recti
6. Enlargement or tenderness of inguinal lymph nodes
7. Rectal examination, done at the time of the pelvic examination. See Chapter 44 for observations, examination, and significance of findings.

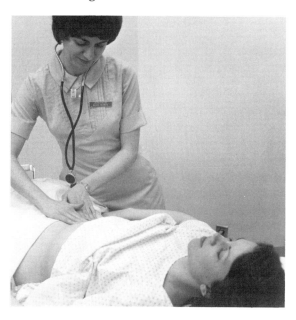

FIGURE 3-3. A nurse-midwife palpating a woman's abdomen.

Genitourinary System
ROS:
1. Urinary
   a. frequency
   b. urgency
   c. dysuria
   d. hematuria
   e. nocturia
   f. suprapubic, flank, or low back pain
   g. polyuria or oliguria
   h. pyuria (pus in urine)
   i. incontinence
   j. known history of urinary tract infections or kidney stones
2. Adrenal (endocrine system)
   a. changes in melanin pigmentation of skin
   b. weakness
   c. symptoms suggesting hypoglycemia
   d. postural hypotension
3. Genitals
   a. lesions
   b. discharge — character, color, odor, pruritis
   c. venereal disease
   d. douching
   *e. menstrual history
   *f. sexual history
   *g. obstetrical history
   *h. family planning history
   i. date and results of last Pap smear
4. Endocrine system
   a. hirsutism
   b. known history of gonadal insufficiency; hormone therapy

Observation and examination:
1. Urinary
   CVA tenderness (see Chapter 42 for methodology and significance of findings)
2. Genitals
   See Chapter 44 for observations, examin-

ation, and significance of findings

Muscular-Skeletal-Vascular Systems

1. Joint pain, stiffness, swelling, redness, heat
2. Muscle weakness, cramps, pain, twitching, tremors, paralysis, paresthesia, atrophy
3. Skeletal pain, injuries, deformities (e.g., scoliosis, lordosis, kyphosis)
4. Limitation of motion in back or range of motion of the extremities
5. Edema of extremities
6. Varicose veins, intermittent claudication (leg or calf muscle pain when walking or exercising), leg heat or tenderness
7. Known history of arthritis, gout, muscular dystrophy, thrombophlebitis, bursitis, osteomyelitis, fractures, disk disease, sciatica

Observation and examination:
1. Curvature and mobility of spine
2. Spinal column vertebral tenderness
3. Radial and pedal pulses
4. Skeletal deformities
5. Range of motion of extremities
6. Edema — finger, fascia, ankle (pedal), pretibial
7. Varicosities; calf heat and/or tenderness
8. Heat, swelling, or redness of joints
9. Homan's sign
10. Length, size, edema, lesions, redness, skin temperature, tenderness or pain, muscle atrophy, contractures, color, scars, or involuntary movements of the extremities
†11. Deep tendon reflexes
†12. Clonus
13. Clubbing, cyanosis, or other abnormality of nails

---

* Do not repeat if this information was already obtained as special sections of the history or under the past medical history.

† See Chapter 43 for observation, examination, and significance of findings.

14. Needle marks or tracks
15. Tremors of fingers

Review of Other Systems
1. Central nervous system
    a. General
        (1) Syncope, loss of consciousness, convulsions, vertigo
        (2) Known history of meningitis, encephalitis, stroke
    b. Mental Status
        (1) Speech disorders, memory disorders
        (2) Emotional status, nervousness, mood; orientation to time, place, and person
        (3) Change in sleep pattern, insomnia, activity pattern
        (4) History of "nervous breakdown"
    c. Motor
        (1) Clumsiness of movement (ataxia), weakness (paresis), paralysis
        (2) Tremor or muscle twitching
    d. Sensory
        (1) Radicular or neuralgic pain (head, neck, trunk, extremities)
        (2) Paresthesia (burning or crawling skin sensation)
        (3) Hypesthesia (decrease in tactile sensation)
        (4) Anesthesia (loss of sensation)
        (5) Hyperesthesia (excessive sensitivity of skin or special senses)
2. Lymphatic and hematopoietic systems
    a. Lymphatic
        (1) Lymph node swelling
    b. Hematopoietic
        (1) Unusual or excessive bruising or bleeding; bleeding tendencies of skin or mucous membranes
        (2) Known history of anemia and treatment, blood transfusion and reaction, blood dyscrasias, exposure to radiation or toxic agents.

REFERENCES

1. University of Mississippi Medical Center, Nurse-Midwifery Education Program. *Management Process*, 1972–1973.
2. College of Medicine and Dentistry of New Jersey, New Jersey Medical School, Nurse-Midwifery Education Program. *Management Process*, 1975.
3. Wiedenbach, E. *Clinical Nursing — A Helping Art.* New York: Springer Publishing, 1964.

BIBLIOGRAPHY

Bates, B. *A. Guide to Physical Examination, 3rd.* Philadelphia: Lippinocott, 1983.

Brown, M. S. et al. *Student Manual of Physical Examination, 2nd.* Philadelphia: Lippincott, 1984.

College of Medicine and Dentistry of New Jersey, New Jersey Medical School, Nurse-Midwifery Education Program. *Curriculum Module: Physical Assessment*, 1975.

Haire, D. Improving the outcome of pregnancy through increased utilization of midwives. *J. Nurse-Midwifery* 26(1):5–8 (January/February) 1981.

Judge, R. D., and Zuidema G. D. (Eds.). *Physical Diagnosis: A Physiological Approach to the Clinical Examination, 4th.* Boston: Little, Brown, 1982.

Malasanos, L. et al. *Health Assessments, 2nd.* St. Louis: Mosby, 1981.

Netter, F. H. *The Ciba Collection of Medical Illustrations. Volume 2, Reproductive System.* Summit, N. J.: Ciba Pharmaceutical Co., 1965.

Patient Assessment Series. New York: American Journal of Nursing Company, 1974–1977.

Prior, J. A., and Silberstein, J. S. *Physical Diagnosis: The History and Examination of the Patient, 6th.* St. Louis: Mosby, 1981.

Reedy, N. J. Nurse-midwife in complicated obstetrics: Trend or treason? *J. Nurse-Midwifery* 24(1):11–17 (January/February) 1979.

Sherman, J., Jr., and Fields, S. K. *Guide to Patient Evaluation, 4th.* Flushing, N.Y.: Medical Examination Publishing, 1982.

University of Mississippi Nurse-Midwifery Education Program. *Curriculum Module: Physical Assessment*, 1973–1975.

Yale University School of Nursing Maternal-Newborn Nursing/Nurse-Midwifery Program. *Curriculum Module: Health Assessment of Women*, 1984.

II Management of the Antepartal Period

4

The Antepartal Period, Diagnosis of Pregnancy, and Abortion

The antepartal period covers the time of pregnancy from he first day of the last menstrual period (LMP) to the start of true labor, which marks the beginning of the intrapartal period. This is in contrast to the prenatal period, which covers the time of pregnancy from the first day of the last menstrual period to the birth of the baby, which marks the beginning of the postnatal period.

The antepartal period is divided into 3 trimesters each consisting of approximately 13 weeks or 3 calendar months. This derives from consideration of the duration of pregnancy as being approximately 280 days, 40 weeks, 10 lunar months, or 9 calendar months from the first day of the last menstrual period. In reality, gestation is not that long. Fertilization takes place at the time of ovulation, approximately 14 days after the last menstrual period. This makes actual gestation approximately 266 days

or 38 weeks in length. Adding 14 days gives a total of 280 days from the last menstrual period. In practice, the first trimester is generally considered to be weeks 1 to 12 (12 weeks), the second trimester to be weeks 13 to 27 (15 weeks), and the third trimester to be weeks 28 to 40 (13 weeks).

DATA BASE FOR DIAGNOSIS OF PREGNANCY

Diagnosis of pregnancy in the first trimester and early second trimester is based on a combination of presumptive and probable signs of pregnancy. Pregnancy is self-evident later in gestation, when the positive signs of pregnancy are readily observed.

Presumptive signs of pregnancy are maternal physiological changes which the woman experiences and which in most cases indicate to her that she is pregnant. *Probable signs* of pregnancy are maternal physiological and anatomical changes other than presumptive signs, which are detected upon examination and documented by the examiner. *Positive signs* are those directly attributable to the fetus as detected and documented by the examiner.

The history, physical, pelvic, and laboratory findings that constitute the data base used in making a diagnosis of pregnancy are specifically related to the presumptive, probable, and positive signs of pregnancy. These signs do not make up the nurse-midwife's total data base, only the part needed to make a diagnosis of pregnancy.

Following is an outline of all the presumptive, probable, and positive signs of pregnancy as they are located within the framework of the history, physical, pelvic, laboratory tests, and adjunctive studies conducted and ordered by the examiner:

History
1. Abrupt cessation of menstruation (presumptive)
2. Nausea and vomiting (presumptive)
3. Tingling, tenseness, nodularity, and enlargement of the breasts and enlargement of the nipples (presumptive)
4. Increased frequency of urination (presumptive)
5. Fatigue (presumptive)
6. Color changes of the breasts, i.e., darkening of the nipples and primary and secondary areolar changes (presumptive)
7. Appearance of Montgomery's tubercles or follicles (presumptive)
8. Continued elevation of the basal body temperature in the absence of an infection (presumptive)
9. Expression of colostrum from nipples (presumptive)
10. Excessive salivation (presumptive)
11. Chadwick's sign (presumptive)
12. Quickening (presumptive)
13. Skin pigmentation and conditions, e.g.,

chloasma, breast and abdominal striae, linea nigra, vascular spiders, palmar erythema (presumptive)

Physical Examination
1. Expression of colostrum from nipples (presumptive)
2. Color changes of the breasts (presumptive)
3. Nodularity, tenseness, and enlargement of breasts and enlargement of the nipples (presumptive)
4. Appearance of Montgomery's tubercles or follicles (presumptive)
5. Enlargement of the abdomen (probable)
6. Palpation of the fetal outline (probable)
7. Ballottement (probable)
8. Fetal movement (positive or probable; authorities vary)
9. Fetal heart tones (postive)

Pelvic Examination
1. Enlargement of the uterus (probable)
2. Change in the shape of the uterus (probable)
3. Piskacek's sign (probable)
4. Hegar's sign (probable)
5. Goodell's sign (probable)
6. Palpation of Braxton Hicks' contractions (probable)
7. Chadwick's sign (presumptive)

Laboratory and adjunctive studies
1. Positive pregnancy test (probable)
2. Sonographic evidence of pregnancy — not routinely done (positive)

There is one other positive sign of pregnancy; this is visualization of the fetal skeleton by roentgenography (x-ray films). The fetal skeleton can first be visualized by the twelfth week of pregnancy because centers of ossification have formed in most of the bones. The skeleton can be clearly visualized by the sixteenth week. However, because of its danger to the fetus, roentgenography is not used for diagnosis of a viable pregnancy.

It is not always appropriate to seek findings

regarding all of the signs of pregnancy outlined here when examining a woman who thinks she is pregnant. This is because not all of the signs are manifested at the same time. For example, if a woman is approximately 2 months pregnant there is no value in attempting to elicit the following signs, as they either are not yet clinically evident or have not yet occurred:

Expression of colostrum
Secondary areolae
Skin pigmentations
Enlarged abdomen
Palpation of a fetal outline
Ballottement
Quickening
Fetal movement
Fetal heart tones by auscultation

Note that this listing includes all of the clinically elicited positive signs of pregnancy.

All of the presumptive and probable signs of pregnancy are evidences of physiologic changes taking place in the woman who is pregnant. However, since the majority of these signs can be due to other conditions, a diagnosis of pregnancy can be made only in the presence of several of these signs.

Maternal Physiologic and Anatomic Changes Indicative of Pregnancy

Physiologic and Hormonal Changes

Knowledge of the physiology of early pregnancy is necessary for understanding the presence of the presumptive and probable signs of pregnancy. It is also important, for purposes of screening for abnormality, to know what other conditions may cause the presence of particular sign.

At the time of ovulation the ovum is extruded from a mature graafian follicle in the ovary. The ruptured follicle undergoes a number of changes to become the corpus luteum of menstruation, which progressively degenerates and completely regresses during the subsequent menstruation. If the ovum is fertilized, the corpus luteum is maintained by the production of chorionic gonadotropin by the syncytiotrophoblast surrounding the blastocyst and becomes the corpus luteum of pregnancy.

The continued production of progesterone by the corpus luteum of pregnancy maintains the uterine lining for implantation and the earliest stages of pregnancy; shortly after implantation the placenta begins producing enough progesterone to take over this function. Progesterone from the corpus luteum of pregnancy also causes the mother's *basal body temperature* to continue at its elevated level following ovulation. With the uterine lining maintained there is no menstruation; this usually is the first indication of pregnancy for women with regular menstrual periods. *Amenorrhea*, however, may also be caused by certain chronic diseases, pituitary tumors, environmental factors or changes, malnutrition, and, most commonly, by emotional upset, especially that caused by the fear of being pregnant.

The placenta produces several hormones. These hormones cause a number of the physiologic changes that aid in the diagnosis of pregnancy.

The high levels of estrogen and progesterone produced by the placenta are responsible for breast changes, skin pigmentations, and uterine enlargement in the first trimester. Chorionic gonadotropin is the basis for the immunologic pregnancy tests. Chorionic somatomammotropin (human placental lactogen — HPL) stimulates the growth of the breasts, has lactogenic properties, and effects a number of metabolic changes.

Specifically, estrogen promotes development of the ductal system of the breasts as well as mammary growth, and progesterone stimulates the development of the alveolar system of the breasts and contributes to mammary growth. Together with chorionic somatomammotropin these hormones are responsible for the presumptive signs of *breast enlargement*, causing the breasts to feel *tense and tingling* during the first 2 months of pregnancy, *enlargement of the nipples*, and the presence of *colostrum* in the breasts, which usually can be expressed by the twelfth week of pregnancy. Hypertrophy of the mammary alveoli causes the breasts to feel *nodular*, starting during the first 2 months of pregnancy. *Montgomery's tubercles* or *follicles* are actually hypertrophied sebaceous glands in the areolae and are prominently noticeable by the second month of pregnancy. Excessive enlargement of the breasts causes *striations*. A *tracing of delicate veins* may be seen just beneath the skin as the breasts enlarge. Many of these breast changes are seen also in women taking oral contraceptive pills, may occur in women with brain or ovarian tumors or taking certain tranquilizers, and sometimes are seen in pseudocyesis (imaginary pregnancy).

While the cause of skin pigmentation is not certain it is thought that estrogen and progesterone have a melanocyte-stimulating effect. This would account for the *darkening of the nipple* and the *primary areolae* (darkening of the areola around the nipple), both of which occur around the third month of pregnancy. It also would account for the *secondary areolae* (mottling of the skin around and beyond the primary areolae); the *linea nigra* (a narrow line of dark skin pigmentation in the midline of the abdomen from the symphysis pubis to the umbilicus); the *striae* (stretch marks) of the abdomen (striae gravidarum), excessively enlarged breasts, and occasionally buttocks and upper thighs; and *chloasma* (the mask of pregnancy — irregular brownish discolorations of the forehead, nose, cheeks, and neck). All of these occur around the fifth or sixth lunar months of pregnancy. The pigmentation of the nipples and breasts varies with the woman's complexion. It is a pronounced pink in blondes, dark brown in brunettes, and black in the black race. Chloasma is most noticeable in brunettes. Although skin pigmentations are

fairly common in pregnant women, they may be absent. Chloasma is seen sometimes in women taking oral contraceptive pills. All skin pigmentations may also be associated with a variety of tumors of different origin. Most of the pigmentation changes of pregnancy regress and disappear after pregnancy has ended, with the exception of the striae, which lose their reddish brown pigmentation but remain as fine silvery white lines of glistening fibrous tissue.

Vascular spiders and *palmar erythema* during pregnancy possibly are due to the hyperestrogenemic state of the woman while pregnant. These conditions, which occur around the fifth to sixth lunar months of pregnancy, usually disappear after pregnancy has ended and have no clinical significance. However, palmar erythema in the first trimester indicates the possibility of hepatitis, with which it is also associated. Vascular spiders generally appear on the face, neck, upper chest, and arms and are minute reddened elevations of the skin with each being a central body from which there is branching of radicles. Many women do not experience either of these conditions during their pregnancy.

Anatomical Changes/Uterine Enlargement

Estrogen and perhaps progesterone are thought to be primarily responsible for the hypertrophy of the uterine wall during the early months of pregnancy. *Uterine enlargement* is the result of a considerable increase in the size and stretching of already existing muscle cells. The uterine wall is strengthened rather than weakened by this development since the hypertrophy of the muscle cells is accompanied by a marked increase in elastic tissue and an accumulation of fibrous tissue. After the third month of pregnancy uterine enlargement is due also, in part, to the mechanical effect of inside pressure on the uterine wall by the growing products of conception. During hypertrophy of muscle cells in the early months of gestation there is a marked increase in the size of the uterine blood vessels and lymphatics. The resulting vascularity, congestion, and edema most likely account for the overall softening of the uterus and, combined with hypertrophy of the cervical glands, give rise to Chadwick's, Goodell's, and Hegar's signs. *Chadwick's sign* is the bluish or purplish discoloration of the vulva and vaginal mucosa, including the vaginal portion of the cervix. *Goodell's sign* is the softening of the cervix from a nonpregnant state of firmness similar to the tip of a nose, to the softness of lips in the pregnant state. *Hegar's sign* is the softening and compressibility of the uterine isthmus. These three signs are evident by about 6 weeks' gestation.

The softness and compressibility of the uterine isthmus (Hegar's sign) has the effect of nonsupport to the enlarging body of the uterus with its increasing heaviness in the fundus. The result is exaggerated uterine anteflexion during the first 3 months of pregnancy while the uterus is still a pelvic organ. This causes the fundus to press on the bladder and *urinary frequency* ensues. Urinary frequency is relieved early in the fourth month of pregnancy as the uterus rises out of the pelvis, thereby no longer causing bladder pressure.

As the uterus enlarges it changes from its nonpregnant pear-shape to a globular form in the early months of pregnancy and becomes an ever larger ovoid after the third month of pregnancy. As it enlarges it can be contained no longer within the pelvis and rises out of the pelvis to become an abdominal organ. The uterus rotates slightly to the right as it rises out of the pelvis. This dextrorotation is thought to be due to the rectosigmoid's occupying the left side of the pelvic cavity. The uterus may enlarge at slightly different rates (1 to 2 weeks' variation) for the primigravida and the multigravida. This variation may create some differences in early sizing and again when the uterus reaches anatomical landmarks such as the umbilicus.

Early uterine enlargement may not be symmetrical. The ovum normally implants in the upper uterine wall, more frequently on the posterior side. This may not be a central implantation but may be located closer to one cornual area. Therefore the cornual area where the ovum implants enlarges first from the embryological development taking place at that site. Such implantation may be detected during pelvic examination by the asymmetry of the uterus and a rough, irregular contour in one of the cornual areas. This uterine irregularity occurs around the eighth to tenth weeks of pregnancy and is called *Piskacek's sign*.

Uterine enlargement contributes to two other maternal signs of pregnancy. The first is based on the hypothesis that the *Braxton Hicks contractions* may, in part, be due to the stretching of the uterine muscle cells. An increase in the concentration of actomyosin in the muscle cells is also thought to contribute to this contractility of the uterus. Braxton Hicks contractions are nonrhythmic, sporadic, painless uterine contractions that start about the sixth week of pregnancy but are not detectable during bimanual pelvic examination until the second trimester and during abdominal examination in the third trimester. They increase in frequency, duration, and intensity as well as attain some degree of rhythm and regularity close to term at which time they are frequently misinterpreted as labor contractions. They are the major culprit of false labor.

The other sign of pregnancy brought about by uterine enlargement is that of *abdominal enlargement*. This begins at the fourth month of pregnancy as the uterus becomes an ever-larger abdominal organ. The abdomen is more prominent when the woman is standing than when she is supine. Abdominal enlargement is also more noticeable in multiparas than in primigravidas because of the loss of muscle tone of the abdominal wall, which was not exercised back into shape after each previous pregnancy. A pendulous abdomen results as the uterus sags forward and downward. This can cause problems during labor in extreme cases.

Other Signs of Pregnancy

With the exception of the pregnancy tests, very little is known about the etiology of the remaining signs of pregnancy. It is thought that the basic metabolic rate (BMR) initially falls early in pregnancy and then progressively rises throughout the pregnancy as a direct result of the metabolic activity of the products of conception. The initial fall in the BMR might account for the *fatigue* often encountered during the first trimester. *Nausea* and *vomiting* have been attributed to a number of possible causes (see Chapter 7) but their actual etiology is unknown. "Normal" nausea and vomiting in pregnancy rarely extend beyond the first trimester. *Excessive salivation (ptyalism)* is an unusual occurrence which may be caused either by increased acidity in the mouth or by the intake of starch stimulating the salivary glands in women susceptible to excessive secretion. Women who have ptyalism frequently are also nauseated. This becomes cyclic, for not only does the excessive saliva intensify the nausea but also the desire to avoid nausea causes the patient to swallow less, thus increasing the amount of saliva in the mouth.

Fetal Contributions to the Diagnosis of Pregnancy

Anatomic

As the uterus enlarges, its wall becomes thinner, changing to a thickness of approximately 5 millimeters at term from an almost solid state. The combination of uterine enlargement, thinning of the uterine wall, and the uterus becoming an abdominal organ enable the detection of a number of signs of pregnancy during the second trimester which were previously inaccessible. The precise time, however, when the fetal heart tones are heard and quickening is felt vary not only with the thinness or obesity of the individual woman but also with parity. The uterus and abdominal musculature of a multipara have hypertrophied

and stretched before. They will do so again more easily and thus may be thin enough to facilitate eliciting of these signs of pregnancy a week or two earlier than in a primigravida.

The *fetal heart* starts beating at the beginning of the fourth week post-fertilization (sixth week after the LMP), but it is not until around the twentieth week following the LMP that it can be heard with a head fetoscope during abdominal examination of the mother. However, it can be heard between the twelfth and twentieth weeks after the LMP with ultrasonic instruments. Fetal heart tones must be differentiated from the maternal pulse, maternal bowel sounds, fetal movement sounds, and the uterine souffle. The funic souffle (the sound of blood rushing through the umbilical arteries) is synchronous with the fetal pulse.

Similarly, weak *fetal movements* start in the third month of pregnancy but it is not until around the twentieth week that they are strong enough and the uterine wall is thin enough for them to be felt and properly diagnosed during abdominal examination. The mother may be aware of fetal movements around the eighteenth week following her LMP. These movements increase in intensity over the weeks from gentle flutterings to unmistakable fetal kicks. The time when she first feels fetal movement is called *quickening*, meaning the perception of life. Quickening may be useful as corroborative evidence in dating a pregnancy but is not definitively diagnostic because the early flutterings are akin in feeling to the movement of gas through the intestines.

It is not until after the twentieth week that the *fetal outline* can be *palpated* during abdominal examination. Again, this is not a definitive diagnostic sign since subserous myomas may feel like fetal parts. *Ballottement* can be elicited abdominally around the same time. In this sign, a sudden tap on the uterus causes the fetus to sink in the amniotic fluid and rebound to strike gently against the fingers of the examiner. Ballottement is possible at this time because there is a large volume of amniotic fluid in relation to the size of the still small fetus. This proportion grossly changes later in pregnancy.

Hormonal Pregnancy Tests

Pregnancy tests are based on the production of chorionic gonadotropin by the syncytiotrophoblastic cells during early pregnancy. Human chorionic gonadotropin (hCG) is secreted into the maternal bloodstream where it is present in the plasma. It is then excreted in the mother's urine.

Human chorionic gonadotrophin is first detected in the urine about 26 days after conception and is excreted at rates which increases rapidly between 30 and 60 days into the pregnancy. Peak levels occur between 60 and 70 days of gestation. The level then gradually decreases to a low between 100 and 130 days and is maintained at this level throughout the remaining weeks of gestation. Blood levels are parallel but can be detected in radioimmunoassay tests as early as 1 day after implantation.

Quantitative assays of hCG are of diagnostic significance in pregnancy. They are abnormally low in ectopic pregnancies and threatened abortions (also causing false negative pregnancy tests) and abnormally high in women with multiple pregnancy, hydatidiform mole, or choriocarcinoma. Quantitative values in the serum radioimmunoassay tests are also useful in dating a pregnancy.

Human chorionic gonadotrophin in the urine has been used for pregnancy tests since the late 1920s when Aschheim and Zondek originated biologic assay of its presence. The biologic tests of pregnancy utilize small immature animals (mice, rats, rabbits, frogs, toads) and are based on the response of the animals' ovaries or testes after being injected with either serum or urine of the woman suspected of being pregnant.

These tests have been largely supplanted by the immunologic assays of hCG (Fig. 4–1). The immunologic assays utilize specific antisera

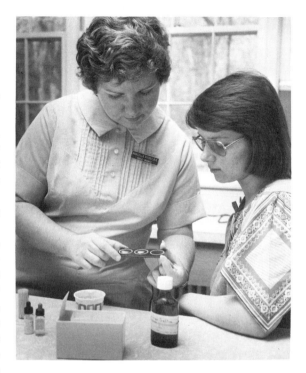

FIGURE 4–1.   Nurse-midwife and woman examining the slide of a pregnancy test.

obtained from animals (rabbits) in which antibody response to hCG has been stimulated. It is based on the fact that hCG is a protein and therefore antigenic. The antisera are mixed with urine from the woman suspected of being pregnant. This mediates the response of the antisera when mixed with either latex particles coated with hCG (latex particle agglutination inhibition tests) or with erythrocytes (from sheep) which have been sensitized to hCG (hemagglutination inhibition tests). If the woman is pregnant her urine contains hCG, which will neutralize the antibodies in the antiserum and inhibit agglutination — a positive pregnancy test. If the woman is not pregnant her urine does not contain hCG, and agglutination will occur — a negative pregnancy test.

The companies that manufacture these pregnancy tests enclose with the necessary materials step-by-step instructions for the performance and interpretation of the test, information pertaining to the period in gestation when the test is most accurate, and data concerning the sensitivity of the test in detecting specific levels of hCG in terms of international units of hCG per liter or milliliter of urine. Because hCG is similar in structure to luteinizing hormone (LH), the antibodies of both these hormones will cross-react with each other. Therefore most tests limit their maximum quantity sensitivity in order to avoid false-positive tests because of cross-reactivity with luteinizing hormone.

False-negative immunologic pregnancy tests occur in about 2 percent of all tests run and usually result from doing the test too early in the pregnancy (i.e., before 6 weeks since the first day of the last menstrual period) or, occasionally, too late in the pregnancy (after the middle of the pregnancy). False-positive results occur in about 5 percent of all immunological tests. This may be caused by the woman's having massive proteinuria or may occur during the onset of menopause in middle-aged women when the levels of pituitary gonadotropins rise while the endocrine function of the ovaries declines. False-positive pregnancy tests may also result from the cross-reaction of pituitary gonadotropins with hCG.

Overall, the immunologic pregnancy tests are as accurate as the biologic pregnancy tests (95 to 98 percent) although accuracy may vary somewhat with the test used and the care taken to assure that the test is being done during the appropriate time of gestation. Since pregnancy tests are not 100 percent accurate, they are considered a probable sign of pregnancy, and the results should be evaluated in relation to the presence or absence of other signs of pregnancy.

More recently, radioreceptorassay and radioimmunoassay tests have become available. Both require expensive equipment and trained technicians. These are extremely sensitive tests able to detect hCG at far lower levels than previous tests. Because the radioreceptorassay test cross-reacts with luteinizing hormone, however, it is more limited in its sensitivity than the radioimmunoassay tests.

Human chorionic gonadotrophin consists of two dissimilar glycoprotein chains designated as an alpha subunit and a beta subunit. The radioimmunoassay blood tests are designed specifically to detect the hCG beta subunit because it has distinctive differences from other glycoprotein beta subunits while the hCG alpha subunit is quite similar, if not identical, to other glycoprotein alpha subunits. This radioimmunoassay test, commonly called beta-preg, can be used as early as one week after conception if the laboratory facilities are available. The laboratory will supply information about the expected levels for the particular week gestation and the sensitivity of the test used. This is a highly accurate test but not 100 percent perfect.

A pregnancy test formerly in use was almost foolproof. It consisted of administering a high dose of a progesterone derivative for 5 days and then observing for withdrawal bleeding, which would not happen if the woman was having a normal pregnancy. Use of this method of pregnancy testing is now in disrepute because there is evidence of an increased possibility of congenital malformations resulting in the fetuses of pregnant women who take this drug.

ABORTION

An increasing number of physicians and hospitals are refusing to perform abortions after the twelfth week or the first trimester of pregnancy. Therefore, if a woman wishes to have an abortion, the early diagnosis of her pregnancy is essential. Although a positive diagnosis cannot be made clinically until around the twentieth week, a tentative diagnosis can be based on the presumptive and probable signs mentioned previously in this chapter. The diagnosis can be confirmed with ultrasound scanning.

A first trimester abortion is done by dilatation and curettage (D&C) or by suction. A second trimester abortion is done by (1) injection of a hypertonic salt solution replacing an equal amount of amniotic fluid ("salting out"), (2) injection of prostaglandin into the amniotic sac, (3) hysterotomy, or (4) hysterectomy for a combined abortion and sterilization procedure. The second trimester methods of abortion carry a higher maternal mortality risk than do the methods of first trimester abortion. Third trimester abortions are not done because the fetus is universally considered to be viable at 28 weeks. In fact, most obstetricians have taken the position of considering termination of pregnancy after the twentieth week as an induced immature or premature birth rather than an abortion. This position is based on standard obstetrical definitions for abortion, immature birth, and premature birth (see Chapter 9).

The 1973 Supreme Court ruling on abortion in effect legalized abortion, although it gave the states regulatory rights on abortion in the second and third trimesters. This ruling voided laws that were restrictive in 31 states, and 15 other states had laws in which revisions had to be made.

The issues are complex, with the central issues being:

1. When does life begin? At conception? Or at the point when the fetus can survive independently of the uterus? This point is much affected today by the life-sustaining technology in neonatal intensive care units.
2. Does the woman have a right to self-determination, including the decision whether or not to be pregnant?
3. Does the fetus, regardless of gestational age, have any rights?
4. Are there any identifiable reasons agreed to by a public majority which might constitute grounds for abortion (e.g., rape; diagnosed genetic defects from heredity, disease, or drugs; contraceptive method failure)?

The proabortion movement stresses the rights of the woman. The antiabortion, or prolife, movement stresses the rights of the fetus to life. In between is the prochoice movement, which is neither proabortion nor antiabortion but instead stresses the right of each individual woman to make her own decision about the choices (alternatives) she has (discussed below). Like all controversial issues, especially those dealing with life, death, and the human body, the subject of abortion is heavily laden with emotion. Irrationality by the extremists on all sides of the issue can result.

All women have an emotional response to learning or having confirmed that they are pregnant. For some it is very happy news, perhaps a much desired and planned-for event; for others the news has all the effect of a catastrophe; for still others the response is that of not caring one way or the other. For all women it requires a number of adjustments. The first trimester is known as the trimester of adjustment, and it is most likely that even the happiest woman in the happiest of circumstances has thought at least once to herself that she wished she was not pregnant. This, however, is quite different from the woman who seriously contemplates an abortion or decides upon and implements her decision to have an abortion. How the woman feels about being pregnant can have far-reaching effects, not only in terms of abortion but also in terms of parent-child relationships if the pregnancy is fulfilled. Therefore, it is vitally important to ask *throughout* the pregnancy how the woman feels about her pregnancy in order to facilitate her coping with the demands of pregnancy and to identify indications of lack of adjustment or precursors to later child abuse.

The legalization of abortion means that every woman, upon being diagnosed as pregnant, now has a choice as to whether or not to carry the pregnancy to its natural conclusion. The woman's decision to have an abortion is not lightly made. In many cases she will turn to the nurse-midwife for counsel, advice, and information. Every woman has the right to know her alternatives and, in the case of first trimester infection (e.g., rubella), her chances of having an affected baby. Her alternatives are three, regardless of circumstances: (1) continue with the pregnancy and keep the baby, (2) continue with the pregnancy and give the baby up for adoption, or (3) terminate the pregnancy with an abortion within the allowable time limits.

If you are a person who in conscience cannot provide abortion counseling, it is only fair that you tell the woman desirous of abortion information that this is the situation and to seek the desired information from someone else. Most professionals in this category will call in a colleague who will provide the information. Clinicians who are not restricted by conscience in the provision of information should be intimately familiar with the local resources for abortion counseling, the procedures for obtaining an abortion, and how to make appropriate referrals.

While nurse-midwives may do abortion counseling, provide abortion information, and give nursing care to the woman having an abortion, the nurse-midwife is professionally prohibited from performing the actual abortion. This is clearly stated in the position of the American College of Nurse-Midwives in a statement adopted in 1971:

The American College of Nurse-Midwives fully supports the statement of the American College of Obstetricians and Gynecologists issued in August, 1970, which states, "abortion is an operative procedure and should only be performed by a physician who has hospital privileges for the care of obstetric-gynecologic patients." The nurse-midwife may, however, at her discretion, be involved in patient care before and after the operative procedure [1].

REFERENCE

1. American College of Nurse-Midwives. *Statement on Abortion*. Washington, D.C., 1971.

BIBLIOGRAPHY

Alpern, D. M. Abortion and the law. *Newsweek* March 3, 1975.

APHA Recommended Program Guide for Abortion Services. Washington, D.C.: American Public Health Association, 1973.

Batzer, F. R. et al. Landmarks during the first forty-two days of gestation demonstrated by the B-subunit of human chorionic gonadotropin and ultrasound. *Am. J. Obstet. Gynecol.* 146(8):973–979, 1983.

Baudry, F., and Wiener, A. The pregnant patient in conflict about abortion: A challenge for the obstetrician, *Am. J. Obstet. Gynecol.* 119:705, 1974.

Braunstein, G. et al. First-trimester chorionic gonadotrophin measurements as an aid in the diagnosis of early pregnancy disorders. *Am. J. Obstet. Gynecol.* 131:25, 1978.

Clark, M. et al. A new doctors' dilemma. *Newsweek* March 3, 1975.

Danforth, D. N. (Ed.). *Obstetrics and Gynecology, 4th*. Philadelphia: Harper & Row, 1982.

Greenhill, J. P., and Friedman, E. A. *Biological Principles and Modern Practice of Obstetrics*. Philadelphia: Saunders, 1974.

Hall, R. E. The supreme court decision on abortion. *Am. J. Obstet. Gynecol.* 116:1, 1973.

Hibbard, B. M. Pregnancy diagnosis. *Br. Med. J.* 1:593, 1971.

Keller, C., and Copeland, P. Counseling the abortion patient is more than talk. *Am. J. Nurs.* 72:102, 1972.

Nichols, C. Clinical management of size/dates discrepancy. *J. Nurse-Midwifery* 30(1):15–24 (January/February), 1985.

Palomaki, J. F. Abortion techniques: What are their risks and complications? *Contemporary OB/GYN* 9:73, 1977.

Pritchard, J. A., MacDonald, P. C., and Gant, N. F. *Williams Obstetrics, 17th*. Norwalk, Conn.: Appleton-Century-Crofts, 1985.

Reid, D. E., Ryan, K. J., and Benirschke, K. *Principles and Management of Human Reproduction.* Philadelphia: Saunders, 1972.

Schwartz, R. O., and Di Pietro, D. L. B-hCG as a diagnostic aid for suspected ectopic pregnancy. *Obstet. Gynecol.* 56(2):197–203 (August) 1980.

Speroff, L., Glass, R. H., and Kase, N. G. *Clinical Gynecologic Endocrinology and Infertility.* Baltimore: Williams & Wilkins, 1973.

Taylor, E. S. *Beck's Obstetrical Practice, 10th.* Baltimore: Williams & Wilkins, 1971.

Tietze, C., and Lewit, S. Joint program for the study of abortion (JPSA): early medical complications of legal abortion. *Studies in Family Planning* 3:97, 1972.

Van der Vlugt, T. H. History, present status, and applications of menstrual regulation. *J. Obstet. Gynecol. Neonat. Nurs.* 3:34, 1974.

Wiedenbach, E. *Family-Centered Maternity Nursing, 2nd.* New York: Putnam's, 1967.

5

Antepartal Examinations

THE INITIAL EXAMINATION

The initial antepartal examination occurs at any point in pregnancy when the woman makes an appointment for her continuing health care. It consists of a complete history, physical and pelvic examinations, and a number of laboratory and adjunctive studies. This chapter describes the details of this examination. It is assumed that the woman's pregnancy has already been diagnosed either by prior examination and a pregnancy test (early in her pregnancy) or, later, by being self-evident. The details of this initial antepartal examination are basically the same regardless of what time in pregnancy it takes place. There are obvious differences depending on where the woman is in the pregnancy, e.g., the size of the uterus.

Data Base

History
In addition to the identifying information; past medical history; family history; menstrual history; obstetric history; gynecologic history; and sexual, contraceptive, and douching history (outlined in Chapter 3), a present pregnancy history needs to be taken. In planning the sequence of information to be obtained during a visit, it is often best to start with the present pregnancy history. This is what most women are interested in and expect to talk about. Your interest in the woman's first interest facilitates obtaining all the other information afterwards. Emphasis also needs to be placed on obtaining the date of her last menstrual period, calculation of her estimated date of delivery, determination of the present number of weeks gestation, and calculation of her gravida and para status.

Gravida/Para. Gravida refers to the number of times a woman has been pregnant. It does not matter at what point during pregnancy the pregnancy was terminated. Nor does it matter how many babies were born from the pregnancy. It is the pregnancy that counts, not the number of babies. A woman who has had one pregnancy from which issued triplets would still be a Gravida 1 until pregnant again, at which time she would be a Gravida 2. A woman who is pregnant for the first time is called a *primigravida*. A woman pregnant for the second time is called a *secundigravida*. Thereafter, if pregnant again, she is called a *multigravida*. A woman who has never been pregnant is called a *nulligravida*.

Para refers to the number of pregnancies that terminated in the birth of a fetus or fetuses that reached the point of viability. This point is still considered to be 28 weeks gestation or 1000 grams, even though a number of babies weighing less than this can now survive with the aid of expert neonatal care and technology. A woman's para designation is achieved only if the pregnancy produces a fetus that has reached the point of viability. For example, a woman who has been pregnant twice and had two first trimester abortions is a Gravida 2, Para 0. On the other hand, it is not the number of fetuses reaching the point of viability but the number of pregnancies carried to the point of the fetus or fetuses' reaching the point of viability that determines parity. So the woman who has had one pregnancy that resulted in 4-pound triplets is a Gravida 1, Para 1. Para is not affected by whether or not the fetus or fetuses are actually born alive or are stillbirths. The woman who has been pregnant twice with one of those pregnancies ending in a full-term stillbirth and the other in a full-term livebirth would be a Gravida 2, Para 2.

A *primipara* is a woman who has had one pregnancy in which the fetus or fetuses reached the point of viability. Unfortunately, primipara is often used interchangeably with primigravida, but it is not possible for a primigravida to be a primipara until after the birth of a baby which reached the point of viability. A *multipara* is a woman who has had two or more pregnancies in which the fetus or fetuses reached the point of viability. It is possible for a multigravida not to be a multipara since, in this system, the para number can be less, but never more, than the gravida number. A

woman who has not carried a pregnancy to the point of viability is called a *nullipara*.

Para does not provide much information about the pregnancies a woman has had. For this reason the two-digit system of Gravida/Para is rarely used. Instead a four- or five-digit system is used in place of para although, in practice, the digits are misnamed as para. This is confusing because, in this system, each baby born is counted rather than counting the number of pregnancies carried to viability, which is the basis for determining para. The digits follow a precise sequence:

First digit: the number of term babies the woman has delivered. *Term* refers to any baby of 36 weeks or 2500 grams or more.
Second digit: the number of premature babies the woman has delivered. *Premature* refers to any baby born between 28 and 36 weeks or weighing between 1000 and 2499 grams.
Third digit: the number of pregnancies ending in abortion (either spontaneous or induced). *Abortion* refers to any baby born before 28 weeks gestation or weighing less than 1000 grams. Even though there is now an *immature* classification for babies born between 20 and 28 weeks or weighing between 500 and 999 grams, for purposes of this system of summarizing a woman's obstetric history these are counted as abortions.
Fourth digit: the number of children currently alive.
Fifth digit: the number of pregnancies that resulted in multiple births. The fifth digit is not commonly used but is useful when there is a history of multiple births.

Following are examples of the four- or five-digit system in use:

Example 1: a Gravida 2 delivered a full-term baby with each pregnancy, both of whom are currently alive. She is a Para 2002.
Example 2: a Gravida 2 delivered a full-term

baby who died at six months of age, and aborted during her second pregnancy. She is a Para 1010.

Example 3: a Gravida 1 delivered premature twins, one of whom died. She is a Para 0201.

Example 4: a Gravida 6 has delivered one full-term livebirth, one full-term stillbirth, one premature livebirth, and premature triplets of whom two lived and one died, and has had two abortions. She is a Para 2424. In this instance it would be useful to use the fifth digit for the number of pregnancies which resulted in multiple births in order to clarify the first four numbers. Using five digits, she is a Para 24241.

In any of the above examples, if the woman is pregnant at the time of this summarizing of her obstetric history, her gravida number would increase by one to account for her present pregnancy. When doing the obstetric history during the initial antepartal examination, if the woman is pregnant for the first time, simply write *primigravida* across the space provided for this history on the chart.

Last Menstrual Period. Because the date of the first day of the last normal menstrual period (LMP) is used as the baseline for determining gestational age and the estimated date of delivery (EDD), it is important to obtain as accurate a date of this event as possible. Unfortunately many women do not keep a record of their menstrual periods. They do, however, have a pretty good general idea of the regularity of their periods and when during the month they occur. A little detective work is often indicated. The success of your detective work will most likely depend on the questions you ask.

The first thing to determine about the date a woman gives for her LMP is to ascertain whether or not this was a normal period for her. To do this, correlate her description of her last menstrual period with her description of her regular menstrual periods, obtained while taking her menstrual history. For example, if she says her last period was scanty and lasted 1 or 2 days, while her usual periods are moderately heavy for the first 2 days and taper off to scanty around the fourth or fifth day, then you know that her last menstrual period was not "normal" for her. Therefore, ask about the period before the one she has given as her last one. If this preceding period is "normal" for her, then this is the one you count as her LMP. It is not uncommon for a woman to experience some spotting at the time of implantation of the blastocyst as a result of the invasive activity of the chorionic villi in the uterine lining. Since the timing of implantation in a woman with a 28-day cycle is close to the time she would be expecting a menstrual period (ovulation at day 14 prior to the next menstrual period, 3 to 4 days to transport the fertilized ovum down the fallopian tube to the uterus [day 17 or 18], 3 days in the uterine cavity before implantation [day 20 or 21], and then several days for implantation), a woman often misinterprets this spotting from implantation as a menstrual period even though distinctly different from her usual period. If you do not explore the normality of her last menstrual period you can make the error of misdating the pregnancy by one month. This can cause undue concern when clinical findings and gestational age do not correlate throughout the pregnancy. Remember, LMP refers to the first day of her last *normal* menstrual period.

Occasionally you will run into the woman who professes no idea of the date of her last menstrual period. To get some idea of when this might have occurred it is useful to use the national holidays or other dates which might be significant to her. Such women often will remember if they had a menstrual period around Christmas, New Year's Day, Easter, Fourth of July, Halloween, Thanksgiving, their birthday, the beginning or end of school, and so forth.

At times a woman is simply a poor historian and accuracy in pinpointing the LMP is impossible. This should be so noted on her chart. If the last menstrual period is unknown, an estimated date of delivery is based on many parameters (see "Size-Dates Discrepancy" in Chapter 9).

Estimated Date of Confinement. The expected date of the end of pregnancy by delivery of a full-term baby is called the *estimated date of confinement* (EDC). This term has been changed by a number of health care professionals to *estimated date of delivery* (EDD). The change was introduced because of a feeling that the word confinement connotes illness, limitation, and a passive role rather than a normal event, a healthy process, and active participation. The estimated date of delivery (EDD) will be used throughout this book.

The EDD is calculated by Naegele's rule, in which 7 days are added to the date of the first day of the LMP and then 3 months subtracted from that date. This is easiest to calculate by substituting numbers for months and days so that the first number stands for the month and the second number stands for the day. One must be careful to use the actual number of days in the month of the LMP when crossing over to another month. This is illustrated in the following example of calculating the EDD by Naegele's rule:

<pre>
  5/28 (LMP of May 28)
+   7 days
  6/4   (June 4 — May has 31 days)
- 3   months
= 3/4   (March 4 — of the next year, as 9
        months have been added)
</pre>

The EDD is at best a "guesstimate" because several variables may alter the actual date of delivery. First, calculation of the EDD is dependent on an accurate recollection by the woman of the date of the first day of her last normal menstrual period. Second, the actual period of

gestation is from the time of fertilization. Since ovulation is generally considered to occur approximately 14 days before the *next* menstrual period, the length of a woman's menstrual cycle will affect the accuracy of the EDD. A woman with a longer menstrual cycle (more than 28 days) will actually begin her pregnancy later in relation to the LMP and subsequently will deliver at a correspondingly later date. The reverse is true for the woman with a shorter menstrual cycle. Third, not all women with 28-day menstrual cycles ovulate 14 days before the next menstrual period; this individual variation as to ovulation time will affect the accuracy of the EDD. Therefore, the woman should be told she probably will not have her baby on the exact date of the EDD. The majority of women deliver within 10 to 14 days, either earlier or later, of their EDD, and this range is considered physiologically normal.

The addition of 7 days in Naegele's rule attempts to counterbalance some of the difference between the LMP and the time of fertilization. The remaining 7 days (to total 14 in a 28-day cycle) are picked up over the 9-calendar-month period of gestation because 7 calendar months have 31 days. However, no single pregnancy would cover the period of time to include all these 7 months.

It is useless to calculate the EDD by Naegele's rule in the presence of any of the following situations:

1. Irregular menstrual periods in which 1 or more months are amenorrheic
2. Conception occurring while the mother is breast-feeding and ovulating but amenorrheic
3. Conception occurring before regular menstruation is established after termination of a pregnancy or discontinuation of oral contraceptive pills

In such instances an estimated date of delivery is based on clinical findings and subsequent projections and, if indicated, an ultrasound scan between 18 and 26 weeks of gestation. The same clinical measurements are used during any pregnancy to double-check the accuracy of the EDD and to detect possible intrauterine growth retardation and other complications. These are discussed in detail in the content relating to fetal evaluation measures in Chapter 7 and in "Size-Dates Discrepancy" in Chapter 9.

Determination of the weeks of gestation according to dates is done most easily and quickly by using one of the gestational calendars or calculators put out by the pharmaceutical companies. However, since there is sometimes an element of slight inaccuracy in using these calculators to determine the EDD, most clinicians calculate the EDD from the LMP by Naegele's rule and use the resulting EDD in setting the calculator to determine the week of gestation.

Present Pregnancy History. The present pregnancy history is designed to detect complications, some of the discomforts, and any complaints about the pregnancy the woman has experienced since her LMP. You may see the woman for her initial antepartal examination at any time during the pregnancy; therefore the present pregnancy history given here covers symptoms of possible problems in all three trimesters. Following is an outline of the present pregnancy history:

1. Headaches
2. Dizziness
3. Visual disturbances
4. Syncope
5. Fever
6. Fatigue
7. Nausea
8. Vomiting
9. Heartburn
10. Breast changes
11. Leakage of colostrum
12. Shortness of breath
13. Abdominal pain
14. Back pain
15. Dyspareunia
16. Vaginal discharge
17. Vaginal bleeding
18. Dysuria
19. Urinary frequency
20. Constipation
21. Hemorrhoids
22. Leg cramps
23. Varicosities
24. Edema (ankle, pretibial, face, hands)
25. Infections (e.g., measles, flu, other viruses)
26. Drugs and medications
27. Roentgenography (exposure to x-rays)
28. Accidents
29. Any complaints, discomforts, or concerns other than those already discussed
30. Sexual satisfaction — sexual changes and the feelings of both partners towards any changes
31. Feelings about her pregnancy — effect on her life, her body image, feelings about the baby
32. Quickening (date of)

A positive response to any of 1 through 29 requires further exploratory history taking to ascertain the following:

1. When during the pregnancy this has occurred; duration; recurrences
2. Specific location (when indicated)
3. Severity (when indicated)
4. Associated symptoms
5. Factors influencing the problem, either aggravating or relieving
6. Medical help (whom); diagnosis and treatment (when indicated)
7. Treatment or relief measures (self or medically initiated) and their effectiveness

Physical Examination
A complete screening physical examination is done during the initial antepartal examination in order to ascertain whether the woman has any medical abnormalities or disease. This

physical examination was outlined in Chapter 3. Variations in findings for the pregnant woman during breast examination are discussed in Chapter 4.

An abdominal examination of the pregnant woman should be done in addition to the physical examination outlined. The following is included in the abdominal examination of the pregnant woman:

1. Observation of any scars and inquiry to obtain explanation of them
2. Observation of linea nigra
3. Observation of abdominal striae
4. Determination of the lie, presentation, position, and variety of the fetus
5. Measurement of fundal height
6. Auscultation of fetal heart tones
7. Estimation of fetal weight
8. Observation or palpation of fetal movement

Each of these items provides informative data useful either in diagnosis of pregnancy, in evaluation of fetal well-being and growth, or as indicators of possible problems. See "Antepartal/Intrapartal Abdominal Examination" in Chapter 41.

Any *scars* on the abdomen must be noted and their reason for being there explored. The scar of a former cesarean section is of particular importance (see Chapter 14). It is useful to know if the woman has had an appendectomy so that this possibility is ruled out in the event of right-sided abdominal pain during the pregnancy.

Observation of *linea nigra* and *abdominal striae* are presumptive signs of pregnancy. Observation or palpation of *fetal movement* and hearing the *fetal heart tones (FHT)* are positive signs of pregnancy. The normal range of fetal heart tones is 120 to 160 per minute. Whether the FHT are in the lower or upper end of this range is *not* an indication of whether the baby will be a boy or a girl.

Determination of the *lie, presentation, position,* and *variety* of the fetus varies in importance

with the length of pregnancy. Prior to the twentieth week it is nearly impossible to ascertain this information because of a combination of the smallness of the fetus, the thickness of the uterus, and the still high ratio of amniotic fluid to baby in the amniotic sac. The baby will continue to turn and somersault in the amniotic sac until the bulk of the baby's body is far greater than the amount of amniotic fluid and there is no longer room for the fetus to turn easily. Consequently information about fetal placement in the uterus has little meaning for labor and delivery management until around the thirty-sixth week of gestation. By this time most babies have settled into what will be their lie and presentation for the intrapartal period. This is not absolute, however, as some babies will turn again. Malpresentation prior to thirty-six weeks gestation is not cause for concern because the baby is still turning. Malpresentation after this time, however, may be cause for concern and possible intervention. This is useful information for planning the management of the intrapartal period, the first step of which is to determine carefully at the beginning of labor if the problem still exists. Lie, presentation, position, and variety are information obtained from doing Leopold's maneuvers of abdominal examination by palpation. The procedure for doing Leopold's maneuvers is in Chapter 41.

Measurement of the fundal height is of greatest value when it is measured the same way by the same examiner throughout pregnancy. It provides information regarding the progressive growth of the fetus and serves as a gross screening tool for detection of problems related to a fundal height which is too large or too small for the presumed gestational age by dates (see Chapter 9). A fundal height that is not increasing but remains the same over a period of time is ominous. Signs and symptoms of possible intrauterine fetal growth retardation or fetal death must be looked for and these possibilities ruled out.

There are four major ways of measuring

fundal height. These are described in Chapter 41, and the norms for different points in pregnancy are given.

Estimated fetal weight (EFW) requires concentrated practice on the part of the examiner in order to develop enough accuracy for the EFW to have any meaning. EFW is important in the intrapartal period, when this figure is compared with the clinical evaluation of the pelvis for ascertaining the adequacy of a given mother's pelvis for the size baby she will be delivering. During the antepartal period EFW is used as one clinical measurement in evaluating gestational age and progressive fetal growth.

Learning to evaluate EFW accurately is difficult because there is no precise measuring tool for checking the accuracy of your estimate during the antepartal period. You can ask an experienced clinician to give you an EFW on your patient but the accuracy of even seasoned clinicians is highly variable. The literature describes the inaccuracy of EFW by clinicians, especially for the smaller and larger babies, but reports greater accuracy for the middle range of average-sized babies. It is important to feel as much of the fetus as possible, to ascertain accurately what proportion of the fetus you have felt, and mentally to envision the remainder. Following are some suggestions for learning how to translate what you feel into an estimated weight:

1. Palpate as many women in the labor and delivery unit as possible. Compare your EFW with the actual weight of the baby at birth.
2. Undress, put into the fetal position, and palpate as many babies as possible (one at a time) in the normal newborn nursery. Compare your estimated weight of the baby against the actual weight of the baby. Remember to redress and, if necessary, calm any crying babies you palpate in order to be fair to and maintain good relationships with the nursery staff.
3. Visualize and study the size of premature newborns in relation to their weights.
4. Visualize and study the size and corresponding weights of fetal specimens at different gestational ages.

The only other addition to the physical examination outlined in Chapter 3 to be done during the initial antepartal examination is to obtain from the woman her prepregnant weight at the time of her last menstrual period as well as the actual measurement of her weight at the time of this examination.

Pelvic Examination

A complete pelvic examination is done during the initial antepartal examination. This includes not only the speculum, bimanual, and rectovaginal examination (see Chapter 44) but also evaluation of the bony pelvis by clinical pelvimetry (see Chapter 47).

Occasionally you may have a woman who refuses to have a pelvic examination. Such women are usually either young adolescents who are primigravidas with minimal sexual experience or women who have had traumatic experiences during pelvic examinations in the past. These women are quite frightened and will be both mentally and physically hurt if an attempted examination is forced upon them. This problem is rarely encountered in women who have had at least one vaginal delivery. Understanding and patience on the part of the examiner are required (Fig. 5-1), and venting of frustration and anger on the woman should be scrupulously avoided. Exploration of the meaning of the woman's behavior to her is mandatory for identification of the problem in order to begin to work through it. Why is she objecting to this procedure? Precisely what is it she is afraid of, if she is afraid? It may be necessary to arrange for this patient to be examined by someone who is skilled in working with such women and known to be especially gentle in doing pelvic examinations. It may

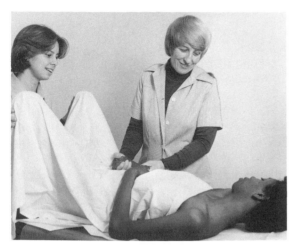

FIGURE 5-1. Nurse-midwives supporting a woman for pelvic examination.

take several antepartal visits before the woman is willing to be examined.

Time is on your side inasmuch as relaxation of the pelvic ligaments occurs as pregnancy progresses. The cause for this pelvic relaxation is unknown, although it has been attributed in the past to the hormone relaxin. However, since a pure substance for definitive study has not been isolated, it cannot be said that relaxin is the causative factor. The relaxation of the pelvic ligaments makes a pelvic examination around the thirty-sixth week of gestation easier to do than during the first or second trimester. The value of earlier examinations must be weighed against patient trauma and a potential breakdown of patient trust and cooperation which could affect all other aspects of her pregnancy. In the absence of clinical symptoms requiring a diagnostic pelvic examination, the pelvic can be delayed until later in pregnancy in order to do clinical pelvimetry.

Laboratory Tests and Adjunctive Studies
The laboratory tests and adjunctive studies ordered during the initial antepartal examination vary by policy from clinical setting to clinical setting. Some tests and studies also vary with the gestational age of the fetus at the time of the examination and with the woman's history. Exactly which tests are used for the same information also varies from setting to setting. The following list encompasses the most common variations; these tests, unless otherwise noted, are routine for all antepartal patients. Additional laboratory tests would be done in the event of pathological findings; these tests, which would be specific to the patient and not routine for all, are covered in the discussion of complications and are not included in this list.

1. Pap smear (done during speculum examination — see Chapter 45)
2. Gonococcal (GC) culture (done during speculum examination — see Chapter 46)
3. Blood type (ABO)
4. Rh factor
5. Indirect Coombs' test/antibody titer if the woman is Rh negative
6. Rubella titer
7. Sickle cell prep or hemoglobin electrophoresis — done in an increasing number of clinical settings
8. Tuberculin test (PPD) except for women with a known previous positive test (see Chapter 9); this test is done in all public health department settings
9. Venereal Disease Research Laboratories (VDRL), rapid plasma reagin (RPR), or other serology test for syphillis
10. Hemoglobin and hematocrit: some settings order a broader spectrum of blood counts and tests such as those included in a SMA-4, SMA-12, or CBC (e.g., WBC, RBC, differential); the hemoglobin and hematocrit, however, are minimal in all settings
11. Urinalysis for protein, glucose, and routine microscopic examination; in addition, some clinical settings also routinely order a urine culture

In some settings it may be your responsibility to draw or otherwise obtain the blood needed for some tests. These procedures are found in Chapters 33 and 34.

A case study of patient management based on the data base obtained during an initial antepartal examination is given later in this chapter. The case study continues by following the woman through an antepartal revisit.

THE REVISIT

The antepartal revisits transpire when the woman returns, after her initial antepartal examination, for prenatal care throughout the remainder of her pregnancy until her entry into true labor. Each revisit consists of a chart review, a history and physical examination geared toward evaluation of the well-being of the mother and the fetus, speculum and/or pelvic examination when indicated, laboratory and adjunctive studies when indicated, and explanations and teaching appropriate to the patient's needs and her baby's gestational age.

Data Base

Chart Review
The chart is reviewed immediately before seeing the woman, for the following information:

1. Name
2. Age
3. Parity
4. Weeks gestation by dates
5. Any significant finding from her:
   a. obstetrical history
   b. past medical history
   c. family history
   d. social history
   e. present pregnancy history
   f. initial physical examination
   g. initial pelvic examination
6. Any previously identified problems, treatment, and evaluation of the effectiveness of the treatment

7. Any particular concerns and desires, plans made, and patient instruction done
8. Specific medications, treatments, and dietary requirements for which the woman is presently responsible
9. Laboratory reports:
   a. normality of results
   b. need to repeat any lab tests
   c. need for further investigation and lab tests

This comprehensive chart review serves the purposes of (1) reacquaintance with the findings, problems, concerns, and unique aspects related to this individual woman, (2) evaluation of the thoroughness of the data base, and (3) evaluation of the thoroughness and effectiveness of the preceding management.

History
The basic revisit history is designed to detect any symptoms or subjective indications of complications or discomforts that may occur at any time during pregnancy, which the woman may be presently experiencing since her last visit. The woman is thus questioned about the following:

1. Any concerns, complaints, questions, or problems she has
2. Headaches
3. Visual disturbances
4. Dizziness
5. Fever/chills
6. Nausea/vomiting
7. Fetal movement
8. Abdominal pain
9. Back pain
10. Dysuria
11. Vaginal discharge
12. Vaginal bleeding
13. Constipation/hemorrhoids
14. Varicosities/leg ache
15. Leg cramps
16. Edema — ankle, pretibial, face, hands
17. Exposure to any infectious diseases

18. Use of any medicines other than those prescribed (e.g., aspirin)
19. Any medical care since last visit (e.g., doctor, emergency room) — what for, diagnosis, treatment, continuing care

In addition, the woman is questioned about possible discomforts, concerns, and desires for information common for the weeks gestation at the time of the revisit (e.g., discomforts and concerns common to this trimester, development of the baby during this month; see subsequent chapters). Inquiry is also made regarding any significant findings identified during the chart review.

Physical Examination
A complete screening physical examination was done during the initial antepartal visit. At each antepartal revisit the following physical examination is done to detect any signs of complications and to evaluate fetal well-being:

1. Blood pressure (compare with baseline blood pressure obtained at the time of the initial visit; note blood pressure readings throughout pregnancy to date)
2. Weight (compare with prepregnant weight; note the number of pounds for the number of weeks since the last visit; note weight gain pattern)
3. Abdominal examination for:
   a. lie, presentation, position, and variety
   b. engagement
   c. measurement of fundal height (compare with measurement at the preceding visit; note pattern of uterine growth)
   d. estimated fetal weight (compare with estimated weight at preceding visit)
   e. fetal heart tones (note rate and location); see Chapter 41
4. CVA tenderness (see Chapter 42)
5. Examination of the upper extremities for finger edema — note if any rings are tight and ask if they are tighter than usual; also ask if woman is not wearing any rings that

she used to wear because they became too tight, or if she has changed the fingers on which she is wearing her rings
6. Examination of the lower extremities for:
   a. ankle and pretibial edema
   b. quadriceps (knee-jerk) deep tendon reflexes (see Chapter 43)
   c. varicosities and Homan's sign when indicated (See page 490)

After the initial physical examination a breast examination for adequate support and for any crusting of leakage should be conducted approximately once a month. If the woman plans to breast-feed, her nipples need to be reevaluated at the thirty-sixth week of gestation to ascertain the need for measures to help bring out flat or inverted nipples.

Pelvic Examination
Part or all of the components of a pelvic examination are done when indicated after the initial examination. Indications include the following:

1. Perform a speculum examination for:
   a. complaint of vaginal discharge: visualize signs of vaginal infection and obtain material for a diagnostic wet smear slide
   b. evaluation of treatment for vaginal infection (some clinicians do not do this if the woman is now asymptomatic)
   c. repeat Pap smear if needed
   d. repeat GC culture in the third trimester
   e. ruling out or confirming premature rupture of membranes (see Chapter 14)
2. Perform clinical pelvimetry late in the third trimester if this needs to be reevaluated or if it was not possible to obtain this information during the initial examination due to patient refusal to be examined (discussed earlier in this chapter)
3. Perform a vaginal examination to assess:
   a. engagement/station
   b. effacement

c. dilatation

Some clinicians do this routinely at the fortieth week of gestation by dates and thereafter to determine cervical "ripeness" (readiness) for labor.

Many, although not all, clinicians believe in performing a 36-weeks pelvic evaluation including a repeat of clinical pelvimetry, GC culture, and evaluation of cervical status. They view this as part of an overall total reevaluation of the woman at this time. This total reevaluation also includes evaluation of laboratory tests done during the thirty-fourth week revisit, such as repeats of the hemoglobin and hematocrit, VDRL, and indirect Coombs (if Rh negative).

Laboratory and Adjunctive Studies

A voided urine specimen is obtained at each revisit; a dipstick tests for the presence of protein and glucose. Laboratory tests and adjunctive studies ordered during the initial antepartal examination are reviewed for results as stated under "Chart Review" earlier in this chapter. Diabetic screening of all women should occur at 28 weeks (see Chapter 9). Some laboratory tests are routinely repeated during the third trimester, usually at the thirty-fourth or thirty-sixth week of gestation. These include the GC culture, hemoglobin and hematocrit, and VDRL. In addition, women who are Rh negative have an indirect Coombs' test drawn every 4 weeks up to 28 weeks (if the preceding titer was negative). At this time, if the titers are still negative, RhoGam is a considered possibility (see Chapter 9) and subsequent antibody screening depends on whether or not RhoGam is administered. Other laboratory tests and adjunctive studies are done if the findings of the history, physical, pelvic, and laboratory examinations suggest a need for further diagnostic workup.

Management

Collection of the data base is the first step in the management process. The remaining steps of the management process are dependent on the data base and its interpretation. Interpretation of the data base (Step 2) includes:

1. Determining normality
2. Differentiating between common discomforts of pregnancy and a possible complication
3. Identifying signs and symptoms of possible deviations from normal or complications
4. Identifying areas of possible learning needs

Anticipation of related potential problems (Step 3) is important in the development of a comprehensive plan of care. The fourth step — evaluation for immediate nurse-midwife intervention, and/or physician consultation and collaborative management, and/or physician referral — applies only when there is deviation from normal with or without an emergency situation.

Development of a comprehensive plan of care includes the following components:

1. Determination of need for laboratory tests or adjunctive studies to rule out, confirm, or differentiate between possible complications
2. Determination of need for consultation with the physician
3. Determination of need for dietary reevaluation and intervention
4. Instructional measures for meeting learning needs
5. Determination of need for any discomfort relief or treatment measures
6. Determination of need for medication or other measures for treatment of minor complications (e.g., vaginitis, asymptomatic bacteriuria, initial urinary tract infection, borderline anemia)
7. Determination of need for consultations with or referrals to other health professionals (e.g., nutritionist, social worker, public health nurse)

8. Determination of need for more active inclusion of significant others
9. Determination of need for specific counseling or anticipatory guidance
10. Scheduling the next revisit; revisits for a woman who is progressing normally through her pregnancy are usually scheduled as follows:
    a. up to 28 weeks gestation: every 4 weeks
    b. between 28 and 36 weeks gestation: every 2 weeks
    c. between 36 weeks gestation and delivery: every week

The revisit appointment data is indicated on the woman's chart with the notation "RTC _____ weeks". *RTC* (return to clinic) is an abbreviation universally used to mean the return appointment time even though the visits may not be to a clinic per se.

CASE STUDY

The following case study is designed to illustrate how management is based on interpretation of the data base starting with the findings obtained during an initial examination and continuing during the subsequent revisit. Because the case study is being presented for a specific purpose, and in order to facilitate clarity in the presentation, parts of the data base which would normally be detailed will instead be either omitted as insignificant for this woman or summarized as "within normal limits (WNL)" so that the parts of the data base which will be used will be obvious. The first part of Chapter 3, discussing the first five steps of the management process, should be reviewed because those steps are utilized in this presentation.

Initial Antepartal Examination
(February 22)

Step 1. Data Base

Ms. Oceana is a 21-year-old, black, Gravida 1 Para 0 at 24 weeks gestation by dates, with an LMP of September 5 and an EDD of June 12.

Present pregnancy history. Experienced quickening in mid-January. This is a planned pregnancy both she and her husband are happy about. They desire natural childbirth. Body changes are seen as evidence of the pregnancy and welcomed. Have continued sexual intercourse without problems. Has been having occasional right-sided pain for the past month, complains of a recurrent malodorous vaginal discharge, and has also felt tired throughout her pregnancy although this has not affected her activities. Otherwise her pregnancy has been uneventful. She is not taking any drugs or medications.

Past medical history. UCHD. Had both rubeola and rubella as a child. Appendectomy at age 17 — no blood transfusion. Otherwise insignificant.

Family history. Paternal grandmother a diabetic controlled by diet and oral medication. Maternal aunt and uncle are twins. Otherwise insignificant.

Obstetric history. Primigravida.

Menstrual history. Menarche at age 11, every 28 days × 5 days with a heavy flow for the first 3 days. No dysmenorrhea.

Sexual, contraceptive, and douching history. Successful and satisfied with use of a diaphragm for past 2 years without any side effects; douches in connection with removal of the diaphragm, has also douched two to three times a week during her pregnancy because of malodorous vaginal discharge; sexual frequency is twice a week with no problems.

Social History. High school graduate; working as a secretary in an insurance office. Husband in final year of college; living in married student housing with high population of children and pets (dogs and cats) although they have no pets of their own. Does not drink or smoke.

Physical Examination. Temperature: 98.6°F, pulse: 84, respirations: 16
Blood pressure: 120/80
Height: 5'6"
Weight: prepregnant, 150 lb; present, 164 lb
General: woman appears her age, well nourished, and in good physical and emotional health
Hair and Skin: WNL
HEENT: WNL
Neck: WNL
Breasts: WNL; nipples erect; plans to breast-feed
Heart and Lungs: WNL
Abdomen: WNL;
scar in right lower abdomen from appendectomy.
Area of right-sided pain identified as being in the right lower quadrant of the abdomen and into the right inguinal region
Fundal height: 26 cm. ? Breech presentation.
FHT: 132 RLQ.
EFW: 700 gm.
No CVAT
Extremities: WNL

Pelvic examination. Thick, white, malodorous discharge with plaques on the vaginal walls and cervix; wet smear slide shows branching hyphae and budding spores; otherwise WNL
Clinical pelvimetry:
  Inlet:
    diagonal conjugate — more than 11.5 cm
    forepelvis — slightly narrowed
  Midplane:
    ischial spines — prominent
    sciatic notch — quite wide, 3-4 fb
    sidewalls — parallel
    sacrum — flat, posterior inclination, and long
Outlet:
    intertuberous diameter — more than 8 cm

public arch — tight 2 fb
coccyx — movable

Laboratory. Urine negative for protein, 2+ glucose by dipstick (no immediate possible explanation)

Step 2. Interpretation of the Data Base
The basis (information from the data base) for each interpretation will be given.

1. Monilial vaginal infection. Basis:
   a. patient complaint of a malodorous vaginal discharge
   b. patient history of douching during pregnancy because of a malodorous vaginal discharge
   c. speculum examination revealing thick, white, malodorous discharge and plaques on the vaginal walls and cervix
   d. visualization of branching hyphae and budding spores on a wet smear slide
2. Need for diabetic screening to rule out diabetes. Basis:
   a. family history shows paternal grandmother is a diabetic controlled by diet and oral medication
   b. history of recurrent malodorous vaginal discharge; known diagnosis of monilia at this time, and most likely the previous episodes were also monilial
   c. glycosuria: 2+ glucose by dipstick
3. Right-sided round ligament pain. Basis:
   a. patient complaint of occasional right-sided pain for the past month
   b. area of pain identified as the right lower quadrant of the abdomen and into the right inguinal region; no s/s of preterm labor
   c. had appendectomy at age 17
4. Borderline pelvis with anthropoid tendency. Basis:
   a. clinical pelvimetry findings:
      (1) slightly narrow forepelvis
      (2) prominent ischial spines
      (3) wide sciatic notch

(4) sacrum long and flat with posterior inclination

(5) pubic arch a tight 2 fb

5. ? Breech presentation. Basis: abdominal examination of a ? breech presentation; this has no significance at this time

6. Teaching needs:

   a. re douching, to discontinue this practice. Basis: patient history of douching two to three times a week during her pregnancy because of a malodorous vaginal discharge

   b. breast care and plans for breast preparation. Basis:
   plans to breast-feed

   c. regarding the relationship between cats and toxoplasmosis and the need to avoid any contact with their excrement, care, or handling. Basis:
   lives in a housing complex with a high population of cats

   d. re rest periods and positioning while resting, during the day and while at work. Basis:
   works as a secretary in an insurance office

   e. relief measures for her right-sided round ligament pain. Basis:
   see 3 above

   f. re use of the vaginal medication prescribed for treatment of her monilial infection. Basis:
   see 1 above and Step 5, item 11

   g. re preparation for childbirth and parenthood classes and the La Leche League. Basis: desires natural childbirth, plans to breast-feed

   h. re diabetic screening (why and how). Basis: see 2 above

   i. re her pelvic measurements and question of pelvic adequacy. Basis:
   see 4 above and Step 3

Step 3. Anticipation of Related Potential Problems

1. Possible cephalopelvic disproportion (CPD)

yielding possible cesarean section. Basis: borderline pelvis with anthropoid tendency

Step 4. Need for Immediate Nurse-Midwife Intervention and/or Physician Consultation and Collaborative Management and/or Physician Referral

None of these are indicated at this visit.

Step 5. Management Plan Based on the Interpretation of the Data Base and Anticipated Related Problems

Each item in the management plan will be correlated with the related interpretation of the data base and subsequent anticipated problems, or marked with an asterisk to connote that this is a routine item of management of the woman at the initial antepartal visit.

*1. Pap smear done during pelvic examination

*2. GC culture done during pelvic examination

*3. PPD test for tuberculosis

*4. ABO and Rh

*5. Indirect Coombs' test

*6. Rubella titer

*7. Sickle cell prep or hemoglobin electrophoresis

*8. VDRL or RPR

*9. Hemoglobin and hematocrit

*10. Routine microscopic urinalysis and urine culture

11. Mycostatin vaginal suppositories, one intravaginally b.i.d. × 15 days (treatment of monilial vaginal infection — correlates with interpretations 1 and 6.f.)

12. Schedule and instruct for a fasting blood sugar (FBS) test and a 1-hour glucose challenge test (see Chapter 9); (diabetic diagnostic screening tests that correlate with interpretations 2 and 6.h.) — repeat in third trimester

13. Reevaluate pelvis upon entry into labor in relation to estimated size of the baby (correlates with interpretation 4 and anticipated problem of CPD)

*14. Ferrous sulfate 300mg tab i t.i.d. p.c.
15. Teaching re the following (correlates with interpretation 6):
   a. not douching
   b. breast care and plans for breast preparation in her last month of pregnancy
   c. cats and toxoplasmosis
   d. rest periods and positioning
   e. round ligament pain relief measures
   f. how to insert and use the Mycostatin vaginal suppositories
   g. names and telephone numbers for making contact with teachers of preparation for childbirth and parenthood classes and the La Leche League
   h. diabetic screening and test instructions
   i. her pelvic measurements, pelvic adequacy, CPD, and possible C-section
*16. RTC for dietary history and calculation of nutritional intervention in 1 week
*17. RTC for antepartal revisit in 4 weeks

First Antepartal Revisit (March 22)

Step 1. Data Base
Chart review. See initial antepartal examination for name; age; parity; significant findings; identified problems and treatment; patient desires, plans made, and patient teaching done; medications; and dietary requirements determined at her nutritional visit on March 1.

Results from the laboratory tests and adjunctive studies ordered at the initial visit are as follows:

1. Pap smear: class 1
2. GC culture: no *Neisseria gonorrhoeae* seen
3. PPD: negative
4. Blood group O, Rh positive
5. Indirect Coombs' test: negative
6. Rubella titer: more than 1:30
7. Hemoglobin electrophoresis:
   Hemoglobin A_1: 98%
   Hemoglobin A_2: 2%

8. VDRL: negative
9. Hemoglobin 9.8 mg, hematocrit 29%
10. Microscopic urinalysis: negative; urine culture: less than 50,000 colony count
11. FBS: 98 mg/100 ml; 1-hour glucose challenge test: 120 mg/100 ml

Today Ms. Oceana is 28 weeks gestation by dates.

History:
Basic revisit history (see earlier in this chapter) is negative.
Accuracy of LMP and EDD reconfirmed with Ms. Oceana.
Complains of continuing fatigue. Is resting midmorning, noon, and midafternoon at work, and when first arrives home after work, as discussed at her last visit.
Relief measures for round ligament pain have been helpful and this is not keeping her awake any more.
Used full regimen of Mycostatin suppositories and is no longer having malodorous vaginal discharge.
No douching since her last visit.
Avoiding cats.
Has contacted both a teacher of Lamaze classes and a local member of the La Leche League. She and her husband attended their first Lamaze class last night and enjoyed it. Is realistic, but hopeful, re pelvic adequacy.
Faithfully taking her iron pills — her stools are black and tarry.
No problems with her dietary requirements; appetite good.

Physical examination:
Blood pressure: 130/84
Weight: 167 lb
Breasts: adequate support, no crusts on nipples
Abdominal examination:
   vertex presentation, ? position, not engaged
   fundal height: 32 cm
   fetal heart tones: 132 RLQ
   estimated fetal weight: 1600 gm

many small parts easily felt
abdomen soft
No CVAT
No edema of the upper or lower extremities
Knee-jerk reflexes: 2+

Pelvic examination: Speculum examination
done to evaluate treatment for vaginal
infection: vaginal walls and cervix clean of any
discharge; wet smear slide negative

Laboratory: Urine negative for protein and
glucose

Step 2. Interpretation of the Data Base
The basis (information from the data base) for
each interpretation will be given.

1. Monilial infection cured. Basis:
   a. no further patient complaint of mal-
      odorous vaginal discharge
   b. no evidence of monilial infection visua-
      lized during speculum examination
   c. wet smear slide negative
2. Not diabetic. Basis:
   FBS and 1-hour glucose challenge test results within normal limits.
3. Measures for round ligament pain effective.
   Basis: patient statement of effectiveness
   during history
4. Anemia — ? iron deficiency anemia. Basis:
   a. hemoglobin 9.8 mg
   b. hematocrit 29%
   c. fatigue throughout pregnancy (from
      initial and revisit history)
   d. heavy menstrual periods (from initial
      history)
   e. hemoglobin electrophoresis normal, thus
      ruling out sickle cell anemia and other
      abnormalities of hemoglobin
5. Need to rule out multiple gestation or a
   single large-for-dates fetus. Basis:
   a. fundal height of 32 cm is greater than
      expected for 28 weeks gestation
   b. fundal height of 26 cm at 24 weeks
      gestation (early sign of trend?)

c. estimated fetal weight in accord with 31
   to 32 weeks gestation rather than
   with 28 weeks gestation
d. many small parts easily felt — indicative
   of multiple gestation if not a posterior
   position
e. unsure of fetal position — indicative of
   multiple gestation
f. soft abdomen and ease in feeling small
   parts rule out polyhydramnios as a possible explanation of the discrepancy
   between gestational age by dates and
   by clinical findings
g. LMP and EDD confirmed, which rules
   out inaccuracy in determining gestational age by dates
h. only one fetal heart heard, which is
   indicative of a single large-for-dates
   fetus
i. family history of fraternal twins on
   maternal side

*Step 3. Anticipation of Related Potential
Problems*
Need diagnoses before further potential pro-
blems can be identified.

*Step 4. Need for Immediate Nurse-Midwife
Intervention and/or Physician Consultation
and Collaborative Management and/or
Physician Referral*
None of these are indicated at this time.
   Consultation/collaboration with a physician
may be indicated later in this visit, or at the
next visit, depending on the ultrasonography
findings.
   Consultation or collaboration with a physician will be indicated at the next visit with
regard to interpretation of the laboratory tests
and management of Ms. Oceana's anemia.

*Step 5. Management Plan Based on the
Interpretation of the Data Base and
Anticipated Related problems.*
Each item in the management plan will be
correlated with the related interpretation of
the data base.

1. Interpretation 1:
   share speculum examination and wet smear slide findings with Ms. Oceana.
2. Interpretation 2:
   share results of diabetic screening tests with Ms. Oceana. Rescreen at 34 weeks.
3. Interpretation 4:
   a. hemoglobin and hematocrit
   b. serum iron concentration level
   c. total iron-binding capacity
   d. reticulocyte count
   e. serum folate level
   f. cell indices (WBC and RBC counts)
   g. platelets
   h. stool examined for ova and parasites
   i. assure adequate supply of iron medication
   j. vitamin C 250 mg b.i.d.
   k. folic acid 1 mg b.i.d.
   l. hold discussion with Ms. Oceana regarding findings, concerns, probable reason for her fatigue, and need for further tests and faithful adherence to medication regimen
4. Interpretation 5:
   a. ultrasound scan to rule out multiple gestation and to determine fetal position
   b. discussion with Ms. Oceana about findings, possible reasons for discrepancy between gestational age by dates and by clinical findings, and ultrasound
5. RTC in 2 weeks

6

Normal Data Base
of Pregnancy

The data base for normal pregnancy consists of the following components:

1. Maternal anatomic and physiologic changes
2. Maternal psychologic adjustment and processes
3. Fetal growth and development
4. Placental development, circulation, and functioning

MATERNAL ANATOMIC AND PHYSIOLOGIC CHANGES

Information concerning the maternal anatomic and physiologic changes is dispersed throughout Part II on Management of the Antepartal Period and in the chapters in Part VII related to antepartal care. This method of presentation was chosen in order to provide the information when it is applicable to understanding particular aspects of the antepartal period and related patient management. Thus, anatomic and physiologic changes are not repeated here with the exception of reproducing the Schuchardt

charts published by Maternity Center Association in New York City. These charts (Fig. 6-1) illustrate the changing position of the abdominal organs and contents as the abdominal space is increasingly filled with the enlarging uterus. Positional changes of the abdominal structures accounts for a number of the normal discomforts of pregnancy discussed in Chapter 7.

MATERNAL PSYCHOLOGIC ADJUSTMENT AND PROCESSES

Pregnancy generally is considered a time of crisis with a defined end point when the baby is born. This end point is a type of resolution to the crisis, but whether or not the woman is ready for this end point depends on her working through the psychologic processes that normally are present during pregnancy. These physiologic processes often seem to be interrelated with the biologic changes taking place at any given point in pregnancy. Pregnancy is a time of transition between what life

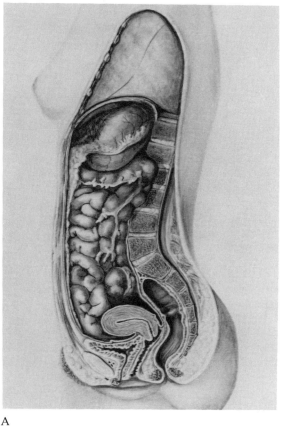
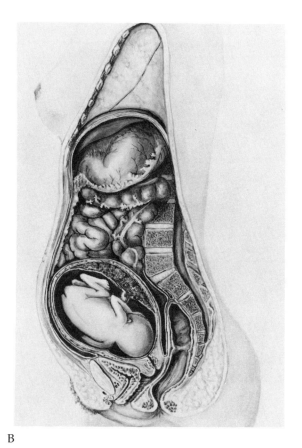

A   B

FIGURE 6-1.   Schuchardt charts. A. nonpregnant; B. fifth lunar month; C. ninth lunar month; D. just before labor. (Reproduced by permission from Maternity Center Association, New York.)

was like without this child and what life will be like with this child.

The emotions of a woman while pregnant are quite labile. She may have extreme reactions with rapidly changing mood shifts. Her emotional reactions and perceptions of the world may change. She is extremely sensitive and tends to overreact. A pregnant woman is far more open both to her internal self and to sharing this with others. She ruminates on her sleeping dreams, daydreams, fantasies, and the meanings of words, objects, events, and abstract concepts such as death, life, fertility, fulfillment, and happiness. She may identify with physical forms which signify being filled with life, food, or childbearing.

The pregnant woman is extremely vulnerable. She fears death for both herself and her baby. She is frightened of the unknown because her body seems out of her control and her life is in the process of being changed irreversibly. This makes many women more dependent and some women more demanding. It is a time of being more susceptible to suggestion as she searches for new supports that might help direct her during this time of trying to project new role requirements, life changes which presently are vague and unknown, and what all this will mean to her.

There is a definable occurrence and sequence of specific psychologic processes throughout pregnancy. Again these interrelate to some

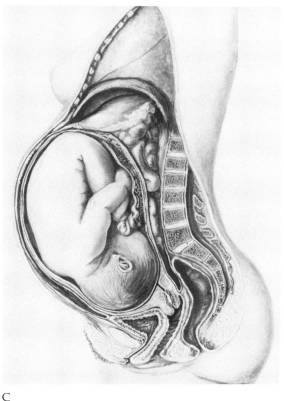

C

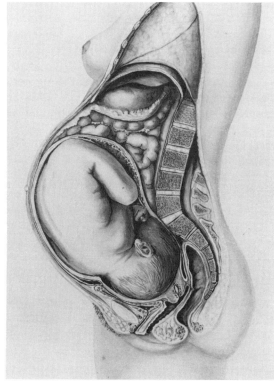

D

extent with the biologic changes taking place. These psychologic events and processes are identifiable by trimester of gestation and this division is used in the following discussion. Both the general psychologic response to pregnancy just discussed and the more specific psychologic processes and events to be discussed recur with each pregnancy for each woman.

First Trimester

The first trimester is often referred to as the period of adjustment. The adjustment the woman is making is to the fact that she is pregnant. The acceptance of this reality and all it means is the most important psychologic task of the first trimester.

Most women are upset and ambivalent about being pregnant. Approximately 80 percent go through a period of disappointment, rejection, anxiety, depression, and unhappiness. It is doubtful that there is a single woman who hasn't said to herself at least once that she wished she were not pregnant — even including those who have planned for and want the pregnancy or have struggled to become pregnant. This universality needs to be discussed with the woman since she will tend to hide her ambivalent or negative feelings because they are in conflict with what she thinks she should be feeling. If she is not helped to understand and accept these ambivalent and negative feelings as normal for this period of time during pregnancy, she most likely will have overwhelming guilt feelings if the baby should subsequently either die or be deformed or abnormal. She will remember the thoughts she had during the first trimester and, unless they are accepted, may also feel herself the cause of any tragedy.

The woman's focus is on herself. From this self-concern arises much of her ambivalence about the pregnancy as she deals with any previous bad experience with pregnancy, the effect the pregnancy will have on her life (especially if she has a career), new or additional responsibilities she will have to assume, anxieties regarding her capability to be a mother, financial and housing concerns, and acceptance of the pregnancy by significant others. Ambivalence normally ends spontaneously as she accepts the pregnancy. This acceptance usually occurs by the end of the first trimester and is facilitated by her feeling safe enough to express the feelings which are creating conflict within her. In the meantime, some of the discomforts of the first trimester — nausea, fatigue, appetite changes, emotional irritability — may reflect her conflict and depression and at the same time serve as a reminder of her pregnancy.

The first trimester is also often an anxious time of waiting for the pregnancy to be "well established." This is particularly true for women who have had previous miscarriages and for female health care professionals who worry about miscarriages and teratogens. These women impatiently await the end of the first trimester as a milestone after which they can relax and believe in their pregnancy.

Weight has particular significance to the woman during the first trimester. It may become a part of the reality testing the woman is doing as she looks to her body for tangible evidence of being pregnant. For many women an early weight gain may be seen as proof that the baby is growing even though the baby is not yet physically evident. The woman sees gaining weight as being within her control and contributing to the growth of her abdomen, which means being pregnant to her. Conversely, females who are pregnant and trying to hide it

(e.g., some unwed adolescents) may starve themselves to prevent "showing" while trying to cope with and make decisions to resolve some of their problems.

Validation of the pregnancy is done over and over as the woman scrutinizes any bodily change for evidence of the pregnancy. The most evident is the cessation of menses. Breast changes are repeatedly studied. This makes your sharing of pelvic findings, especially those indicative of pregnancy, very important. During the first trimester her pregnancy is her own secret to share with whomever she chooses. Her thoughts largely relate to what is happening to her, her body, her life. At this point the baby is not yet perceived as a separate being.

Women vary widely in their sexual desire during the first trimester. While some women experience an increase in desire, generally speaking it is a time of impaired libido, and this creates the need for open and honest communication with mates. Many women feel a need for much love and loving without sex. Libido is heavily influenced by fatigue, nausea, depression, sore and enlarged breasts, worries, anxieties, and concerns — all of which may be a normal part of the first trimester.

Second Trimester

The second trimester is often referred to as the period of radiant health. This is because it is during this trimester that the woman generally feels good and is largely free from normal discomforts of pregnancy. However, it is also the time of the most regressed and inward phase of pregnancy. The second trimester actually subdivides into two phases: prequickening and postquickening. Quickening heralds the fact of a separate life, thereby adding impetus to the woman's primary psychologic task of the second trimester, that of developing her own mothering identity distinct from that of her own mother's.

Towards the end of the first trimester and during the prequickening portion of the second trimester, the woman undergoes a complete reliving and reevaluation of all aspects of her relationship with her own mother. The total range of these feelings is scrutinized and the basis for them relived. All the interpersonal problems the woman and her mother had or have are analyzed. The potential that can exist in the mother-child relationship is examined. With this comes understanding and acceptance of her own mother's qualities which she values and respects. The other qualities of her mother, those that are negative, unwanted, or do not engender respect, are rejected. This may cause guilt and inner conflict unless she is helped to understand the normality of this process and that rejection of specific qualities of her mother in developing her own mothering identity is not equivalent to rejection of her mother as a person.

Included in this total process is the evolution of the woman from a care receiver (from her mother) to a caregiver (preparatory to being a mother). Into this enters possible conflict over competing with her mother to be seen as a "good" mother. The actual resolution of all this does not occur until long after the baby is born, but the preoccupation with her own mother and related processes diminish as the transfer to her self-identity as caregiver is made. At the same time she is demanding attention and love (being a receiver) which, in effect, she is storing for her baby in her role as caregiver.

With quickening comes a number of changes as the pregnancy is unquestionably verified in the woman's mind. Her social contacts increasingly become other pregnant women or brand new mothers and her interests and activities focus on pregnancy, childbearing, and preparation for a new role. This creates the need for a certain amount of grief work, which in turn serves as a catalyst for assumption of her new role. The grief involves letting go of former relationships, attach-

ments, and significant aspects and events of the former self-role. They will be affected by the forthcoming baby and new role. This does not mean discarding all these relationships and ties but does involve a change in and toward them. For a multipara this includes a certain disengagement from established ties with her other children as she prepares her home and family for the changes a new baby will create. Much of the woman's new or changed role is tried out, developed, and refined in fantasy, imagination, and day dreaming.

Quickening also enables the woman to conceptualize her baby as an individual separate from herself. This new awareness starts a change in her focus from herself to the baby. Frequently this change is manifested by dreams that someone else, usually a stranger, is being injured. These dreams generally are interpreted as the mother's concern about harm to her baby. At this point the sex of the baby is unimportant. The concern is for the baby's well-being and welcome into the family group.

Most women feel more erotic during the second trimester; approximately 80 percent of pregnant women experience a significant improvement in their sexual relationships as compared with both their first trimester and before pregnancy. The second trimester is relatively free of physical discomforts; the size of her abdomen is not yet an insurmountable problem; vaginal lubrication is greater; the related anxieties, worries, and concerns causing the woman's previous ambivalence and depression have subsided; and her shift for caretaking from her mother to her husband all contribute to an increase in libido and sexual satisfaction.

Third Trimester

The third trimester is often referred to as the period of watchful waiting. Now that the woman is aware of the baby's presence as a separate being, she becomes impatient for the baby's arrival. There is an uneasy sense that the baby could arrive at any time, a fact that places the woman on edge as she watches and waits for the signs and symptoms of labor.

The third trimester is a time of active, visible preparation for childbirth and parenthood as the woman's attention focuses on the forthcoming baby. Both fetal movement and the size of the enlarging uterus are constant reminders of the baby. People around her are now making plans for the baby. She becomes protective of the baby by avoiding crowds or anyone or anything she perceives as dangerous. She fantasizes that danger lurks in the outside world. The choosing of names for the baby is a preparatory activity for the baby's arrival. Preparation for childbirth and parenthood classes are attended. Layettes are made or bought. Rooms are rearranged. Much thought is given to care of the baby. There is much speculation as to the baby's looks and sex.

A number of fears surface during the third trimester. Some of these fears are for her own and the baby's lives, an abnormal baby, labor and delivery (pain, loss of control, the unknown), whether or not she will know when she is in labor, the ability of the baby to emerge since her abdomen is already unbelievably large in size, and concern that her own vital organs will be injured by the baby's kicking. Her dreams reflect her interests and her fears. She dreams mostly about babies, children, delivery, losing a baby, or being trapped in a small place and unable to squeeze out. She keeps busy so she will not think of what frightens her and of all the unknowns.

She also undergoes another grief process as she anticipates the loss of attention and special prerogatives of being pregnant, the inevitable separation of her baby from her body, and the feeling of loss of her full abdomen as it becomes a collapsed and empty vessel. Slight depression is not uncommon, and there may be further increased dependency and introversion with a feeling of vulnerability.

Once again the woman experiences physical discomfort, which increases as pregnancy nears completion (see Chapter 10). She may feel awkward, ugly, sloppy, and in need of large and frequent doses of reassurance from her mate. By the middle of the third trimester, the heightened sexuality of the second trimester diminishes as her abdomen becomes an obstacle. Alternate positions for sexual intercourse and alternate methods of achieving sexual satisfaction may help — or may create guilt if she is not comfortable with them. The honest sharing of feelings is essential between the couple and in their consultation with you.

FETAL GROWTH AND DEVELOPMENT

The processes which make possible the beginning and early development of a human being involve entire fields of study. Included are the subjects of genetics, gamete maturation (spermatogenesis and oogenesis), ovum and sperm transport, sperm capacitation and acrosome reaction, fertilization, cellular division (specifically meiotic and mitotic), zygote changes and transport during the first week of life, implantation, embryology (which covers roughly the period of life from the second through seventh week of life post-fertilization), fetology (which covers from the eighth week of life after fertilization to birth), and congenital malformations and abnormalities. It is not within the scope of this book to discuss these topics in any detail. Students interested in perusing these subjects are encouraged to explore textbooks and courses relevant to their interests. This book zeros in on the minimal knowledge needed by the practicing nurse-midwife in the area of fetal growth and development. Basically this includes an appreciation of the intricate and vulnerable stages of cellular differentiation, reorganization, division, and proliferation, and structural beginnings occurring during the embryonic period; an ability to describe for the mother-to-be what her baby looks like during each month of the fetal period; and an understanding of the causes of congenital malformations.

First Trimester

In relation to the three trimesters of pregnancy, the entire zygotic and embryonic period and the first 2 weeks of the fetal period (total of 10 weeks of life after fertilization) are within the first 12 weeks of pregnancy (counting from the last normal menstrual period) constituting the first trimester.

Figure 6-2 is a summary by days and weeks of the events in fetal growth and development that occur during the first trimester. While it ends with the tenth week of age it is equivalent with the twelfth week of gestation as calculated from the last normal menstrual period (LMP). It is important to make this correlation and to check when reading other sources of literature as to whether they are dating fetal development from the LMP or from the assumed time of fertilization 2 weeks later. Otherwise you may be 2 weeks off in your understanding of what is happening.

Growth and development begins with the moment of fertilization and the fusing of the female and male pronuclei from the ovum and sperm respectively. This fusion produces what is called a zygote. At this moment a new individual is created with his or her own unique makeup as determined by this totally new combination of chromosomes and genes. This unique combination results because the pronucleus of each gamete (sex cell, i.e., ovum and sperm) contains only half (23 or the haploid number) of the total number (46 or the diploid number) of chromosomes in human beings. This halving of the chromosome number is a result of gametogenesis, the process by which

mature ova and spermatozoa are developed. At the moment of fertilization the fusion of the pronucleus of the two gametes restores the diploid number of chromosomes, which is subsequently reflected through mitotic cellular division in every cell in an individual's body except those which later undergo gametogenesis. Also determined at the moment of fertilization, as a result of this fusion and restoration of the diploid number, is the sex of this new individual. Sex is determined by the male gamete, which carries either an X or a Y chromosome. The female gamete carries only an X chromosome. Upon fusion an XX combination normally develops into a female, while an XY combination normally develops into a male.

Immediately following fertilization the resulting zygote begins to undergo mitotic cellular division called cleavage. Going through sequential stages, the dividing cellular mass is called a morula; with cellular reorganization and the entry of fluid, the morula becomes a blastocyst. It is the blastocyst which implants in the uterine lining. By the time the process of implantation is completed on the tenth or eleventh day after fertilization, the embryonic period has begun.

At the time of implantation the embryo is known as a bilaminar embryo because the embryonic disc arising from the inner cell mass consists of two layers of cells: (1) the embryonic ectoderm and (2) the embryonic endoderm. The embryonic endoderm is the first of the three germ layers from which all tissues (e.g., bone, muscle, connective, skin), organs, and structures derive. These germ layers are also responsible for the fetal membranes, the umbilical cord, and, in part, the placenta.

At the beginning of the third week the primitive streak, arising from the embryonic disc, is the growth center for the embryo for approximately 2 weeks, after which it becomes insignificant and eventually disintegrates. A trilaminar embryo develops during the third

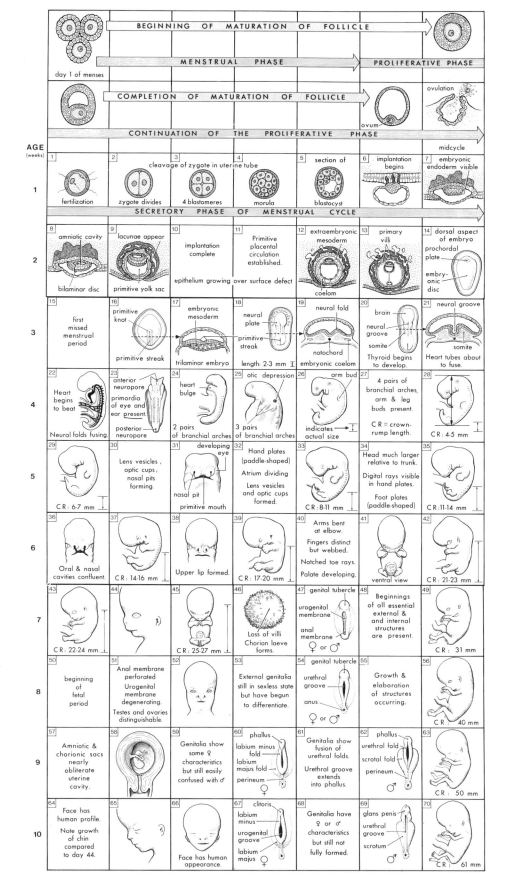

BEGINNING OF MATURATION OF FOLLICLE

day 1 of menses

MENSTRUAL PHASE | PROLIFERATIVE PHASE

COMPLETION OF MATURATION OF FOLLICLE

ovulation

ovum

CONTINUATION OF THE PROLIFERATIVE PHASE

midcycle

AGE (weeks)

cleavage of zygote in uterine tube

1 fertilization | 2 zygote divides | 3 4 blastomeres | 4 morula | 5 section of blastocyst | 6 implantation begins | 7 embryonic endoderm visible

1

SECRETORY PHASE OF MENSTRUAL CYCLE

2

8 amniotic cavity — bilaminar disc | 9 lacunae appear — primitive yolk sac | 10 implantation complete epithelium growing over surface defect | 11 Primitive placental circulation established. | 12 extraembryonic mesoderm — coelom | 13 primary villi | 14 dorsal aspect of embryo prochordal plate — embryonic disc

3

15 first missed menstrual period | 16 primitive knot — primitive streak | 17 embryonic mesoderm trilaminar embryo | 18 neural plate — primitive streak length: 2-3 mm | 19 neural fold notochord embryonic coelom | 20 brain neural groove somite Thyroid begins to develop. | 21 neural groove somite Heart tubes about to fuse.

4

22 Heart begins to beat Neural folds fusing. | 23 anterior neuropore primordia of eye and ear present. posterior neuropore 2 pairs of branchial arches | 24 heart bulge 3 pairs of branchial arches | 25 otic depression indicates actual size | 26 arm bud | 27 4 pairs of branchial arches, arm & leg buds present. CR = crown-rump length. | 28 CR: 4-5 mm

5

29 CR: 6-7 mm | 30 Lens vesicles, optic cups, nasal pits forming. | 31 developing eye nasal pit primitive mouth | 32 Hand plates (paddle-shaped) Atrium dividing Lens vesicles and optic cups formed. | 33 CR: 8-11 mm | 34 Head much larger relative to trunk. Digital rays visible in hand plates. Foot plates (paddle-shaped) | 35 CR: 11-14 mm

6

36 Oral & nasal cavities confluent. | 37 CR: 14-16 mm | 38 Upper lip formed. | 39 CR: 17-20 mm | 40 Arms bent at elbow. Fingers distinct but webbed. Notched toe rays. Palate developing. | 41 ventral view | 42 CR: 21-23 mm

7

43 CR: 22-24 mm. | 44 | 45 CR: 25-27 mm | 46 Loss of villi Chorion laeve forms. | 47 genital tubercle urogenital membrane anal membrane ♀ or ♂ | 48 Beginnings of all essential external & and internal structures are present. | 49 CR: 31 mm

8

50 beginning of fetal period | 51 Anal membrane perforated Urogenital membrane degenerating. Testes and ovaries distinguishable. | 52 | 53 External genitalia still in sexless state but have begun to differentiate. | 54 genital tubercle urethral groove anus ♀ or ♂ | 55 Growth & elaboration of structures occurring. | 56 CR: 40 mm

9

57 Amniotic & chorionic sacs nearly obliterate uterine cavity. | 58 | 59 Genitalia show some ♀ characteristics but still easily confused with ♂ ♀ | 60 phallus labium minus fold labium majus fold perineum | 61 Genitalia show fusion of urethral folds. Urethral groove extends into phallus. | 62 phallus urethral fold scrotal fold perineum | 63 CR: 50 mm

10

64 Face has human profile. Note growth of chin compared to day 44. | 65 | 66 Face has human appearance. | 67 clitoris labium minus urogenital groove labium majus ♀ | 68 Genitalia have ♀ or ♂ characteristics but still not fully formed. | 69 glans penis urethral groove scrotum ♂ | 70 CR: 61 mm

week with the appearance of the third germ layer, the embryonic mesoderm, located between the preceding two layers of cells. Figure 6-3 specifies what each germ layer is responsible for in the makeup of the body. Towards the end of this week somite development begins, which will ultimately result in 42 to 44 pairs of somites. Arising from the mesoderm, the somites are responsible for most of the skeleton of the head and trunk, its related musculature, and much of the dermis of the skin. They are also useful in dating early embryos that are recovered up to approximately 30 days after fertilization. During the third week the neural tube (rudiment of the brain and spinal cord), notochord (rudiment of the vertebrae), coelomic spaces (rudiment of the body cavities), and a primitive cardiovascular system and primitive blood cells develop.

The heart starts to beat at the beginning of the fourth week. It is during the fourth week that rapid growth causes both longitudinal and transverse folding of the embryonic disc. Longitudinal folding, involving a head fold and a tail fold, converts the embryo from a straight form to a curved form. Transverse folding, involving right and left transverse folds folding toward the midline, converts the embryo from a flat form to a cylindrical form. By the end of the fourth week the embryo has assumed its often-called salamander look, has the rudiments of ears (otic pit), arms (arm buds), legs (leg buds), and facial and neck structures (the first four branchial arches).

During the fifth week rapid development of the brain results in extensive growth of the head and makes it much larger in relation to the rest of the body. Development is from cephalic to caudal, with development of the legs almost a week behind development of the arms. The eyes begin development with lens vesicles, optic cups, and retinal pigment.

The nose, mouth, and palate begin to take form during the sixth week and the eyelids become visible. Arms and legs undergo extensive development ending during the seventh week with well-differentiated regions (e.g., wrist, elbow, knee), increased length, and clearly defined fingers and toes.

During the seventh week the neck region is established, the abdomen is less protuberant (although the intestines to some degree are still herniated into the proximal portion of the umbilical cord), and urogenital development is beginning. The external ears are evident although they are not fully developed with elevation to their proper position. The embryo by the end of the seventh week has distinctly human characteristics.

The end of the seventh week also marks the end of the embryonic period. All essential internal and external structures are present and are undergoing further elaboration and growth, including the replacement of cartilage with bone cells. The embryonic period obviously is a critical period during which any teratogen (e.g., drugs, x-rays, viruses) may either be lethal or cause major congenital malformations (see Fig. 6-4).

The first trimester of pregnancy also includes the first 2 weeks of the fetal period. By the end of the tenth postfertilization week or the twelfth gestational week calculated from the LMP, the intestines are fully into the abdomen and out of the umbilical cord, the external genitalia have male or female characteristics but neither

FIGURE 6-2 (facing page).   Summary by days and weeks of events in fetal growth and development during the first trimester. Development of a follicle containing an oocyte, ovulation, and phases of the menstrual cycle are illustrated. Development begins at fertilization, about 14 days after the onset of the last menstruation. Cleavage of the zygote in the uterine tube, implantation of the blastocyst, and early development of the embryo are also shown. The main features of the developmental stages during the embryonic period and the first 2 weeks of the fetal period are illustrated. (Reproduced by permission from K. L. Moore. *The Developing Human: Clinically Oriented Embryology, 2nd.* Philadelphia: Saunders, 1977.)

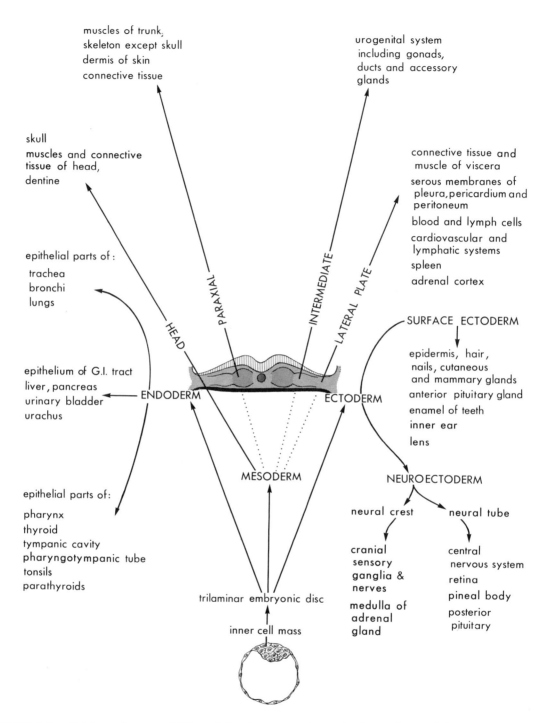

muscles of trunk,
skeleton except skull
dermis of skin
connective tissue

urogenital system
including gonads,
ducts and accessory
glands

skull
muscles and connective
tissue of head,
dentine

connective tissue and
muscle of viscera

serous membranes of
pleura, pericardium and
peritoneum

blood and lymph cells

cardiovascular and
lymphatic systems

spleen

adrenal cortex

epithelial parts of :

trachea
bronchi
lungs

PARAXIAL   INTERMEDIATE   LATERAL PLATE

HEAD

SURFACE ECTODERM

epidermis, hair,
nails, cutaneous
and mammary glands
anterior pituitary gland
enamel of teeth
inner ear
lens

epithelium of G.I. tract
liver, pancreas
urinary bladder
urachus

ENDODERM   ECTODERM

MESODERM   NEUROECTODERM

epithelial parts of:

pharynx
thyroid
tympanic cavity
pharyngotympanic tube
tonsils
parathyroids

neural crest   neural tube

cranial
sensory
ganglia &
nerves

medulla of
adrenal
gland

central
nervous system
retina
pineal body
posterior
pituitary

trilaminar embryonic disc

inner cell mass

FIGURE 6-3. Origin and responsibilities of the three germ layers in the makeup of the body. (Reproduced by permission from K. L. Moore. *The Developing Human: Clinically Oriented Embryology, 2nd.* Philadelphia: Saunders, 1977.)

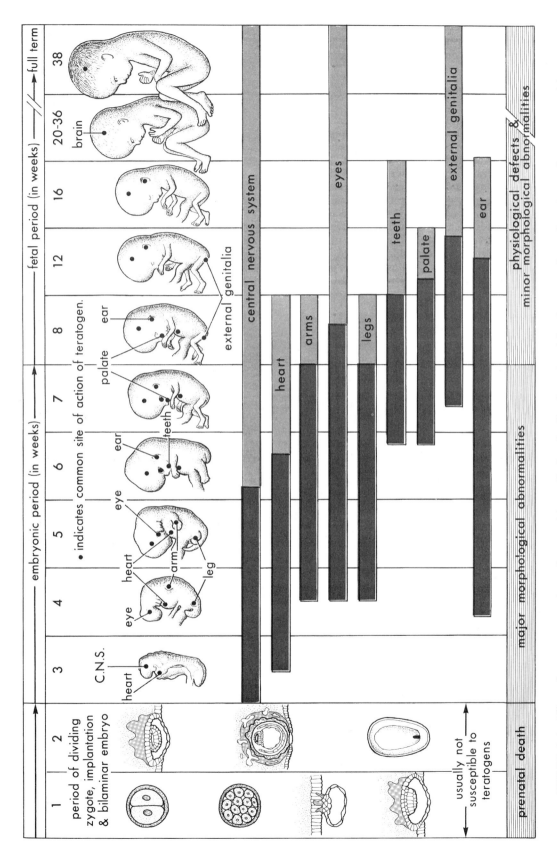

FIGURE 6-4 Effect of teratogens on the embryo and fetus. During the first 2 weeks of development, the embryo is usually not susceptible to teratogens. The darker areas denote highly sensitive periods; the lighter areas indicate less sensitive stages. (Reproduced by permission from K. L. Moore. *The Developing Human: Clinically Oriented Embryology, 2nd.* Philadelphia: Saunders, 1977.)

are yet fully formed, the anus has formed, and the facial characteristics of the fetus now look undeniably human. The fetus, now weighing approximately 0.5 to 1 ounce, can swallow, make respiratory movements, urinate, move the specific parts of the limbs, squint, frown, and open and shut his or her mouth. The head is about a third of the crown-rump length, which is approximately 56 millimeters (2.2 inches).

Second and Third Trimesters

The second trimester, 15 weeks long, includes weeks 13 through 27 by gestational age based on the LMP. This is equivalent to weeks 11 through 25 by postfertilization age. The third trimester, of 13 weeks, includes weeks 28 through 40 by gestational age based on the LMP. This is equivalent to weeks 26 through 38 by postfertilization age. *The following discussion is dated on the basis of gestational age.*

Weeks 13 to 16 (Fourth Lunar Month)
The eyelids are fused and head growth slows, while the ears move to a higher elevation on the sides of the head and the chin becomes evident with development of the mandible. Body growth accelerates with the legs again being slower in growth than the arms as the cephalic to caudal direction of growth continues. The arms but not the legs have reached their full length. Fingernails have started to develop but the toenails have not. Reflex response and muscular activity begin. The uterus is too thick and the activity too slight to yet be felt by the mother. Sex is clearly distinguishable during the fourteenth week (twelfth week after fertilization). By the sixteenth week there has been rapid progress in bone development. Centers of ossification of the skeleton are sufficiently established that they could be seen with roentgenography. The average crown-rump length is 4.5 inches, and the fetus weights between 3.5 and 4 ounces by the end of the sixteenth week.

Weeks 17 to 20 (Fifth Lunar Month)
Rapid body growth continues. The legs reach their total length and toenails develop. The eyelids remain fused. The fetus moves freely inside the uterus without the confinement that later growth imposes. Stronger fetal movement and a thinner uterine wall result in the mother's experiencing quickening around the eighteenth week. The fetus hiccups, and the mother may feel this as a rhythmic series of slight jerks or jolts. By the end of the month the vernix caseosa covers the entire body. Vernix caseosa, a mixture of sebum (secretion from the sebaceous glands) and surface epithelial cells, is a thick, cheesy substance that is protective to the delicate skin of the fetus. The fetal heart may be heard with a fetoscope by the end of the month. By the end of the twentieth week the average crown-rump length of the fetus is about 6.5 inches and the average weight is almost 0.75 pound.

Weeks 21 to 24 (Sixth Lunar Month)
Hair growth is prominent during the sixth lunar month. The fetus is completely covered with lanugo, a fine downy hair. Eyebrows, eyelashes, and head hair are present. The head remains large compared to the rest of the body. The skin is wrinkled, translucent, and red, giving an aged appearance to the fetus, which is also thin and lean due to a lack of subcutaneous fat. Both capillary blood and the red myohemoglobin of the muscles show through the skin. Buds for the permanent teeth are present. The fetus still has room in the uterus to somersault and can make the motions of crying and sucking. The hands make fists and also grip. Brown fat, which is a source of energy, heat production, and heat regulation in the newborn, forms. By the end of the month the average crown-rump length of fetus is just over 8 inches and the weight is approximately 1.25 pounds.

Weeks 25 to 28 (Seventh Lunar Month)
Although a little fat storage begins and the contours start to round out, the fetus still is

lean and continues to look old and wrinkled during this month. A substantial weight gain makes the body better proportioned by the end of the month. The hair on the baby's head is longer, the sucking motions are stronger, the eyes begin to open and shut, and the fingernails are present. The average crown-rump length of the fetus is approximately 9 inches and the weight is about 2.25 pounds by the end of the twenty-eighth week.

Weeks 29 to 32 (Eighth Lunar Month)

Subcutaneous fat deposits begin to smooth out some of the wrinkles but the fetus has not totally lost its wrinkled, old appearance. The body is filling out and is not quite so lean. Thick vernix caseosa covers the entire fetus. The hair on the head continues to grow and the lanugo is plentiful except on the face, from which it has now disappeared. Fingernails reach the ends of the fingers; toenails are present but do not reach the ends of the toes. The fetus has control of rhythmic breathing motions and body temperature. The eyes are open. The average crown-rump length is about 11 inches and weight is approximately 3.75 pounds.

Weeks 33 to 36 (Ninth Lunar Month)

By the end of this month the skin is smooth without wrinkles as the subcutaneous fat becomes thicker from additional deposits. The body is rounder, with the arms and legs taking on a somewhat chubby appearance. The hair is longer, the toenails have reached the ends of the toes, and the left testicle has usually descended into the scrotum. The average crown-rump length is a little over 12.5 inches and the weight is approximately 5.5 pounds during the thirty-sixth week.

Weeks 37 to 40 (Tenth Lunar Month)

The tenth lunar month provides the necessary finishing touches. Full growth and development are attained. The fetus is now well rounded with a prominent chest and protuberant mammary glands in both sexes. Both testes

are in the scrotum. The lanugo has disappeared from most of the body. The nails project beyond the ends of the tips of both the fingers and the toes. The skin varies in color from white to pink to bluish-pink regardless of race because the melanin that colors the skin is produced only after exposure to light. The crown-rump length now averages 14 inches. The weight depends on a number of variables but has a general average of 7.5 pounds.

PLACENTAL DEVELOPMENT, CIRCULATION, AND FUNCTIONS

Development and Circulation

The placenta is partly fetal and partly maternal in origin. The fetal contribution derives from the chorion; the maternal contribution derives from the decidua at the site of implantation.

The outer layer of cells forming the wall of the blastocyst is called the trophoblast. As the trophoblast begins to invade the epithelium of the endometrium it differentiates into two layers: (1) cytotrophoblast, which is the inner layer, and (2) syncytiotrophoblast, which is the outer layer. This differentiation occurs as the trophoblast comes into contact with the endometrium.

The syncytiotrophoblast is a multinucleated protoplasmic mass without intercellular boundaries. From this mass project an amorphous type of fingerlike projections, which penetrate through the endometrial epithelium into the endometrial stroma (see Fig. 6-5). The endometrial stroma contains both glands and capillaries. Lacunae, which are hollow spaces, form around the eighth day in the syncytiotrophoblast as it invades the stroma. As a result the endometrial glands are eroded and the capillaries rupture to fill the lacunae with embryotroph. Embryotroph is a mixture of glandular secretions and maternal blood which is nutritive to the embryo and reaches it by diffusion from the syncytiotrophoblast.

After the embryo is completely imbedded

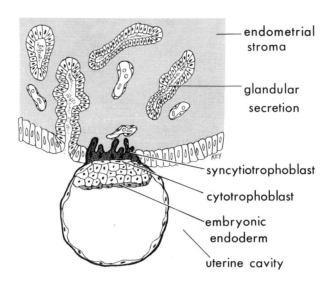

FIGURE 6-5. Early stage of implantation. The syncytiotrophoblast has penetrated the endometrial epithelium and started to invade the endometrial stroma. (Reproduced by permission from K. L. Moore. *The Developing Human: Clinically Oriented Embryology, 2nd.* Philadelphia: Saunders, 1977.)

within the endometrium around the twelfth day after fertilization, the lacunae in the syncytiotrophoblast join together to form intercommunicating lacunar networks. These give the syncytiotrophoblast a spongelike structure. At the same time the endometrium undergoes what is called the decidual reaction, in which the stromal cells enlarge with an accumulation of glycogen and lipid to become known as the decidual cells, and the capillaries become dilated with congestion to form sinusoids. Erosion of these sinusoids by the trophoblast fills the lacunar networks with maternal blood and establishes a primitive circulatory system.

Decidua is the name for the uterine endometrium during pregnancy. It differs from the nonpregnant endometrium because of the following decidual reaction. With the exception of the zona basalis, the decidua is shed after birth, giving rise to the Latin origin of the word *deciduus* meaning "a falling-off." As Moore points out, the shedding of the decidua is akin to the falling of leaves from deciduous trees in the fall [1]. There are three areas of decidua:

1. Decidua basalis — the decidua beneath the site of implantation of the embryo which becomes the maternal contribution to the placenta.
2. Decidua capsularis — the decidua surrounding the remainder of the embryo, thereby serving as a covering between the embryo and the uterine cavity. With fetal growth the decidua capsularis bulges into the uterine cavity and fuses with the decidua parietalis. The uterine cavity is thus obliterated. This occurs by the end of the fourth lunar month of gestation.
3. Decidua parietalis (also called the decidua vera) — the decidua lining the rest of the uterus:

The decidua basalis and parietalis consist of three layers as follows:

1. Zona compacta — the surface layer, which is compact in structure.
2. Zona spongiosa — the middle layer, which is spongy in structure due to the decidual cells and capillaries.

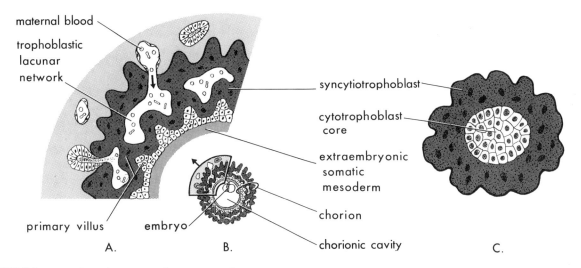

FIGURE 6-6. Development of primary villi. A. detail of the section of the wall of the chorionic sac outlined in B. B. sketch of a 14-day conceptus illustrating the chorionic sac and the shaggy appearance created by the primary villi (X6). C. drawing of a transverse section through a primary villus (X300). (Reproduced by permission from K. L. Moore. *The Developing Human: Clinically Oriented Embryology, 2nd.* Philadelphia: Saunders, 1977.)

3. Zona basalis — the bottom or base layer, which will remain to regenerate a new endometrium when the rest of the decidua is shed postpartally.

Around the fourteenth day after fertilization, chorionic villi begin to form when cytotrophoblastic cells reorganize into columns of cells extending into the core of the syncytiotrophoblast (see Fig. 6-6). These are known as the primary villi and form around the outer surface of the embryonic sac. Shortly thereafter these villi branch and develop central cores of mesenchyme; at this point they are called secondary villi. The mesenchymal cells develop into blood vessels within the villi that connect with the blood vessels of the chorionic sac, also arising from the mesenchyme, and thus with the embryo via the forerunner of the umbilical cord, the connecting stalk. The villi are now called true villi or tertiary villi. Cytotrophoblastic cells at the end of the villi proliferate and extend still further into and through the syncytiotrophoblast into the endometrial stroma

to firmly attach and anchor the embryonic or chorionic sac to the decidua.

Until approximately the eighth week after fertilization, the villi cover the surface of the entire chorionic sac. After that, as the sac grows, the blood supply in the area of the decidua capsularis diminishes, thereby causing the villi in the area of the decidua capsularis to degenerate. The result is a denuded chorionic sac called the chorionic laeve or smooth chorion. At the same time, the villi in the area of the decidua basalis proliferate, branch, and enlarge in the rich blood supply there. This results in a multiple treelike or tufted structure called the chorionic frondosum or villous chorion. The chorionic frondosum is the fetal contribution to the placenta.

As the chorionic villi invade and attach to the decidua basalis, remnants of the decidua covered with trophoblast form the placental septa (refer again to Fig. 6-6). The placental septa separate, incompletely, the irregular-shaped placental cotyledor.s. Each placental cotyledon consists of the main stem of a chori-

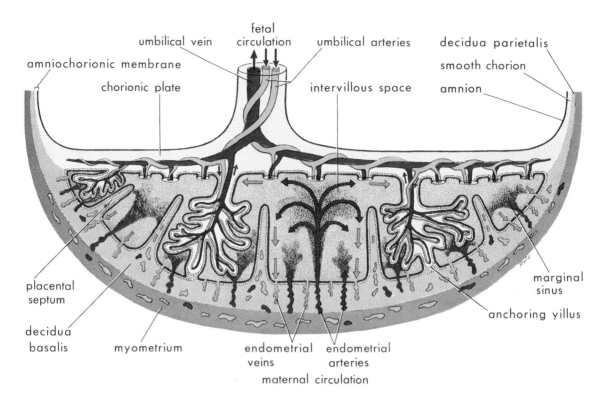

FIGURE 6-7. Placental circulation. Schematic drawing of a section through a mature placenta showing (1) the relation of the villous chorion (fetal placenta) to the decidua basalis (maternal placenta); (2) the fetal placental circulation; and (3) the maternal placental circulation. Maternal blood is driven into the intervillous space in funnel-shaped spurts, and exchanges occur with the fetal blood as the maternal blood flows around the villi. The inflowing arterial blood pushes venous blood out into the endometrial veins which are scattered over the entire surface of the decidua basalis. The umbilical arteries carry deoxygenated fetal blood to the placenta and the umbilical vein carries oxygenated blood to the fetus. Note that the cotyledons are separated from each other by decidual septa of the maternal portion of the placenta. Each cotyledon consists of two or more main-stem villi and their many branches. In this drawing only one main-stem villus is shown in each cotelydon, but the stumps of others are indicated. (Based on Ramsey, 1965.) (Reproduced by permission from K. L. Moore. The Developing Human: Clinically Oriented Embryology, 2nd. Philadelphia: Saunders, 1977.)

onic villus and all its numerous branches and infinite further subbranches. There are between fifteen and thirty cotyledons. The septa restrict the exchange of blood between the cotyledons in the intervillous space. This means that infarcting or pathology in one cotyledon remains a localized problem (see Fig 6-7).

The intervillous space is an elaboration of the earlier lacunar networks. The spaces of the lacunar networks enlarge with further invasion of the decidua by the trophoblast to form one large blood sinus called the intervillous space. Located between the chorionic plate on one side and the decidua basalis on the other, the intervillous space is incompletely partitioned by the placental septa that extend from the decidua but do not reach the chorionic plate. The chorionic plate consists of trophoblast externally (next to the intervillous space) and mesoderm internally. The internal mesoderm of the chorion fuses with the amnion around the end of the first trimester. Together the amnion and chorion constitute the fetal membranes, which enclose and contain the fetus and the amniotic fluid. Branches of the umbilical arteries and the umbilical vein run between the internal and external layers of the chorionic plate before they enter the chorionic villi that extend into the intervillous space.

Placental circulation, thus, consists of two separate circulations — fetal and maternal — with provision of a large area for exchange of materials between the two circulations as determined by the placental membrane or "barrier." The placental membrane is composed of the layers of fetal tissue between the circulating fetal and maternal blood. These layers are trophoblast, connective tissue in the chorionic villi, and the endothelium of the fetal capillaries. Regardless of how thin this membrane becomes as the placenta matures, neither the functions of the placental membrane nor the effectiveness of these functions change.

Fetal circulation to the placenta comes from the two umbilical arteries by which deoxygenated blood leaves the fetus. These arteries subdivide and branch in the chorionic plate and enter the chorionic villi where further subdivision occurs within the branching villi to form an extensive capillary-venous network at the terminal divisions. At this point placental transfer occurs, that is, the transfer of materials between the fetal and maternal circulations takes place across the placental membrane. The return circulation to the fetus is by way of the branching of the umbilical vein, which corresponds with the branching of the umbilical arteries, to the chorionic plate and then, with further converging, into the umbilical vein through which the oxygenated blood is carried to the fetus (see Fig. 6-7).

Maternal circulation in the placenta is actually outside of the maternal circulatory system. It consists of entry of oxygenated blood into the intervillous space by way of spiral arteries of the endometrium and exit of deoxygenated blood from the intervillous space by way of venous openings into the endometrial veins. The arterial entrances and venous exits supplying each cotyledon are randomly scattered throughout the placenta. While the numbers vary with authorities, there may be as many as 120 spiral artery entrances into the intervillous space of the mature placenta. The blood enters the intervillous space from the spiral artery under tremendous pressure as dictated by the maternal blood pressure. This results in a rhythmic spurting of a fountain of blood into and across the intervillous space to the chorionic plate. The blood is then dispersed laterally by this boundary and flows over the surfaces of the multitudinous branches of the chorionic villi. This flow is slow enough to allow for the exchange of materials between the fetal and maternal circulations across the placental membrane. Eventually the now deoxygenated maternal blood exits through the venous portals (see Fig. 6-7).

Functions of the Placenta

The placenta truly is an organ of life with a number of functions designed to provide for and protect the fetus. The placenta provides the fetus with oxygen—carbon dioxide exchange, essential nutrients, excretion of metabolic waste products, and needed metabolic processes. It also protects the fetus by transferring maternal antibodies to the fetus and by its synthesis of hormones essential to the maintenance and well-being of the pregnancy. The placenta thus has three functions: (1) metabolism, (2) as an organ of transfer, and (3) as an endocrine organ in the synthesis, production, and secretion of both protein hormones and steroid hormones.

During early pregnancy the placenta synthesizes glycogen. This function declines as the fetal liver develops. The placenta also synthesizes cholesterol and fatty acids and has other metabolic processes which most likely provide the needed energy and allow for the other functions of transfer and endocrine biosynthesis.

As an organ of transfer, the placenta has a number of mechanisms by which to transfer materials between the fetal and maternal circulations in the intervillous space across the placental membrane. These include the following:

1. Simple diffusion — the transfer of substances across a membrane from an area of higher concentration to an area of lower concentration. Low molecular weight substances diffuse readily across the placental membrane. This probably is the mechanism involved in the transfer of oxygen, carbon dioxide, many electrolytes, water, drugs, and analgesic and anesthetic agents.
2. Facilitated diffusion — materials diffusing from a higher concentration to a lower concentration are facilitated across the placental membrane to allow for more rapid or more specific transfer. Substances essential for rapid fetal growth but in low concentration in the maternal blood (e.g., glucose) is an example.
3. Active transport — transfer is against usual physiological principles. This is a metabolic process requiring energy. Active transport includes the transfer of substances from the mother to the fetus which are in low concentration in the maternal blood and in high concentration in the fetal blood. The transport of iron and ascorbic acid from the mother to the fetus are examples.
4. Pinocytosis — a substance is taken into and moved across the cells of the fetal membrane to the fetal blood stream by invaginations of the chorionic villi simply engulfing the material. This may be the mechanism involved in the transfer of large protein molecules with a high molecular weight such as immune gamma globulin G.
5. Breaks between cells — a break in the chorionic villi allows for the direct transfer of cells. The prime example of this is the sensitization of an Rh-negative woman from receipt of erythrocytes from her Rh-positive fetus. These breaks, or leaks, are occasional and do not negate the general truth of the statement that the two circulations of the fetus and the mother are separate without gross intermingling of the blood.
6. Placental infection — condition in which the placenta is infected and the lesions in the placenta caused by the infectious organisms serve as a means of access into the fetal bloodstream. Protozoal and bacterial infections are transferred this way. Viral infections may pass through the placental membrane and infect the fetus without infecting the placenta.

Substances which have been identified as being transferred across the placental membrane include the following:

1. Oxygen from mother to fetus
2. Carbon dioxide from fetus to mother
3. Water
4. Vitamins
5. Glucose
6. Electrolytes
7. Amino acids
8. Whole proteins
9. Lipids
10. Minerals
11. Waste products, e.g., urea, uric acid, bilirubin
12. Hormones
13. Maternal antibodies to selected diseases
14. Most drugs and pharmacologic agents
15. Selected viral, protozoal, and bacterial infections

The hormones which the placenta synthesizes, produces, and secretes include the following:

1. Human chorionic gonadotropin (hCG). A protein hormone most likely produced early in the pregnancy by the syncytiotrophoblast primarily in order to maintain the corpus luteum and thus the endometrium and the pregnancy.
2. Human placental lactogen (hPL). A protein hormone most likely produced early in the pregnancy by the syncytiotrophoblast. It is involved in lactogenic and metabolic processes. It has also been called chorionic growth hormone and chorionic somatomammotropin.
3. Estrogens. Steroid hormones elaborated by the placenta to the extent of causing a hyperestrogenic state. The precursor for the production of these estrogens is the adrenal cortex of both the mother and the fetus, with greater emphasis on the latter.
4. Progesterone. A steroid hormone elaborated by the placenta utilizing blood cholesterol as a precursor.

See Chapter 4 for the effect of these hormones in relation to the woman and the diagnosis of pregnancy.

The placenta may also synthesize a thyroid-stimulating hormone (chorionic thyrotropin) and adrenocorticosteroids (chorionic ACTH) although there is as yet no direct evidence of the latter.

REFERENCES

1. Moore, K. L. *The Developing Human: Clinically Oriented Embryology, 2nd.* Philadelphia: Saunders, 1977.

BIBLIOGRAPHY

Caplan, G. Psychological aspects of maternity care. *Am. J. Pub. Health* 47:25, 1957.

Colman, A. D., and Colman, L. L. *Pregnancy: The Psychological Experience.* New York: Seabury, 1973.

Flanagan, G. L. *The First Nine Months of Life.* New York: Simon and Schuster, 1965.

Friederich, M. A. Psychological changes during pregnancy. *Contemporary OB/GYN* 9:27, 1977.

Gillman, R. D. The dreams of pregnant women and maternal adaptation. *Am. J. Orthopsychiatry* 38:688, 1968.

Harding, P. G. R. The metabolism of brown and white adipose tissue in the fetus and newborn. *Clin. Obstet. Gynecol.* 14:685, 1971.

Lederman, R. P. *Psychosocial Adaptation in Pregnancy.* Englewood Cliffs, N. J.: Prentice-Hall, 1984.

Light, H. K., and Fenster, C. Maternal concerns during pregnancy. *Am. J. Obstet. Gynecol.* 118:46, 1974.

Malnory, M. E. A prenatal assessment tool for mothers and fathers. *J. Nurse-Midwifery* 27(6):26−34 (November/December) 1982.

Masters, W. H., and Johnson, V. E. Pregnancy and sexual response. In *Human Sexual Response.* Boston: Little, Brown, 1966.

Moore, D. S. The body image in pregnancy. *J. Nurse-Midwifery* 22:17, 1978.

Moore, K. L. *The Developing Human: Clinically Oriented Embryology, 3rd.* Philadelphia: Saunders, 1982.

Pritchard, J. A., MacDonald, P. C., and Gant, N. F. *Williams Obstetrics, 17th.* New York: Appleton-Century-Crofts, 1985.

Reid, D. E., Ryan, K. J., and Benirschke, K. *Principles and Management of Human Reproduction.* Philadelphia: Saunders, 1972.

Rubin, R. Attainment of the maternal role. *Nurs. Research* 16:237, 1967.

Rubin, R. Cognitive style in pregnancy. *Am. J. Nurs.* 70:502, 1970.

Rubin, R. *Maternal Identity and the Maternal Experience.* New York: Springer, 1984.

Rubin, R. Maternal tasks in pregnancy. *Maternal-Child Nursing J.* 4:143−154, 1975.

Snell, R. E. *Clinical Embryology for Medical Students, 2nd.* Boston: Little, Brown, 1975.

Stichler, J. F., Bowden, M. S., and Reimer, E. D. Pregnancy: A shared emotional experience. *Am. J. Mat. Child Nurs.*, 3:153, 1978.

Management Plan for Normal Pregnancy

PHILOSOPHY AND SCOPE

Care of the pregnant woman and the inclusion of those persons significant to her in her care are both exciting and challenging. To share in and facilitate a woman's or couple's growth as they open themselves to new feelings and the exploration of these is to be allowed to participate in one of life's great experiences. Each woman or couple and each childbearing experience is unique. Management of the pregnancy and the corresponding focus on how the woman and her partner are experiencing this condition, therefore, must be in accord with the uniqueness of their experience.

Management of the care of the pregnant woman, as at all other times in the childbearing cycle, incorporates basic philosophical beliefs of nurse-midwifery as discussed in the first chapter of this book. These include facilitation of natural processes, family-centered care, continuity of care, and the woman's right to

participate knowledgeably in her own childbearing experience. Because of this, nurse-midwives most likely subscribe to the listing of rights contained in "The Pregnant Patient's Bill of Rights," prepared by Doris Haire in 1974 and distributed by the Committee on Patients' Rights in New York City.* These are as follows:

The Pregnant Patient has the right to participate in decisions involving her well-being and that of her unborn child, unless there is a clearcut medical emergency that prevents her participation. In addition to the rights set forth in the American Hospital Association's "Patient's Bill of Rights," (which has also been adopted by the New York City Department of Health) the Pregnant Patient, because she represents TWO patients rather than one, should be

---

* Reprinted here in part with permission of Doris Haire.

recognized as having the additional rights listed below.

1. *The Pregnant Patient has the right*, prior to the administration of any drug or procedure, to be informed by the health professional caring for her of any potential direct or indirect effects, risks or hazards to herself or her unborn or newborn infant which may result from the use of a drug or procedure prescribed for or administered to her during pregnancy, labor, birth or lactation.

2. *The Pregnant Patient has the right*, prior to the proposed therapy, to be informed, not only of the benefits, risks and hazards of the proposed therapy but also of known alternative therapy, such as available childbirth education classes which could help to prepare the Pregnant Patient physically and mentally to cope with the discomfort or stress of pregnancy and the experience of childbirth, thereby reducing or eliminating her need for drugs and obstetric intervention. She should be offered such information early in her pregnancy in order that she may make a reasoned decision.

3. *The Pregnant Patient has the right*, prior to the administration of any drug, to be informed by the health professional who is prescribing or administering the drug to her that any drug which she receives during pregnancy, labor and birth, no matter how or when the drug is taken or administered, may adversely affect her unborn baby, directly or indirectly, and that there is no drug or chemical which has been proven safe for the unborn child.

4. *The Pregnant Patient has the right*, if cesarean section is anticipated, to be informed prior to the administration of any drug, and preferably prior to her hospitalization, that minimizing her and, in turn, her baby's intake of nonessential pre-operative medicine will benefit her baby.

5. *The Pregnant Patient has the right*, prior to the administration of a drug or procedure, to be informed of the areas of uncertainty if there is NO properly controlled follow-up research which has established the safety of the drug or procedure with regard to its direct and/or indirect effects on the physiological, mental and neurological development of the child exposed, via the mother, to the drug or procedure

during pregnancy, labor, birth or lactation — (this would apply to virtually all drugs and the vast majority of obstetric procedures).

6. *The Pregnant Patient has the right*, prior to the administration of any drug, to be informed of the brand name and generic name of the drug in order that she may advise the health professional of any past adverse reaction to the drug.

7. *The Pregnant Patient has the right* to determine for herself, without pressure from her attendant, whether she will accept the risks inherent in the proposed therapy or refuse a drug or procedure.

8. *The Pregnant Patient has the right* to know the name and qualifications of the individual administering a medication or procedure to her during labor or birth.

9. *The Pregnant Patient has the right* to be informed, prior to the administration of any procedure, whether that procedure is being administered to her for her or her baby's benefit (medically indicated) or as an elective procedure (for convenience, teaching purposes or research).

10. *The Pregnant Patient has the right* to be accompanied during the stress of labor and birth by someone she cares for, and to whom she looks for emotional comfort and encouragement.

11. *The Pregnant Patient has the right* after appropriate medical consultation to choose a position for labor and for birth which is least stressful to her baby and to herself.

12. *The Obstetric Patient has the right* to have her baby cared for at her bedside if her baby is normal, and to feed her baby according to her baby's needs rather than according to the hospital regimen.

13. *The Obstetric Patient has the right* to be informed in writing of the name of the person who actually delivered her baby and the professional qualifications of that person. This information should also be on the birth certificate.

14. *The Obstetric Patient has the right* to be informed if there is any known or indicated aspect of her or her baby's care or condition which may cause her or her baby later difficulty or problems.

15. *The Obstetric Patient has the right* to have her and her baby's hospital medical records complete, accurate and legible and to have their records, including Nurses' Notes, retained by

the hospital until the child reaches at least the age of majority, or, alternatively, to have the records offered to her before they are destroyed.

16. *The Obstetric Patient*, both during and after her hospital stay, has the right to have access to her complete hospital medical records, including Nurses' Notes, and to receive a copy upon payment of a reasonable fee and without incurring the expense of retaining an attorney.

It is the obstetric patient and her baby, not the health professional, who must sustain any trauma or injury resulting from the use of a drug or obstetric procedure. The observation of the rights listed above will not only permit the obstetric patient to participate in the decisions involving her and her baby's health care, but will help to protect the health professional and the hospital against litigation arising from resentment or misunderstanding on the part of the mother.

Management of the care of the woman throughout the antepartal period includes the following components:

1. Diagnosis of the pregnancy
2. Evaluation of the well-being of the woman
3. Evaluation of the well-being of the fetus
4. Relief measures for the common discomforts of pregnancy
5. Anticipatory guidance and instruction
6. Screening for maternal and fetal complications

The diagnosis of pregnancy was discussed in Chapter 4. Evaluation of the well-being of the woman and of the fetus is detailed in Chapters 5 and 8. Further evaluation of the well-being of the fetus by adjunctive tests and studies is elaborated upon in this chapter.

FETAL EVALUATION MEASURES

The fetal evaluation measures discussed in this chapter are used when the fetus is suspected of being at risk. Because many of them are expensive, or carry with them an element of risk in the procedure involved, or both, the value of their use must be weighed against any possible risk and the expense in each given situation.

Ultrasonography

Ultrasound is the generation of high frequency sound waves which, when beamed into the body, are reflected or echoed when an interface is encountered between different types of tissues or structures with different densities. These echoes can be translated into a visible image of the tissues or structures encountered.

The advantages of ultrasound include that the procedure is simple and painless. Prior to 20 weeks gestation, it is necessary to have a full but not overdistended bladder for the procedure. Obstetrically ultrasonography has a number of diagnostic uses which may be ordered by the nurse-midwife:

1. Localization of intrauterine contraceptive devices (IUDs). IUDs made of all present-day materials reflect sound waves. Ultrasound, thus, is invaluable in locating IUDs when there is a question as to whether or not they are in the uterus. It serves the double function of determining whether the woman is pregnant (if 5 weeks since her LMP) and eliminates the possibility of exposing an early pregnancy to either roentgenography or intrauterine probing with a sound.
2. Early pregnancy. Pregnancy can be diagnosed by ultrasound by 5 weeks gestation based on the LMP.
3. Abortion prediction. This requires serial observation over a period of weeks for failure of growth in the gestational sac. One ultrasound observation may be misleading. A gestational sac low in the uterus does not necessarily presage an abortion. There is a correlation only if there is also bleeding.
4. Ectopic pregnancy.

5. Hydatidiform mole. This has such a characteristic image of multiple scattered echoes that diagnosis is reliable to the exclusion of other tests.

6. Gestational age and fetal maturity. An estimated fetal age is determined between approximately 5 and 10 weeks by measuring the gestational sac, between approximately 8 and 14 weeks by measuring the crown-rump length, between approximately 14 and 20 weeks by measuring femur length, and between approximately 18 and 26 weeks by measuring the biparietal diameter. The fetal head is demonstrable by ultrasound by about the twelfth week of gestation. The growth of the fetal head is almost linear until approximately the thirtieth week of gestation. The weeks given here for each entity are when the measurements correlate most closely with the gestational age. There are other (thus far less useful) fetal measurements which at certain points in time have a higher correlation with gestational age than at other times, such as abdominal circumference (34 to 36 weeks) and head-abdomen ratio (35 to 36 weeks).

   While tables correlating the fetal biparietal diameter by ultrasound with gestational age considered to be accurate within 11 to 14 days have been developed, each institution utilizing ultrasound generally establishes its own growth curves based on its decisions regarding measurement procedures. These include the calibration velocity and how the biparietal diameter is measured on the table of the skull (e.g., outer table to outer table, inner table to inner table, etc.). Whatever the methodology, it must be consistent for accuracy and meaning in the interpretation of resulting growth curves. This information must be known in using tables developed elsewhere so that either their procedures are used or so their data can be interpolated to match the data at your own institution.

7. Multiple gestation. Multiple gestation has been diagnosed as early as the first trimester with ultrasound.

8. Localization of the placenta. Knowing the location of the placenta is invaluable in aiding diagnosis of third trimester bleeding. Since the placenta can be localized early in the second trimester, its position is also useful to physicians preparatory to performing amniocentesis.

9. Fetal anomalies. A number of fetal anomalies can be identified, including, abnormalities of the head and spine and of the genitourinary tract; gastrointestinal defects; and cardiac, thoracopulmonary, and musculoskeletal anomalies.

10. Fetal death. Fetal movement, respiratory movements, and movement of the fetal heart will not be present. Separation and overlapping of the skull bones (Spalding's sign) will be evident.

11. Estimated fetal weight.

12. Fetal lie and presentation.

13. Intrauterine growth retardation (IUGR). Total intrauterine volume (TIUV) is thought to be an accurate predictor of IUGR. TIUV, obtained by measuring the dimensions of the uterine cavity and applying them to a geometric formula, is the total volume of all the intrauterine products. The correlation of a diminished TIUV with IUGR is due to the smaller size of the IUGR fetus and associated oligohydramnios (see Chapter 9).

14. Polyhydramnios is indicated by a large intrauterine space that projects a clean image because there are no echoes.

15. Oligohydramnios.

16. Placental grading. Placental grading (grades 0 to III) is used for evaluating fetal maturity, predicting potential perinatal problems in a preterm pregnancy, and estimating fetal pulmonary maturity. The latter has not proved accurate enough to be useful.

17. Biophysical profile. A biophysical profile is used to evaluate fetal well-being (e.g.,

in a postdates pregnancy) and consists of the following:

a. biparietal diameter
b. fetal movement
c. respiratory movements
d. muscle tone
e. amniotic fluid volume
f. placental grade
g. ponderal index (a height-weight ratio)
h. heart rate pattern

Ultrasonography is still in its developmental period. Even now it is reliably replacing former diagnostic methods, especially roentgenography, as a far safer methodology. With experience and refinement the uses will further expand and the technology improve. Ultrasound does not carry the known risks that accompany irradiation.

Questions are being raised, however, about the unknowns of ultrasound and if there might be any adverse long-term effects which would develop or evidence themselves years later. Data are inconclusive. The methodology of the research thus far on the safety of ultrasound can be criticized. There is evidence of in vitro cellular damage and genetic alterations with exposure to ultrasound at higher level output intensities than are used in vivo. These findings have not been demonstrated in vivo and thus application to the clinical situation and obstetric diagnostic ultrasound is anything but clear. Issues in the controversy include safety, risk-benefit ratios, routine use of ultrasound versus indicated use of ultrasound and the effect of either on outcomes, lack of valid research on latent or long-term effects, and informed consent.

The nurse-midwife should perform an exhaustive, comprehensive assessment of the woman and fetus (history, physical, pelvic, and laboratory findings) and think through how the information ultrasonography will provide will be used *before* determining the need for an ultrasound. The nurse-midwife then explains the risk-benefit ratio to the woman *before* ordering the ultrasound. A reasonable path for pregnant women and health care professionals during this controversy is outlined in a position paper by the International Childbirth Education Association (ICEA) as recommendations for the use of diagnostic ultrasound [1]:

- Pregnant women should avoid ultrasound exposure unless there is a documented medical reason for its use and/or disease is suspected.
- Pregnancy is a normal physiological process which does not, by itself, constitute a medical reason for ultrasound exposure.
- Participation in an ultrasound examination must be voluntary.
- Pregnant women should be specifically informed that the Doptone and electronic fetal monitor are both ultrasound devices. Written informed consent should accompany the use of electronic fetal monitoring.
- Ultrasound examination should not be withheld when there are valid indications of potential psychological and physical benefit.
- The desire of a healthy pregnant woman to know the baby's sex or "see the baby move" should not, by itself, be considered a valid reason for exposure to ultrasound.
- Before an ultrasound examination, expectant parents should be given information about the procedure, its benefits and known risks, gaps in knowledge about biological effects, and alternative tests which might be done and their benefits and risks.
- The pregnant woman's partner (i.e., support person of her choice) should be offered the opportunity to accompany her during the scanning procedure to allay anxiety and promote family involvement.
- Pregnant women should be given the opportunity to view the ultrasound screen during the procedure.
- Pregnant women should not undergo an ultrasound examination for commercial demonstration of equipment.
- Ultrasound examinations should be conducted and interpreted only by skilled personnel trained in ultrasound use and interpretation. The pregnant woman has the right to inquire about the training in ultrasonography of her physician and operators of the equipment. Physicians should be able to verify qualifications on request.

- Public health agencies and medical and scientific organizations have an obligation to publicize information on the biological effects of ultrasound, known risks, areas of uncertainty, and availability of guidelines for ultrasound use.

Amniocentesis and Amniotic Fluid Studies

Amniocentesis is the aspiration of amniotic fluid by way of a needle passed transabdominally into the gestational (amniotic) sac. The technique of amniocentesis can also be used for the injection of solutions into the amniotic sac. It is generally not possible to perform an amniocentesis until the second trimester, when the uterus has enlarged sufficiently to become a readily accessible abdominal organ and the entire uterine cavity is filled with the amniotic sac. This latter change occurs when the chorionic laeve fuses with the decidua parietalis around the uterine cavity other than at the site of implantation, at approximately the third to fourth month of gestation.

The ratio of amniotic fluid to fetus is high in the first trimester, about 3:2 by 20 weeks gestation, and decreases thereafter as the fetus grows. The average fluid volume during the third trimester is around 800 ml; this quantity decreases to around 450 ml by term and further decreases postterm.

Amniocentesis is performed only by physicians and usually is indicated only when a fetus is in jeopardy or suspected of being high risk. The physician weighs the reason for performing an amniocentesis against the risks involved in the technique. These risks include the following:

1. Perforation of the placenta or fetal placental vessels, which may result in:
   a. hemorrhage
   b. transfer of fetal cells which could cause or aggravate isoimmunization and hemolytic disease in the fetus
   c. fetal death
2. Infection, which may result in:
   a. maternal morbidity or mortality
   b. fetal or neonatal morbidity or mortality

3. Abortion
4. Premature labor or premature rupture of membranes
5. Fetal trauma resulting from needle puncture
6. Trauma to the umbilical cord or umbilical vessels

The risk of amniocentesis is reduced when performed after the twentieth week of gestation. Many authorities are recommending giving RhoGam to Rh-negative women when the amniotic fluid is bloody and there is the possibility of an Rh-positive fetus.

Early in pregnancy amniotic fluid is light yellow or straw-colored with slight turbidity. It then becomes essentially colorless and clear, reflecting light and containing white particulate matter (vernix caseosa). The color of the amniotic fluid thus may indicate conditions or diseases even before definitive testing is done. The following are examples:

1. Opaque fluid with green-brown discoloration — may be thick, depending on the amount of meconium in the amniotic fluid. May indicate fetal distress.
2. Yellow with slight turbidity — colored by products of hemolysis, especially bilirubin. The deeper and brighter the yellow, the worse the hemolytic disease of the fetus.
3. Opaque with some degree of dark red — indicates the presence of blood in the amniotic fluid. May indicate perforation of a placental vessel.
4. Opaque, yellow-brown fluid — referred to as "tobacco juice." Characteristic of fetal intrauterine death.

A number of studies and diagnostic procedures are possible because of the technique of amniocentesis. These include the following:

1. *Diagnosis of genetic disorders or abnormalities.* Amniocentesis for diagnosis of genetic disorders or abnormalities resulting from chromosomal aberrations usually is done

sometime between the fourteenth and eighteenth weeks of gestation, when there is a sufficient number of shed fetal cells in the fluid. For diagnosis of chromosomal abnormality the amniotic fluid is centrifuged, the cells cultured, and karyotyping done. Because of the small but definite risks of amniocentesis, stringent criteria generally govern its use for the purpose of diagnosing genetic disorders or abnormalities. Amniocentesis for diagnosis of genetic disorders or abnormalities caused by biochemical disorders usually is done around the twentieth week of gestation, which is when these problems can best be diagnosed. A large number of metabolic disorders can be diagnosed on the basis of identifying the biochemical characteristics of cultured amniotic fluid cells or the metabolites in the amniotic fluid.

2. *Diagnosis of the sex of the fetus.* This is often done when amniocentesis is being performed for another reason. Determination of fetal sex alone is not generally considered a valid reason to risk the possible complications of amniocentesis. Sex can be determined by studies conducted on either cultured or uncultured amniotic fluid cells.

3. *Measurement of the lecithin-sphingomyelin (L/S) ratio.* The L/S ratio is used to determine fetal maturity. The determination of fetal maturity is sometimes an essential part of the data base entering into a decision making process regarding artificial termination of pregnancy (e.g., repeat cesarean section, diabetes, postmaturity, small-for-gestational-age [SGA], and so forth). It should be noted that, while the L/S ratio generally is considered an excellent predictor of fetal maturity, the converse is not true; that is, it is neither accurate nor reliable as an indicator of fetal immaturity.

The L/S ratio predicts the potential development of respiratory distress syndrome (RDS), since lecithin is essential to preventing collapse of the alveoli during respiratory expiration after birth. Prior to the thirty-fourth week of gestation, lecithin and sphingomyelin are present in the amniotic fluid in approximately equal amounts. Thereafter, this balance changes as the amount of lecithin increases in relation to sphingomyelin. When the proportion of lecithin to sphingomyelin becomes twice as much (2 to 1, or an L/S ratio of 2.0), the chance of RDS is slight unless the mother is diabetic. An L/S ratio of 2 or above is considered indicative of a mature fetus. An L/S ratio between 1.50 and 1.99 is considered an intermediate range in which nearly half will develop RDS. An L/S ratio of less than 1.50 is considered indicative of an immature fetus with a high probability of developing RDS. If the amniotic fluid is contaminated with red blood cells or if the the initial centrifuging of the amniotic fluid was too vigorous, the L/S ratio will be inaccurate.

4. *Determination of fetal maturity by the "shake test."* The shake test is also called the rapid surfactant test, the foam stability test, and the foam test. It is generally considered as reliable as the L/S ratio for determining fetal maturity, more accurate (though also unreliable) than the L/S ratio as an indicator of fetal immaturity, and simpler, less time-consuming, and cheaper than the L/S ratio. The shake test is used to determine the amount of surfactant properties of lecithin present as an indicator of fetal maturity. This is determined by whether or not there is a complete circle of foam or bubbles around the circumference of a test tube in which amniotic fluid has been shaken with ethanol and isotonic saline for 15 seconds and then allowed to sit for 15 minutes. A complete ring of bubbles is interpreted as fetal maturity. An incomplete ring of bubbles indicating fetal immaturity may be a false-negative test and is not reliable as an indication of fetal immaturity and the probability that RDS would develop if the baby were delivered at this time. A positive

shake test is fairly reliable for fetal maturity.

5. *Determination of fetal maturity by measurement of the creatinine level in the amniotic fluid.* This test is based on the fact that the concentration of creatinine in the amniotic fluid increases noticeably during the last trimester. Before the thirty-fourth week of gestation there is nearly always less than 2 milligrams creatinine for 100 milliliters of amniotic fluid. After the thirty-seventh week it is rare for the creatinine level to be less than 2 milligrams per 100 milliliters and it may be as high as 3 to 4 milligrams per 100 milliliters. However, creatinine is not necessarily a measure of immature pulmonary function nor of fetal maturity because the concentration level may be altered by maternal disease (e.g., preeclampsia, renal disease). Therefore the measurement of creatinine for evaluation of fetal maturity is presently thought by many experts to be unreliable. Others feel it may contribute to a total picture when used as one of a battery of tests and methods for evaluating fetal well-being.

6. *Other tests of fetal maturity using amniotic fluid.* These tests are listed here merely for general information. Authorities consider them even less reliable than those already discussed. These tests include the following:
   a. increase in fetal fat cell percentage or lipid staining of amniotic fluid cells
   b. decreasing osmolality of the amniotic fluid
   c. decreasing concentration of bilirubin in the amniotic fluid

7. *Determination of the severity of fetal hemolytic disease (erythroblastosis fetalis).* This evaluation is done by spectrophotometric analysis using optical density values for hemolysis pigments (mostly bilirubin) in the supernatant of amniotic fluid which has been centrifuged. It is done when the results of a maternal indirect Coombs' test is positive and an antibody titer indicates the possibility of severe hemolytic disease in the fetus (1 to 16 or higher)

8. *Amniography and fetography.* For both of these studies the technique of amniocentesis is used to inject a radiopaque water soluble agent into the amniotic sac. Amniography is used to outline the fetal soft parts and gastrointestinal tract, demonstrate abnormal amounts of amniotic fluid, and to locate the placenta. Fetography is used to outline the fetus and to diagnose some external soft-tissue anomalies and hydrops fetalis. The dangers of amniography and fetography (e.g., exposure to radiation, the risks of amniocentesis, and the possible harmful effects of the chemical agents) combined with the fact that most of this information can now be obtained by ultrasound has rendered these studies largely obsolete.

Alphafetoprotein (AFP) Testing

Alphafetoprotein testing is done to identify women at risk for having a baby with a neural tube defect (e.g., spina bifida, anencephaly) or a number of other congenital defects. Alphafetoprotein is a normally occurring fetal protein. It is found in abnormally concentrated amounts in the amniotic fluid of a fetus with a neural tube defect and in the mother's blood. Neural tube defects occur in about 2 in 1000 births in the United States. Ninety-five percent of women who bear a child with a neural tube defect have no family history of neural tube defects and previously have delivered an unaffected child.

AFP testing is most accurate between 15 and 18 weeks gestation. Testing at that time also allows for a second test if necessary before 20 weeks gestation, after which the test is invalid. AFP testing is actually a sequence of tests. The first test is of maternal serum. Approximately 5 percent of all women tested will have a positive initial AFP test. These women are retested with another maternal serum AFP test within 1 week. About 3 percent of all women undergoing AFP screening will have two positive blood tests. Of these women, 5 percent will have a baby with a neural tube defect. Other reasons for elevated AFP levels include multiple gestation, erroneous determination of gestational age (pregnancy further along than expected), and fetal demise. Ultrasonography is done after two positive maternal serum AFP tests to rule out twins, identify anencephaly, and detect fetal demise. From 45 percent to 55 percent of the time no explanation is found for the elevated serum AFP level. The final test, if twins and other causes are ruled out with ultrasound, is amniocentesis. Approximately one or two of every hundred women who enter an AFP testing program will have amniocentesis. Approximately one of fifteen women undergoing amniocentesis will have an elevated amniotic fluid AFP level which is indicative of significant fetal pathology. While almost 100 percent accurate for picking up anencephaly, AFP testing detects only four out of five cases of open spina bifida. Women who undergo AFP testing and learn that they are carrying an affected child with a neural tube defect must then decide whether to have an abortion or to carry the child to term with the opportunity to prearrange and plan for optimal circumstances for the delivery and special care for the baby. AFP testing can not identify how severe the defect is.

Approximately 2 percent of women who have delivered one child with a neural tube defect will have a second child similarly affected. Thus, every woman who has had such a child should have ultrasound and amniocentesis in any subsequent pregnancy.

Although AFP testing is not yet considered an obstetrical routine it should be offered to all pregnant women for their consideration and decision. A more recent finding is that a low maternal serum AFP level may be associated with Down's syndrome. The logistics of including screening for Down's syndrome with AFP screening are under consideration.

Amnioscopy and Fetoscopy

Amnioscopy and fetoscopy both involve direct visualization through the fetal membranes. In amnioscopy, the amniotic fluid is viewed through the fetal membranes at the cervical os. In fetoscopy, the fetus and placenta are visualized through the fetal membranes with an endoscope inserted through a small abdominal incision.

Of the two techniques amnioscopy is better developed but has a number of drawbacks: (1) it is not possible to perform until the cervix is sufficiently dilated, (2) the cervical os may not be accessible (e.g., because of a posterior cervix), (3) the membranes may be inadvertently ruptured during the procedure, (4) it may be uncomfortable to the woman, and (5) the internal manipulations may predispose to genital tract infection. Amnioscopy may be done during late pregnancy in multiparas with patulous cervices, or during labor. Detection of meconiumstained amniotic fluid indicates a probable episode of fetal hypoxia and need for a closely monitored delivery.

Estriol Level Determinations

Normal estriol production is dependent on a physiologically normal fetus and placenta since the fetal adrenal gland provides the precursor for the production of estrogens by the placenta. Measurement of estriols in either blood or urine and comparison of the findings with the established normal values for the time in gestation, therefore, gives an indication of the functioning of the fetoplacental unit. The level of estriols increases throughout pregnancy, especially in the last trimester, to a peak at term. This curve, however, has a great deal of latitude in it because there is a wide range of normal values between women and, further, variation in the daily values of the same woman. Accordingly, a single measurement of estriol level is essentially useless for attaching any significance to the finding.

A series of values, therefore, is needed in order to assess the well-being of the fetus and to determine whether there is any compromise in fetoplacental functioning. Compromise is determined by a decrease in estriol as reflected in a curve of descending values from a series of measurements. Measurements need to be done daily in order to detect a decrease or fall in values. Between 30 percent to 50 percent of cases with a significant decline may be missed if the measurement is done even every other day or every third day. Estriol values within the average normal range indicate that the fetus is probably not in jeopardy or immediate danger. Estriol values falling below normal range or significantly decreased values indicate fetal compromise, distress, or even death, depending on the severity of the fall. The following rules of thumb are in use by different clinicians in various settings:

1. A sudden decrease of:
   a. 40% from a previous measurement
   b. 50% from the mean of previous measurements
   c. 35% from the mean of the values of the preceding 3 days;
   is considered a significant decrease warranting immediate further assessment.
2. A value below:
   a. 12 milligrams
   b. 10 milligrams
   is significant, even if a single value, warranting immediate further assessment.
3. A value above 12 milligrams indicates probable fetal well-being; values between 4 and 12 milligrams may indicate fetal jeopardy if late in pregnancy, with the probability of jeopardy being higher the closer the value is to 4 milligrams; values below 4 milligrams indicate severe fetal jeopardy, impending death, or fetal death.

While there is some variation in these interpretations of values, it is clear when a nurse-midwife should consult with a physician regarding reports of estriol levels on her or his patients.

An estriol series may be ordered whenever possible compromise of fetoplacental function is suspected or when there is a potential concern such as in the following conditions:

1. Postmaturity by dates
2. Unsure dates and the possibility of postmaturity
3. Elderly primigravida
4. Toxemia/hypertensive disorders of pregnancy
5. Diabetes
6. Intrauterine growth retardation
7. Suspected fetal death
8. Fetal abnormality such as anencephaly

While there is a greater body of literature about urinary estriol measurement, it is generally agreed that measurement of plasma estriols is equally valid. In fact, measurement of plasma estriols may be more accurate because plasma estriol concentration is not affected by diurnal patterns or bed rest; urinary estriol concentration is affected by these factors. Certainly, obtaining a blood specimen for plasma estriols is much easier and introduces less chance for improper collection of the specimen than is true for collecting a refrigerated 24-hour urine for urine estriols. The latter requires not only a reliable patient but also one who will be able to work out a method for collection and refrigeration of her urine in relation to the demands and responsibilities of her daily life.

Specimen collection is only one problem. There are over twenty factors and conditions, many of them normal or unrelated to fetal well-being, which decrease the estriol level but do not mean fetal jeopardy. There are also several factors and conditions which will spuriously increase the estriol level or for which estriol determination is of little to no value in management of the patient. There are some authorities who think estriol level determinations are of little or no value anyway and that no decisions should be based on these values alone. This places the onus for decision making on clinical judgment and the utilization of other studies.

Fetal Movement

Fetal movement is generally thought to be an indication of fetal well-being. Recent studies have attempted to ascertain the normal amount of movement in order to develop tools for counting fetal movements to detect fetal distress. The obvious and ideal person to count fetal movements is the mother, but two difficulties have been encountered. First is the variation in maternal sensitivity to fetal movement. Some women are not always aware of fetal movement, especially of short duration, and other women mistake fetal hiccups or Braxton Hicks contractions for fetal movement. Secondly, there is a lack of agreement on the normal number of fetal movements at any given time. This is further complicated by the wide range of non-threatening factors which affect fetal movement (e.g., sound, nutritional intake, touch, external stimulation).

Nonetheless, parameters have been set for the lower limits of normal within established time periods during which the mother counts and records daily fetal movement. The lower limit of normal is generally agreed to be ten movements in 12 hours. Fewer than this constitutes a movement alarm signal (MAS). If the mother's count results in an MAS, she immediately reports this and is immediately seen for a nonstress test and/or contraction stress test. The absence of MAS correlates well with good outcomes (>90%). When there is an MAS, special note must be made of any progressive decrease in fetal movement: progressive decrease is ominous. Moreover, a sudden or progressive fall in the movement count, even if it stays within normal range,

may not be normal for this fetus and instead may be an indicator of fetal distress and impending death.

Contraction Stress Test

The contraction stress test (CST) assesses fetal-placental functioning and the fetus's projected ability to cope with the continuation of a high-risk pregnancy and the stress of labor. It aids the physician in selecting the optimal time for delivery of a high-risk fetus.

The underlying physiological and technological bases for the CST are as follows:

1. Contractions decrease the blood flow through the intervillous space.
2. If the uteroplacental reserve is normal this intermittent decrease in blood flow by contractions will not negatively affect the fetus.
3. If the uteroplacental reserve is diminished or suboptimal, the intermittent decrease in blood flow by contractions will affect the fetus.
4. This negative effect on the fetus is reflected as a fetal heart rate pattern of late deceleration. Depending on the equipment used, a decreased or absent fetal heart rate variability may also be present. (See Chapters 12 and 14 for a discussion of fetal heart rate patterns.)
5. A fetal heart rate pattern of late deceleration is thought to be due to uteroplacental insufficiency in the presence of a decreased blood flow through the intervillous space produced by a contraction.

Thus a CST is a test that ascertains the fetus's response to contractions — naturally occurring or induced by nipple stimulation or oxytocin — by using external fetal monitoring to record simultaneously the fetal heart rate and the uterine contractions. Uterine activity is increased after an amniocentesis; this is an example of a time when a CST could probably be obtained without using oxytocin or nipple stimulation.

Some of the conditions in which a CST might be helpful in selection of an optimal time for delivery include the following:

1. Postmaturity — suspected or actual
2. Intrauterine growth retardation as suspected by a small-for-gestational-age fetus
3. History of a previous stillbirth
4. Meconium-stained amniotic fluid obtained at amniocentesis
5. Falling or abnormal estriol value determinations
6. Diabetes
7. Toxemia/hypertensive disorders of pregnancy
8. Chronic hypertension
9. Chronic lung disease
10. Cyanotic heart disease
11. Chronic renal disease
12. Hyperthyroidism
13. Collagen disease
14. Severe isoimmunization
15. Sickle cell disease or other hemoglobinopathies

The CST is conducted in either an inpatient or outpatient setting. The woman's bladder should be empty (to promote comfort and avoid disruption); she should be in either a semi-Fowler's, left lateral, or lateral recumbent position (to avoid supine hypotensive syndrome); and her blood pressure should be checked every 10 to 15 minutes (to assure that the woman is normotensive). A baseline recording is obtained and, if uterine contractions are naturally occurring at a rate of three in a 10-minute period, induction of contractions is not necessary.

There are two methods for inducing the contractions needed for a contraction stress test — nipple stimulation and intravenous oxytocin. Nipple stimulation causes the neurohypophysis to release endogenous oxytocin.

This method of producing naturally occurring oxytocin avoids the risks, discomfort, and expense associated with the intravenous infusion of oxytocin. At the beginning of the test, warm washcloths are applied to the breasts. A&D Ointment or K-Y Lubricating Jelly is applied to the nipples to prevent soreness. The woman then stimulates her nipples by either rolling them or gently pulling them. Stimulation is initially unilateral. If contractions are inadequate (fewer than three contractions occur in the first 10 minutes), the woman then simultaneously stimulates both nipples for another 10 minutes. If contractions are still inadequate, intravenous oxytocin is used. Nipple stimulation provides adequate contractions in approximately 75 percent of women using this method.

The administration of oxytocin to induce contractions is called an oxytocin challenge test or oxytocin contraction test (OCT). A venipuncture is done, an intravenous line is established, and a very dilute solution of oxytocin controlled by an infusion pump is administered via a piggyback setup to another bag of intravenous solution. The rate of infusion is increased at intervals until the contractions are occurring at a frequency of at least three in a 10-minute period and lasting at least 30 seconds (preferably 40 to 60 seconds). The recording is then interpreted and the oxytocin stopped. If, during the test, there are three late decelerations, the test should be considered finished and the oxytocin infusion stopped, regardless of the frequency of the uterine contractions. Both the monitoring and the intravenous solution without oxytocin in it are continued until the contractions have diminished to their baseline activity. This is to assure that the OCT has not put the woman into labor without your knowing about it.

Two methods to test for cord compression can be used during an oxytocin challenge test. These are the Hillis maneuver and the Mueller maneuver. The Hillis maneuver is done by exerting fundal pressure in order to exaggerate the fetal position. This forces the fetal chin against the chest. If the umbilical cord is around the baby's neck it will be compressed as evidenced by a severe variable deceleration for the length of time pressure is exerted. The Mueller maneuver is done by exerting suprapubic pressure against the fetal head to push it against the pelvic brim. A cord in the area, which would have the potential for prolapse, will be compressed between the fetal head and the pelvic brim as evidenced by a severe variable deceleration until the pressure is released. The fetal heart rate then immediately returns to its baseline.

A negative CST is one in which no late decelerations occur with contractions as frequent as three in a 10-minute period. A negative CST indicates fetal well-being and predicts that the fetus will continue to be all right for another week without needing the intervention of delivery if the woman's clinical status does not change. However, an occasional intrauterine death has been reported within a week of a negative CST test meeting this criterion. By and large, though, authorities agree that a negative CST is a valuable piece of information for aiding in decision making. Negative CSTs are repeated weekly or sooner depending on the continuing clinical status.

A positive CST is one in which there have been repeated late deceleration fetal heart rate patterns during the test. A positive CST indicates that the fetus may not withstand continuation of the pregnancy. Thus, serious consideration needs to be given to immediate termination of the pregnancy by delivery. However, a positive CST is not a reliable finding due to the fact that there is a 25 percent rate of false-positive results. Again, most authorities agree that a positive CST is a valuable piece of information in decision making but urge caution and encourage use of a total picture of assessment methods and clinical judgment. In other words, the decision to terminate a pregnancy should not be made only on the basis of a positive CST.

There are three other categories of interpretation of a CST. These are as follows:

1. *Hyperstimulation*, in which the contractions are more frequent than every 2 minutes or have a duration of more than 90 seconds. This is more apt to occur with the use of oxytocin than with nipple stimulation. Hyperstimulation renders the test invalid; it cannot be interpreted and may be misinterpreted as a positive test. In other words, late decelerations in the presence of hyperstimulation may be due to this phenomenon itself and not to uteroplacental insufficiency. The test should be repeated within 24 to 48 hours with an even more dilute solution of oxytocin.
2. *Suspicious*, in which there has been an occasional late deceleration but this is not repetitive and does not occur with continued contractions. The CST should be repeated within 24 to 48 hours.
3. *Unsatisfactory*, in which the recording (tracing) is not of good enough quality to be interpreted. This may be due to the problems inherent with external fetal monitoring (see Chapter 12).

Nonstress Test

The nonstress test (NST) monitors the fetal heart rate in response to fetal movement in order to assess fetal well-being. It has the advantage of involving no external stimulation (e.g., oxytocin infusion) in the conduct of the test. Because of this it can be done for women for whom the CST might be contraindicated. Such women include those with previous cesarean section, placenta previa, or threatened premature labor. Otherwise, the indications for an NST are the same as those for a CST. The other advantage is that its simplicity and absence of risk factors allow it to be done in an outpatient setting.

The preparation and positioning of the

woman are the same as for the CST. The fetal heart rate is then externally monitored for approximately 20 to 30 minutes. It is important that the fetus not be in a fetal sleep state for the entirety of this time as sleep may cause decreased fetal heart rate variability. If necessary, abdominal palpation can be used to rouse the fetus. During the test the woman presses a button whenever she feels fetal movement; this marks the monitor strip so fetal movement and the fetal heart rate pattern can be correlated.

Interpretation of the nonstress test is based on fetal heart rate patterns (described in Chapters 12 and 14) and on patterns of fetal heart rate reactivity to fetal movement. Normally, the fetal heart rate decreases (within the normal range of 120 to 160 beats per minute) and variability increases with gestational age, probably in relation to the development of the central nervous system. The fetus normally has a transient accelerated heart rate with average baseline variability when moving or in response to external stimuli such as abdominal palpation. Abnormal fetal heart rate reactivity response to fetal movement is evidenced by a persistent reduction in baseline variability with an absence of fetal heart rate acceleration. This pattern may indicate a distressed fetus and occurs when the fetal central nervous sytem is depressed by drugs, hypoxia, or acidosis.

A *reactive* test is one in which a normal fetal reactivity pattern is demonstrated. This is evidenced by fetal heart rate accelerations of 15 beats per minute above the baseline lasting for 15 to 30 seconds in association with fetal movement (two or more occurrences of this acceleration pattern within a 10-minute period or five or more accelerations within a 20-minute period). A normal fetus near term will also evidence a baseline fetal heart rate between 120 and 160 beats per minute, a variability between 10 and 25 beats per minute, and no decelerations of any type.

A *nonreactive* test is one in which there is a persistent decreased variability with an absence of accelerations in fetal heart rate in response to fetal movement. This is evidenced by fetal heart rate accelerations of less than 15 beats per minute above the baseline or lasting less than 15 seconds in association with fetal movement (fewer than two such accelerations within a 10-minute period or fewer than five accelerations within a 20-minute period); or an absence of accelerations associated with fetal movement.

A *suspicious* nonstress test is one in which there are definite fetal heart rate accelerations associated with fetal movement but the number of them, the increase in beats per minute above the baseline, or the length of their duration does not meet the criteria for being either reactive or nonreactive.

A reactive test indicates fetal well-being and predicts a good outcome if birth were to occur within 1 week. If the test is nonreactive, further assessment of fetal status should be initiated to aid in determining fetal well-being and the wisdom of pregnancy continuation. If the test is suspicious, it should be repeated in 24 to 48 hours. The nonstress test can be repeated or continued at any desired frequency without concern for adverse effects to the fetus.

COMMON DISCOMFORTS OF PREGNANCY AND THEIR RELIEF MEASURES

Not all women experience all of the following common discomforts of pregnancy but many women experience a few to a great number of them. Relief from these discomforts can make a significant difference in how a woman views her pregnancy experience. Insofar as is known or commonly accepted, the physiologic, anatomic, and psychologic bases for each discomfort are given to stimulate your thinking of further possible relief measures. Relief measures are predicated on the causes of the discomfort and are geared towards symptomatic management.

Nausea

Nausea, with or without vomiting, is known as morning sickness but frequently occurs during the day or evening. It is more apt to occur when the stomach is empty, so it is usually worse in the morning. The cause of morning sickness are not really known, although a number of ideas have been advanced. These include hormonal changes of pregnancy, gastric overloading, slowed peristalsis, enlarged uterus, and emotional factors. Nausea is a common problem occurring in over half of pregnant women — so common, in fact, that it is a presumptive sign of pregnancy. Fortunately, it is a limited discomfort; as it is normal only during the first trimester. Nausea eases as the first trimester ends, about the same time the uterus is becoming an abdominal organ. Persistent nausea and vomiting beyond the first trimester may indicate a severe emotional problem, hyperemesis gravidarum, or hydatidiform mole.

The relief measures for morning sickness are numerous. Any one or all or any combination or none may be effective for each individual. It gives most women some comfort and relief just to be trying something to ease the problem. The relief measures are as follows:

1. Small, frequent meals, even as often as every 2 hours, as these are more apt to be retained than three large meals a day
2. Dry crackers before getting up in the morning
3. Something sweet to eat or drink (e.g., fruit, fruit juices) before going to bed at night and before getting up in the morning
4. Avoidance of foods with strong or offensive odors
5. Restriction of fats in her diet
6. Acupressure wristbands
7. Reassurance that nausea will end sometime during the fourth month of pregnancy
8. Considerate, understanding, loving treatment of the woman with special attention to the little things that are important to her (this needs to be communicated to her significant others)
9. Vitamin B_6, 50 mg b.i.d. po
10. Medication — opinion varies because of possible teratogenic effects of any drugs on the embryo or fetus during this period of time
11. A formula with an unknown author which is frequently used by nurse-midwives:

$$\frac{t + u}{ph + ps}$$

where t = time
u = understanding
ph = physiologic basis of nausea
ps = psychologic basis of nausea

Fatigue

Fatigue occurs during the first trimester for no known reason. One idea is that it is due to the initial fall in the basic metabolic rate early in the pregnancy but why this happens is not clear. Fortunately, it is a limited discomfort, usually disappearing by the end of the first trimester. It can have the effect of increasing the intensity of the psychological responses the woman is having during this time.

The relief measures are to reassure the woman of its normality and spontaneous remission by the second trimester. It will help her to have frequent rest periods if possible during the day until this passes.

Upper Backache (Nonpathological)

Upper backache is first noticeable during the first trimester due to the increase in size and resulting heaviness of the breasts, which is one of the presumptive signs of pregnancy. This enlargement may produce muscular strain if the breasts are not adequately supported.

The relief measure, then, is a well-fitting and supportive brassiere. The characteristics of a good bra are listed later in this chapter in the discussion of instruction and anticipatory guidance. By decreasing breast mobility, a snug, supportive bra also reduces the discomfort of breast tenderness resulting from their enlargement.

Leukorrhea

Leukorrhea is a profuse, thick, excessive vaginal secretion that begins during the first trimester. The secretion is acidic because of the conversion of an increased amount of glycogen in the vaginal epithelial cells by Döderlein's bacilli into lactic acid. While this serves the function of providing a protection to the mother and fetus against possible harmful infection, it does provide a medium which fosters the growth of the organisms responsible for vaginitis (see Chapter 25). The productivity of the cervical glands in secreting an increased amount of mucus at this time to form the cervical mucus plug may also contribute to leukorrhea. Relief measures are close attention to bodily cleanliness in the area and a frequent change of soft, cotton-crotch panties.

Urinary Frequency (Nonpathological)

Urinary frequency as a nonpathological discomfort of pregnancy often occurs at two different times during the antepartal period. Frequency during the first trimester is due to the increased weight in the fundus of the uterus, with the softening of the isthmus (Hegar's sign) causing increased anteflexion of the enlarging uterus, which exerts direct pressure on the bladder. This is relieved as the uterus continues to enlarge and rises out of the pelvis to become an abdominal organ while the bladder remains a pelvic organ. Urinary frequency during the third trimester occurs most often in primigravidas, after lightening has occurred. The effect of lightening is that the presenting part descends into the pelvis and causes direct pressure against the bladder. The pressure makes the woman feel the need to void. The enlarging uterus or the presenting part also takes up space in the pelvic cavity, thereby allowing less room for distention of the bladder before the woman feels the need to void.

The only relief measures are an explanation of why this is happening and a decrease in fluid intake before bedtime so that the woman is not disturbed with many trips to the bathroom when she is trying to sleep.

Heartburn

Heartburn is a discomfort that may start toward the end of the second trimester and extend through the third trimester. Heartburn is another word for regurgitation or the reflux of acidic gastric contents into the lower esophagus by reversed peristalsis. The gastric contents are acidic by virtue of the hydrochloric acid in the stomach. This causes the material to burn the throat and taste bad. The causes of heartburn are thought to be as follows:

1. Relaxation of the cardiac sphincter of the stomach due to the effects of increased amounts of progesterone
2. Decreased gastrointestinal motility resulting from smooth muscle relaxation which is probably due to increased amounts of progesterone and to uterine pressure
3. Lack of functional room for the stomach because of its displacement and compression by the enlarging uterus

There are numerous relief measures for heartburn. Finding the combination that will help an individual woman is largely a matter of trial and error. The relief measures are as follows:

1. Small, frequent meals, avoiding overloading of the stomach

2. Good posture, to give more room for the stomach to function — slumped posture only adds to the problem by allowing further pressure on the stomach
3. Avoidance of fats with meals — fat depresses both motility of the stomach and the secretion of gastric juices needed for digestion
4. On the other hand, sometimes some form of fat shortly before meals (e.g., a pat of butter ½ hour before) helps some women
5. Avoidance of beverages with meals since this tends to inhibit gastric juices — a dry diet without breadstuffs has helped some women
6. Avoidance of very cold foods with meals, to inhibit gastric juices
7. Drinking cultured milk rather than sweet milk has helped some women
8. Drinking milk and/or eating ice cream has helped some women
9. Antacid preparations such as Maalox, Gelusil, Amphojel, and Milk of Magnesia

Flatulence

Increased flatulence is thought to be due to decreased gastrointestinal motility. This probably results both from the effect of increased progesterone on relaxing smooth muscle and from the displacement of and pressure upon the intestines by the enlarging uterus.

The only relief measures are to encourage a regular pattern of daily bowel movements and to avoid gas-forming foods.

Constipation

Women previously without a problem of constipation may develop this problem during the second or third trimester. This is thought to be due to decreased peristalsis as a result of relaxation of the smooth muscle of the large bowel in the presence of increased amounts of progesterone. The displacement and compression of the bowel by the enlarging uterus or pre-senting part may also contribute to decreased motility in the gastrointestinal tract and thus to constipation. One of the common side effects of iron medication is constipation; this compounds the problem for a large percentage of pregnant women.

The relief measures for constipation are most effective when all are used in combination. Medication should be reserved for use only if the natural methods are not sufficient. Following is the list of relief measures for constipation:

1. An adequate fluid intake — defined as a minimum of eight glasses (drinking-glass size) per day
2. Prunes or prune juice — prunes are a natural mild laxative
3. Adequate rest — this may require rest periods during the day
4. Warm liquids (e.g., water, tea) upon rising
5. Foods in the diet which contain roughage, bulk, and natural fiber (e.g., lettuce, celery, bran)
6. Establishment of regular and good bowel habits — this includes establishing a regular time of day for having a bowel movement and being deliberately conscious of not ignoring the "urge" or delaying when feeling like having a bowel movement
7. General exercise, good posture, good body mechanics, and daily exercise of contracting the lower abdominal muscles — all of these measures facilitate venous circulation, thereby preventing congestion in the large intestines
8. Mild laxatives, stool softeners, and/or glycerin suppositories if indicated

Hemorrhoids

Hemorrhoids often are preceded by constipation. Therefore, all the reasons for constipation have the potential of leading to the development of hemorrhoids. Progesterone also causes relaxation of the vein walls and of the large bowel. In addition, the enlarging uterus causes increasing pressure — specifically in the hemorrhoidal veins as well as generally — interfering with venous circulation and causing congestion in the pelvic veins.

There are a number of relief measures for hemorrhoids. Some solely give comfort and others both numb and reduce the hemorrhoids. The latter are noted in the following listing of relief measures for hemorrhoids:

1. Avoidance of constipation — prevention is the most effective measure
2. Avoidance of straining during defecation
3. Sitz baths — the heat of the water not only gives comfort but also increases circulation
4. Witch hazel compresses — for reduction
5. Ice bag — for reduction
6. Epsom salt compresses — for reduction
7. Reinsertion of the hemorrhoids into the rectum in conjunction with perineal tightening (Kegel's) exercise (see Chapter 23)
8. Bedrest with hips and lower extremities elevated
9. Analgesic ointments and/or topical anesthetics
10. Preparation H

Leg Cramps

The physiologic basis for leg cramps is not clear. For a number of years leg cramps were thought to be due to inadequate or impaired calcium intake or an imbalance in the calcium-phosphorous ratio in the body, but these are no longer stated in current literature. Another school of thought is that the enlarged uterus exerts pressure either on the pelvic blood vessels, thereby impairing circulation, or on the nerves as they course through the obturator foramen on their way to the lower extremities. Relief measures are as follows:

1. Have the woman straighten her affected leg and point her heel, i.e., dorsiflex her foot. If she is in bed she needs strong, steady pressure against the bottom of her foot, either someone's hand or the footboard of the bed, to push against; if she is standing the floor serves this function. This measure is nearly guaranteed to instantly alleviate an acute leg cramp.
2. General exercise and a habit of good body mechanics to improve circulation.
3. Leg elevation periodically throughout the day.
4. A diet which includes both calcium and phosphorous.

Dependent edema

Dependent pedal edema is the result of impaired venous circulation and increased venous pressure in the lower extremities. These circulatory disturbances are caused by pressure of the enlarging uterus on the pelvic veins when sitting or standing and on the inferior vena cava when supine. Any constrictive clothing that inhibits venous return from the lower extremities adds to the problem. Dependent edema is generally evidenced in the ankles and feet and must be carefully differentiated from edema associated with preeclampsia/eclampsia (see Chapter 9). Relief measures include the following:

1. Avoidance of constrictive clothing
2. Elevation of the legs periodically throughout the day
3. Positioning on the side when lying down

Varicosities

A number of factors may contribute to the development of varicosities during pregnancy. Varicose veins are more apt to occur in women who have a familial tendency or congenital predisposition. Varicosities may result from impaired venous circulation and increased venous pressure in the lower extremities; these changes are caused by pressure of the enlarging uterus on the pelvic veins when sitting or standing and on the inferior vena cava when supine. Any constrictive clothing inhibiting venous return from the lower extremities or prolonged periods of standing add to the problem. Progesterone-induced relaxation of the vein walls and valves and surrounding smooth muscle also contributes to the development of varicosities.

Varicosities during pregnancy are most pronounced in the legs and/or vulva. Relief measures specific to vulvar varicosities are so noted in the following listing:

1. Use of support hose, Ace bandages, or elastic stockings — whichever is used, they should be put on after elevation of the legs and before arising
2. Avoidance of constrictive clothing, e.g., knee-high or ankle hose, round garters
3. Avoidance of long periods of standing
4. Rest periods with the legs elevated periodically throughout the day
5. Lying in the right-angle position several times daily (Fig. 7-1)
6. Assuming the incline position several times daily (for vulvar varicosities) (Fig. 7-2)
7. Keeping the legs uncrossed when sitting
8. Sitting whenever possible, preferably with legs elevated, rather than standing
9. Maintaining good posture and good body mechanics, and walking to facilitate increased circulation
10. Providing physical support for vulvar varicosities with a foam rubber pad held in place with a sanitary belt

Dyspareunia

Pain during sexual intercourse may stem from a number of causes during pregnancy. Physiologic changes may be responsible, such as pelvic/vaginal congestion resulting from im-

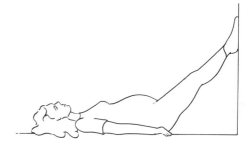

FIGURE 7-1.   Right-angle position.

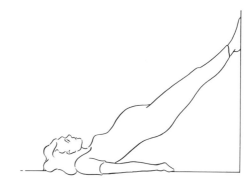

FIGURE 7-2.   Incline position.

paired circulation due to pressure of the enlarging uterus or the presenting part. Physical problems may be posed by an enlarged abdomen or may be encountered in late pregnancy when the presenting part descends into the true pelvis. Psychologic factors may cause dyspareunia because of misconceptions and fears such as hurting the baby when there is no indication for this concern. Appropriate relief measures depend on the causes.

1. Positional changes will alleviate problems with an enlarged abdomen.
2. Accessible congestion may be reduced with ice, but this treatment imposes its own discomforts.
3. Explanation and discussion of misconceptions and fears with substitution of facts and knowledge may be immensely helpful and reassuring.

4. Education of both partners in alternative ways of sexually satisfying each other may be welcomed.

Nocturia

In addition to the urinary frequency of the first trimester and possibly the third trimester, discussed earlier in this chapter, there is thought to be a physiological basis for nocturia. Venous return from the extremities is facilitated when the woman lies in a recumbent lateral position, since the uterus is no longer pressing against the pelvic vessels and inferior vena cava. When the woman lies in this position while sleeping at night, the result is a reversed diurnal pattern, which yields increased urinary output. The only relief measures consist of whatever comfort she derives from an explanation of why this is happening and reduction of fluids after the evening meal so her intake during this time doesn't add to the problem.

Insomnia

Insomnia may be due to any number of causes such as concerns, anxieties, or excited anticipation of an event the next day, akin to insomnia in the nonpregnant state. The pregnant woman, however, has additional, physical, reasons for insomnia. These include the discomfort of the enlarged uterus, the associated discomforts the enlarging uterus and pregnancy cause, as discussed throughout this chapter, and fetal movement, especially if the fetus is active. The relief measures for insomnia are time-honored and may or may not be effective. For many women they are at least something to do.

1. Warm bath
2. Warm drink (milk, tea with milk) before going to bed
3. Nonstimulating activity prior to going to bed

4. Use of relaxation positions
5. Use of the technique of progressive relaxation

Round Ligament Pain

The round ligaments attach on either side of the uterus just below and in front of the insertion of the fallopian tubes; they then cross the broad ligament in a fold of peritoneum, pass through the inguinal canal, and insert in the anterior (upper) portion of the labia majora on either side of the perineum. The ligaments are composed largely of smooth muscle that is continuous with the smooth muscle of the uterus. This muscle tissue enables the round ligaments to hypertrophy during pregnancy and, in essence, stretch as the uterus enlarges. It is anatomically mandatory that the round ligaments be able to increase in length as the uterus rises high into the abdomen. Round ligament pain is thought to be due to this stretching and possibly to the pressure of the increasingly heavier uterus on the ligaments. It is a common discomfort which must be differentiated from gastrointestinal tract and abdominal organ disease, e.g., appendicitis, gallbladder inflammation, and peptic ulcer. One feature that aids in this differentiation is the extension of pain into the inguinal area, which, among the conditions mentioned, is peculiar only to round ligament pain.

Relief measures are few and not always effective. Round ligament pain is one of the discomforts that a woman simply has to put up with. Explanations of why she is having pain will at least alleviate anxieties or fears and may help her to cope. Additional measures include:

1. Flexing her knees onto her abdomen
2. Take warm baths
3. Apply a heating pad to the area — only if sure the pain is not due to any medical complication such as appendicitis

4. Support the uterus with a pillow under it and a pillow between her knees when lying on her side (Fig. 7-3)

Low Back Pain (Nonpathological)

Low back pain is backache in the lumbosacral region. This usually increases in intensity as the pregnancy progresses because it results from a shift in the woman's center of gravity and thus in her posture; these changes are produced by the weight of the enlarging uterus. Unless the woman pays deliberate attention to her posture she will walk with a sway back from increasing lordosis. This curvature strains the back muscles and causes the ache or pain. It has been suggested that students who have not experienced pregnancy should tie a 10-pound bag of sugar or flour around their waists and walk around with it to get an idea of what this localized weight does to the back.

The problem is exaggerated if the woman's abdominal muscles are lax; they fail to give any support to the heavy enlarged uterus. This causes the uterus to sag, a condition that increases the curvature of the back still further. Weakness of the abdominal muscles is more common in grand multiparas who have not exercised and regained their abdominal muscle tone after each pregnancy. Primigravidas usually have excellent muscle tone because their muscles have not been stretched before. Low back pain, thus, generally increases in severity with parity.

Backache may also result from excessive bending, walking without rest periods, and lifting, especially if any or all of these are done while tired. Such activities add strain to the

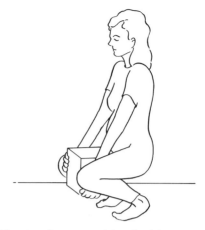

FIGURE 7-4. Proper position for lifting.

back. Proper body mechanics for lifting are essential to avoid this type of muscular strain. There are two principles to be followed:

1. Stoop, rather than bend, to lift an object (e.g., toddler, groceries) so that the legs (thighs) rather than the back bear the weight and strain.
2. Have the feet spread apart and one foot slightly in front of the other when stooping so there is a broad base for balance when arising from the stooped position (Fig. 7-4).

Relief measures for low back pain are as follows:

1. Good posture.
2. Proper body mechanics for lifting.
3. Avoiding excessive bending, lifting, or walking without rest periods.
4. Pelvic rocking.
5. Supportive low-heeled shoes — high heels are unstable and further exaggerate the problem of the center of gravity and lordosis.
6. For resting or sleeping:
   a. a hard mattress.
   b. positioning with pillows to straighten the back and alleviate pulling and strain.

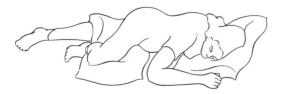

FIGURE 7-3. Sidelying relaxation position.

7. If the problem is severe, external abdominal support is advisable, e.g., a maternity girdle or an abdominal binder.

Nonpathological Hyperventilation and Shortness of Breath

It is thought that the increased amount of progesterone during pregnancy acts directly on the respiratory center to lower the levels of carbon dioxide and increase the oxygen levels. Increased oxygen levels benefit the fetus. The increased metabolic activity which occurs with pregnancy causes an increase in carbon dioxide levels; hyperventilation lowers the levels of carbon dioxide. Women may experience this effect of progesterone early in the second trimester.

Shortness of breath is largely a discomfort of the third trimester. During this time the uterus has enlarged to the point of pressing on the diaphragm. In addition, the level of the diaphragm elevates approximately 4 centimeters during pregnancy. Although there is some widening of the transverse diameter of the thoracic cage it is not sufficient to compensate for the elevation of the diaphragm, and a decrease in both the functional residual capacity and the residual volume of air results. This, combined with the pressure being exerted on the diaphragm possibly decreasing still further the functional residual volume, causes a feeling of slight difficulty (or awareness of difficulty) in breathing and shortness of breath. Many women tend to respond to this by hyperventilating.

The relief measures for hyperventilation are as follows:

1. Explain its physiologic basis.
2. Encourage the woman to deliberately regulate the speed and depth of her respirations at normal rates when she is aware of hyperventilating.
3. Alleviate shortness of breath as a causative factor (described below).

The relief measures for shortness of breath are geared toward providing more room for abdominal contents, thereby reducing the pressure on the diaphragm and facilitating lung functioning. These are as follows:

1. Have the woman periodically stand up and s−t−r−e−t−c−h her arms above her head and take a deep breath.
2. Encourage good posture — no slumping of shoulders.
3. Teach the woman to do intercostal breathing.
4. Instruct her to do the same stretching when in bed as when standing.
5. Explain the reasons for shortness of breath — alleviation of anxieties or fears will reduce a response of hyperventilation.

Tingling and Numbness of Fingers

The change in the center of gravity resulting from the enlarged and heavy uterus may cause the woman to assume a posture in which her shoulders are too far back and her head is anteflexed in an effort to counterbalance her heavy front and curved back. This posture is thought to cause compression of the median and ulnar nerves in the arm, which would cause tingling and numbness of the fingers. Hyperventilation may also cause finger tingling and numbness, but most women do not hyperventilate enough as a result of pregnancy to have this effect. Relief measures include explaining the probable cause and encouraging scrupulous attention to good posture. Some women obtain relief simply by lying down.

Supine Hypotensive Syndrome

Supine hypotensive syndrome causes the woman to feel faint; she may pass out if the problem is not immediately alleviated. Supine hypotensive syndrome occurs when the woman lies in a supine position (such as for sleep or on an examining table) because the full weight of the enlarged uterus and its contents is on the inferior vena cava and other vessels of the venous system. Venous return from the lower half of the body is inhibited, which in turn reduces the amount of blood filling the heart and subsequently lowers cardiac output. Supine hypotensive syndrome is actually obvious arterial hypotension. In addition, the weight of the enlarged uterus compresses the aorta, which also results in deleterious changes in arterial pressure.

Supine hypotensive syndrome is alleviated immediately by simply having the woman either turn on her side or sit up. Reassurance and explanation are essential since she is likely to be frightened.

INSTRUCTION AND ANTICIPATORY GUIDANCE

Anticipatory guidance and instruction during the antepartal period relate largely to the activities of daily life, the common discomforts of pregnancy and their relief measures, preparation for childbirth and parenthood, the danger signs, an understanding of the physical and psychologic changes taking place, and the basics of fetal growth and development. The following is an outline of these topics with the exception of the common discomforts of pregnancy and their relief measures, which were discussed immediately preceding this segment of the chapter.

This material is presented in topical outline with only occasional further notations for several reasons: (1) most nurse-midwifery students will have taught this material as student nurses or in nursing practice, (2) some of the material is elsewhere in this book, and (3) there are innumerable pamphlets, booklets, books, and textbooks that detail this instruction. Those who are unfamiliar with this teaching can use the topical outline to identify areas in which they need instruction, refer to the literature, and observe classes and discussion groups dealing with the information.

Principles of Antepartal Teaching

As in any teaching, be sure you have an audience in your potential learner before talking. Otherwise you may be wasting her time and your time. Common mistakes are to try to teach too much at one time and to try to teach at the end of an exhausting day for her in the clinic or office. An interested learner at such a time would be rare. Some information is mandatory to communicate, e.g., danger signs of critical complications; the use (or, rather, nonuse) of over-the-counter drugs, especially aspirin; the potential dangers of cat care; and so forth. Joyce Roberts [2] advocates the following ranking of priority in information giving:

1. Information given in response to specific questions, problems, or experiences of a woman at the particular time in her pregnancy
2. Information that is essential for a woman to have for her own or her baby's health and safety
3. Anticipatory guidance that will facilitate a woman's efforts to deal realistically with the pregnancy and with issues or aspects of childbirth which she is likely to encounter
4. Additional information regarding pregnancy progress, childbirth, or institutional policies that may be helpful but not related to the immediate needs of the woman

Not all women have learning needs for all of the instruction and anticipatory guidance you have to give. Unvalidated assumptions regarding a woman's learning needs should not be made. Find out first if she wants the information you have to share with her — for each topic that comes up as a potential for discussion. Especially be alert not to make assumptions about professionals (e.g., nurse-midwives, nurses, physicians) and what they want and need to know. Most such women do not like to have to rely upon themselves or to feel they should act as though they know it all — they may know for other women, but this is their own experience which may well be new and fraught with their own unique set of anxieties and joys.

Antepartal Teaching Outline

1. Interpretation of physical findings and laboratory results
2. Value of keeping appointments for antepartal revisits
3. Signs and symptoms of complications that indicate a need to call the nurse-midwife immediately:
   a. vaginal bleeding
   b. facial or hand edema
   c. prolonged nausea and vomiting
   d. fever, chills
   e. sudden, sharp, continuing abdominal pain
   f. sudden gush of fluid from the vagina
   g. continuing severe headache
   h. visual changes, e.g., blurring of vision, dizziness, spots before eyes
   i. any change from normal in urination
4. Perineal and vaginal care
   a. direction of wiping — front to back
   b. cotton-crotch panties
   c. no douching
5. Breast care
   a. daily cleansing with warm water and a soft, clean cloth followed by careful drying
   b. if colostrum is crusted on the nipple, soften with an application of nipple cream or lanolin before trying to remove
   c. gentle handling
   d. good breast support (see 6, below)
   e. preparation for breast-feeding in ninth month of pregnancy (see Chapter 47)
   f. cut the nipple area out of cotton bras or drop the flaps on nursing bras, letting the nipples contact and rub against clothing a few minutes several times a day — this will help desensitize them and make them less tender
   g. if nipples are inverted and the woman plans to breastfeed:
      (1) Woolwich breast shields — worn inside the bra cups and designed to exert pressure which will bring the nipple out; may be purchased through the La Leche League if not available locally
      (2) nipple rolling
6. Breast support. A good brassiere is essential for preventing or alleviating upper backache; gives comfort for tender enlarged breasts; and provides alignment for facilitating ductile functioning. There is little change in breast size for the remainder of the antepartal period after the fourth to fifth lunar month of gestation. Characteristics of a good bra are as follows:
   a. supportive, porous, soft, washable material
   b. shaped to avoid compression and irritation of the breasts and nipples while giving snug support
   c. wide, adjustable shoulder straps
   d. wide back band with a number of available fastening adjustments
   e. support is from below upward and from the sides inward
7. Abdominal support
   a. abdominal muscle tightening exercises, e.g., chin-chest, controlled breathing, sit-ups
   b. maternity girdle, if needed
   c. abdominal binder, if needed
8. Clothing
   a. supportive, washable, loose-fitting (never binding or constrictive of circulation), mood-lifting
   b. adjustable — there is little change in breast size for the remainder of the pregnancy after the fourth to fifth lunar month of gestation
   c. shoes — comfortable with a broad base; avoid high heels which are un-

stable and increase any problem with lordosis

    d. maternity clothes usually not needed until around the fifth calendar month of pregnancy

9. Fetal growth and development appropriate for the period of gestation now and until the next antepartal revisit

10. Bodily and psychologic changes appropriate for the period of gestation now and until the next antepartal revisit

11. Possible discomforts for the period of gestation now and until the next antepartal revisit

12. Explanation of relief measures for any present discomforts.

13. Dental care
    a. appointment with dentist
    b. cleansing of teeth after meals
    c. gum care — will tend to bleed because of hyperemia by midpregnancy

14. Avoidance of cats — explain regarding toxoplasmosis

15. Avoidance of moderate to excessive intake of alcohol — explain regarding fetal alcohol syndrome

16. Smoking. Encourage stopping or at least reduction in smoking if the woman smokes. Women who smoke have an increased risk for perinatal mortality, fetal wastage, premature labor and delivery, and small-for-gestational-age babies.

17. Medicines. Avoid all medicines and drugs, including aspirin and BC Powder, except those prescribed by the nurse-midwife or physician working with the nurse-midwife. Over-the-counter drugs or any prescription obtained from any other physician for any other condition should be discussed with the nurse-midwife before taking.

18. Immunizations. In 1973 the American College of Obstetricians and Gynecologists made recommendations regarding specific immunizations during pregnancy. The following lists a few immunizations women are apt to ask about and gives their recommendations:

    a. rubella — contraindicated
    b. mumps — contraindicated
    c. influenza — only if there is serious underlying disease; refer to a physician
    d. poliomyelitis — only in an epidemic and then it is mandatory
    e. tetanus and diphtheria — only if the woman has never had a series or has not had a booster within ten years. It is not a routine part of antepartal care to bring a woman up-to-date in her immunizations during this time nor is it recommended
    f. immunizations for foreign travel — the nurse-midwife should check with the consulting physician regarding the specific immunization(s) the woman says she needs to meet requirements for wherever she is planning to travel

19. Nutrition. See Chapter 8.

20. Food cravings/pica. Of no concern as long as the diet is otherwise nutritionally adequate and the pica intake is no more than moderate. Food cravings (e.g., pickles and ice cream) are usually transient. Pica, involving a craving for clay or dirt (or laundry starch if the others are not available), is basically sociocultural in origin and is best indulged in limited quantities, if possible, in order to not interfere with a nutritious diet.

21. Rest. In addition to whatever amount of sleep the individual needs, she should have periodic rest periods during the day, preferably with her feet elevated. She should avoid sitting or standing for prolonged periods of time.

22. Exercise and activity. Whatever the woman is *accustomed to*, stopping short of fatigue — never excessive. No other limits if the woman is experienced in whatever form of exercise she wishes to pursue. It is not the time, however, to be learning new

strenuous sports, e.g., skiing, skydiving. Daily exercise such as walking outdoors is good for mental health, relaxation, bowels, and muscle conditioning.

23. Work. At the woman's discretion within the following limits and recommendations:
    a. provision for a rest period approximately every 2 hours (this is the same as a lunch period and a morning and afternoon break on a day shift)
    b. not to the extent of fatigue
    c. avoid severe physical strain
    d. to be reassessed in the event any complications develop

24. Body mechanics
    a. posture
    b. lifting (see low back pain earlier in this chapter)
    c. getting up from a supine position:
       (1) bend knees
       (2) turn to side
       (3) push up with arms to a sitting position

25. Bathing
    a. no hot baths — exhausting
    b. no cold baths — chilling
    c. shower or tub bath a matter of personal preference and choice
    d. later in pregnancy a shower may be safer than a tub bath because of awkwardness from change of center of gravity and balance — be sure the shower has a nonskid floor

26. Sexual intercourse
    a. changes in position to accommodate enlarged abdomen
    b. alternative methods of satisfying male and female sexual needs
    c. alleviation of any unnecessary concerns or fears regarding harming the baby with sexual intercourse
    d. abstinence if necessary, e.g., suspected premature rupture of membranes, bleeding, bleeding and cramps in first trimester

27. Travel
    a. as desired if pregnancy is progressing normally
    b. need for periodic walking (every 2 hours) to encourage circulation and avoid venous stasis
    c. if close to term, have alternative plans for delivery wherever she might be and plans for any emergencies en route

28. Preparation for childbirth and parenthood. Encourage attending classes for this (Fig. 7-5). The general areas of content may include:
    a. reproductive anatomy; bodily changes during pregnancy and related discomforts and relief measures
    b. exercises to promote relaxation (Fig. 7-6), to relieve discomforts, for use during labor, positioning, breathing exercises for working with contractions, for conditioning specific muscle groups, posture, body mechanics
    c. nutrition
    d. fetal growth and development
    e. signs of impending labor; process and progress of labor; comfort measures; where to go, what to do, what to take to the hospital, what to expect
    f. breast preparation for those planning to breast-feed
    g. preparations for baby in the home, what to bring to the hospital for taking baby home, basics of baby care
    h. general hygiene, for example, breast care, perineal care, bowel habits
    i. potential problems: danger signs, what to do, prevention
    j. postpartal course, adjustments, what to expect in the hospital (individualize to the hospital), sibling rivalry, 4- to 6-weeks checkup
    k. response to concerns, questions, and so forth

29. Sibling preparation for birth

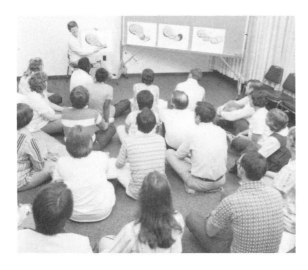

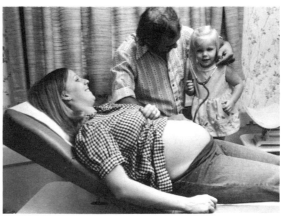

FIGURE 7-7   Sibling listening to fetal heart tones.

FIGURE 7-5. A nurse-midwife teaching childbirth education class.

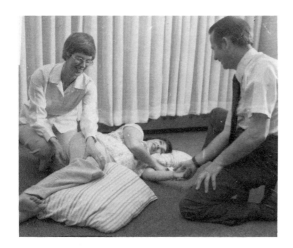

FIGURE 7-6. A nurse-midwife helping a couple with relaxation exercise.

a. select adult sibling attendant
b. attend classes for sibling, sibling attendant, and parents
c. involve sibling in antepartal visits (Fig. 7-7) according to age level (e.g., listen to fetal heart, feel fetal movement, feel baby parts)
d. involve sibling in baby preparations
30. Superstitions and "old wive's tales" — dissuade with facts, reason, and understanding
31. Breathing and relaxation exercises. Teach or reinforce what is learned in the preparation for childbearing and parenthood classes she is attending
32. La Leche League meetings. Encourage attending a series of meetings. This is a particularly good antepartal learning experience for a woman who plans to breast-feed, especially if this will be her first breast-feeding experience. The practical tips and observing of breast-feeding answer many questions as well as provide an opportunity to see individual variations of nursing and mother-baby interactions. La Leche League members also provide a known source of help if needed after birth.
33. Signs and symptoms of labor and when to call the nurse-midwife and/or come to the hospital or birth center
34. Preparations for coming to the hospital

or birth center, for example, what to pack for self and baby, where to go, admissions procedures, what to expect, and so forth

35. What to do in the event of emergency childbirth
36. Baby preparations
    a. supplies, furniture, equipment, clothing
    b. purchase and installation of infant car seat
    c. what to bring to the hospital or birth center for taking baby home
    d. decision regarding method of infant feeding (i.e., by breast or bottle)
    e. preparation of couple for changes in life necessitated by a baby
    f. preparation of siblings for baby's arrival and presence in the home
    g. care of siblings during intrapartal and immediate postpartal period

REFERENCE

1. *ICEA Position Paper: Diagnostic Ultrasound in Obstetrics*. International Childbirth Education Association, March, 1983.
2. Roberts, J. E. Priorities in prenatal education. *J. Obstet. Gynecol. Nurs* (May/June) 1976, pp. 17–20.

BIBLIOGRAPHY

Alexander, D. Prenatal detection of genetic disease by amniocentesis. *Contemporary OB/GYN* 10:44, 1977.

Aladjem, S., and Brown, A. K. (Eds.). *Clinical Perinatology*. St. Louis: Mosby, 1974.

Anderson, G. Conditions which may affect estriol excretion in pregnancy. *PCC (Perinatal Coordinating Center) News* Vol. I, No. 2, February, 1975, p. 2.

Anderson, G. Interpretation of the oxytocin challenge test (OCT). *PCC (Perinatal Coordinating Center) News* Vol. I, No. 7, July, 1975, p. 2.

Anderson, G. The oxytocin challenge test. *PCC (Perinatal Coordinating Center) News* Vol. I, No. 6, June, 1975, p. 1.

Anderson, G. Urinary estriols: frequency and interpretation. *PCC (Perinatal Coordinating Center) News* Vol. I, No. 3, March, 1975, p. 3.

Anderson, G. G. Postmaturity: a review. *Obstet. Gynecol. Surv.* 27:65, 1972.

Atlay, R. D., Gillison, E. W., and Horton, A. L. A fresh look at pregnancy heartburn. *J. Obstet. Gynaecol. Br. Comm.* 80:63, 1973.

Aubry, R. H. et al. The lecithin/sphingomyelin ratio in a high-risk obstetric population. *Obstet. Gynecol.* 47:21, 1976.

Babson, S. G. Benson, M. L., and Benda, G. I. *Management of High-Risk Pregnancy and Intensive Care of the Neonate*. St. Louis: Mosby, 1975.

Betz, G., and Hagerman,D. D. Increased urinary estriol excretion without change in blood estriol concentration resulting from bed rest in the third trimester of pregnancy in the human. *Gynecol. Invest.* 4:288, 1973.

Catz, C. S., and Abuelo, D. Drugs and pregnancy. *Drug Therapy* April, 1974, p. 79.

Chez, R. A. (Moderator). Symposium: sex in pregnancy. *Contemporary OB/GYN* 6:99, 1975.

Coleman, C. A. Fetal movement counts: An assessment tool. *J. Nurse-Midwifery* 26(1):15–23 (January/February) 1981.

Cooper, J., Soffronoff, E., and Bolgnese, R. Oxytocin challenge test in monitoring high-risk pregnancies. *Obstet. Gynecol.* 45:27, 1975.

Cranley, J. J. Managing varicose veins in pregnancy. *Contemporary OB/GYN* 7:139, 1976.

Creasy, R. K., and Resnik, R. *Maternal Fetal Medicine: Principles and Practice*. Philadelphia: W. B. Saunders, 1984.

Danforth, D. N. (Ed.). *Obstetrics and Gynecology, 4th*. Philadelphia: Harper & Row, 1982.

Daniels, M. B. The birth experience for the sibling: Description and evaluation of a program. *J. Nurse-Midwifery* 28(5):15–22 (September/October) 1983.

Diamond, F. High-risk pregnancy screening techniques. *J. Obstet. Gynecol. Neonat. Nurs.* 7:15, 1978.

Doran, T. A. et al. Amniotic fluid tests for fetal maturity. *Am. J. Obstet. Gynecol.* 119:829, 1974.

Doust, B. D. Role of ultrasound in obstetrics and gynecology. *Hosp. Prac.* 8(10):143, 1973.

Ewing, D., Farina, J., and Otterson, W. Clinical application of the oxytocin challenge test. *Obstet. Gynecol.* 45:563, 1974.

Ewy, D., and Ewy, R. *Preparation for Breast Feeding*. Garden City, N. Y.: Dolphin Books, Doubleday, 1975.

Fischer, S., Fullerton, J. T., and Trezise, L. Fetal movement and fetal outcome in a low-risk population. *J. Nurse-Midwifery* 26(1):24–30 (January/February) 1981.

Fitzhugh, M. L., and Newton, M. Posture in pregnancy. *Am. J. Obstet. Gynecol.* 85:1091, 1963.

Freeman, R. K., and Kreitzer, M. S. Current concepts in antepartum and intrapartum fetal evaluation, *Curr. Prob. Ped.* 2(9):3, 1972.

Freeman, R. K. The use of oxytocin challenge test for antepartal clinical evaluation of uteroplacental respiratory function, *Am. J. Obstet. Gynecol.* 121:481, 1975.

Gaziano, E. P., Hill, D. L., and Freeman, D. W. The oxytocin challenge test in the management of high risk pregnancies. *Am. J. Obstet. Gynecol.* 121:947, 1975.

Gohari, F., Berkowitz, R., and Hobbins, J. C. Prediction of intrauterine growth retardation by determination of total intrauterine volume. *Am. J. Obstet. Gynecol.* 127(3):255–260, February 1, 1977.

Gonzalez, F. A. Ultrasound. *J. Nurse-Midwifery* 29(6):391–394 (November/December) 1984.

Grannum, P. A. T., Berkowitz, R. L., and Hobbins, J. C. The ultrasonic changes in the mature placenta and their relation to fetal pulmonic maturity. *Am. J. Obstet. Gynecol.* 133(8):915–922, April 15, 1979.

Haire, D. Fetal effects of ultrasound: A growing controversy. *J. Nurse-Midwifery* 29(4):241–246 (July/August) 1984.

Haire, D. *The Pregnant Patient's Bill of Rights.* New York: The Committee on Patient's Rights, 1974.

Henahan, J. F. What to tell your pregnant patient about drinking: Don't, *Mod. Med.* April 15, 1977, p. 29.

Hobbins, J. C. et al. Ultrasound in the diagnosis of congenital anomalies. *Am. J. Obstet. Gynecol.* 134:331, 1979.

Hobbins, J. C., Winsberg, F., and Berkowitz, R. L. *Ultrasonography in Obstetrics and Gynecology, 2nd.* Baltimore: Williams & Wilkins, 1983.

Hogan, K., and Tcheng, D. The role of the nurse during amniocentesis. *J. Obstet. Gynecol. Neonat. Nurs.* 7:24, 1978.

Holtzman, L. C. Sexual practices during pregnancy. *J. Nurse-Midwifery* 21:29, 1976.

Horger, E. O., III, and McCarter, L. M. Diagnostic ultrasound in obstetrics and gynecology. *J. S. Carolina Med. Assoc.* 71:154, 1975.

ICEA Position Paper: Diagnostic Ultrasound in Obstetrics. International Childbirth Education Association, March, 1983.

Kier, J. *Woman's Guide to a Stress-Free Pregnancy and Creative Childbirth.* Houston, Texas: Butterfly Books, 1985.

Kitzinger, S. *The Complete Book of Pregnancy and Childbirth.* New York: Knopf, 1980.

Kohorn, E. I., and Kaufman, M. Sonar in the first trimester of pregnancy. *Obstet. Gynecol.* 44:473, 1974.

Leader, L. R., Baillie, P., and Van Schalkwyk, D. J. Fetal movements and fetal outcome: A prospective study. *Obstet. Gynecol.* 57(4):431–436 (April) 1981.

Lee, C., Di Loreto, P. C., and Logrand, B. Fetal activity acceleration determination for the evaluation of fetal reserve. *Obstet. Gynecol.* 48:19, 1976.

Lehrman, E. J. Nurse-midwifery practice: A descriptive study of prenatal care. *J. Nurse-Midwifery* 26(3):27–41 (May/June) 1981.

MacLaughlin, S. M., and Johnston, K. B. The preparation of young children for the birth of a sibling. *J. Nurse-Midwifery* 29(6):371–376 (November/December) 1984.

Malnory, M. E. A prenatal assessment tool for mothers and fathers. *J. Nurse-Midwifery* 27(6):26–34 (November/December) 1982.

Mandelbaum, B. Gestational meconium in the high-risk pregnancy. *Obstet. Gynecol.* 42:87, 1973.

May, K. A. Active involvement of expectant fathers in pregnancy: Some further considerations. *J. Obstet. Gynecol. Nurs.* (March/April) 1978, p. 7.

Midwinter, A. Vomiting in pregnancy. *Practitioner* 206:743, 1971.

Moore, D. S. Prepared childbirth: The pregnant couple and their marriage. *J. Nurse-Midwifery* 22:18, 1977.

National Institutes of Health, Consensus Development Panel. The use of diagnostic ultrasound imaging in pregnancy. *J. Nurse-Midwifery* 29(4):235–239 (July/August) 1984.

Noble, E. *Childbirth with Insight.* Boston: Houghton Mifflin, 1983.

O'Brien, G. D. Fetal femur — a new dimension of growth. *Contemporary OB/GYN* pp. 186–192 (April) 1983.

O'Brien, G. D., and Queenan, J. T. Ultrasound fetal femur length in relation to intrauterine growth retardation, Part II. *Am. J. Obstet. Gynecol.* 144(1):35–39, September 1, 1982.

O'Brien, W. D., Jr. Ultrasonic bioeffects: A view of experimental studies. *Birth* 11(3) (Fall) 1984.

An Overview of Ultrasound: Theory, Measurement, Medical Applications, and Biological Effects. U.S.

Department of Health and Human Services Publication, FDA 82–8190, July, 1982.

Parma, S. A family centered event? Preparing the child for sharing in the experience of childbirth. *J. Nurse-Midwifery* 24(3):5–10 (May/June) 1979.

Petitti, D. B. Effects of in utero ultrasound exposure in humans. *Birth* 11(3) (Fall) 1984.

Preparation for Childbearing, 3rd. New York: Maternity Center Association, 1969.

Pritchard, J. A., MacDonald, P. C., and Gant, N. F. *Williams Obstetrics, 17th.* Norwalk, Conn.: Appleton-Century-Crofts, 1985.

Queenan, J. T., Kubarych, S. F., Griffin, L. P., and Anderson, G. D. Diagnostic ultrasound: Determination of fetal biparietal diameters as an index of gestational age. *J. Kentucky Med. Assoc.* 73:595, 1975.

Queenan, J. T. (Moderator). Symposium: Ultrasound: Diagnostic applications in obstetrics, *Contemporary OB/GYN* 9:74, 1977.

Quinlan, R. W., Cruz, A. C., Buhi, W. C., and Martin, M. Changes in placental ultrasonic appearance. I. Incidence of grade III changes in the placenta in correlation to fetal pulmonary maturity. *Am. J. Obstet. Gynecol.* 144(4):468–470, October 15, 1982.

Quinlan, R. W., Cruz, A. C., Buhi, W. C., and Martin, M. Changes in placental ultrasonic appearance. II. Pathologic significance of grade III placental changes. *Am. J. Obstet. Gynecol.* 144(4):471–473, October 15, 1982.

Ray, M., Freeman, R. K., Pine, S., and Hesselgesser, R. Clinical experience with the oxytocin challenge test. *Am. J. Obstet. Gynecol.* 114:1, 1972.

Roberts, J. E. Priorities in prenatal education. *J. Obstet. Gynecol. Nurs.* May/June, 1976, p. 17.

Roberts, N. S. et al. Mid-trimester amniocentesis: Indications, techniques, risks and potential for prenatal diagnosis, *J. Reprod. Med.* 28:167, 1983.

Roehner, J. Fatherhood: In pregnancy and birth. *J. Nurse-Midwifery* 21:13, 1976.

Sabbagha, R. E. et al. Sonar BPD and fetal age. *Obstet. Gynecol.* 43:7, 1974.

Sadovsky, E. What do movements of the fetus tell about its well-being? *Contemporary OB/GYN* 12:59–67 (December) 1978.

Sadovsky, E., Yaffe, H., and Polishuk, W. Z. Fetal movement monitoring in normal and pathologic pregnancy. *Int. J. Gynaecol. Obstet.* 12(3):75–79, 1974.

Schifrin, B., Lapidus, M., Doctor, G. S., and Leviton, A. Contraction stress test for antepartum fetal evaluation. *Obstet. Gynecol.* 45:433, 1975.

Schneider, J. M. Assessment of fetal well-being — Part I: Oxytocin challenge test. *Perinatal Press,* July/August, 1976, p. 8.

Schreier, A. C. The nurse-midwifery management of physiological edema in pregnancy. *J. Nurse-Midwifery* 21:18, 1976.

Shearer, M. H. Revelations: A summary and analysis of the NIH consensus development conference on ultrasound imaging in pregnancy. *Birth* 11:1–14 (Spring) 1984.

Solberg, D. A., Butler, J., and Wagner, N. N. Sexual behavior in pregnancy. *N. Engl. J. Med.* 288:1098, 1973.

Sorokin, Y., and Dierker, L. J. Fetal movement. *Clin. Obstet. Gynecol.* 25(4):719–734 (December) 1982.

Stenchever, M. A. The use of tobacco and drugs in pregnancy. *Contemporary OB/GYN* 8:13, 1976.

Stone, M. L., Weingold, A. B., and Lee, B. O. Clinical applications of ultrasound in obstetrics and gynecology. *Am. J. Obstet, Gynecol.* 113:1046, 1972.

Summers, L. *Nipple Stimulation to Induce Uterine Contractions for Antepartum Fetal Heart Rate Testing.* Unpublished master's thesis, Yale University School of Nursing, May, 1983.

Tejani, N., Mann, L. I., and Weiss, R. R. Antenatal diagnosis and management of the small-for-gestational-age fetus. *Obstet. Gynecol.* 47:31, 1976.

Tucker, S. M. *Fetal Monitoring and Fetal Assessment in High-Risk Pregnancy.* St. Louis: Mosby, 1978.

Wiedenbach, E. *Family-Centered Maternity Nursing.* New York: Putnam's, 1967.

Williams, B. Sleep needs during the maternity cycle. *Nurs. Outlook* 15(2):53, 1967.

The Womanly Art of Breastfeeding. Franklin Park, Ill.: La Leche League International, 1963.

Wonnell, E. B. The education of the expectant father for childbirth, *Nurs. Clin. North Am.* 6:591, 1971.

Umbeck, K., and Diamond, F. An oxytocin challenge test protocol, *J. Obstet. Gynecol. Nurs.* January/February, 1977, p. 29.

Ziegel, E., and VanBlarcom, C. C. *Obstetric Nursing, 6th.* New York: Macmillan, 1972.

8

Nutritional Intervention in Pregnancy

IMPORTANCE OF NUTRITION

The quality of life is inseparably bound not only to prenatal care in general but also to prenatal and postnatal nutrition and environmental influences specifically. Scrupulous attention to postnatal nutrition, if prenatal nutrition has been inadequate, is like locking the barn door after the horse has been stolen — it is at best a salvage job for what remains.

There appears to be a genetic design for fetal growth and development. This design is in accord with the genetic constitution of the individual fetus; however, it is influenced by maternal factors. Maternal factors cannot improve the genetic design, but some factors prohibit fulfillment of the design. Prohibitive factors include prenatal malnutrition, smoking, and maternal disease.

Birth weight is used as the standard evaluative measurement of a newborn all over the world inasmuch as it is the most accurate and routinely obtained measurement. The import-

ance of the newborn's birth weight and the importance of the factors that influence the birth weight have been identified and enumerated in a number of studies.

Maternal disease may affect the fetus in a number of ways. In relationship to birth weight, maternal disease may result in either a small-for-gestational-age infant (e.g., maternal preeclampsia) or in a large-for-gestational-age infant (e.g., maternal diabetes). Smoking has been correlated with significantly smaller babies by birth weight than the babies of nonsmoking mothers. This is due to interference with metabolic processes.

Many studies focus on the effect of malnutrition on pregnancy outcome. This is because nutrition is a factor in all pregnancies, whereas smoking and maternal disease affect only the babies of mothers who smoke or are ill. The concern, therefore, is in the differences in birth weight when these two factors (smoking and maternal disease) are controlled. These differences in birth weight are directly related to nutrition during pregnancy. Maternal nutritional factors which have been shown to relate to birth weight are (1) prepregnancy weight and (2) weight gain during pregnancy.

One other factor which has an obvious direct correlation with birth weight is gestational age. As the length of gestation increases, there is an increase in birth weight (see Chapter 6). It has also been shown that male babies weigh more than female babies by an average of approximately 144 grams (5 oz) and that birth weight increases with parity.

Other maternal factors have been studied but do not correlate with birth weight when prepregnancy weight, weight gain during pregnancy, maternal disease, and smoking are controlled. The maternal factors which do *not* correlate include age, height, marital status, and income.

Low birth weight (whether by prematurity or by small-for-gestational-age) has been shown to correlate with an increased incidence of the following:

1. Perinatal mortality (stillbirth, neonatal death)
2. Small head circumference
3. Mental retardation
4. Cerebral palsy
5. Learning problems/disabilities
6. Visual and hearing defects
7. Neurologic defects
8. Poor infant growth (stunted) and development

Conversely, a high maternal weight gain has been shown to be associated with an increased birth weight and, therefore, with the following:

1. Reduction in the rate of prematurity
2. Better growth (height and weight) as measured at 8 months and better performance (neurological, motor, and mental) as measured at 12 months in the Collaborative Study of Cerebral Palsy [1]
3. Decreased incidence of the detrimental outcomes associated with low birth weight

Furthermore, brain growth may be directly affected by maternal nutrition. There are two types of cellular growth: (1) hyperplasia, in which there is an increase in the number of cells by cell division, and (2) hypertrophy, in which there is an increase in the size of the existing cells. Malnutrition during either type of cellular growth results in a smaller organ. If malnutrition occurs during hyperplastic growth, the damage is irreversible since the smaller size is due to a reduced number of cells. If malnutrition takes place during hypertrophic growth, the damage is reversible at any time with improved nutrition since the smaller size is due to a lack of increase in the size of the cells. While the details of human brain growth are not known, it is generally thought that the bulk of cellular growth of the brain is from 15 weeks gestation to 2 years of age, with a peak from 28 weeks gestation to 6 months after birth. Most likely this peak period of time in brain growth reflects the second of the sequential three phases of growth: (1) hyperplasia only, (2) combination of hyperplasia and hypertrophy, and (3) hypertrophy only.

Thus the profound effect of malnutrition during gestation becomes obvious. However, the impact becomes even greater when one studies the types of intrauterine growth failure. Two have been identified: (1) uteroplacental insufficiency and (2) malnutrition or, specifically, maternal protein deficiency. In uteroplacental insufficiency, fetal growth retardation is asymmetric, that is, the body and body organs are small but the brain is of normal size with its full complement of cells. In malnutrition, fetal growth retardation is symmetric, that is, the body, body organs, and brain are all reduced both in size and in the number of cells by approximately the same percentage amount. Rat studies show that prenatal malnutrition results in a 15 percent reduction in the number of fetal brain cells, that postnatal malnutrition results in a 15 percent reduction in the number of brain cells, and that a combination of prenatal and postnatal nutrition results not in a 30 percent but in a 60 percent reduction in the number of brain cells.

The meaning of low birth weight in relation to malnutrition needs to be redefined. The traditional definition of prematurity is birth weight below 2500 grams (5 lb 8 oz). However, babies between 2500 and 2999 grams (5 lb 8 oz and 6 lb 10 oz) should also be considered at risk by virtue of low birth weight. Considerable focus has been concentrated on the less-than-2500-gram newborn, and miraculous reduction of mortality has been achieved with the technology to be found in neonatal intensive care units. The high perinatal mortality rate for those weighing less than 2500 grams at birth certainly warrants this attention. But the group of babies weighing between 2500 and 3000 grams at birth gets lost in the shuffle.

While this group shows much less perinatal mortality than the below-2500-gram group, it is still three times higher than the rate for babies weighing between 3000 and 3500 grams (6 lb, 10 oz and 7 lb, 12 oz) at birth. Babies in the 2500- to 2999-gram weight group also show an increased incidence in the detrimental conditions listed earlier for low-birth-weight babies. Thus, 3000 grams, or approximately 6½ pounds, seems to be another critical cut off point, as is 5½ pounds.

The statistics improve considerably in the 3000 to 3499 gram (6 lb 10 oz to 7 lb 12 oz) group of babies. However, the optimum birth weight seems to be between 3500 and 4000 grams (7 lb 12 oz to 8 lb 14 oz), since studies show this group to have an increased incidence of higher intelligence and a decreased incidence of physical disabilities. It also represents the upper end of a continuum reflecting steadily better pregnancy outcome.

As little as 120 grams (4 oz) can make a very real difference in pregnancy outcome. In two separate studies (one comparing private and clinic populations, the other comparing whites and blacks), a 120-gram difference in average birth weight accounted for twice as much perinatal mortality and twice the incidence of low birth weight in the clinic babies and in the black babies. Proper prenatal nutrition

eradicates the differences in outcome in these populations.

It seems that the genetic design not only determines fetal growth potential but also limits fetal growth after that potential has been attained. In other words, increased maternal caloric and nutrient (protein) intake will not result in obese, oversized babies incapable of vaginal delivery if this is not the genetic design. While the pregnancy outcome cannot surpass the potential, it can fall considerably short. For all babies, the determinant of whether that potential is met seems to be nutrition. For some babies there are additional superimposed factors such as maternal disease and smoking. Even then, good maternal nutrition can help ameliorate the effects of these factors.

The tragedy thus lies with the 2500-gram to 3000-gram (5 lb 8 oz to 6 lb 10 oz) group of babies, whose mortality is much lower than the below-2500-gram babies but who are more likely not to have met their genetic potential. Mental retardation and physical disabilities are more common in this group than in neonates weighing over 3000 grams. While the ideal is to strive for birth weights between 3500 and 4000 grams, it is probably more realistic, and certainly a worthy goal, to strive for birth weights above 3000 grams.

It is estimated that approximately 10 percent of the population of the United States is born with mental or physical handicaps or both. Since this is directly related to prenatal malnutrition, improving maternal nutrition to the point of raising birth weights to over 3000 grams would have a profound effect on individual and societal quality of life. Its economic effect would also be felt nationally. One need only compare the cost of providing supplementary food, when needed, to a pregnant woman (less than $100 in 1970) and the estimated gain to society if just one individual is prevented from being severely mentally retarded (approximately $900,000 in 1970). Conley [2] describes in great detail the cost factors related to programs for the mentally retarded. The figures mount into billions of dollars spent each year. Between the cost for an optimal outcome and the cost of caring for the severely metally retarded is the cost to society of those individuals who are not severely mentally retarded but who are functioning mentally and/or physically at a level less than they could have been if their genetic potential had been met. Their potential contribution to society is forever lost. And finally, there are the costs of the emotional and economic burdens borne by the families of those born with mental and/or physical handicaps.

NUTRITIONAL NEEDS

With the foregoing information in mind, it suffices to say that nutrition of the mother is a prime concern in prenatal care. Certain aspects of maternal nutritional needs require specific patient instruction: calories, protein, iron, folic acid, and vitamin C.

Caloric and protein needs go hand-in-hand. This is true because calories are needed in order to protect the protein so that it is not burned for energy. When caloric intake is insufficient it is possible to have a protein deficit even if protein intake is adequate, because the protein will be used for meeting metabolic energy requirements of the mother. A measurement of positive nitrogen balance indicates protein storage. If 90 to 100 percent of the protein intake is being utilized, only a small amount is being stored. The result is a smaller baby. If there is a 30 percent utilization of the protein intake, the remainder is stored and a larger baby will result. A positive nitrogen balance is dependent on both the calorie and protein intake and indicates protein storage. Further, if both calorie and protein intake are so inadequate that fat is catabolized to meet the maternal metabolic energy requirements, maternal acetonuria will occur. This may result in neurological damage of the fetus.

The number of calories and the number of grams of protein a pregnant woman should eat per day have been generalized in the Recommended Daily Dietary Allowances (RDA) of the Food and Nutrition Board of the National Academy of Sciences—National Research Council as an additional 300 calories and an additional 30 grams over the recommended intake for non-pregnant females (Table 8-1). The recommended intake for nonpregnant females varies depending on categories of age ranges and average height and weight figures for each category. However, this number of calories is much too generalized to assure adequate caloric intake for the individual woman. Further, the RDA recommendation for protein (total of 74 to 76 grams per day) is less than the amount advocated by many researchers and clinicians. They recommend 85 to 90 grams of protein per day and even more for the pregnant adolescent. The obvious conclusion is that caloric and protein intake needs to be calculated for each individual in order to result in optimal pregnancy outcome. This calculation is described later in this chapter. Gone forever should be the days of dietary restrictions, nagging and scolding of the woman for weight gain, calculations of ideal weight gains based on the weight by trimester of the products of conception and pregnancy components, and reducing diets for maternal obesity.

It also has been shown that protein intake indicates the adequacy of the diet in general. In other words, if the protein intake is adequate most of the other necessary dietary nutrients are also adequate, including vitamins and minerals. The exceptions to this generalization during pregnancy are iron and folic acid.

It is generally accepted that all pregnant women should receive iron supplementation in the form of ferrous iron in the amount of 30 to 60 milligrams daily during the second and third trimesters. This amount of iron is needed to meet the demands for both maternal and fetal hemoglobin synthesis. Most women do not have iron stores adequate to meet this demand, and further dietary intake is insuf-

Table 8-1. Recommended Daily Dietary Allowances

| | Nonpregnant Females | | | | | |
	11–14 yr*	15–18 yr†	19–22 yr†	23–50 yr†	Pregnancy	Lactation
Energy (kcal)	2,200	2,100	2,100	2,000	+ 300	+ 500
Protein (gm)	46	46	44	44	+ 30	+ 20
Vitamin A (μg RE)‡	800	800	800	800	+ 200	+ 400
Vitamin D (μg)§	10	10	7.5	5	+ 5	+ 5
Vitamin E (mg α-TE)‖	8	8	8	8	+ 2	+ 3
Ascorbic acid (mg)	50	60	60	60	+ 20	+ 40
Folacin (μg)**	400	400	400	400	+ 400	+ 100
Niacin (mg NE)***	15	14	14	13	+ 2	+ 5
Riboflavin (mg)	1.3	1.3	1.3	1.2	+ 0.3	+ 0.5
Thiamin (mg)	1.1	1.1	1.1	1.0	+ 0.4	+ 0.5
Vitamin B_6 (mg)	1.8	2.0	2.0	2.0	+ 0.6	+ 0.5
Vitamin B_{12} (μg)	3	3	3	3	+ 1.0	+ 1.0
Calcium (mg)	1,200	1,200	800	800	+ 400	+ 400
Phosphorus (mg)	1,200	1,200	800	800	+ 400	+ 400
Iodine (μg)	150	150	150	150	+ 25	+ 50
Iron (mg)	18	18	18	18	§§	§§
Magnesium (mg)	300	300	300	300	+ 150	+ 150
Zinc (mg)	15	15	15	15	+ 5	+ 10

From the Food and Nutrition Board, National Academy of Sciences–National Research Council, ed. 9, 1980.
* Weight 46 kg (101 lb), height 157 cm (62 in)
† Weight 55 kg (120 lb), height 163 cm (64 in)
‡ Retinol equivalents. 1 retinol equivalent = 1 μg retinol or 6 μg β carotene.
§ As cholecalciferol. 10 μg cholecalciferol = 400 IU of vitamin D.
‖ α-tocopherol equivalents. 1 mg d-α tocopherol = 1 α-TE.
** The folacin allowances refer to dietary sources as determined by *Lactobacillus casei* assay after treatment with enzymes (conjugases) to make polyglutamyl forms of the vitamin available to the test organism.
*** 1 NE (niacin equivalent) is equal to 1 mg of niacin or 60 mg of dietary tryptophan.
§§ The increased requirement during pregnancy cannot be met by the iron content of habitual American diets nor by the existing iron stores of many women; therefore the use of 30–60 mg of supplemental iron is recommended. Iron needs during lactation are not substantially different from those of nonpregnant women, but continued supplementation of the mother for 2-3 months after parturition is advisable in order to replenish stores depleted by pregnancy.

ficient to do so. Some clinicians, however, believe that well-nourished pregnant women do not need iron and vitamin supplementation. Supplemental iron reduces the incidence of iron deficiency anemia. Folic acid supplementation in the amount of an additional 200 to 400 micrograms, or a total of 0.4 to 0.8 milligrams daily, reduces considerably the incidence of megaloblastic anemia. Vitamin C, 250 milligrams daily, taken in conjunction with iron supplements, with enhance iron absorption and may be prophylactic for post-partal hemorrhage.

The long-held practice of routinely restricting sodium intake during pregnancy or as part of the treatment for preeclampsia has been severely questioned and is considered passé. Restriction of sodium intake combined with the use of diuretics is potentially dangerous. Such practice is not considered safe management of pregnant women unless medical complications are present which in the nonpregnant state include this practice as part of the treatment regimen. During pregnancy the body establishes a compensatory mechanism in order to conserve sodium, which would otherwise be excessively lost with resulting electrolyte imbalance because of a 50 percent increase in glomerular filtration rate. If, at the same time the system is trying to conserve sodium from normal physiological processes, it is further insulted by dietary restriction, the mechanism is compromised through overwork.

When a person is overweight, her diet must be analyzed to ascertain if the overweight is due to edema only, fat only, or a combination of the two. Overweight due to fat is caused by too many calories. Overweight as a result of edema most likely is due to inadequate protein and caloric intake. It may well be that increased protein and calories will reduce the incidence of preeclampsia and eclampsia.

INTERVENTION METHODOLOGY*

The method presented here is known as the *Higgins Intervention Method for Nutritional Rehabilitation during Pregnancy.* Its usability has been demonstrated by the staff of the Montreal Diet Dispensary and by others who have been taught the method. Its effectiveness has been clearly shown in studies of the pregnancy outcome of those receiving the services of the Montreal Diet Dispensary both at the Diet Dispensary and at the Royal Victoria Hospital Maternity Clinics in Montreal.

The Higgins Intervention Method uses the 1948 Canadian Dietary Standard (CDS), approved by the Canadian Council on Nutrition (Table 8–2), as a baseline for establishing

---

* This method is presented with the permission of Mrs. Agnes Higgins, (retired) Executive Director of the Montreal Diet Dispersary, Montreal, Quebec, Canada.

what the client's nonpregnant calorie and protein intake should be. The CDS determines caloric and protein intake on the basis of (1) ideal body weight and (2) individual activity level. This method of establishing the recommended intake is more specific than the U.S. RDA and has a profound effect on caloric and protein levels as can be noted by comparing the two. After adding the pregnancy allowance, the resulting total amounts of calories and protein vary much more when using the CDS and are more in accord for the individual. Ideal body weight is determined by using the actuarial tables of the Metropolitan Life Insurance Company for desirable weights of women, based on height and body frame (Table 8-3). Individual activity level is a subjective evaluation.

Determination of Calorie and Protein Requirements

Determination of calorie and protein requirements according to the Higgins Intervention Method consist of the normal requirements plus additional corrective allowances. The method is applied as follows:

1. Collection of baseline data:
   a. age
   b. height
   c. body frame
   d. nonpregnant weight
   e. weeks gestation
   f. present weight
   g. activity level
   h. present dietary intake
   i. existence of any of the following conditions:
      (1) pernicious vomiting
      (2) pregnancy spacing less than 1 year apart
      (3) poor obstetrical history (stillbirths, spontaneous abortions, preterm babies)

Table 8-2. Canadian Dietary Standard for Female Adults*

Ideal Body Weight (lb)	Sedentary Activities		Moderate Activities		Heavy Activities	
	Calories	Protein	Calories	Protein	Calories	Protein
80	1600	40	1900	40	2400	40
85	1650	43	1950	43	2450	43
90	1700	45	2000	45	2500	45
95	1750	48	2050	48	2550	48
100	1800	50	2100	50	2600	50
105	1875	51	2175	51	2675	51
110	1950	53	2250	53	2750	53
115	2025	54	2325	54	2825	54
120	2100	55	2400	55	2900	55
125	2150	57	2450	57	2950	57
130	2200	58	2500	58	3000	58
135	2250	59	2550	59	3050	59
140	2300	60	2600	60	3100	60
145	2350	63	2650	63	3150	63
150	2400	65	2700	65	3200	65
155	2450	68	2750	68	3250	68
160	2500	70	2800	70	3300	70

* 1948

Table 8-3. Desirable Weights for Women*

Height (includes 2-inch heels)	Small Frame (range in pounds and average)	Medium Frame (range in pounds and average)	Large Frame (range in pounds and average)
4'10"	92−98 (95)	96−107 (101.5)	104−119 (111.5)
4'11"	94−101 (97.5)	98−110 (104)	106−122 (114)
5'0"	96−104 (100)	101−113 (107)	109−125 (117)
5'1"	99−107 (103)	104−116 (110)	112−128 (120)
5'2"	102−110 (106)	107−119 (113)	115−131 (123)
5'3"	105−113 (109)	110−122 (116)	118−134 (126)
5'4"	108−116 (112)	113−126 (119.5)	121−138 (129.5)
5'5"	111−119 (115)	116−130 (123)	125−142 (133.5)
5'6"	114−123 (118.5)	120−135 (127.5)	129−146 (137.5)
5'7"	118−127 (122.5)	124−139 (131.5)	133−150 (141.5)
5'8"	122−131 (126.5)	128−143 (135.5)	137−154 (145.5)
5'9"	126−135 (130.5)	132−147 (139.5)	141−158 (149.5)
5'10"	130−140 (135)	136−151 (143.5)	145−163 (154)
5'11"	134−144 (139)	140−155 (147.5)	149−168 (158.5)
6'0"	138−148 (143)	144−159 (155.5)	153−173 (163)

* 1959 Actuarial Tables. Courtesy of the Metropolitan Life Insurance Company.

(4) failure to gain 10 pounds by the twentieth week of gestation

(5) serious emotional upset or problems

2. Determination of normal requirements:

a. If the mother is 20 years of age or more:

(1) The client's height and body frame is applied to the Table of Desirable Weights for Women* (Table 8-3) and the ideal weight based on these data is ascertained.

(2) The client's ideal weight, as determined in (1), and her activity level are now applied to the Canadian Dietary Standard (Table 8-2) and the woman's nonpregnant calorie and protein requirements are ascertained.

(3) After 20 weeks gestation, 500 calories and 25 grams of protein are added to the daily nonpregnant calorie and protein requirements of the woman as determined above. These now become her normal pregnancy calorie and protein requirements. If the pregnancy is a multiple gestation, 500 calories and 25 grams of protein are added for each fetus.

b. If the mother is 19 years of age or less:

(1) The client's age is applied to Table 8-4, taken from the 1958 U.S. RDA. (Note that both the calorie and protein allowance for these ages were higher in 1958 than in the 1980 U.S. RDA reported in Table 8-1.) This determines the woman's nonpregnant calorie and protein requirements. This use of higher nonpregnant calorie and protein requirements as

the baseline for adolescent pregnancy is in keeping with the fact that the dietary requirements for pregnancy are superimposed on the adolescent's own dietary requirements for this period of growth in her life. It must be remembered that the nonpregnant adolescent would normally be gaining weight as a reflection of her own growth; the averages are shown in Table 8-5. Therefore, weight gain during and after the adolescent's pregnancy must be evaluated in view of what she normally would gain if she were not pregnant.

(2) After 20 weeks gestation, 500 calories and 25 grams of protein are added to the daily nonpregnant requirements of the woman as determined above. These now become her normal pregnancy calorie and protein requirements. If the pregnancy is a multiple gestation, 500 calories and 25 grams of protein are added for each fetus.

3. Determination of additional corrective allowances: Additional corrective allowances of calories and protein are given for three categories of identifiable nutritional conditions which may adversely affect pregnancy outcome if not considered: (1) undernutrition, (2) underweight, (3) nutritional stress. Each requires a separate addition to the daily normal pregnancy requirements for protein and calories.

a. Undernutrition — Assessment and Corrective allowance.

Undernutrition is defined as a deficit in protein between the normal pregnancy protein requirements for an individual woman and her actual dietary intake of protein as determined by calculations performed on the data collected from a diet history described later in this chapter. The corrective allowance is as

---

* In using this table be sure to use the height figure 2 inches taller than your client measures in her stocking feet, since the heights in the table include shoes with 2-inch heels. For example, if your client measures 5'4" in her stocking feet, use the line of figures for 5'6" in the table.

follows:

(1) *protein* — the number of grams of protein deficit is added to the daily normal pregnancy requirements for protein

(2) *calories* — for each gram of protein deficit, 10 calories are added to the daily normal pregnancy requirements for calories (i.e., 10 calories × the number of grams of protein deficit = the total calorie addition)

b. Underweight — Assessment and Corrective Allowance.

Underweight is defined as the mother's prepregnant weight being 5 percent or more under the ideal weight as determined above from the Table of Desirable Weights. The corrective allowance is as follows:

(1) *protein* — 20 grams per day

(2) *calories* — 500 calories per day

Both the protein and calorie corrections are added to the daily normal pregnancy requirements for protein and calories. This corrective allowance of protein and calories will permit an additional weight gain of 1 pound per week and should be continued for the number of weeks equivalent to the number of pounds the mother was underweight prior to conception. The allowance may be cut in half if needed for a weight gain of 1/2 pound per week or increased to a maximum addition of 1000 calories and 40 grams protein daily if a weight gain of 2 pounds per week is needed in order to make up the deficit by the time of delivery.

c. Nutritional Stress — Assessment and Corrective Allowance:

Nutritional stress is defined as the existence of one or more of the following conditions:

(1) pernicious vomiting

(2) pregnancy spacing less than 1 year apart

Table 8-4. Calorie and Protein Requirements for Women under 19, U.S. RDA

Age	Calories	Protein
13–15	2600	80 grams
16–19	2400	75 grams

From the Food and Nutrition Board, National Academy of Sciences—National Research Council, 1958.

Table 8-5. Average Nonpregnant Adolescent Female Weight Gain

Age	Average Weight Gain per Year
11–13	11 lb
13–15	8 lb
15–17	3 lb
17–19	1 lb

(3) poor obstetrical history

(4) failure to gain 10 pounds by the twentieth week of gestation

(5) serious emotional upset or problems

The corrective allowance is an additional 200 calories and 20 grams protein for each stress condition present (up to a maximum allowance of 400 calories and 40 grams protein) to be added to the daily normal pregnancy requirements for protein and calories.

4. The foregoing calculations may be summarized as in Table 8-6 for ease in totaling the woman's daily caloric and protein requirements.

Evaluation of Dietary Adequacy, and Nutrition Counseling

In order to evaluate dietary adequacy, a 24-hour recall diet history is taken. This is cross-checked against the client's responses to a list of common foods and food categories (e.g., citrus fruits) and, if necessary, further checked by questioning about food purchasing (i.e., what foods and in what amounts for how

Table 8-6. Summary Format for Calculating Calorie and Protein Requirements during Pregnancy

	Calories	Protein (gm)
Nonpregnant requirements	____	____
Addition for pregnancy (after 20th week)	500	25
Undernutrition corrective allowance	____	____
Underweight corrective allowance	____	____
Nutritional stress corrective allowance	____	____
Total	____	____

many people). The daily number of calories and grams of protein in the woman's diet is then determined by calculations based on the information obtained from the standard food composition table. These figures are then used to compare the woman's usual actual calorie and protein intake against her requirements as discussed earlier in this chapter.

Nutrition counseling is most effective when the dietary patterns and eating habits of the mother are changed as little as possible. Milk primarily is used to make up any deficiency between the woman's intake and her calorie and protein requirements. Peanut butter, cheese, bread, and eggs can also be used to meet calorie and protein requirements. Nutrition counseling includes attempting to motivate the woman to follow her diet. Telling her that she is drinking the supplementary milk to "feed her baby" is helpful in relation to any negative feelings she might have about drinking milk and also in discouraging her from giving it to other children in the family if the milk is obtained through WIC.

Mrs. Higgins suggests that a mother-to-be mark the milk cartons with B for baby. This reinforces the idea of feeding her baby. She knows the baby is fed milk after being born, so it usually makes sense to her that her baby needs milk before being born as well. Mrs.

Higgins has been quite successful in motivating clients at the Montreal Diet Dispensary by promoting the concept of the mother's having "a blue-ribbon baby." The nutritionists at the Montreal Diet Dispensary make a home visit to each client to establish a friendly contact, to evaluate the home situation as to food storage and preparation facilities (e.g., refrigerator, stove, running water), and to ascertain the response of other family members to the pregnancy.

After the initial visit and calculations the woman's diet is periodically reviewed utilizing a 24-hour recall diet history. The nurse-midwife, at the very least, should completely reevaluate the woman nutritionally at critical nutritional points during the pregnancy. For example, a woman first seen during the first trimester should have a nutritional reevaluation as follows:

1. 20 weeks gestation — the diet is recalculated at this time so the pregnancy allowance of 500 calories and 25 grams protein can be added.
2. 28 weeks — the peak in cellular growth of the brain is starting.
3. 36 weeks — for encouragement through the last critical month of pregnancy and to provide a total evaluation of the woman's well-being since she is also being reevaluated obstetrically at this time.

REFERENCES

1. Singer, J. E., Westphal, M., and Niswander, K. Relationship of weight gain during pregnancy to birth weight and infant growth and development in the first year of life: A report from the collaborative study of cerebral palsy. *Obstet. Gynecol.* 31:417, 1968.
2. Conley, R. W. *The Economics of Mental Retardation.* Baltimore: Johns Hopkins University Press, 1973.

BIBLIOGRAPHY

Brewer, G. S. *What Every Pregnant Woman Should Know: The Truth about Diets and Drugs in Pregnancy.* New York: Random House, 1977.

Brewer, T. H. Human maternal-fetal nutrition. *Obstet. Gynecol.* 40:868, 1972.

Brewer, T. H. *Metabolic Toxemia of Late Pregnancy.* Springfield, Ill.: Thomas, 1966.

Calloway, D., and King, J. University of California (Berkeley) study, In *Nutritional Supplementation and the Outcome of Pregnancy,* Proceedings of a Workshop, November 3–5, 1971. Washington, D.C.: National Academy of Sciences, 1973.

Chesley, L. C. *Hypertensive Disorders in Pregnancy.* New York: Appleton-Century-Crofts, 1978.

Churchill, J. A. et al. Birth weight and intelligence. *Obstet. Gynecol.* 28:425, 1966.

Committee on Nutrition. *Nutrition in Maternal Health Care.* Chicago: American College of Obstetricians and Gynecologists, 1974.

Conley, R. W. *The Economics of Mental Retardation.* Baltimore: Johns Hopkins University Press, 1973.

Corbett, M. A., and Burst, H. V. Nurse-midwives and adolescents: The South Carolina experience. *J. Nurse-Midwifery* 21(4):13–17 (Winter) 1976.

Corbett, M. A., and Burst, H. V. Nutritional intervention in pregnancy. *J. Nurse-Midwifery* 28(4): 23–29 (July/August) 1983.

Dobbing, J. Effects of malnutrition on learning and behavior in experimental animals. In Scrimshaw, N. S., and Gordon, J. E. (Eds.), *Malnutrition, Learning, and Behavior.* Cambridge, Mass: MIT Press, 1968.

Dobbing, J. Undernutrition and the developing brain, *Am. J. Dis. Child.* 120:411, 1970.

Gazella, J. G. *Nutrition for the Childbearing Years.* Wayzata, Minn.: Woodland, 1979.

Harvie, F. H. (Ed.). *Pediatric Methods and Standards,* 4th. Philadelphia: Lea and Febiger, 1972.

Higgins, A. C. A preliminary report of a nutrition study on public maternity patients: 1963–1972, unpublished report, 1973.

Higgins, A. C. Montreal diet dispensary study, In *Nutritional Supplementation and the Outcome of Pregnancy,* Proceedings of a Workshop, November 3–5, 1971. Washington, D.C.: National Academy of Sciences, 1973.

Higgins, A. C. Nutritional status and the outcome of pregnancy. *J. Can. Diet. Assoc.* 37:17, 1976.

Institute of Medicine. *Preventing Low Birthweight.* Washington, D.C.: National Academy Press, 1985.

Jacobson, H. N. Current concepts in nutrition: Diet in pregnancy. *N. Engl. J. Med.* 297:1051, 1977.

Jeans, P. C. et al. Incidence of prematurity in relation to maternal nutrition. *J. Am. Diet. Assoc.* 31:576, 1955.

Love, E. J., and Kinch, R. A. H. Factors influencing the birth weight in normal pregnancy. *Am. J. Obstet. Gynecol.* 91:342, 1965.

Maternal Nutrition and the Course of Pregnancy: Summary Report. Committee of Maternal Nutrition, Food and Nutrition Board, National Research Council, National Academy of Sciences. Washington, D.C.: U.S. Department of Health, Education and Welfare, 1970.

Nutritional Supplementation and the Outcome of Pregnancy, Proceedings of a Workshop, November 3–5, 1971. Committee on Maternal Nutrition, Food and Nutrition Board, National Research Council. Washington, D.C.: National Academy of Sciences, 1973.

Piechnik, S. L., and Corbett, M. A. Reducing low birth weight among socioeconomically high-risk adolescent pregnancies: Successful intervention with certified nurse-midwife-managed care and a multidisciplinary team. *J. Nurse-Midwifery* 30(2):88–98 (March/April) 1985.

Pipes, P. L. *Nutrition in Infancy and Childhood.* St. Louis: Mosby, 1977.

Pitkin, R. M. et al. Maternal nutrition: A selective review of clinical topics. *Obstet. Gynecol.* 40:773, 1972.

Primrose, T., and Higgins, A. A study in human antepartum nutrition, *J. Reprod. Med.* 7:251, 1971.

Problems of Nutrition in the Perinatal period. Report of the Sixtieth Ross Conference on Pediatric Research. Columbus, Ohio: Ross Laboratories, 1970.

Robinson, M. Salt in pregnancy, *Lancet* 1:178, 1958.

Sameroff, A. J., and Chandler, M. J. Reproductive risk and the continuum of caretaking casualty , In Horowitz, F. (Ed.). *Review of Child Development Research.* Chicago: University of Chicago Press, 1975.

Singer, J. E., Westphal, M., and Niswander, K. Relationship of weight gain during pregnancy to birth weight and infant growth and development in the first year of life: A report from the collaborative study of cerebral palsy, *Obstet. Gynecol.* 31:417, 1968.

Smoking and pregnancy, In *Health Consequences of Smoking: A Report of the Surgeon General*. Washington, D.C.: U.S. Department of Health, Education and Welfare, 1971.

Subcommittee on Nutrition, Brain Development, and Behavior of the Committee on International Nutrition Programs. *The Relationship of Nutrition to Brain Development and Behavior*. Food and Nutrition Board, National Research Council. Washington, D.C.: National Academy of Sciences, 1973.

Susser, M., and Rush, D. New York—Columbia University study, In *Nutritional Supplementation and the Outcome of Pregnancy*, Proceedings of a Workshop, November 3–5, 1971. Washington, D.C.: National Academy of Sciences, 1973.

Tanner, J. M. Physical growth and development, In Forfar, J. O., and Arneil, G. C. (Eds.). *Textbook of Paediatrics*. London: Churchill Livingstone, 1973.

Tompkins, W. T., and Wiehl, D. G. Nutrition and nutritiona deficiencies as related to the premature. *Ped. Clin. North Am.* 1:687, 1954.

Underwood, P. B. et al. Parental smoking empirically related to pregnancy outcome. *Obstet. Gynecol.* 29:1, 1967.

Warkany, J. The importance of prenatal diet, In *New Steps in Public Health*. Milbank Medical Foundation, 1945.

Weathersbee, P. S., Olsen, L. K., and Lodge, J. R. Caffeine and pregnancy: A retrospective survey. *Postgrad. Med.* 62:64, 1977.

Weigley, E. S. The pregnant adolescent. *J. Am. Diet. Assoc.* 66:588, 1975.

Williams, P. S. *Nourishing Your Unborn Child*. New York: Avon, 1974.

Winick, M. et al. Effects of prenatal nutrition upon pregnancy risk. *Clin. Obstet. Gynecol.* 16:184, 1973.

The Working Group on Nutrition and Pregnancy in Adolescence. Relation of nutrition to pregnancy in adolescence. *In Maternal Nutrition and the Course of Pregnancy*. Committee on Maternal Nutrition, Food and Nutrition Board, National Research Council. Washington, D.C.: National Academy of Sciences, 1970.

Wynn, M., and Wynn, A. *Nutrition Counselling in the Prevention of Low Birth-Weight*. London: The Foundation for Education and Research in Child-Bearing, 1975.

9

Coauthored by Therese A. Dondero, C.N.M.
Director, Midwifery Service
North Central Bronx Hospital
Bronx, New York

Screening for and Collaborative Management of Antepartal Complications

In this chapter the numerous possible antepartal complications are discussed from the viewpoint of screening and collaborative management. The signs and symptoms, nurse-midwifery management, and collaborative management of the more common or well-known complications are presented. Other complications rarely seen in practice or resulting from another complication are not included, e.g., genital tract developmental abnormalities, choriocarcinoma, hypofibrinogenemia and fibrinogenopenia, disseminated intravascular coagulation, urinary calculi, and gastrointestinal diseases (e.g., gastric ulcers, gallbladder disease, liver diseases, pancreatitis, intestinal obstruction). Also not included are a number of other medical (e.g., respiratory), endocrinologic (e.g., hypothyroidism, hyperthyroidism), and surgical (e.g., appendectomy) problems further complicated by the fact of pregnancy. Students interested in the study of these and other complications are encouraged to consult standard medical and obstetrical textbooks and journals.

The nurse-midwife is an expert on normal childbearing and detection of complications. In order to detect abnormality a thorough knowledge of the range of normal is essential. Knowledge of the signs and symptoms of the more common or well-known complications enables the nurse-midwife to identify possible complications and initiate the process of differential diagnosis and physician consultation at the earliest indication of a problem.

There are a few conditions and complications which have a "gray zone" of minimal severity when detected early and which nurse-midwives do manage. These include some urinary tract infections, anemias, gestational diabetes, and incipient toxemias. Still other conditions/complications are diagnosed and treated by the nurse-midwife, such as vaginal infections, gonorrhea, and the minor discomforts of pregnancy (see Chapter 7).

The conditions and complications in this chapter are those the nurse-midwife will either manage, consult the physician about, contribute to the management of care in collaboration with the physician, or refer to the physician. The nurse-midwife assumes any one of these roles either initially, after diagnostic laboratory work, or in the event of increasing severity of the problem.

ABORTION

Definitions

1. *Abortion*: the termination of pregnancy by expulsion of the products of conception prior to the ability of the fetus to survive if born. This is generally accepted to be up to 20 weeks gestation or 500 grams in weight.
2. *Spontaneous abortion*: abortion that occurs naturally, without having been induced. Also known as "miscarriage."
3. *Habitual abortion*: spontaneous abortion that has terminated the course of three or more consecutive pregnancies.

Categories of Spontaneous Abortion

There are four categories of spontaneous abortion. Their definitions, signs and symptoms, and nurse-midwifery disposition are discussed here. The possibility of ectopic pregnancy should also be considered for any woman with first trimester bleeding or pain. Regardless of category of spontaneous abortion, all postabortal Rh-negative mothers with negative antibody titers should receive RhoGam within 72 hours of the abortion.

Threatened Abortion
The pregnancy is considered threatened any time there is vaginal bleeding during the first half of pregnancy. The bleeding may be fresh (bright red) or old (dark brown). It may be slight and persist for several days. Approximately one-third of women who have painless vaginal bleeding during the first half of pregnancy abort. Other possible causes of bleeding include postcoital bleeding from severe cervicitis or cervical lesions, spotting during implantation, hydatidiform mole, and choriocarcinoma. A threatened abortion may or may not be accompanied by lower abdominal cramping pain or low backache.

If the woman calls the nurse-midwife during the first trimester and her bleeding is slight without low abdominal or back pain, the nurse-midwife may simply advise the woman as follows:

1. Bedrest — some clinicians believe bedrest is beneficial; others think it has no effect on outcome and therefore advise continuation of normal activity; still other clinicians believe that limiting activity either has a therapeutic physiologic influence or helps the woman psychologically by making her feel she has done all that is possible to maintain the pregnancy
2. Pelvic rest (no sexual intercourse, no douching, no insertion of anything into the vagina)
3. Notification of nurse-midwife immediately if woman starts to have:
   a. an increase in bleeding
   b. lower abdominal cramps or back pain
   c. a gush of fluid from her vagina (indicative of rupture of the membranes)
4. Attendance at the next clinic or office day for:
   a. gentle speculum examination of the vagina and cervix and screening for vaginitis and cervicitis
   b. gentle bimanual examination for size of uterus, effacement, dilatation, and status of membranes

c. hemoglobin and hematocrit determination

d. evaluation of blood pressure, temperature, pulse, and respirations

The nurse-midwife should then consult with a physician. If the bleeding is heavy the woman should be evaluated immediately by a physician. If the bleeding is slight but accompanied by lower abdominal or back pain, or if the woman is febrile, the nurse-midwife should consult with the physician. The prognosis for continuation of a pregnancy is poor when there is a combination of bleeding and pain.

Inevitable Abortion

When an abortion is almost certain to occur and cannot be stopped, it is classified as inevitable. This happens when there is cervical dilatation and/or rupture of the membranes in addition to vaginal bleeding and lower abdominal or back pain.

If you have never seen the woman before, refer her to a physician. If the woman is your patient, however, have her come to your office or to the clinic in order to assess the following:

1. Gestational age
2. Amount of bleeding
3. Amount of abdominal pain
4. Emotional status
5. Previous and/or *stat.* hematocrit
6. Degree of dilatation
7. Vital signs

If the woman is in the first trimester, does not have excessive bleeding or pain, has normal vital signs, is not severely emotionally distressed, and has a previous hematocrit of at least 30%, you may offer her two choices. One choice is to be assisted in the abortion by your consulting physician by terminating the pregnancy now with a suction D&C. The other choice is to return home to await the inevit-able spontaneous evacuation of the products of conception. With either decision, apprise your consulting physician of the situation.

If the woman chooses to remain at home during the abortion, instruct her to take her temperature every 4 hours (unless asleep) or more often if she has chills, and to call you if she soaks through a regular sanitary napkin in an hour or less, passes clots larger than 2½ centimeters (50-cent piece), or has a fever of 100°F (37.8°C) or above, and when she aborts. If she has had two or more consecutive spontaneous abortions ask her to save, if possible, the products of conception in a container for genetic studies.

If any of the assessment data are outside the limits given in the aforesaid situation, then arrange for your consulting physician to assist the woman in completing this spontaneous abortion. If the woman has had two or more consecutive spontaneous abortions, the products of conception should be analyzed for genetic abnormalities.

Follow-up care of the woman includes support through the grieving process, counseling regarding contraception and resumption of sexual intercourse within 2 to 4 weeks, and future pregnancy counseling. Genetic counseling and an endocrinologic workup should be considered if there have been repeated abortions. Developmental abnormalities of the genital tract (e.g., becornuate uterus, vaginal septum) should be ruled out in any woman having multiple spontaneous abortions or second trimester losses.

Incomplete Abortion

Incomplete abortion occurs when the placenta is not expelled with the fetus at the time of the abortion. The retained placenta (all or part) will eventually be the cause of bleeding, which may be profuse, or infection, especially if the abortion occurred during the second trimester. Physician management of the woman will include evacuation of the uterus.

Missed Abortion

In missed abortion there is fetal death but the products of conception are retained for a prolonged period of time (weeks.) Signs and symptoms of a missed abortion include the following:

1. Normal early pregnancy with accompanying presumptive and probable signs of pregnancy
2. Vaginal spotting or bleeding or lower abdominal or back pain at the time of death of the fetus (may or may not occur)
3. Fundal height not only ceases to increase but after a while the uterus becomes smaller (due to maceration of the fetus and absorption of the amniotic fluid)
4. Regression of mammary changes of pregnancy
5. The woman often loses a few pounds in weight
6. Persistent amenorrhea
7. No fetal heart tones when anticipated by dates

When a woman presents with these signs and symptoms, order a sonogram for confirmation of fetal death. If fetal death has occurred, notify your consulting physician and order the following baseline coagulation studies:

1. Prothrombin
2. Partial prothrombin
3. Fibrinogen
4. Platelets

Further management of the missed abortion is by the physician while the nurse-midwife provides continuing supportive care. Follow-up care of the woman by the physician/nurse-midwife team includes support through the grieving process; and counseling regarding contraception, resumption of sexual intercourse within 2 to 4 weeks, and future pregnancy. Genetic counseling, endocrinologic workup, and screening for uterine anomalies should be done.

Severe blood coagulation problems may develop when there is prolonged retention of the dead products of conception. The psychological effects on the woman are often immense because her grief process over the loss of her pregnancy is compounded by having to deal with the concept of carrying a dead fetus inside herself.

INCOMPETENT CERVIX

An incompetent cervix is almost impossible to diagnose in a primigravida. It is also rare in primigravidas who have not had any cervical operations (e.g., cervical cone biopsy).

Evidence of an incompetent cervix occurs in the second trimester. Painless dilatation of the cervix results in rupture of the membranes and expulsion of a fetus not yet of viable age. This sequence of events is repeated in subsequent consecutive pregnancies regardless of pregnancy interval.

An identifiable history suspicious of incompetent cervix includes a previous history of fetal loss at 14 weeks gestation or more, or a previous history of cervical operations, or both. The nurse-midwife should do the following additional assessment of a woman in early pregnancy with a suspicious history:

1. History
   a. description of signs and symptoms surrounding previous loss, (e.g., bleeding, abdominal cramping, suprapubic pain, low back pain, ruptured membranes) and when they occurred in relation to bleeding and dilatation
   b. any congenital abnormalities of previously aborted fetuses
   c. family history of early fetal loss
   d. previous suction abortion (three or more) or one or more second trimester abortions
   e. history of cervical trauma with previous delivery

2. Pelvic examination
   a. speculum exam — visualization for:
      (1) cervical discharge
      (2) cervical length
      (3) evidence of previous cervical laceration
   b. bimanual exam — digital examination for:
      (1) consistency and length of the cervix
      (2) dilatation of the internal and external cervical os
      (3) palpable membranes
      (4) position and station of the presenting part

If upon vaginal examination you find that the cervix is effaced or dilated up to 4 centimeters, arrange with your consulting physician for a cerclage procedure. If the cervix is dilated 4 or more centimeters and the membranes are bulging, physician consultation is obtained for a threatened abortion. Some obstetricians may try a cerclage procedure on a woman who is dilated 4 or 5 centimeters if effacement is such as to allow a suture to be placed.

The woman who has only a history of cervical trauma should be followed with vaginal speculum and digital examinations every 2 weeks until viability of the fetus in order to ascertain any changes in the cervix. Many physicians may perform an immediate cerclage procedure for women with a history of two or more spontaneous second trimester losses not due to either fetal or uterine congenital anomalies.

Follow-up care after discharge from the hospital of a woman who has had a cerclage procedure may be done by the nurse-midwife. This care includes the following:

1. Emotional support. This is especially important for women with repeated losses. These women walk a fine balance between hope, fear of another loss, and the potential for disappointment. Cultural attitudes towards the ability to bear children may strongly affect the psyche of such women.
2. Vaginal speculum and digital examination

every 2 weeks until viability of the fetus to ascertain:
   a. intactness of the suture
   b. length of the cervix
   c. cervical dilatation
   d. cervical consistency
   e. position of the cervix
   f. station of the presenting part
   g. vaginitis or cervicitis
   h. vaginal odor
3. Patient education to report:
   a. signs and symptoms of premature labor (abdominal cramping, suprapubic pain, low back pain, contractions)
   b. vaginal bleeding
   c. ruptured membranes
   d. signs and symptoms of vaginitis
   e. foul vaginal discharge (may be indicative of an infected suture)

The suture is removed in the following circumstances:

1. If the suture is not intact, consult regarding possible replacement or removal.
2. If the suture is lacerating the cervix, consult regarding possible removal.
3. Rupture of the membranes with or without labor. The incidence of amnionitis significantly increases when rupture of the membranes occurs and the suture is not removed immediately (within hours).
4. Anticipation of labor. Some obstetricians prefer to remove the cerclage suture routinely at 38 weeks gestation.
5. When the woman has started labor.

Removal of the suture and spontaneous vaginal delivery is preferable to an elective cesarean section.

HYDATIDIFORM MOLE

Hydatidiform mole is a developmental anomaly of the placenta in which a degenerative process in the chorionic villi causes all or part of the villi to become a mass of cystlike clear vesicles hanging in clusters from thin pedicles, thereby resembling a bunch of grapes. While a hydatidiform mole usually is a benign neoplasm, it has the potential for becoming malignant and often precedes the extremely malignant but fortunately rare trophoblastic neoplasm known as choriocarcinoma. The incidence is 10 times higher in women over 45, indicating that hydatidiform mole is much more common in pregnancies at the end of the childbearing cycle. Signs and symptoms include the following:

1. Apparently normal first trimester of pregnancy
2. Persistent nausea and vomiting
3. Uterine bleeding evident by the twelfth week of pregnancy — spotting or profuse bleeding but usually just a bloody discharge, usually more brown than red, occurring intermittently or continuously over time
4. Possible anemia as a result of blood loss or poor nutritional intake
5. A large-for-dates uterus clearly out of proportion to presumed gestational age (occurs in about one-third of cases)
6. Shortness of breath
7. Often enlarged, tender ovaries (theca lutein cysts)
8. No fetal heart tones
9. No fetal activity
10. Palpation of fetal parts impossible
11. Pregnancy-induced hypertension, preeclampsia, or eclampsia *before* 24 weeks gestation

These findings indicate that the nurse-midwife should obtain a specimen for a serum chorionic gonadotrophin titer and a sonogram. Hydatidiform mole has a characteristic pattern upon ultrasonography. A persistently high, or even rising, level of chorionic gonadotrophin after 100 days from the first day of the last menstrual period is indicative of abnormal trophoblastic

growth or a multiple gestation. The woman is referred to the physician.

ECTOPIC PREGNANCY

Ectopic pregnancy occurs whenever the blastocyst implants anywhere except in the endometrium lining the uterine cavity. Possible sites for ectopic pregnancy include the cervix, fallopian tubes, ovaries, and abdomen. The signs and symptoms for each type of ectopic pregnancy are given in this section. For all women with a suspected ectopic pregnancy, the nurse-midwife should draw a quantitative human chorionic gonadotrophin (see Chapter 4) and refer the woman to the physician. The importance of drawing the hCG when an ectopic pregnancy is first suspected is early diagnosis; if a tubal pregnancy can be diagnosed before rupture, microsurgery is more likely to save the fallopian tube.

Cervical Pregnancy

Cervical pregnancy is rare and seldom lasts beyond the twentieth week of gestation. Signs and symptoms include the following:

1. Painless bleeding appearing soon after the time of implantation
2. Palpation of a cervical mass with distention and thinning of the cervical wall, partial dilatation of the external cervical os, and a slightly enlarged uterine fundus

Tubal Pregnancy

Tubal pregnancy accounts for 95 percent or more of ectopic pregnancies. Signs and symptoms are those of tubal rupture or abortion and may vary widely from woman to woman. The classical case involves a woman who may or may not realize she's pregnant because slight vaginal bleeding or spotting has substituted for menstrual periods. Without warning, she suddenly has a sharp, stabbing, tearing, severe lower abdominal pain. Hypotension and other signs of shock may or may not quickly develop. Her abdomen is tender and vaginal examination is quite painful. Movement of the cervix elicits exquisite pain. A tender, boggy mass may be felt to one side of the uterus. The cul-de-sac may be full of blood thereby causing the vaginal posterior fornix to bulge. Pain in the neck or shoulder, especially upon inspiration, may be present as a result of diaphragmatic irritation from blood in the peritoneal cavity.

Signs and symptoms which may presage the full-blown classical case described above include the following:

1. Uterine changes are not diagnostic because the uterus grows to the same size and consistency as a pregnant uterus for the first trimester due to the influence of the placental hormones. It may be displaced to one side by the tubal pregnancy.
2. Pelvic examination may be quite painful and exquisitely so upon movement of the cervix — or may not be painful at all.
3. A soft, pliable pelvic mass can be palpated posterior or lateral to the uterus. The mass may be firm if distended with blood.
4. The woman may have vaginal bleeding or spotting that is scanty and dark brown. It may be continuous or intermittent. Infrequently, it is profuse. There won't be any bleeding as long as the placenta is functional.
5. The entire decidual lining of the uterus (decidual cast) may be expelled.
6. A history of amenorrhea may or may not be obtained since the bleeding and spotting described above may be mistaken for a menstrual period. Careful history taking in comparison to the woman's normal menses may yield a more accurate and useful history.
7. Neck or shoulder pain may occur as a result of diaphragmatic irritation.
8. The woman experiences acute abdominal pain in the upper or lower abdomen — may be unilateral, bilateral, or generalized.
9. Vital signs (blood pressure, pulse, and temperature) may remain normal.
10. Diarrhea (more common) and nausea and vomiting (less common) may occur.
11. The woman has very low chorionic gonadotropin levels or negative pregnancy tests.
12. White blood cell count may be normal or may range up to 30,000.

The ambiguity of the symptoms obviously makes diagnosis difficult. This problem is compounded because differential diagnosis from salpingitis, threatened or incomplete abortion, appendicitis, a twisted ovarian cyst, and a ruptured corpus luteum or follicular cyst must be made.

Ovarian Pregnancy

Ovarian pregnancy is rare. Signs and symptoms are:

1. Enlarged ovary or ovarian mass
2. Other symptoms relating to rupture into the peritoneal cavity and similar to that of tubal rupture

Abdominal Pregnancy

Abdominal pregnancy is almost always the result of an early tubal pregnancy rupture or abortion into the peritoneal cavity. In a few exceedingly rare cases the fertilized ovum makes the abdomen the site of its primary implantation. In addition to the signs and symptoms of a ruptured tubal pregnancy the following may exist:

1. Gastrointestinal disturbances — diarrhea, constipation, flatulence, abdominal pain, nausea, and vomiting
2. High frequency of a transverse lie
3. Marked pain from fetal movements late in pregnancy
4. Ease in palpating small parts
5. Ease in hearing fetal heart tones
6. Lack of ability to stimulate contraction of the musculature surrounding the fetus
7. Palpation of the uterus on vaginal examination and of small parts outside of it
8. Cervical displacement
9. Dilatation (up to 2 centimeters) but *no* effacement of the cervix as a result of spurious labor

HYPEREMESIS GRAVIDARUM

Hyperemesis gravidarum is excessive nausea and vomiting during pregnancy. This pernicious vomiting is differentiated from the more common and more normal morning sickness by the fact that it is of greater intensity and extends beyond the first trimester. Hyperemesis gravidarum may occur in any of the three trimesters. The following are signs, symptoms, and effects:

1. Pernicious vomiting
2. Poor appetite
3. Poor nutritional intake
4. Weight loss
5. Dehydration
6. Electrolyte imbalance
7. Extreme response to underlying psychosocial problems
8. Failure of vomiting to be controlled by treatment measures for morning sickness (see Chapter 7)
9. Acidosis due to starvation
10. Alkalosis resulting from loss of hydrochloric acid in the vomitus
11. Hypokalemia

The nurse-midwife should do the following additional workup for a woman suspected of having hyperemesis gravidarum:

1. History
   a. frequency of vomiting episodes
   b. relationship of vomiting to food intake (amount and type)
   c. dietary history
   d. elimination — frequency, amount, constipation, diarrhea
   e. foul, bilious material or feces in vomitus (intestinal obstruction)
   f. blood in vomitus (peptic ulcer)
   g. fever or chills
   h. exposure to viral infection
   i. exposure to contaminated food
   j. abdominal pain
   k. history of diabetes
   l. previous abdominal surgery
2. Physical examination
   a. weight
   b. temperature, pulse, respirations
   c. skin turgor
   d. moistness of mucous membranes
   e. condition of tongue — swollen, dry, cracked
   f. abdominal palpation for:
      (1) organomegaly
      (2) tenderness
      (3) distention
   g. bowel sounds
   h. sweet odor to breath
   i. assessment of fetal growth
3. Laboratory
   a. BUN and electrolytes
   b. urine dipstick for acetone and glucose
   c. arterial blood gases and serum pH (physician consultation needed) in the presence of acidosis or alkalosis

If the woman is spilling glucose as well as acetone, call your physician consultant and immediately measure the blood glucose to assess for diabetes. If a woman diagnosed as having hyperemesis gravidarum is only dehydrated, intravenous fluid administration may be done on an outpatient or inpatient basis following consultation with the physician. A woman who is severely dehydrated or who continues to vomit while receiving IV therapy should be admitted to the hospital.

Measures used to stop the vomiting include:

1. Admission to the hospital to remove the woman from stressful home and family situations
2. Correction of fluid and electrolyte imbalance
3. Phenergan 25 to 50 mg IM or rectally every 4 hours
4. Social service or psychological assistance with any existing psychosocial problems

INFECTIONS

Infections are caused by microorganisms, primarily those in the following categories: viruses, bacteria, fungi, rickettsias, protozoons, and animal parasites. The danger of these microorganisms in pregnancy is twofold. One is the direct effect on the mother and subsequent indirect effect on the fetus (e.g., maternal dehydration, poor nutritional intake, and electrolyte imbalance). Colds and influenza with the possible sequelae of pneumonia are examples of disease entities with this type of effect. The other danger is the direct effect on the fetus since certain microorganisms are known to cause congenital malformations.

Tuberculosis

Tuberculosis (TB) is an infection caused by *Mycobacterium tuberculosis* and, rarely, *Mycobacterium bovis*. Inoculation with the tubercle bacillus occurs through droplet inhalation. Once inoculation has occurred, an initial lesion develops in the lung with formation of a localized inflammatory exudate combined with necrosis of the surrounding lung tissue. The infection spreads to the lymphatic nodes and can then be disseminated throughout the body. Because of this dissemination, tuberculosis can be extrapulmonary (e.g., genital, skeletal).

In the majority of individuals infected, the primary (pulmonary) lesion is arrested by encapsulation, fibrosis, and calcification. These individuals may never suffer from active tuberculosis. A chest x-ray examination in such individuals will reveal evidence of calcification of the primary lesion. Usually this calcification represents host resistance at the time of the initial infection and indicates that the local and systemic progression of the disease has been arrested. There is evidence that the process of encapsulation affects the immune system thereby allowing reinfection to occur at any time. Most adults in whom active tuberculosis is found do not have new cases of TB but rather, reinfection has occurred.

The incidence of tuberculosis appears to be affected by geographical location and the socioeconomic status of a given population. Tuberculosis remains one of the more common infectious diseases in the childbearing age group. It is endemic in certain countries, such as those in southeast Asia.

The diagnosis of active tuberculosis is made through history, physical examination, and laboratory testing as follows:

1. History
   a. previous history of tuberculosis evidenced either by symptoms or by a positive chest x-ray
   b. exposure to other individuals with tuberculosis
   c. fever — one of the earliest symptoms; initially minimal to moderate temperature elevation occurs daily in the late afternoon or evening, usually accompanied by a feeling of euphoria and well-being; temperature elevations reach 103°F (39.5°C) or higher as disease progresses
   d. weight loss — minor weight loss with anorexia early in the disease; increased

weight loss, fatigue, and irritability as the disease progresses

e. persistent colds and a chronic cough which is worse in the morning

f. chronic, productive cough with large amounts of purulent, greenish-yellow sputum and hemoptysis

g. pleurisy with effusion — in young child-bearing women the findings indicative of pleurisy should lead you to suspect active tuberculosis since pleurisy in this age group is uncommon

h. spontaneous atelectasis, especially in a young person, may be a sign of active tuberculosis

2. Physical examination
   a. crepitant rales on auscultation, heard best after coughing
3. Diagnostic tests
   a. sputum culture (looking for acid-fast organisms)
   b. chest x-ray

If you suspect that a woman has active tuberculosis, obtain a chest x-ray and sputum for culture, and refer her to your consulting physician for immediate evaluation.

Screening test

The screening test most commonly used is the PPD (purified protein derivative). Screening tests will detect hypersensitivity to the tuberculin protein.

The purpose of screening for tuberculosis is to detect those individuals who have inactive disease, those who have converted from no infection to infection, and those in whom it is not known whether they have been infected with tuberculosis. Do *not* give PPD to someone with signs or symptoms of active tuberculosis; a chest x-ray and sputum culture are diagnostic for such an individual.

PPD is administered intradermally on the forearm in the amount of 5 tuberculin units. Production of a palpable area of induration greater than 10 mm in diameter after 48 to 72 hours is diagnostic of infection with the tubercle bacillus. This positive PPD may indicate active or clinically inactive tuberculosis. The diagnosis of active tuberculosis is made through the history, physical, sputum culture, and chest x-ray described earlier. A negative PPD rules out tuberculosis.

Many individuals from countries outside the United States (e.g., England, Carribean Islands) receive bacillus Calmette-Guérin (BCG) vaccine in childhood to prevent tuberculosis infection. These individuals should not be screened with PPD since they will almost always have a positive PPD secondary to the BCG vaccine and PPD can cause serious localized damage to the forearm. Individuals who have received BCG should be screened with a chest x-ray every 2 years. Since many people who received BCG vaccine as a child may not have been informed that this was given, look for the scar caused by the vaccine before giving PPD.

Before screening for tuberculosis with PPD, determine whether the woman has been screened previously and, if so, the results. If she had a negative screening test in the past, administer the PPD. If this PPD is positive, the woman is a converter representing new disease which may or may not be currently active.

All women with a positive skin reaction should have a chest x-ray, and you should inform your consulting physician. The woman's abdomen should be shielded during the x-ray procedure.

Some clinicians recommend prophylactic chemotherapy with isoniazid (INH) during pregnancy for all women under 35 with a positive PPD and negative chest x-ray and for all women who are recent converters regardless of age. Treatment with INH is also recommended for women with an abnormal chest x-ray and a positive PPD who do not have active tuberculosis. Some clinicians will not prescribe prophylactic INH during pregnancy but commence treatment following delivery. INH, although safe, is not approved for use during pregnancy. If a woman is receiving INH for either prophylaxis or treatment of active disease and becomes pregnant, most clinicians recommend continuing treatment since discontinuation and restarting of INH causes development of drug resistance.

You should inform your consulting physician about all women with a positive PPD and those women in whom you suspect active disease. The families of women with a positive PPD and of women in whom you suspect active TB should be evaluated for active disease and, if TB is not evident, then screened with PPD.

Hepatitis

Hepatitis is an inflammation of the liver. There are many types of hepatitis, noninfectious and infectious. Noninfectious hepatitis is often drug induced, for example, in individuals receiving INH. Infectious hepatitis can be part of a more generalized illness caused by many different infectious agents, such as cytomegalovirus and the virus producing mononucleosis.

This section discusses only acute infectious viral hepatitis. There are two clearly defined types of viral hepatitis: types A and B. All other forms of viral hepatitis are grouped together as non-A, non-B.

Hepatitis Non-A, Non-B
The hepatitis non-A, non-B category includes an unknown number of as yet uncharacterized diseases. There are presently no tests available to diagnose non-A, non-B hepatitis. It is a diagnosis made by excluding hepatitis A and B.

Hepatitis non-A, non-B is transmitted through blood transfusions and contact with contaminated blood, saliva, vaginal secretions, and semen. Hepatitis non-A, non-B has a carrier state and a chronic form. The precautions to be taken with women who are diagnosed as having non-A, non-B hepatitis are similar to those used in instances of hepatitis A and B.

Viral Hepatitis A
Viral hepatitis A is transmitted through fecal contamination since the virus is shed through the feces. At the time the virus enters the bloodstream it is infectious, but only for a relatively short period of time. Hepatitis A can be spread by ingestion of contaminated food or water or by contact with blood during the time it is infectious.

The disease is of short duration and there is no carrier state or chronic state. Diagnosis is made by history, symptoms, and a blood test for hepatitis A antibody.

Viral Hepatitis B
Viral hepatitis B is transmitted through blood, blood by-products, saliva, vaginal secretions, and semen. Viral hepatitis B has a carrier state, although most individuals with hepatititis B become disease-free noncarriers.

The incidence of hepatitis B is highest among the following:

1. Intravenous drug abusers and their contacts
2. Bisexual men
3. Sexual partners of individuals with hepatitis B
4. Native-born Chinese, Southeast Asians, sub-Sahara Africans, and Eskimos
5. Individuals with a history of hepatitis
6. Individuals who have received blood or blood by-products
7. Health care personnel in obstetrics, surgery, laboratory, and housekeeping

Screening is done by drawing a blood specimen for hepatitis B surface antigen (HBsAg). This test becomes positive within 2 weeks of exposure and before the appearance of jaundice.

Women who are HBsAg-positive and hepatitis B *e* antigen-positive have a 90-percent chance of transmitting their disease to their infants. Of the infected infants, 90 percent will become carriers and the female carriers will transmit the hepatitis B virus to their offspring. Twenty-five percent of the infants will die of cirrhosis or primary hepatocellular carcinoma. Health care providers are at risk to contract hepatitis when they take care of hepatitis B carriers or patients with active or chronic disease.

Infectious viral hepatitis may be detected through history, physical examination, and laboratory data as follows:

1. History
   a. blood transfusion within the past year
   b. exposure to someone who has hepatitis or is jaundiced
   c. intravenous drug use or addiction
   d. country of origin
   e. occupation
   f. previous hepatitis or jaundice
   g. malaise
   h. gastrointestinal discomfort
   i. anorexia
   j. nausea
   k. vomiting
   l. fatigue
   m. arthralgia (achy joints)
   n. sudden dislike for coffee and cigarettes
2. Physical examination
   a. tender, enlarged liver
   b. jaundice (sclerae or body)
3. Laboratory tests
   a. positive screening test (HBsAg)
   b. elevated liver function tests (SGOT, SGPT, LDH, and bilirubin)

Any evidence or suspicion of hepatitis should be immediately reported to your consulting physician. A pregnant woman with active disease should be hospitalized. Any hepatitis is significant in a pregnant woman because the anorexia, nausea, and vomiting interfere with her nutritional status. Family members should be screened. All cases are reported to the health department.

Maternal-newborn transfer of hepatitis B can occur at the time of delivery through contact with the infected maternal blood, or during close maternal-infant contact in the postpartal period. The transfer can occur regardless of route of delivery. Hepatitits B virus is present in all the body fluids except breast milk of an infected individual and is transmitted parenterally. Breast-feeding is not contraindicated except during periods of cracked nipples or breast abscesses because of the presence of blood.

Precautions need to be taken during the antepartal course, labor and delivery, and postpartum period to avoid contamination with any of the woman's body fluids. Precautions include the following:

1. Antepartum
   a. careful technique with speculum and bimanual examinations
   b. careful handling of specimens (e.g., blood, urine, vaginal discharge)
2. Labor
   a. careful technique with vaginal examinations
   b. careful disposal of used bed linens and chux
   c. careful handling of bedpans, soiled chux, and urine or stool specimens (wear gloves)
   d. no internal electronic fetal monitoring
   e. no scalp pH assessments
3. Delivery
   a. protective eyeglasses (hospital should provide these)
   b. mask, gown, and gloves
   c. careful technique with DeLee suctioning
   d. careful delivery technique
   e. careful handling of needles
   f. careful disposal of linens

4. Postpartum
   a. stool and blood precautions

Newborn infants of HBsAg-positive mothers should receive 0.5 milliliter of HBIG (hepatitis B immune globulin) intramuscularly within 1 hour of birth. The pediatrician should be notified when birth is imminent for attendance at birth and administration of the HBIG. The pediatrician will do further follow-up during the first year of life.

Health care providers who work with populations at high risk for hepatitis B have the option of obtaining hepatitis B vaccine. Taking the vaccine is not without theoretical risk of contracting AIDS (autoimmune deficiency syndrome), however, and this danger should be explored if the vaccine option is considered. Health care providers who have been contaminated should consult their own health care provider. Their options are to obtain hepatitis B immune globulin or to do nothing; each has its own set of risks that should be carefully weighed and discussed with the health care provider.

Rubella

The virus that causes rubella, or German measles, is particularly virulent during pregnancy. If the woman contracts rubella during the first trimester there is approximately a 20 percent chance that her baby will be born with congenital malformations. This figure is as high as 50 percent during the first month of pregnancy. The most common malformations are cataracts, cardiac defects, and deafness. There may also be glaucoma, microcephaly and other defects involving the eye, ear, heart, brain, and central nervous system. The most severely affected fetuses may abort spontaneously.

A rubella antibody titer for immunity (hemagglutination inhibition) is done routinely as part of the initial antepartal examination by many practitioners or in many practice settings. An antibody titer of 1:10 or above is generally accepted as indicative of immunity. Below 1:10 indicates lack of immunity and a note should be made on the woman's record to offer rubella immunization postpartally. However, high antibody titers of 1:64 or above may indicate present disease since there is a prompt antibody response with infection. Such a situation requires searching for signs and symptoms of the disease, ordering a series of antibody titers, and consulting with the physician.

Diagnosing rubella is difficult because the disease may be subclinical, thereby infecting the fetus but not exhibiting itself clinically in the mother. If the mother knows she has been exposed to rubella and has an antibody titer below 1:10 (not immune), a blood specimen should be obtained for serologic testing (IgG and IgM) and the woman referred to a physician. Authorities differ on the administration of hyperimmune gamma globulin in such a situation. Clinical signs and symptoms of rubella, when they are present, include the following:

1. Low-grade fever
2. Drowsiness
3. Sore throat
4. Rash — pale or bright red on the first or second day, spreading rapidly from the face over the entire body, and fading rapidly
5. Swollen neck glands
6. Duration of 3 to 5 days

Women who are not immune and contract rubella during the first trimester of pregnancy are faced with the decision of whether or not to obtain a therapeutic abortion. There is no chemotherapeutic agent to prevent the disease once contracted. There are effective vaccines available but these are contraindicated for pregnant women because attenuated rubella virus may be teratogenic — even when given up to 2 months before becoming pregnant.

Cytomegalovirus

Cytomegalovirus is another microorganism that may cause congenital malformations if contracted by the mother while pregnant. In contrast to the other damaging organisms, cytomegalovirus has its effect during the fetal period (10 to 40 weeks post-LMP) rather than during the organogenesis of the embryonic period.

Fortunately cytomegalovirus, causing cytomegalic inclusion disease, is rare. The infection is usually asymptomatic in the mother and the disease is not suspected until birth. Possible malformations include microcephaly or hydrocephaly, microphthalmia (abnormally small eyes), and congenital predisposition to seizures, blindness, encephalitis, and learning disabilities. There is no vaccine and no effective treatment of the infection.

Toxoplasmosis

Toxoplasmosis is a protozoal infection caused by the intracellular parasite *Toxoplasma gondii*. It causes severe congenital malformations when the mother acquires the infection while pregnant because it crosses the placenta to the fetus. It, too, has its effect during the fetal period rather than during organogenesis in the embryonic period. The effect on the fetus may be death, prematurity, central nervous system defects, anencephalus, hydrocephalus, and destructive changes in the eye or brain. The signs and symptoms of toxoplasmosis in the pregnant woman are vague when present and include the following:

1. Fatigue and malaise
2. Muscle pain
3. Swollen lymph nodes

Usually the disease is asymptomatic. Virology testing is available. Consultation with a virologist is indicated for women with a history of handling cat feces or eating raw meat.

Toxoplasmosis is contracted through eating infected meat that is raw or undercooked or through contact with infected cat feces. Accordingly, the history taken at the initial antepartal visit should include specific inquiries about (1) how well cooked the woman likes her meat and (2) whether there is a cat in her household and, if so, who takes care of it.

Genital Herpesvirus

Herpesvirus may be transmitted to the fetus systemically during pregnancy if the mother has herpes viremia, or it may be transmitted to the neonate during vaginal delivery. Spontaneous abortion or fetal death may result from the former.

The occurrence of congenital defects from herpesvirus during pregnancy is rare. Herpesvirus infection contracted by the neonate during delivery may result in neonatal death or severe central nervous system or ocular damage. All neonatal herpesvirus infections (disseminated and localized varieties) induce death in some of their victims. The most severe forms of neonatal herpesvirus infections are disseminated. Disseminated neonatal herpesvirus infection without central nervous system involvement approaches 90 percent mortality but usually produces no sequelae for those who survive. Disseminated neonatal herpesvirus infection with CNS involvement has a mortality rate of about 70 percent but the survivors usually are left with sequelae. Less than 1 percent of infants are born with a herpes infection.

Herpesvirus lesions are thin-walled vesicles which occur singly or in clusters. They may rupture and become secondarily infected. Specific ulcers or diffuse inflammation, or both, may be noted over the cervix, vagina, or vulva. The vulvar lesions in the initial infection are extremely painful; lesions inside the vagina or on the cervix do not hurt. Subsequent occurrences of external lesions are usually less painful. A woman may have prodromal signs of an impending recurrence such as tingling, neuralgia, the sensation of pressure, or increased vaginal discharge (heavy, clear, sticky, nonodorous) if the cervix or vaginal wall is involved.

It is important to make a definitive diagnosis of herpesvirus at the time the woman develops symptoms in order not to misdiagnose benign conditions of the genitals such as pimples, infected hair follicles, or nabothian cysts. Diagnosis is made by history and culture.

1. History
   a. symptoms at onset of current episode
   b. history and symptoms of previous occurrences
   c. contact with sexual partner(s) who have or have had herpes
   d. precipitating factors in recurrences
   e. increased vaginal discharge: characteristics
2. Laboratory tests
   a. Lesions are scraped and cultured with a specific commercially prepared medium for definitive diagnosis; a cytological smear for giant inclusion cells may be used if the viral culture media are not available.
   b. Women without lesions may be cultured weekly from 32 weeks gestation on for asymptomatic shedding of herpesvirus. One swab is taken of the cervix, vagina, and labia. A second swab is taken of the rectum. This is done in conjunction with a virology laboratory.

A woman who is diagnosed to have herpesvirus during pregnancy will need considerable emotional support as she deals with associated anger, guilt, and concern for herself and for her baby. She should be counseled and educated regarding situations which increase the likelihood of recurrence, the possibility of cesarean section, and the reporting of signs and symptoms of a recurrence.

A woman who has had two negative cultures a week apart immediately prior to onset of labor and is lesion-free at the time labor begins may deliver vaginally. If the services for viral cultures are not available, a woman who gives a history of being lesion-free and free of any signs or symptoms of a nonvisible painless genital lesion for two weeks before labor may deliver vaginally.

A woman with premature rupture of membranes should be evaluated immediately and a decision made regarding mode of delivery. Most experts agree that when a woman with active herpesvirus has had ruptured membranes for longer than 4 to 6 hours without delivery, the risk of neonatal herpesvirus infection is significantly increased. Cesarean section of such women for the prevention of neonatal herpesvirus, therefore, is not considered warranted.

A woman with either a positive culture or a lesion within 2 weeks of the onset of labor should have a cesarean section to avoid neonatal herpesvirus infection. Regardless of route of delivery, internal electronic fetal monitoring should not be done as application of the scalp clip increases the likelihood of transmission of the herpesvirus.

The nurse-midwife and consulting physician should agree upon a protocol for the diagnosis, monitoring, and management of women with herpesvirus. This protocol should be developed in conjunction with available laboratory resources and specialists and should include the following:

1. Type of cultures
2. Transporation of cultures
3. Reporting of results
4. Nurse-midwifery consultation with consulting physician

The cost-benefit ratio of weekly herpesvirus

cultures should be considered in the development of this protocol.

Herpes Gestationis

Herpes gestationis is a rare and serious dermatologic disease peculiar to pregnancy. It should not be confused with *Herpesvirus* infections. It has a high incidence of associated congenital abnormalities. Symptomatology is as follows:

1. History of herpes gestationis in previous pregnancies
2. Usually develops during the second trimester
3. Lesions which are of varying shape and form, and fairly generalized over the body, usually involving the face, forearms, trunk, and legs
4. Reddened, blisterlike lesions of varying shape and form which are filled with fluid (lymph or pus) and cause excruciating burning and itching

Gonorrhea

Gonorrhea is a venereal disease caused by gram-negative intracellular diplococcal bacteria called *Neisseria gonorrhoeae*. Infection may involve the urethra, Skene's glands, Bartholin's glands, vulva, vagina, cervix, endometrium, fallopian tubes, ovaries, peritoneum, rectum, conjunctiva of the eyes, oral mucosa, and joints (yielding gonococcal arthritis). In the female, it is most commonly found in the lower genital tract. During pregnancy the adherence of the membranes to the decidua provides a barrier to ascending infection. However, if not treated or if treated inadequately, the infection will ascend rapidly after delivery with resulting gonorrheal endometritis, salpingitis, oophoritis, and pelvic peritonitis.

Signs and symptoms of a gonorrheal infection range from none (asymptomatic) to any or all of the following:

1. Lower abdominal pain
2. Urethritis with tenderness, urinary frequency, and dysuria
3. Expression of purulent discharge from Skene's or Bartholin's glands or the urethra
4. Tenderness in the area of Skene's or Bartholin's glands (skenitis or bartholinitis)
5. Acute PID (pelvic inflammatory disease) in the nonpregnant woman
6. Yellowish, purulent vaginal discharge

Specimens for culture are routinely obtained from the cervix (see Chapter 46). Also, any exudate expressed from the urethra and Skene's or Bartholin's glands is cultured. Many authorities also advocate collecting specimens from the vaginal fornices and the rectum.

Failure to detect and treat gonorrhea in pregnant women may result in neonatal gonorrheal ophthalmia which may, in turn, result in blindness. For this reason, prophylactic treatment of the newborn's eyes is essential (and mandated in most states by law) shortly after birth of the baby.

The standard treatment for uncomplicated gonococcal infections is 4.8 million units of procaine penicillin G given intramuscularly. Other drugs may be used if the woman is allergic to penicillin or her strain of gonorrhea is resistant to penicillin. These include ampicillin, erythromycin, spectinomycin, and for nonpregnant women, tetracycline.

A series of three follow-up cultures should be initiated 1 to 2 weeks after treatment. Treatment of the infection is considered effective only after three successive negative cultures.

The signs and symptoms of *anaphylactic shock* are given here because this disastrous event may occur as a reaction in individuals who are unknowingly allergic to penicillin. A careful history of any previous evidence of sensitivity to penicillin is obtained prior to both prescribing and administering this drug. These signs and symptoms include the following:

1. Marked pallor
2. Cyanosis
3. Rapid, shallow respirations
4. Rapid, weak pulse
5. Pupil dilatation
6. Decreased blood pressure
7. Venous collapse
8. Cardiac arrest

Syphilis

The spirochete *Treponema pallidum* is the organism responsible for syphilis. Syphilis is an infectious venereal disease which is transmitted by direct contact and which crosses the placental barrier to the fetus of an infected mother. Untreated syphilis results in 40 percent fetal or neonatal loss due to spontaneous abortion, stillbirth, and perinatal death. Another 40 percent results in congenital syphilis in the newborn. Congenital syphilis is a destructive disease ranging from crippling lesions in the internal organs and long bones to fetal death.

Because the symptoms of both primary and secondary syphilis often are unnoticed, a screening test for syphilis is required by law in most states. Obtaining a specimen of blood for a VDRL (Venereal Disease Research Laboratory) is a routine part of the initial antepartal examination and often is repeated at the 36-weeks visit. The test usually is positive 4 to 6 weeks after the individual is infected. An occasional false-positive report occurs during pregnancy. This can be upsetting to a couple if it is ascertained that the man has a negative VDRL. This aspect of concern should be included in the plan of management and involve both partners in careful explanations.

Primary syphilis is evidenced by single or multiple lesions, usually in the genital area. It starts as a red papule, develops into an ulcer, and then becomes a chancre filled with spirochete-laden purulent discharge. Immediate diagnosis can be obtained by arranging with a bacteriologist to perform a dark-field examination. This consists of scraping the lesion and observing the spirochete under a specialized polarized light microscope. The chancre is painless and heals spontaneously without a scar. There also may be enlarged lymph nodes.

Symptoms of secondary syphilis appear approximately 6 weeks after the primary stage, usually in the form of a skin rash or lesions such as condylomata lata. There may or may not be systemic symptoms such as malaise, headaches, and fever. The rash may be so slight and limited to the genital areas as to be unnoticed.

All positive VDRLs should be followed by fluorescent treponemal antibody tests (FTAs) for definitive diagnosis. A positive FTA calls for evaluation by the consulting physician, treatment as indicated, and monthly VDRL titers until a 1:2 ratio is reached. The FTA will remain positive for the rest of the woman's life. Syphilis is usually treated with benzathine penicillin G given intramuscularly. Sensitivity to penicillin must first be ascertained. Several broad-spectrum antibiotics are also effective, including erythromycin and tetracycline (contraindicated for pregnant women).

Condylomata Lata

Condylomata lata are highly infectious primary syphilitic lesions. They occur on the external genitalia and look like a grouping of small, flat warts covered with a gray exudate. *Treponema pallidum* can be cultured from them.

Condylomata Acuminata

Condylomata acuminata are not to be confused

with condylomata lata as they are not venereal in origin and are in no way associated with syphilis. They are wartlike growths which may appear in one small clump or in innumerable clumps of varying size. The size of the clump may be much larger than its attachment to the genitalia. The growth of condylomata acuminata seems to be stimulated by the leukorrhea of pregnancy. They often appear first on the vulva and perineum.

If delivery occurs while they still are present, care must be taken to avoid tearing or cutting into any of them because they may bleed excessively. It is far better to cut an episiotomy of unusual direction than to cut through condylomata acuminata. The pediatrician should be notified when a baby is born vaginally to a woman with condylomata acuminata because these babies have an increased risk of developing vocal cord polyps.

Condylomata acuminata may extend into the vagina and cover the vaginal mucosa and cervix. Extensive growth may necessitate delivery by cesarean section.

Treatment in pregnant women is difficult for the following reasons:

1. Continuing excessive vaginal secretions
2. Increased vascularity that occurs with pregnancy may contraindicate excision
3. Contraindication during pregnancy of the standard treatment of applying podophyllin to the lesions

Certainly it helps to treat any existing vaginal infection which adds to the volume and character of vaginal discharge (see Chapter 25). Large clumps of external condylomata acuminata create hygenic and psychosocial-sexual difficulties. Vaginal discharge and feces may be entrapped in the clump and cause a foul odor. Careful cleaning, a sitz bath after each bowel movement and when needed, and frequent change of underwear will help control the problem of odor. The aesthetics of having large, uncomfortable condylomata negatively affects the woman's self-image and sexual life.

URINARY TRACT INFECTIONS

There are a number of urinary tract infections and diseases. The three most common ones are discussed in this chapter: asymptomatic bacteriuria, cystitis, and acute pyelonephritis.

Pregnant women are susceptible to urinary tract infections because the hydronephrosis that normally occurs during pregnancy may cause uninary stasis. Women can help prevent urinary tract infections due to urinary stasis by drinking at least eight large glasses daily of water and apple or cranberry juice and frequently emptying their bladder. As always, good hygiene also contributes to the prevention of urinary tract infections.

Asymptomatic Bacteriuria

As the name states, there are no symptoms associated with this infection. Its importance lies in the fact that 25 percent of women exhibiting asymptomatic bacteriuria at their initial antepartal examination will later develop a symptomatic urinary tract infection during their pregnancy.

The presence of bacteria in the urine (bacteriuria) is considered significant when the urine is a clean catch specimen and it contains 100,000 bacteria of the same species per milliliter. This most often indicates an infection, and authorities agree that the presence of 100,000 organisms per milliliter should be treated. However, judgment should be used. A colony count of 100,000 nonpathogenic (contaminant) organisms per milliliter of urine (e.g., lactobacillus) does not represent infection nor indicate treatment. It does indicate a grossly contaminated specimen; and another specimen should be obtained and the test repeated. Mixed bacteria counts which total more than

100,000 organisms per milliliter of urine also indicate contamination, not infection, and another specimen should be obtained and the test repeated.

Some clinicians believe that women whose specimens contain more than 50,000 pathogenic organisms of the same species per milliliter of urine should also be treated. This caution is again with the viewpoint of lessening the incidence of symptomatic urinary tract infections and in case it is finally proved that there is indeed a relationship between bacteriuria and low birth weight or prematurity. These women should receive patient education on reporting the signs and symptoms of premature labor (see Chapter 14). This is especially important when the woman has sickle cell trait since a correlation has been shown between sickle cell trait and bacteriuria. Black women with urinary tract infections who have not been screened for sickle cell disease should be so screened.

Organisms are pathogenic or nonpathogenic dependent on where they are located in the body. Following is a listing of the more common pathogenic organisms that may be found in urine:

Escherichia coli — colon bacteria normally non-pathogenic in the intestinal tract and highly pathogenic outside it

Neisseria gonorrhoeae — treat for gonorrhea

Proteus — normally found in the intestinal tract but pathogenic in the urinary tract

Klebsiella — more frequently associated with respiratory infections but may also cause urinary tract infections

Pseudomonas aeruginosa — a bacteria usually found in soil or decaying organic matter but pathogenic in humans including causing urinary tract infections

Corynebacterium — usually from a vaginal infection caused by *Corynebacterium vaginale* (Gardnerella *vaginalis*), which may also cause cystitis or pyelitis

Staphylococcus aureus — commonly present on the skin and mucous membranes of the nose and mouth; pathogenic in the urinary tract

Beta-hemolytic streptococcus — these bacteria comprise the majority of pathogenic streptococci

Enterococcus — any species of streptococcus normally inhabiting the intestinal tract and pathogenic in the urinary tract

Some laboratory reports simply report a coliform group. As this is a general term encompassing *E. coli*, enterococci, and *Klebsiella*, the report of coliforms would be of pathogenic bacteria.

The most common nonpathogenic (contaminant) organisms seen on urine reports include the following:

alpha-hemolytic streptococcus — generally not pathogenic in the urinary tract

Staphylococcus epidermis — common on the mucous membranes and skin including the genital area, and a major source of urine specimen contamination

Lactobacillus — normal in the mouth, intestinal tract, and vagina

The treatment of asymptomatic bacteriuria is best based on a report of the sensitivity of the microorganisms present to which antimicrobial agents. Most, however, are sensitive to sulfa drugs (e.g., Gantrisin), nitrofurantoin (e.g., Macrodantin), and ampicillin. The safest of these is ampicillin. The sulfa drugs are contraindicated late in pregnancy and may be a factor in kernicterus of the newborn, and the nitrofurantoin drugs are contraindicated in women with glucose-6-phosphate dehydrogenase (G6PD) deficiency since drug-induced hemolysis may occur and cause hemolytic anemia. Ampicillin, 500 milligrams four times daily for 7 to 10 days, is considered a standard treatment and may be the treatment of choice.

Nurse-midwives often diagnose and treat aymptomatic bacteriuria in accord with their medical protocols and standing orders. A follow-up urine culture should be performed within 2 weeks of treatment as a test of the effectiveness of the prescribed therapy.

Cystitis

Cystitis by definition is inflammation of the bladder. Usually this is due to a bacterial infection. Cystitis does not involve the upper urinary tract but may presage such an infection as the infection ascends. Signs and symptoms of cystitis include the following:

1. Urinary urgency
2. Urinary frequency
3. Dysuria
4. Lower abdominal (suprapubic) pain
5. Hematuria (possible)

Laboratory findings from microscopic urinalysis and urine culture and sensitivity include the following:

1. Bacteriuria
2. Abnormally increased number of white blood cells in the urine
3. Red blood cells in the urine

Treatment is the same as that stated for asymptomatic bacteriuria. Treatment also is usually instigated if there is a WBC count of 50 or more per milliliter of urine. Some clinicians treat if there is a WBC count above 25 per high-power field of spun clean-catch urine. Treatment on the basis of a WBC count and symptomatology may be initiated prior to obtaining and interpreting a urine specimen for culture and sensitivity of bacteria. A follow-up urine culture should be performed within 2 weeks of treatment as a test of the effectiveness of the prescribed therapy.

Acute Pyelonephritis

Pyelonephritis by definition is inflammation of one or both kidneys. The infectious agent is bacterial. The frequency of pyelonephritis in pregnancy, including the puerperium, is approximately 2 percent. Occurrence is due, in part, to a number of naturally occurring physiologic and anatomic events associated with pregnancy. These include the following:

1. Compression of the ureters at the pelvic brim by the uterus
2. Dilatation and decreased tone of the ureters due to hormonal effects (probably progesterone)
3. Urine stasis favorable to microorganisms, caused by 1 and 2 above
4. Decreased bladder tone and urine stasis in the immediate puerperium (see Chapter 24)

Signs and symptoms of acute pyelonephritis are as follows:

1. Fever and shaking chills
2. Hematuria
3. History of loss of appetite, nausea, and vomiting
4. History of asymptomatic bacteriuria or cystitis
5. Urinary urgency due to associated cystitis
6. Urinary frequency due to associated cystitis
7. Dysuria due to associated cystitis
8. Temperature — usually 100°F or above
9. Low back (lumbar) pain
10. CVA tenderness (if infection is unilateral, it will most often involve the right side)
11. Lower abdominal (suprapubic) pain

Laboratory findings from microscopic urinalysis and urine culture and sensitivity include the following:

1. Bacteriuria

2. Abnormally increased number of white blood cells in the urine
3. Red blood cells in the urine
4. Proteinuria (depending on the extent of renal damage)

Physician consultation is obtained by the nurse-midwife. Hospitalization may be required.

ANEMIAS AND HEMOGLOBINOPATHIES

There are a large number of anemias and hemoglobinopathies which may complicate or be complicated by pregnancy, including the following:

1. Iron deficiency anemia
2. Megaloblastic anemia
3. Anemia resulting from blood loss
4. Anemia associated with infection
5. Acquired hemolytic anemia
6. Macrocytic anemia
7. Microcytic anemia
8. Aplastic or hypoplastic anemia
9. Sickle cell disease (hereditary)
10. Sickle cell — hemoglobin C disease
11. Sickle — thalassemia
12. Thalassemia (hereditary anemia)

The interested student is encouraged to read in depth regarding these anemias in the medical and obstetric textbooks and journals.

The working definition of anemia is generally accepted to be when the hemoglobin is less than 12.0 grams per 100 milliliters blood in nonpregnant women and less than 10.0 grams per 100 milliliters blood in pregnant women. Naturally occurring physiologic changes in pregnancy affect normal hemoglobin levels in pregnant women. The increase in maternal blood volume is due more to an increase in plasma than in red blood cells. Although there is an increase in the number of erythrocytes in circulation it is not proportionate to the increase in plasma volume. The disproportion of erythrocytes to plasma exhibits itself in a lowered hemoglobin. The increase in the number of erythrocytes also is one of the factors in the increased need for iron during pregnancy, along with fetal demand. This disproportion is greatest during the second trimester because toward the end of pregnancy the increase in plasma volume ceases while increased erythrocyte production continues.

The need for iron and vitamin supplements during pregnancy is generally accepted universally and prescribed routinely for pregnant women. Many clinicians feel the same about folic acid supplementation, 1 milligram per day, and others specifically prescribe vitamin C in addition because this is thought to enhance iron absorption. It has been shown that the incidence of iron deficiency anemia and megaloblastic anemia is thus reduced or the disease at least minimized. Iron deficiency anemia constitutes approximately 95 percent of anemias related to pregnancy. Some clinicians believe that iron and vitamin supplementation is not necessary for well-nourished pregnant women.

In addition to prescribing routine iron, folic acid, and vitamin supplements, the nurse-midwife must be able to screen for anemia. Although often asymptomatic, anemia may evidence the following signs and symptoms:

1. Fatigue, malaise, drowsiness
2. Dizziness, weakness
3. Headaches
4. Sore tongue
5. Skin pallor
6. Pale mucous membranes, e.g., conjunctivae
7. Pale fingernail beds
8. History of heavy menses, especially of several days duration
9. History of closely spaced pregnancies
10. History of anemia ("low blood") with preceding pregnancies
11. Loss of appetite, nausea, and vomiting
12. Pica, i.e., excessive craving for and inges-

tion of food substances, or such things as clay or dirt, starch, ice

The nurse-midwife should take a careful dietary history and analyze it (see Chapter 8). Included in this history should be thorough investigation into the possibility of pica. Pica is excessive craving and ingestion either of food substances or of clay or dirt, starch, ice, and so forth. Such ingestion of nonnutritive substances is filling. Thus nutritive foodstuffs are neglected, resulting in malnutrition and its sequelae.

Women with between 10 and 12 grams hemoglobin per 100 milliliters blood should be started on iron, folic acid, and vitamin supplements if not already taking all of these. They should also be counseled on high-iron foods for their diet as iron is more readily absorbed from foodstuffs than from oral iron medication. High-iron foods include green leafy vegetables, collard greens, egg yolks, raisins, prunes, liver, oysters, and some fortified cereals.

If hemoglobin levels do not stabilize or continue to drop, a careful history should be taken to ascertain whether or not the woman is taking her pills and following her diet. The possibility of pica should be reinvestigated.

If the hemoglobin falls to between 9 and 10 grams per 100 milliliters blood then the nurse-midwife should order the following laboratory tests:

1. *Stat.* hemoglobin or hematocrit to rule out possible laboratory error if indicated by previous lab results
2. Sickle cell prep (if not already done) or hemoglobin electrophoresis if the sickle cell prep is positive
3. Serum iron concentration level
4. Iron binding capacity
5. Serum folate levels
6. Cell indices (WBC and RBC counts)
7. Reticulocyte count (measures the production of erythrocytes)
8. Platelet count
9. Stool culture for ova and parasites

The nurse-midwife consults with the physician upon receipt of the results. If the hemoglobin is below 9 grams per 100 milliliters, the nurse-midwife should apprise the consulting physician of the problem while initiating the preliminary laboratory workup just listed.

HEART DISEASE

A woman with any form of cardiac disease is referred to the physician for medical and obstetric management. Indications for such referral include a history of rheumatic fever or any of the following history, signs, and symptoms:

1. a diastolic, presystolic, or continuous heart murmur, especially one that ends in a loud first sound
2. a loud (Grade II or III/VI), harsh, apical systolic murmur
3. severe arrhythmia
4. cardiac enlargement beyond that normal for pregnancy
5. history of heart disease, heart failure, or cardiac surgery
6. signs and symptoms of congestive heart failure:
   a. persistent rales at the base of the lungs, with or without a cough, and still audible after the woman takes two to three deep breaths
   b. increased inability to carry out usual physical activity
   c. increasing dyspnea with exertion (differentiate from normal dyspnea in pregnancy due to the hyperventilation caused by elevated progesterone levels)
   d. hemoptysis
   e. cyanosis
   f. edema in the lower extremities (differentiate from normal pregnancy dependent pedal edema)

A woman with a history of rheumatic fever who has no signs or symptoms of heart disease should be evaluated by an internist or cardiologist and a recommendation obtained for antibiotic prophylaxis at the time of delivery. Due to the special needs of these women throughout pregnancy and labor, a collaborative approach by the nurse-midwife, physician, and childbirth educator is most beneficial.

DIABETES MELLITUS

A woman with diabetes who requires insulin for the management of her blood glucose levels is referred to the physician for medical and obstetric management. The role of the nurse-midwife is to screen for possible diabetes in pregnant women who are not obviously diabetic. Diabetes is a disease that may be precipitated by the endocrinological and hormonal changes of pregnancy.

All pregnant women for whom there are no initial risk factors for diabetes mellitus should be screened at 28 weeks gestation. If the screening test is normal, no further testing is needed. A woman who exhibits any of the following should be screened three times during the course of her pregnancy: in the first trimester or at the first visit, at 28 weeks, and at 34 to 36 weeks.

1. Family history of diabetes mellitus (parents, siblings, grandparents).
2. History of previous unexplained stillbirth.
3. Poor obstetrical history (e.g., spontaneous abortions, congenital anomalies).
4. Previous delivery of newborn weighing 9 pounds or more.
5. Nonpregnant weight greater than 180 pounds (may vary depending on height and body build).
6. Recurrent monilial infections (if this alone, screen only at 28 weeks).
7. Recurrent (two positive tests) glycosuria in clean-catch specimens, not explained by dietary intake; if glycosuria occurs

early in pregnancy and does not recur, do not repeat the screen later in pregnancy. Glycosuria secondary to dietary intake illustrates the lowered renal threshold for glucose which is a normal physiologic change during pregnancy.

8. Signs and symptoms of diabetes:
   a. polyuria (excessive urine output).
   b. polydipsia (excessive thirst).
   c. polyphagia (excessive eating).
   d. weight loss.
   e. poor healing.
9. Preeclampsia or chronic hypertension.
10. Polyhydramnios.
11. Age 25 or older.
12. Gestational diabetes in a previous pregnancy.

A woman with secondary risk factors such as preeclampsia, polyhydramnios, or a large-for-gestational-age fetus should be screened when these risk factors are first noted, regardless of any previous screening with negative results, and again at 34 to 36 weeks gestation.

There is a seemingly unending controversy as to which test combines the epitomy in simplicity and reliability. The fasting blood sugar should not be used alone for diabetic screening purposes because the fasting blood sugar in gestational diabetics is normal. Postprandial screening has generally been replaced with glucose load challenge screening tests. The 1-hour glucose challenge screen has an exceptionally high incidence of false-positive outcomes, which means that a larger number of unnecessary 3-hour glucose tolerance tests (GTTs) will be done. No woman with diabetes, however, will be missed. The 2-hour glucose challenge screening test has a lower rate of false positives. Some women with diabetes, however, may be missed.

The most efficacious diabetic screening is done by a combination of the fasting blood sugar and either the 1-hour or 2-hour post-glucose challenge. A combination of the fasting blood sugar and the 1-hour screen gives the greatest sensitivity for abnormal glucose tolerance. A combination of the fasting blood sugar and the 2-hour postglucose challenge eliminates unnecessary use of the GTT for those women who don't need this diagnostic workup, thereby also making it cost-effective.

A properly done glucose challenge requires that the woman have nothing to eat or drink from the previous midnight. She should drink the entire glucose mixture (flavored glucose) within 10 minutes. While she waits the 1 or 2 hours for the second blood test, she should not eat or drink (other than water) and should not moderately or vigorously exercise, nor smoke.

Most laboratories have established their laboratory values on the basis of using 100 grams of the glucose mix (contains 100 grams of glucose). However, norms have now been established for use of 50 grams or 75 grams of the glucose mixture. The normal range of blood glucose levels for any screening test is dependent upon the amount of glucose mixture used and whether plasma or whole blood levels are used by an individual laboratory. It is necessary, therefore, to check the methods and resulting lab values being used in each institution with which you work. However, generally speaking, a fasting plasma blood sugar of 105 milligrams or greater per 100 milliliters of blood, a 1-hour 50-gram glucose challenge plasma blood sugar of 135 milligrams or greater per 100 milliliters of blood, and a 2-hour 75-gram glucose challenge plasma blood sugar of 120 milligrams or greater per 100 milliliters of blood are abnormal values.

Table 9-1 shows when a GTT should be done as a follow-up to screening. A woman who is a known or obvious diabetic (abnormal fasting blood sugar *and* abnormal 1- or 2-hour glucose challenge) should *not* be subjected to a GTT. An abnormal fasting blood sugar has particular significance because the normal fasting state of a pregnant woman is relative hypoglycemia, which means that the woman's fasting blood value is that of hypoglycemia although she herself is not in a hypoglycemic state.

The next disagreement is whether administration of the glucose in a GTT should be done orally or intravenously. The intravenous GTT has a high incidence of false-negative outcomes — approximately a third again as many as for the oral GTT. On the other hand, the oral GTT involves drinking a 100-gram glucose mixture that is often poorly tolerated during pregnancy causing nausea and vomiting (which affects the test), and the absorption rate from the intestine is highly variable. In the nonpregnant state the oral GTT is considered more sensitive than the intravenous GTT.

An oral GTT is considered abnormal, or diagnostic for diabetes, if two or more of the following glucose values are met or exceeded:

1. Fasting — 90 milligrams of glucose per 100 milliliters of whole blood
2. 1 hour — 165 milligrams of glucose per 100 milliliters of whole blood
3. 2 hours — 145 milligrams of glucose per 100 milliliters of whole blood
4. 3 hours — 125 milligrams of glucose per 100 milliliters of whole blood

The above are glucose values for whole blood. If plasma rather than whole blood is analyzed for glucose, then the values are approximately 15 percent higher, as follows:

1. Fasting — 105 milligrams of glucose per 100 milliliters of plasma
2. 1 hour — 190 milligrams of glucose per 100 milliliters of plasma
3. 2 hours — 165 milligrams of glucose per 100 milliliters of plasma
4. 3 hours — 145 milligrams of glucose per 100 milliliters of plasma

Table 9-2 shows how the diagnosis is derived from a combination of the screening tests and a GTT. Note that a woman with a normal fasting blood sugar, an abnormal 1- or 2-hour glucose challenge, and two abnormal values on a GTT is a gestational diabetic.

Table 9-1.   Management Schematic for Diabetic Screening

Fasting Blood Sugar	(plus)	One- or Two-hour Glucose Challenge	(equals)	Indicated Action
Positive		Negative		Do GTT
Negative		Positive		Do GTT
Positive		Positive		Do *not* do GTT; woman is diabetic. Refer to physician.
Negative		Negative		Rescreen at 34–36 weeks gestation if has risk factors; if no risk factors, not necessary to screen again.

Table 9-2.   Diagnostic Schematic Based on Laboratory Tests

Fasting Blood Sugar	(plus)	One- or Two-hour Glucose Challenge	(plus)	Glucose Tolerance Test	(equals)	Diagnosis
Positive		Negative		Two abnormal values		Diabetic
Negative		Positive		Two abnormal values		Gestational diabetic
Positive		Positive		Not done		Diabetic
Negative		Negative		Not done		Not diabetic

A percentage of women who have a negative screening test at 28 weeks may convert to an abnormal test at 34 to 36 weeks. This is probably due to an even more increased placental hormone production as well as a further stressed pancreatic reserve. The late onset (after 34 weeks) of gestational diabetes may account for some of the macrosomic infants born to women whose earlier screening test at 28 weeks was negative. A woman who demonstrates abnormal glucose tolerance on the initial or 28-week screening tests and a normal diagnostic GTT should have another GTT at 34 to 36 weeks gestation.

Women with known diabetes mellitus or nongestational diabetes detected by screening should be referred to the physician for medical and obstetric management of care. Gestational diabetes (class A, controlled by diet) may be collaboratively managed by the nurse-midwife and physician, depending upon the clinical practice setting and individual practice protocols.

Most women with gestational diabetes can achieve diabetic control by diet. Careful explanation of the exchange food list and instructions can best be accomplished by a collaborative arrangement with a nutritionist. The diet is calculated on the basis of 30 calories per kilogram of body weight. The calories are distributed as 45 percent carbohydrate, 20 percent protein, and 35 percent fat. The goal of management is to maintain a normal fasting blood sugar (less than 105 milligrams per 100 milliliters of plasma) and a 2-hour postprandial test at less than 120 milligrams per 100 milliliters plasma.

Home glucose monitoring by finger stick is now available and should be taught to every woman with diabetes. She should be instructed to bring her record to each prenatal visit. Serum glucose determinations performed in a laboratory to confirm the home monitoring values are necessary. A fasting plasma level and a 1-hour or 2-hour postprandial determination should be performed every 2 weeks through the 28th week of gestation and weekly thereafter.

If one or both values are elevated (fasting blood sugar of 105 milligrams or more per 100 milliliters plasma; 1-hour blood sugar of 135 milligrams or more per 100 milliliters plasma; 2-hour blood sugar of 120 milligrams or more per 100 milliliters plasma), further investigation is important. Dietary intake, adherence to the prescribed diet, signs of infection (recent or current upper respiratory infection, symptoms of a urinary tract infection), and unusual stress at home — any of these can affect glucose metabolism. Urine analysis and culture and sensitivity can be done either monthly or in each trimester to detect asymptomatic bacteriuria. The presence of a urinary tract infection will adversely affect the woman's glucose values despite strict adherence to the prescribed diet. If none of the aforementioned conditions are present to explain the elevated glucose values, the physician should be contacted immediately.

If the plasma glucose values remain normal, and there is no other underlying disease such as preeclampsia or hypertension or a history of previous unexplained stillbirths, the woman on a prescribed diet can be managed without induction until 40 to 42 weeks gestation. Perinatal mortality does not increase with gestational diabetes unless complicated by preeclampsia, hypertension, or a history of previous unexplained stillbirths. Because of this, the woman should be carefully screened for development of preeclampsia throughout pregnancy; this screening should include kidney function and uric acid tests at least once in the third trimester.

Careful abdominal palpation should be performed to detect polyhydramnios. If this condition is detected, consult with your physician. Once the pregnancy has exceeded 40 weeks gestation, the woman should be followed according to the postdates protocol (applied at 40 weeks gestation for gestational diabetics) with fetal movement charts and nonstress testing. (See "Postdates Pregnancy" later in this chapter.)

Management of labor in women with diet-controlled gestational diabetes is no different from that for any other woman. If intravenous fluids are necessary, a glucose mixture should *not* be used. Since the incidence of macrosomia is higher, the nurse-midwife should carefully evaluate the estimated fetal weight and progress of labor with a higher level of suspicion for shoulder dystocia. The pediatrician should be informed upon admission of the woman to labor. Some of these women's babies may develop hypoglycemia following birth, especially if the infant is macrosomic.

A woman with a diagnosis of gestational diabetes in one pregnancy will not necessarily be a gestational diabetic in another pregnancy. An abnormal glucose tolerance test in pregnancy, however, may be predictive of later nonpregnant glucose intolerance. Approximately 60 percent of these women may develop glucose intolerance by 16 years later. Therefore, the nurse-midwife should inform the woman with gestational diabetes of the potential problem and advise her to seek periodic testing as part of her routine, ongoing health care.

MULTIPLE PREGNANCY

It is essential that a multiple pregnancy be identified as early as possible. There are a number of complications associated with the pregnancy, labor and delivery, and puerperium of a woman pregnant with more than one fetus. No woman receiving antepartal care should enter labor with undiagnosed multiple gestation. This statement, however, does *not* mean advocacy of routine ultrasound screening. Rather, it emphasizes the importance of clinical skill and judgment.

The following are signs and symptoms indicative of a possible multiple pregnancy:

1. Large-for-dates uterine size, fundal height, and abdominal girth associated with rapid uterine growth during the second trimester
2. Familial history of twins (in and of itself not indicative)
3. History of recent infertility problem treated with Clomid (in and of itself not indicative)
4. Abdominal palpation reveals three or more large parts and/or multiple small parts, especially in the third trimester when these are more readily felt
5. Auscultation of more than one fetal heart tone clearly distinct from another fetal heart tone (differing by more than 10 beats per minute) and from the maternal pulse

Diagnosis is made on the basis of clinical findings. If you suspect that there are more than twins, then order an ultrasound scan for diagnosis of the number and size. Ultrasound may be used to screen for discrepancy in the size of the fetuses (discordance). The risk-benefit ratio of ultrasound, however, must be considered and presented to the woman in making the decision about serial ultrasound assessments for diagnosing discordance.

Antepartal management of multiple gestation includes monitoring the pregnancy for early signs of premature labor (see Chapter 14), signs and symptoms of preeclampsia (discussed later in this chapter) and fetal growth (see Chapter 7); and prevention of a baby that is small for gestational age, intrauterine growth retardation, and premature labor. Maternal nutrition is critical to the development of the fetuses. As stated in Chapter 8, protein and calories should be added to the diet for each fetus. Women are seen every week for the duration of their pregnancy for evaluation of weight gain, fetal growth, premature labor, and preeclampsia. They are also evaluated weekly up to 34 weeks

for cervical changes. After that time tocolytic agents to stop premature labor cannot be given.

In multiple gestation the physical discomforts of pregnancy are more extreme, body image may be even more distorted, preparations for baby care are multiplied, and finances may be more strapped. All these factors pose additional stress requiring additional time on the part of the nurse-midwife in counseling and patient education.

Management also includes limiting activity and increasing rest periods throughout pregnancy. Instruction regarding sexual activity should be based on cervical findings, previous obstetrical history, and strength of Braxton Hicks contractions. Advice may include the use of condoms because of the prostaglandins in the semen that cause uterine irritability. The woman should also be instructed in the signs and symptoms of premature labor.

Ultrasound or abdominal x-ray is used by some clinicians to determine the presentation and position of the second twin. Other clinicians point out that if the first fetus has a vertex presentation then there is no need for a sonogram or x-ray to determine the presentation and position of the second fetus as there is no possibility of locked (conjoint) twins. Regardless, the presentation and position of the second twin can easily change after delivery of the first twin, and the nurse-midwife needs to be prepared for all eventualities.

When diagnosis of a multiple gestation is made, the nurse-midwife informs the physician of this finding and keeps the physician apprised of the progress of the pregnancy. Plans should be made for physician attendance at the delivery.

ABO AND RH DISEASE

Screening for blood incompatibility between the mother and the fetus is limited to Rh incompatibility because there is no generally accepted method for detecting and diagnosing ABO incompatibility during pregnancy.

History taking which may be relevant to ABO or Rh incompatibility includes the following:

1. History of previous blood transfusion
2. History of previous "yellow baby" or a baby needing a blood transfusion
3. History of stillbirth or neonatal death resulting from causes unknown to the mother
4. History of RhoGam after previous deliveries or abortions

Determination of the Rh type is made through routinely obtained laboratory work ordered during the initial prenatal visit. If the woman is Rh negative, an indirect Coombs' test is ordered. The indirect Coombs' test is a screening test for Rh antibodies. If the test is positive, thereby indicating the presence of Rh antibodies, Rh antibody titers are then obtained. In the interests of conserving time and being practical, many clinicians simply order Rh type, indirect Coombs' test, and antibody titers at the initial antepartal visit.

A woman who is Rh negative with a negative indirect Coombs' should have the indirect Coombs' test repeated every 4 weeks up to 28 weeks. If the antibody titers are negative at 28 weeks, 300 micrograms of Rh immune globulin (e.g., RhoGam) should be considered and offered as an option to the woman. In offering this option, the benefit and possible risk should be explained. The benefit is the decreased risk of developing antibody titers during the antepartal period in the event of a maternal-fetal transfusion which may occur with a placenta previa or abruptio placentae and during the intrapartal period. The possible risk is dependent upon the sex of the fetus. If the fetus is female and Rh negative, there is a theoretical risk that she will develop antibodies, which has implications for her reproductive future in the event she carries an Rh positive fetus. If the fetus is male then there is no need for concern.

If the woman chooses to have Rh immune globulin, no further antibody screening tests are then indicated prior to delivery, as protection against developing antibodies is provided for approximately 12 weeks. If a blood sample is taken during this time (e.g., upon admission in labor) there may be titers of anti-D present due to passive immunity as a result of the RhoGam. These titers should be less than 8 by 38 to 40 weeks gestation. Titers greater than 8 suggest that active immunization due to Rh incompatibility has occurred.

If the indirect Coombs' test is positive, the nurse-midwife consults with the physician for collaborative management or referral, depending on the antibody titers and severity of the problem.

HYDRAMNIOS (POLYHYDRAMNIOS)

Polyhydramnios is an excessive amount of amniotic fluid. There is a higher incidence of polyhydramnios in women with the following conditions:

1. Multiple pregnancy (especially with monozygotic twins)
2. Diabetes
3. Erythroblastosis
4. Fetal malformations (especially of the gastrointestinal tract or central nervous system, e.g., anencephaly, meningomyelocele)

Hydramnios may produce the following further complications:

1. Fetal malpresentations complicating delivery
2. Premature separation of the placenta (abruptio)
3. Uterine dysfunction during labor
4. Immediate postpartum hemorrhage as a result of uterine atony from overdistention
5. Cord prolapse

The signs and symptoms of polyhydramnios are clinical and include the following:

1. Uterine enlargement, abdominal girth, and fundal height far beyond that expected for gestational age
2. Tenseness of the uterine wall making it difficult or impossible to:
   a. auscultate fetal heart tones
   b. palpate the fetal outline and large and small parts
3. Elicitation of a uterine fluid thrill
4. Mechanical problems, if polyhydramnios is severe, such as:
   a. severe dyspnea
   b. lower extremity and vulvar edema
   c. pressure pains in the back, abdomen, and thighs
   d. nausea and vomiting
5. Frequent change in lie (unstable lie)

If you suspect a woman of having polyhydramnios, the following workup should be done:

1. Obtain a sonogram to confirm the diagnosis and identify any coexisting conditions or complications.
2. Screen for diabetes (see pages 177–180).
3. Screen for ABO/Rh disease (see pages 181–182).

When a diagnosis of polyhydramnios is made, consultation with your physician is indicated. Collaborative management is appropriate if the screening tests for related or coexisting complications are negative. Otherwise the woman is referred to the physician. Emotional support is especially needed if congenital anomalies are present. Women with severe polyhydramnios have a number of mechanical difficulties and discomforts (listed under signs and symptoms) which require attention by the nurse-midwife for relief measures (see pages 126 to 135).

OLIGOHYDRAMNIOS

Oligohydramnios is an abnormally small amount of amniotic fluid. There is a higher incidence of oligohydramnios in women with the following conditions:

1. Congenital anomalies (e.g., renal agenesis, Potter's syndrome)
2. Intrauterine growth retardation
3. Early rupture of the fetal membranes (24 to 26 weeks)
4. Postmature syndrome

Oligohydramnios may lead to the following further complications:

1. Lung hypoplasia
2. Limb deformities

The clinical signs and symptoms of oligohydramnios include the following:

1. "Molding" of the uterus around the fetus
2. Fetus easily outlined
3. Fetus not ballotable

These clinical signs and symptoms are based on the fact that the amniotic fluid volume is below what is normally found for that particular gestational age. At term, the normal amniotic fluid volume is approximately 2 cups (480 cc). Detection of oligohydramnios involves careful palpation and comparison with normal at each examination. The clinical impression of oligohydramnios can be refined by including the evaluation of amniotic fluid value in every abdominal palpation.

Amniotic fluid volume detection by sonography is a part of the biophysical profile. The significance of the measurements for oligohydramnios is not clear in the literature. Some authors suggest a measurement of 1 centimeter or less of amniotic fluid is indicative of oligohydramnios. Clinical decisions based on this criterion are not conclusive. Some authors consider a pocket of fluid less than 2 centimeters significant.

The management of oligohydramnios is to do a workup to exclude congenital anomalies, intrauterine growth retardation, and premature rupture of the membranes. Oligohydramnios is a significant finding in diagnosing postmaturity syndrome in a postdates pregnancy.

FETAL DEATH

Signs and symptoms of fetal death include the following:

1. Cessation of uterine growth or decrease in uterine size — fundal height stationary or decreasing over time
2. Cessation of fetal movement
3. Cessation of fetal heart tones — not heard with a Doptone: items 2 and 3 constitute the so-called silent uterus, which gives rise to an ominous feeling of fetal death
4. Cessation of maternal weight gain or decrease in weight
5. Retrogressive breast changes
6. Collapsed fetal skull felt upon examination
7. Sonographic signs:
   a. Spalding's sign — excessive overlapping of the skull bones; occurs several days after death as a result of liquefaction of the brain
   b. no heart movement
   c. no fetal movement
8. Radiologic signs (x-ray ordered if ultrasonography is not available)
   a. Spalding's sign
   b. exaggerated curvature of the fetal spine — occurs several days after death due to maceration of the spinous ligaments
   c. gas formation in the circulatory system of the fetus

The nurse-midwife consults with the physician when suspicious of the possibility of fetal death. Management options are twofold and should be discussed with the woman. Expectant management involves awaiting the onset of labor. Labor can be anticipated to start within 2 to 3 weeks of fetal death; onset of labor is thought to be due to cessation of placental functioning. The risk involved in expectant management is the potential development of disseminated intravascular coagulation (DIC). Coagulation studies are done every week as screening tests for DIC. These consist of prothrombin, partial prothrombin, fibrinogen, and platelets. If these tests remain within normal range, waiting for spontaneous labor to ensue may continue. If there is a drop in platelets or fibrinogen, and/ or an increase in the partial prothrombin or prothrombin, consultation with the physician is indicated for induction of labor.

Emotional support is extremely important antepartally, intrapartally, and during the postpartal course. The nurse-midwife should help the woman explore feelings, first trimester ambivalence (see pages 95–96), beliefs about possible causes of the death, and her own and other family members' guilt feelings. Information should be supplied to counteract "old wives' tales" concerning possible causes of the fetal death (e.g., falling down stairs, raising arms over head, lifting heavy object). The nurse-midwife may need to initiate this discussion in order to elicit specific beliefs held by the woman or family members or significant others.

Support during labor will be difficult if the nurse-midwife does not examine her own personal feelings and reactions to an intrauterine death. If you keep in mind that this is still the child of this woman then your approach to labor will not be to block out the experience for the woman and her family with drugs. The woman, the baby's father, and other supportive family members should be encouraged to view, touch, and hold the infant. This may be difficult for the woman to do for a variety of reasons including drowsiness secondary to medication or emotional reasons. The option to view the baby should be kept open and arrangements made with the morgue to allow viewing whenever and as often as it is required by the woman, baby's father, and family. This reality orientation is an essential ingredient to facilitating the grief process.

You should avoid making a false diagnosis of the cause of death but do need to point out to the parents even the smallest deviations from normal, if any, (e.g., nuchal cord, twisted cord). Most intrauterine deaths have no known cause even after autopsy. These are the most difficult for the woman to handle.

The nurse-midwife should assist the family in decisions regarding autopsy and burial. If an autopsy is performed, arrange to meet with the woman and significant others as soon as the preliminary results are available. Inform them that the final results usually take 6 weeks to 3 months.

The nurse-midwife must evaluate and assess her own value system and responses to death and grieving before she can begin to understand and be able to assist a woman through the grief process. The first stage of grief manifests itself in extreme emotion. These emotions should not be denied or hampered by well-intentioned but inappropriate and often destructive platitudes (e.g., "It's all right, you can have another baby"; "It's God's will, just accept it"; "Aren't you fortunate to have other children?"). For a discussion of the grief process, see Chapter 24.

The determination if or when a woman or couple should have another child should be based on the resolution of the grief process and ability to see a subsequent child as a separate individual, not a replacement. If another pregnancy occurs, you will need to do anticipatory guidance regarding the woman's fears of a repeated disastrous outcome.

HYPERTENSIVE DISORDERS OF PREGNANCY

More is written and less is known about the hypertensive disorders of pregnancy than any other obstetric complication. The interested student is referred to obstetrics textbooks and journals. The hypertensive disorders of pregnancy include the following:

1. Preeclampsia — the development of an elevated blood pressure *with* proteinuria due to pregnancy. It is primarily a complication of primigravidas occuring after 20 to 24 weeks gestation except in the presence of trophoblastic disease.
2. Eclampsia — same as preeclampsia with the addition of one or more convulsions with their sequelae.
3. Chronic hypertensive vascular or renal disease with or without superimposed preeclampsia or eclampsia.
4. Gestational hypertension (pregnancy-induced hypertension: PIH) — the development of an elevated blood pressure *without* proteinuria during pregnancy or within the first 24 hours postpartum in a previously normotensive woman who has no evidence of hypertensive vascular disease.
5. Gestational proteinuria — the presence of proteinuria *without* coexisting hypertension during pregnancy, with no evidence of any urinary tract infection or history of intrinsic renovascular disease.
6. Gestational edema — the development of a *general* and excessive accumulation of fluid in the tissues (measured as greater than 1+ pitting edema after 12 hours rest in bed) *without* coexisting hypertension or proteinuria.

The role of the nurse-midwife in relation to the hypertensive disorders of pregnancy lies in meticulous screening, in prevention, and in knowing when to consult with and/or refer the woman to the physician.

The classical clinical signs of preeclampsia are the triad of hypertension, proteinuria, and edema. Definitions of these three clinical signs are as follows:

1. Hypertension:
   a. blood pressure of 140/90 or higher, or
   b. a rise of 30 millimeters of mercury in the systolic pressure and/or rise of 15 millimeters of mercury in the diastolic pressure over the woman's baseline blood pressure, or
   c. mean arterial pressure equal to or more than 105 millimeters of mercury for two readings taken 6 hours apart
      (1) in reality, the second reading is often taken the next day
      (2) mean arterial pressure is calculated as follows:

$$MAP = \frac{(D \times 2) + S}{3}$$

   where MAP = mean arterial pressure
   D = diastolic blood pressure
   S = systolic blood pressure
2. Proteinuria:
   a. protein in the urine at a concentration of more than 0.3 gram in a 24-hour specimen, or
   b. protein in the urine in excess of 1 gram per liter (1+ to 2+ by standard turbidimetric methods)
      (1) in random clean-catch, midstream voided specimen (eliminates protein contamination from vaginal infection), and
      (2) on two or more occasions at least 6 hours apart when there is no known urinary tract infection
3. Edema:
   a. fluid retention first evidenced by a sudden excessive weight gain (2 to 5 pounds or more in a week),
   b. differentiated from dependent edema in the lower extremities,
   c. evaluated in relation to the overall pattern of weight gain, and
   d. unquestionably significant when in the hands and face

Conditions associated with or which predispose to the development of preeclampsia include the following:

1. Trophoblastic disease
2. Multiple pregnancy
3. Chronic hypertensive vascular disease
4. Chronic renal disease
5. Diabetes mellitus
6. Familial tendency — a woman has double the risk of developing preeclampsia if her mother had preeclampsia
7. Previous history of preeclampsia — one-third of women with preeclampsia in a previous pregnancy develop hypertension (although not necessarily preeclampsia) in a subsequent pregnancy

The signs and symptoms of preeclampsia form the base of a routine history, physical, and laboratory screening that is done on each prenatal visit. This is as follows:

1. History
   a. headaches, dizziness, blurring of vision, spots before the eyes, or scotomata
   b. hand, face, or general body edema
2. Physical examination
   a. blood pressure (compare to baseline blood pressure either before pregnancy or prior to 24 weeks gestation)
   b. weight (compare to prepregnant weight and to weight at last visit — note visit interval)
   c. ankle, pretibial, hand, face, or abdominal edema (note amount)
   d. reflexes (note degree of reflex response)
3. Laboratory test
   a. urine for protein

A history of unremitting headaches and visual problems, or an elevated blood pressure, or a sudden excessive weight gain, or hand or face edema, or proteinuria, or a combination of any of these indicates the need for further investigation. This includes:

1. History
   a. careful history regarding the headaches and visual disturbances to rule out migraine headaches, need for glasses, and stress and tension in the woman's personal life
   b. evaluation of dietary intake (see Chapter 8)
   c. evaluation of the overall weight gain pattern to differentiate edema from good nutritional intake
2. Physical examination
   a. ophthalmic examination — papilledema, A–V nicking, vessel narrowing, hemorrhagic areas
3. Laboratory tests
   a. hematocrit
   b. liver function tests
   c. kidney profile:
      (1) BUN
      (2) serum creatinine
      (3) serum electrolytes
      (4) serum uric acid

As precise ranges vary from laboratory to laboratory it is necessary to check the laboratory values for the institution or laboratory from which you obtain laboratory results. If any laboratory tests come back with abnormal values, consult with your physician.

Many nurse-midwives use the labels "mild" preeclampsia, "early" preeclampsia, or "borderline" preeclampsia to indicate the presence of signs and symptoms which may portend the development of preeclampsia but which do not yet meet criteria for the diagnosis of preeclampsia. Unfortunately, these labels are often considered diagnoses. Such misdiagnoses may channel women into unnecessary and expensive tests and interventions and skew nurse-midwifery statistics. A "tentative" diagnosis, however, of preeclampsia in a woman who actually exhibits one or more of the classical clinical signs of preeclampsia is an appropriate diagnosis until the "pure" diagnosis can be made or disproved 6 or more hours later.

For women who are "tending toward" preeclampsia but don't yet meet criteria for diagnosis, the nurse-midwife may prescribe bedrest — at least 2 hours in the morning and afternoon on her left side (for diuresis) — and a high protein, high caloric diet. Restriction of salt and the use of diuretics have no place in the management of impending or actual preeclampsia or eclampsia. In fact, it has been shown that preeclampsia and eclampsia can largely be prevented by a diet high in protein with the protein intake adequately protected with calories and normal sodium intake (see Chapter 8).

Signs and symptoms of progressively severe preeclampsia when associated with hypertension, proteinuria, or edema include the following:

1. Hyperreflexia (reflects central nervous system irritability) — extremely severe when clonus is present
2. Headaches (frontal or occipital) — usually resistant to customary effective treatment
3. Visual disturbances — blurring of vision, scotomata, flashing lights, spots before the eyes, and the like
4. Epigastric pain
5. Oliguria — less than 500 milliliters urine output in 24 hours
6. Increasingly elevated blood pressure — 160/110 and above is considered severe
7. Increasingly greater proteinuria — 3+ or 4+ is considered severe

A woman who meets criteria for a diagnosis of preeclampsia will have one or more of the classical clinical signs of preeclampsia. A nurse-midwife should consult with a physician about any woman who demonstrates hypertension by itself, or a combination of any two of the signs, or any one of the signs and hyperreflexia (3+ or greater) with or without clonus.

The nurse-midwife should listen to her inner hunches — it is the adolescent with a rise in blood pressure not yet elevated to critical levels and evidencing no other symptoms, but "not feeling good," who may convulse the next day. If uncomfortable or unsure, order the laboratory tests and consult with the physician. Share with the physician your inner uneasiness as well as the factual data base.

Collaborative management in the hospital includes the following:

1. Bed rest
2. Decreased environmental stimulation
3. Screening for diabetes
4. 24-hour record of intake and output
5. High protein, high calorie diet
6. Continuing monitoring of liver and kidney function — in addition to repeating the previously listed laboratory tests, 24-hour urine for protein and creatinine should also be collected

Continued monitoring of the woman includes evaluation for uteroplacental insufficiency and assessment for possible intrauterine growth retardation (IUGR). If the woman develops preeclampsia before 36 weeks gestation, ultrasound is indicated for detection of IUGR. Careful fundal height measurements and estimated fetal weights should be recorded. The status of the fetus should also be evaluated by fetal movement and nonstress test, contraction (nipple stimulation) stress test, oxytocin stress test, or a combination of these.

Timing of delivery is based on the condition of the fetus or the severity of the disease. In other words, a woman may not have severe preeclampsia but the uterine environment may be so hostile for the baby that delivery is advisable. Delivery may also be indicated if the woman's condition is worsening. Preeclampsia is not a disease that can be treated and cured. The process will continue until the baby is born.

It is important to differentiate chronic hypertension from preeclampsia. It is even more important to recognize when preeclampsia is superimposed on chronic hypertension. Chronic hypertension, by strict definition,

either precedes pregnancy or occurs before the 24th week of gestation. A chronically hypertensive woman may be receiving antihypertensive drugs or a low salt diet or both. Her blood pressure should remain stable during pregnancy. If the blood pressure rises above what is normal for her or if proteinuria suddenly appears, these should be recognized as signs of superimposed preeclampsia or renal disease and not as part of the course of chronic hypertension. Collaborative management of these patients is indicated. A baseline set of liver and kidney function tests (listed before) and a diabetic screen should be obtained on the initial visit. A careful ophthalmic examination adds to the data base regarding the severity of this disease process.

ANTEPARTAL BLEEDING

There are multiple causes of antepartal bleeding, most of which are not life threatening. Placenta previa and abruptio placentae, however, are life threatening and will be discussed in this chapter.

Following is a list of possible causes of antepartal bleeding. Differential diagnosis between them is imperative and is based on history, physical, pelvic, and laboratory findings.

Vaginitis	Rectal polyps
Cervicitis	Rectal cancer
Cervical erosion	Urethritis
Cervical cancer	Hemorrhagic cystitis
Cervical polyps	Extrachorial placentas
Recent cone biopsy	Ruptured vasa previa
Ruptured vaginal septum	Spontaneous abortion
Ruptured vaginal or vulvar varicosities	Implantation bleeding
	Ruptured uterus (see Chapter 14)
Vaginal trauma	Bloody show
Condylomata acuminata	Placenta previa
Rectal hemorrhoids	Abruptio placentae

Placenta Previa

Placenta previa is malposition of the placenta in the lower uterine segment, either anteriorly or posteriorly, instead of in the uterine fundus, so that the fully developed placenta either covers (totally or partially), or is at the margin or in close proximity to, the internal cervical os (Fig. 9-1). Except in total placenta previa, the degree of occlusion of the cervical os may depend on the degree of cervical dilatation.

Placenta previa may be a serious cause of antepartal hemorrhage in the third trimester. It is more common in women with the following conditions:

1. Multiparity
2. Maternal age greater than 35
3. Multiple pregnancy (larger placenta)
4. Erythroblastosis (larger placenta)
5. Uterine surgery scars

The cardinal sign of placenta previa is *painless* bleeding or hemorrhage which is usually sudden in onset and without warning. It occurs during the third trimester and may be accompanied or precipitated by uterine irritability. A woman with painless vaginal bleeding in the third trimester, not in labor, with an unengaged presenting part or a malpresentation must be suspected of having placenta previa.

The nurse-midwife does *not* do a vaginal examination. The diagnosis can be confirmed with ultrasonography. In the phenomenon of the so-called migrating placenta, a sonogram in early pregnancy indicates a low-lying placenta; on ultrasound examination later in gestation, when the uterus has further enlarged, the placenta is found to be normally situated in the uterus. If a low-lying placenta is an incidental finding on an early ultrasound prior to 26 weeks and there was not and has not been any vaginal bleeding, a repeat ultrasound is not necessary. However, if the ultrasound was done for vaginal bleeding, or there is vaginal bleeding now, a repeat ultrasound is indicated.

A woman with a total placenta previa should be hospitalized for the duration of her preg-

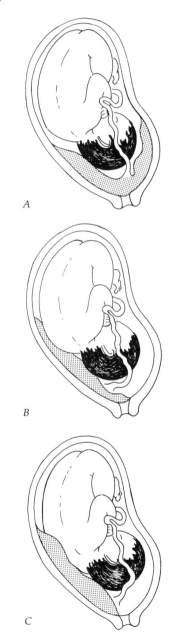

FIGURE 9-1.   Placenta previa. A. total; B. partial; C. marginal.

nancy. Components of management of care include serial hematocrits, blood type, cross-match, Rh, antibodies, indirect Coombs' test, and coagulation studies (prothrombin, partial prothrombin, fibrinogen, platelets); and blood replacement if indicated. For monitoring of the fetus, management of care includes assessing continued growth, nonstress tests, and fetal movement records.

A woman who has been admitted with vaginal bleeding from partial or marginal placenta previa is given the same laboratory tests and, if needed, blood replacement. She may be discharged if the bleeding stops and her hemoglobin and hematocrit are at acceptable levels. Pelvic precautions should be prescribed for women with all types of placenta previa: nothing should be inserted into the vagina, for example, vaginal therapeutics, douches, penis.

Total placenta previa is accompanied by an unexplained increased fetal mortality which is not secondary to bleeding. Because of this fact, most clinicians will deliver the baby prior to term. Other indications for delivery include uncontrollable hemorrhage, fetal distress, and maternal distress.

The decision for delivery of a woman with partial or marginal placenta previa is based on the gestational age of the fetus and the severity of the bleeding. This is not an issue if the pregnancy is at term. Many women with partial or marginal placenta previa can deliver vaginally because the presenting part acts as a tamponade.

Abruptio Placentae

Abruptio placentae (Fig. 9-2) is a shorter name for "premature separation of the normally implanted placenta" which differentiates it by definition from placenta previa. It may be a serious cause of antepartal hemorrhage in the third trimester. Hemorrhage may be concealed or obvious or both. Obvious hemorrhage may

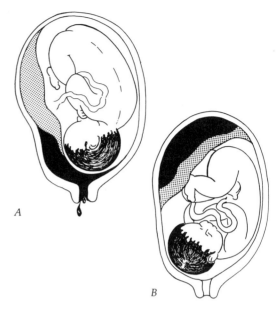

FIGURE 9-2. Abruptio placentae. A. marginal separation with obvious bleeding; B. central separation with concealed bleeding.

result from either a marginal or partial separation.

Etiological factors are unknown but hypotheses associate abruptio placentae with the following conditions:

1. Maternal hypertension
2. Preeclampsia
3. Folic acid deficiency
4. Severe abdominal trauma
5. Short umbilical cord
6. Malnutrition
7. Sudden decrease in uterine volume or size, for example, with rupture of the membranes in polyhydramnios, between delivery of babies in multiple gestation
8. Maternal age over 35
9. Rough or difficult external version

The signs and symptoms of abruptio placentae are dependent upon the position of the placenta in the uterus (anterior or posterior) and the degree of separation. The major difference of signs and symptoms between a placenta that is located on the posterior wall (posterior placenta) and a placenta located on the anterior wall (anterior placenta) is that of uterine activity and the feel of the uterus. The well-known boardlike abdomen may *not* occur when the placenta is located on the posterior wall because you will not be able to feel the portion of the uterine wall into which blood is being extravasated. It may not occur even if the placenta is on the anterior wall if the separation is small or marginal.

Uterine activity with a posterior placenta is not unlike labor: the woman has back pain and there is colicky, discoordinate uterine activity interspersed with relaxation of the uterus. Bleeding may be either concealed or obvious. Uterine activity with an anterior placenta is not unlike hypertonic uterine dysfunction: the woman's perception of pain is out of proportion to what the examiner feels, there is increased uterine tone between what feel like contractions, and the woman experiences painful localized or generalized uterine tenderness. The classical hypertonic, boardlike uterus and uterine rigidity will occur with a large abruption.

Other signs and symptoms vary according to the degree of separation. The fetal heart rate pattern may be normal with a small degree of abruption. A greater degree of separation will produce abnormal fetal heart rate tracings of variable or late decelerations, loss of beat-to-beat variability, or a sinusoidal pattern. There may be decreased or absent fetal movements for up to 12 hours prior to any obvious signs of an abruption. Other women may have violent fetal movement when there is a large abruption and massive hemorrhage. If a cesarean section is done within minutes of this occurrence, a live baby may issue. Otherwise, fetal movement ceases.

Other signs and symptoms of a significant abruption include uterine enlargement (concealed hemorrhage only) and the signs and symptoms of maternal shock. The severity of maternal shock depends on the severity of the abruption. You should not make the mistake of thinking the blood loss from obvious bleeding is always the total actually lost, because there may be concomitant concealed hemorrhage. Uterine enlargement from concealed hemorrhage is measured by marking the abdomen at the level of the fundus, checking every 15 minutes for an increase, and remarking accordingly. Ultrasonography for a retroplacental clot will yield information only if the placenta is anterior or in the fundus. This procedure is most useful when there has been a traumatic blow to the abdomen. A negative finding on ultrasound does not preclude the diagnosis of an abruption.

The management for abruptio placenta is delivery. If the woman is stable and there is no evidence of deterioration in the fetal or maternal condition, delivery may be vaginal. Management includes rupture of the membranes, internal monitoring of the fetus, and pitocin induction or stimulation.

The diagnosis of abruptio placentae should be considered for any woman who presents with back pain and colicky uterine activity. This woman should be observed for at least 3 to 4 hours. Cervical findings, fetal movement history, fetal heart rate pattern, monitoring of uterine activity by palpation, vital signs, urine for proteinuria, and maternal vital signs should be obtained. If an abruption is occuring it should become apparent during this period of observation.

Management of Hemorrhage in Placenta Previa and Abruptio Placentae

Management of a woman who is hemorrhaging from either diagnosis is the same and consists of the following:

1. Call for help. This includes requesting notification of your physician consultant.
2. Start 5% dextrose in Ringer's lactate intravenously with a 16-gauge intracatheter.

3. When starting the IV, obtain blood for type and cross-match for three or more units, CBC, platelets, prothrombin, partial prothrombin, fibrinogen, and a tube for clotting time to hang on the wall.
4. Place the woman in Trendelenburg position.
5. Monitor the woman's vital signs (blood pressure, pulse).
6. Monitor the fetal heart tones (put on an external monitor).
7. Administer oxygen to the woman.
8. Place warm blankets on the woman's body.
9. Start a second IV. Two intravenous infusion routes are needed: one for electrolyte solutions and the other for blood transfusion. The IV line for blood transfusion is kept open until the blood is obtained.
10. Have the operating room set up for an emergency cesarean section.
11. Insert a Foley catheter to measure output and in preparation for possible surgery.

SIZE-DATES DISCREPANCY

A size-dates discrepancy exists when there is reasonable knowledge of the date of a woman's last menstrual period, an estimated date of delivery has been determined, and the size of the uterus is either larger or smaller than expected for the gestational age as determined by the estimated date of delivery.

The most common cause of size-dates discrepancy, especially in the third trimester, is a big baby. The next most common cause is an inaccurate date for the last menstrual period. Size-dates discrepancies in the first or second trimesters have causes which are different from those in the third trimester. Congenital anomalies, chronic maternal disease, or viral infection contribute to first or second trimester discrepancies in size (usually size smaller than expected for dates).

It is the responsibility of the nurse-midwife to obtain as accurate a data base as is possible on the *first* prenatal visit.

1. History
   a. history of the last menstrual period and the previous menstrual period
      (1) ascertain the first day of the last menstrual period — determine whether of usual cycle length and usual amount of bleeding and length of menses
      (2) previous menstrual period — determine whether of usual cycle length and usual amount of bleeding and length of menses
      (3) bleeding after the last menstrual period — find out when it occurred in relation to the last menstrual period. Implantation bleeding is common and many times misinterpreted by a woman as her last menstrual period. Usually the interval from the last menstrual period is shorter and the type, amount, and length of bleeding are different.
   b. careful history of menstrual cycles for 6 months to 1 year prior to the last menstrual period in order to determine current normal length of cycles. Cycle length other than 28 days will render invalid gestational age determination based on dates. This is because the standard calculation of dates is based on 28-day lunar months. For example, a woman with 35-day cycles will probably ovulate 7 days later than the woman with a 28-day cycle, thereby making her estimated date of delivery 287 days from her last menstrual period instead of 280 days.
   c. contraceptive history, especially related to oral contraceptives: last month taken, history of vaginal bleeding patterns after discontinuation, interval method after discontinuation. Pregnancy occurring because of missed pills gives an irregular bleeding pattern which complicates accurate dating.
   d. coital history
   e. extenuating psychosocial situations which may influence accuracy of the

reported last menstrual period. For example, a woman who becomes pregnant during her partner's absence presents a difficult situation. This information may not be forthcoming on a first prenatal visit, but the possibility should be kept in mind if a size-dates discrepancy occurs.

f. history of quickening. If the prenatal visit, takes place before 16 weeks gestation, instruct the woman to mark a calendar when quickening occurs. Discuss trying to distinguish fetal movement from gas movement. If the prenatal visit occurs after 16 weeks, try to ascertain when the woman first felt quickening.

2. Physical and pelvic examinations
   a. fundal height measurement — this may vary according to prepregnancy weight, current weight, height, overall body type, and different examiners (see Chapter 41). Contrary to popular practice, the use of fundal height measurement as the single parameter to determine that size is appropriate for dates is inadequate and misleading. Fundal height gives a rough estimation of size and shows whether the fetus is or is not growing. The diagrams and charts in Chapter 41 which correlate fundal height with weeks of gestation have value as a guide but should not be used as a rigid, literal interpretation of whether or not size equals dates. Therefore, obtaining a fundal height measurement 2 centimeters greater or less than expected for the estimated gestational age does *not* indicate the need for an ultrasound exmination.
   b. estimated fetal weight — note size of head, buttocks, and general body proportions.
   c. abdominal girth palpation to gain an impression of the size of the uterus. Some women carry their babies entirely anterior, while other babies "fill out"

the sides of the woman's abdomen and occupy posterior space. Fundal height may not reflect this, which is another reason why fundal height by itself may be misleading.

d. evaluation of amniotic fluid volume by palpation for normalcy.
e. date at which first fetal heart tone is heard with a fetoscope — bring back all women at or before the estimated twentieth week of gestation.
f. bimanual examination for uterine size and position. Evaluate uterine position as this may affect fundal height. Even experienced clinicians may be off by 2 weeks. A single size, rather than a range, however, should be recorded.

If attention is paid to all of these clinical evaluation techniques for every woman at every visit, clinical acumen will increase, detection of a true size-dates problem becomes more accurate, and normal variations will not be misinterpreted as size-dates discrepancies.

Size-dates discrepancy is suspected when the size of the uterus does not match the gestational age based on dates. The reference point used for making this determination is the approximate expected location of the fundal height at various weeks of gestation (see Table 14-1 in Chapter 41). This reference point has to be evaluated in relation to other findings, including how the woman is carrying the baby (e.g., anteriorly, posteriorly), station, estimated fetal weight, lie and presentation, and obstetrical or medical conditions which would make the uterine size larger or smaller, as all these factors affect fundal height.

When you suspect a size-dates discrepancy, differential diagnosis is necessary in order to determine the cause of this discrepancy. Possibilities include:

1. Erroneous dates
2. Large baby (size greater than expected for dates)
3. Intrauterine growth retardation (size smaller than expected for dates)

4. Multiple pregnancy (size greater than expected for dates)
5. Diabetes:
   a. gestational to class B (size greater than expected for dates due to a macrosomic infant)
   b. classes C and above (size smaller than expected for dates)
6. Thyroid disease (size smaller than expected for dates)
7. Inadequate nutritional intake or inadequate weight gain pattern (size smaller than expected for dates)
8. Polyhydramnios (size greater than expected for dates)
9. Oligohydramnios (size smaller than expected for dates)
10. Fetal lie:
    a. transverse lie or oblique lie (size smaller than expected for dates)
    b. breech lie (size greater than expected for dates)
11. Congenital anomalies
12. Station of presenting part (size smaller than expected for dates if the presenting part is deep in the pelvis)
13. Hypertension or preeclampsia
14. Psychosocial factors, for example, death in family, severe emotional shock
15. Viral infection such as toxoplasmosis, rubella, cytomegalic inclusion disease

Further evaluation of a size-dates discrepancy is based on the potential differential diagnosis and consists of the following:

1. Review the data base obtained on the first prenatal visit (described earlier in this section).
2. Review fundal height growth pattern.
3. Review maternal weight gain pattern.
4. Reevaluate the estimated fetal weight — size of palpated head and buttocks, amount of amniotic fluid, relationship of the uterus to the size of the woman.
5. Perform abdominal palpation to determine:

   a. fetal lie.
   b. station of presenting part.
   c. multiple gestation.
6. Ascertain whether there have been any intervening psychosocial factors affecting nutrition and sleep patterns.
7. Ascertain existence of upper respiratory infection, influenza, or other viral infections since last visit.
8. Review smoking and use of alcohol and other drugs.
9. Review diet (24-hour recall and 3- or 7-day diet history).
10. Evaluate blood pressure and screen for signs and symptoms of preeclampsia if size is smaller than expected for dates.
11. Screen for diabetes mellitus (if screening was not done previously) if size is larger than expected for dates.
12. Evaluate thyroid function if clinical symptoms are present (increased pulse, dry skin, enlarged thyroid gland, tremors, etc.).
13. Schedule return visit to ascertain fetal growth pattern, weight gain, and diet intake.
14. Ultrasonography, if used for dating, should be done early in pregnancy, between 18 and 26 weeks of estimated gestational age. An ultrasound can be helpful in determining gestational age between 18 and 26 weeks. A later ultrasound is of little value, may add confusion to the clinical picture, and can give a false sense of knowledge of the date of delivery. Ultrasound may be done at other times, however, to rule out multiple pregnancy, intrauterine growth retardation, congenital anomalies, polyhydramnios, and oligohydramnios if the clinical picture indicates the need.

Management of size-dates discrepancy consists of either consulting with the physician for management of a complication or determining a new estimated date of delivery if the pregnancy is normal and all the above data have been gathered (except 13) and evaluated. Particular care needs to be taken, however, not to change the dates if you suspect a normal so-called lag period early in the third trimester. This may occur around 28 to 32 weeks of gestation and is a period when there is little to no increase in fundal height. Careful palpation, however, reveals growth that is being accommodated posteriorly in the woman's abdomen.

If the pregnancy is normal and an ultrasound has been done, use the originally estimated date of delivery if the sonogram is within 2 to 3 weeks of agreement with the estimated date of delivery by dates. This will avoid the *very serious* problem of later missing a true post-dates pregnancy. If the date of the last menstrual period is unknown or the woman is a late registrant, an estimated date of delivery based on many parameters is usually more accurate than an estimated date of delivery based on one ultrasound, especially after 26 weeks.

INTRAUTERINE GROWTH RETARDATION/ SMALL-FOR-GESTATIONAL-AGE

Intrauterine growth retardation (IUGR) and small-for-gestational-age (SGA) are terms used interchangeably to describe a fetus or newborn whose size is smaller than the norm. IUGR, as a term, is used most often to describe intrauterine impaired growth and is a pathologic prenatal process. Small-for-gestational-age is a neonatal diagnosis and describes an infant who falls below the tenth percentile for birth weight. It is not possible to distinguish between IUGR and SGA prior to delivery. The majority of SGA infants are small because of IUGR. SGA, however, may also reflect (1) the genetic design of constitutionally small babies or (2) low birth weight caused by failure to achieve genetic potential due to inadequate maternal nutrition during pregnancy.

Intrauterine growth retardation is subdivided into two categories: symmetrical and asymmetrical. Infants with symmetrical IUGR are found to have compromised growth of body length and head circumference as well as have a low birth weight. Infants with asymmetrical IUGR have decreased body weight and body length but the head circumference is normal or relatively normal in size. This phenomenon is termed *head sparing*.

Risk factors associated with IUGR include poor nutrition, poor maternal weight gain, vascular disease, heart disease, preeclampsia, renal disease, infection, genetic abnormalities, multiple gestation, previous obstetrical history of IUGR, drug use, prepregnancy weight less than 90 pounds, anemia, diabetes (class C and above), alcohol abuse, and hypoglycemia (low fasting blood sugar and a flat GTT). Epidemiologically, low birth weight has been associated with late onset of prenatal care and factors related to low socioeconomic status.

Maternal weight gain and weight gain pattern often give early signs of possible impaired growth of the fetus. Early nutritional intervention can improve fetal growth if undernutrition is the only detectable cause and you have ruled out underlying infection, anomalies, and obstetric and medical diseases which cause uteroplacental insufficiency and thus contribute to poor growth of the fetus.

Prenatal detection of IUGR or SGA is made through an awareness of slow, inadequate growth of the pregnancy. Diagnosis of IUGR and SGA during pregnancy is difficult to make even with the sophisticated ultrasound equipment available today. The diagnosis of IUGR is often missed because the lack of growth is not recognized or if recognized is assumed to be a size-dates discrepancy due to inaccurate dates. Furthermore the diagnosis of IUGR by ultrasound is missed in approximately 30 percent of cases, although this may vary in accord with the experience and accuracy of the sonographer. In order to entertain a diagnosis of suspected IUGR or SGA, you must obtain various pieces of clinical information from the prenatal examinations. Specifically, it is necessary to determine the presence or absence of maternal risk factors which might contribute to the development of IUGR or SGA.

Evaluation of the pregnancy for progressive growth is a key factor in detecting possible IUGR or SGA. The operative word here is *progressive*. In order to make a diagnosis of IUGR or SGA, or of suspected IUGR or SGA, there should be less than a 2-centimeter growth of the uterus in 4 weeks. One single measurement that indicates the uterus is 2 centimeters smaller than expected for the estimated gestational age is *not* an indication of IUGR and does not warrant a workup for IUGR. Even if the uterine size remains consistently 2 centimeters smaller throughout the pregnancy, this in itself does not indicate IUGR. It is the lack of progressive growth over time which should lead you to entertain the possibility of a diagnosis of IUGR or SGA.

In evaluating uterine size the following should be considered: maternal height, weight, and body build; the estimated fetal weight; presentation and position; station of the presenting part; and the number of different previous examiners. (Also see Physical and pelvic examination in "Size-Dates Discrepancy" on page 193.) The number of different previous examiners alone can confuse your evaluation of the growth pattern in a particular pregnancy. Measurements of fundal height and abdominal girth by the same examiner are quite specific for detecting a growth lag or lack of growth, especially if the uterus grew less than 2 centimeters in 4 weeks.

Confirmation of your clinical suspicions is accomplished by obtaining two ultrasounds at least 4 weeks apart. These ultrasound examinations should include head circumference, abdominal circumference, head-abdomen ratio, crown-rump length, femur length, total intrauterine volume, and amniotic fluid volume. One single measurement, such as the biparietal diameter alone, will not confirm asymmetrical IUGR. Abdominal circumference by ultrasound is reliable since the measurement includes the fetal liver, which is always compromised in a fetus with IUGR. During normal fetal development, the head-abdomen circumference ratio

is greater than unity until 36 weeks, after which the ratio falls below unity.

Amniotic fluid volume should be determined to assist you in evaluating the severity of growth impairment. Oligohydramnios is found with severe growth impairment. Oligohydramnios may be due to the decrease in urine output by the fetus. The inability to detect by ultrasound at least one pocket of amniotic fluid of at least 1 centimeter correlates well with the diagnosis of IUGR. Perinatal morbidity also correlates with the amount of amniotic fluid: morbidity increases as fluid decreases. Amniotic fluid volume may also be assessed clinically by abdominal palpation for "molding" of the uterus around the fetus, being able to outline the fetus easily, and finding the fetus not ballottable.

Management of IUGR involves not only attempting to control the medical process which may be contributing to the problem but also surveillance of the fetus to identify a compromised uteroplacental unit or fetal deterioration. Once a diagnosis of IUGR has been made, the woman should be screened for underlying medical causes such as hypertension, preeclampsia, renal disease, and diabetes. Management includes limited activity with periods of bed rest in the left lateral position throughout the day, no smoking, no alcohol, and aggressive nutritional intervention. Even if the first ultrasound does not confirm your diagnosis, trust your clinical judgment and institute this management plan anyway.

The woman whose pregnancy is complicated by IUGR requires additional emotional support from you, especially if eating and smoking habits need to be changed. Bed rest improves uteroplacental blood flow and is helpful in IUGR. However, this activity restriction places additional stress on the family unit by requiring a shift of traditional roles related to household duties and to child care, if there are other children. Social service intervention may be necessary to arrange for child care or a homemaker to assist with household chores if there is no other support system available for the woman. You may find it helpful to prepare the woman, before labor ensues, for the possibility of following her labor with electronic fetal monitoring and fetal scalp pH measurements as well as the possibility of cesarean birth. All of these issues should be clarified before labor begins so there are no surprises causing increased stress for the woman.

Fetal surveillance is comprised of a number of tests to detect fetal compromise. Any single test carries a high number of false-positives which will not help you decide accurately when delivery should be accomplished. The decision regarding delivery should be made on the basis of a combination of test results, maternal condition, and fetal maturity factors.

Continued collaboration with your consulting physician is important to assess the antepartum testing results as well as to plan for the delivery. Timing of the delivery of a fetus with IUGR depends on the maturity of the fetus as well as the intrauterine environment. Delivery of a premature infant with IUGR carries a higher morbidity and mortality. The goal of any management plan is to continue the pregnancy while carefully following the fetus for signs of stress.

Oligohydramnios, decreased fetal movements, and a nonreactive nonstress test are indicators of a compromised fetus. Oligohydramnios in a fetus with normal kidneys indicates decreased fetal urine production secondary to chronic fetal stress; decreased fetal movements reflect dysfunction of the central nervous system; and a nonreactive nonstress test is an indicator of central nervous system depression which may be related to chronic hypoxia.

Contraction stress tests should be done when the nonstress test indicates fetal compromise. The absence of variability and accelerations with fetal movements is ominous as is the occurrence of spontaneous decelerations during a nonstress test or a contraction stress test.

If all testing parameters remain normal, the pregnancy should not be terminated. When the surveillance tests demonstrate a compromised fetus, you should discuss when delivery should occur with your consulting physician. Otherwise, spontaneous labor is awaited. Pediatric consultation during the prenatal period is helpful in planning for the delivery. A pediatrician's attendance at the delivery should be arranged since infants with IUGR are at a very high risk for developing meconium aspiration, hypocalcemia, hypoglycemia, and polycythemia.

The timing and method of delivery depend on the status of the fetus. In a woman with IUGR and a reactive nonstress test, caution should be observed once there are uterine contractions. A reactive nonstress test does not guarantee absence of fetal distress once labor begins. The incidence of fetal distress (such as hypoxia from cord compression secondary to oligohydramnios, or late decelerations secondary to uteroplacental insufficiency) is much higher in the growth-retarded fetus. Therefore, you should instruct the woman with IUGR to call and proceed to the hospital as soon as labor begins. Vaginal delivery is the recommended route except when electronic fetal monitoring and scalp pH indicate fetal acidosis.

Collaborative managment of a labor complicated by IUGR or SGA includes maintenance of optimal psychologic and physiologic functioning for this labor. Maternal positions which facilitate uteroplacental blood flow as well as promote the progress of labor should be used (left lateral, sitting, standing). Emotional support and thorough explanations of procedures will assist the woman through a potentially stressful labor and birth.

Pediatric and nursing assistance are needed for the birth, which should take place in a setting equipped to manage the neonatal complications of IUGR. Birth may be accomplished in bed, preferably in a delivery room fully equipped for neonatal resuscitation. If meconium is present in the amniotic fluid, oronasal suctioning with a DeLee catheter as soon as the head is delivered reduces the incidence of meconium aspiration. Likewise, slow delivery of the shoulders to allow chest compression will permit any excess meconium-stained fluid to be spontaneously expressed.

You should provide continued emotional support of the mother over and above the usual if the baby's neonatal course is complicated. Coordination with the pediatric staff facilitates communication with the mother and is an important role of the nurse-midwife.

LARGE-FOR-GESTATIONAL-AGE

The term large-for-gestational-age (LGA) is used to describe newborn infants whose birth weights exceed the established upper limits of normal for a given population. The established norm in the United States for a diagnosis of LGA is 4000 grams (8 pounds 13 ounces) or over the ninety-fifth percentile in weight at birth for gestational age. Nationality of the pregnant woman plays an important role in the size of her infants. For example, women from a Scandinavian background tend to have larger babies, which is normal for that particular population.

The most common reason for an LGA infant is a large mother. Diabetes accounts for only a small number of LGA infants. If you suspect an LGA infant, however, the woman should be screened for diabetes mellitus if this has not already been done. Another group of women who have large babies are those whose pregnancies continue beyond term, since the fetus continues to gain weight in prolonged pregnancies.

LGA is suspected and evaluated through the following data base:

1. History
   a. previous obstetric history:
      (1) birth weights of previous infants
      (2) previous shoulder dystocia
   b. size (height, weight, body build) of the father of the baby
   c. birth weight of both the mother and father of the baby
   d. presence of diabetes or gestational diabetes during a previous pregnancy
   e. nationality
   f. previous uterine myomata
2. Physical examination
   a. size (height, weight, body build)
   b. fundal height
   c. estimated fetal weight (becomes more evident in third trimester)
   d. abdominal girth
   e. fetal head or buttocks feel larger than expected on palpation
   f. palpation for uterine myomata

The differential diagnoses for a uterus which is larger than expected for dates are:

1. Wrong dates
2. Polyhydramnios
3. Multiple gestation
4. Uterine myomata
5. Right dates and large baby
6. Diabetes (gestational or class B)

Once you have ruled out the other differential diagnoses and have determined that the dates are correct and this is a large baby, a diet history should be done. This history should be evaluated for appropriate nutritional intake (see Chapter 8) and any necessary counseling done. Discussion should also take place with the woman about the possible difficulties she might have in labor due to having a large baby (arrest of labor, arrest of descent, shoulder dystocia).

Labor management should include a high suspicion for relative cephalopelvic disproportion (CPD). A pelvis which might be adequate for an average size baby may not be adequate for a large baby despite what appear to be adequate pelvic dimensions. When the woman enters labor and the estimated fetal weight indicates a large infant, careful assessment of the pelvis by clinical pelvimetry is necessary. If you anticipate a large baby, notify your consulting physician when the woman is in labor. The pediatrician should also be notified of a possible LGA infant since these babies tend to have a more complicated neonatal course.

The descent pattern as well as the progress of labor should be carefully followed. Because of the higher incidence of failure to progress in labor the mother should be monitored for adequate pelvis, contraction pattern, position of the presenting part, presence of caput or molding, and maternal pushing efforts. When there has been no progress in descent and in the mechanisms of labor in second stage with good maternal pushing effort and good contractions over a period of time, cesarean section rather than an instrument delivery is the delivery route of choice. An LGA baby with arrested descent is arrested for a reason, and the most likely reason is that the shoulders are caught on the symphysis pubis.

The complications involved in the vaginal delivery of an LGA infant include shoulder dystocia with fractured clavical or Erb's palsy in the newborn and severe lacerations of the vagina secondary to manipulations to accomplish the delivery. Preparations for delivery should include anticipation for shoulder dystocia (see Chapter 15).

POSTDATES PREGNANCY

Postdates pregnancy is based on a 28-day cycle and occurs when pregnancy exceeds 42 weeks (294 days) from the first day of the last menstrual period. Cycle length other than 28 days will invalidate gestational age determination based on dates. The incidence of postdates pregnancy is 2.2 percent to 10.4 percent of all term pregnancies.

Postdates pregnancy needs to be delineated from the postmaturity syndrome, which occurs in approximately 25 percent of postdates pregnancies. Postmaturity syndrome is a diagnosis that can be made only after delivery; it is postdates pregnancy accompanied by a combination of the following:

1. Oligohydramnios
2. Meconium-stained amniotic fluid
3. Newborn with:
   a. loss of subcutaneous fat
   b. long fingernails
   c. wrinkled, peeling skin
   d. alert facies
   e. absence of lanugo
   f. absence of vernix caseosa

The postmaturity syndrome is most likely due to decreasing uteroplacental function. These babies are stressed, as evidenced by often having respiratory distress syndrome, hypoglycemia, polycythemia, and temperature instability. Meconium aspiration is a real danger.

The major difficulties in the management of a postdates pregnancy are making the diagnosis and determining whether postmaturity syndrome is also present. Of critical importance in diagnosing postdates pregnancy is an accurate dating of the pregnancy. This depends on the collection of an accurate data base on the *first* prenatal visit.

Management of postdates pregnancy begins at the first prenatal visit with an accurate determination of the estimated date of delivery based upon the parameters outlined in the history and physical and pelvic examinations in the section entitled "Size-Dates Discrepancy" (see pages 192–195). Once the estimated date of delivery has been established, it should never be changed unless the evaluation for differential diagnosis as described in "Size-Dates Discrepancy" is done (see pages 193–194). Changing the estimated date of delivery of any woman is potentially harmful, especially when done with an inaccurate data base such as one ultrasound performed after 26 weeks or by equating only fundal height measurement to expected gestational age. By making a change without adequate rationale, the nurse-midwife runs the real risk of missing the diagnosis of postdates pregnancy or postmaturity syndrome.

Once a woman has passed her due date, surveillance of the pregnancy for signs of uteroplacental insufficiency and a compromised fetus becomes the objective. Consult your physician in the event of any abnormal parameters. Surveillance consists of the following:

1. Fetal movement record. You can have the woman begin recording fetal movements at 40 weeks. This will give you sufficient time to teach her how to keep this record and also to establish a pattern of fetal movement on which to base clinical impressions. Instructions vary as to how often and when to count the fetal movements and when the woman should notify you. One method is to have her count fetal movements starting 1 hour after eating breakfast, lunch, and dinner and continuing for a period of 1 hour. If four or fewer fetal movements occur in an hour, have her count for another hour and if still four or fewer fetal movements occur in the second hour to either notify you or come to the hospital.

2. Nonstress testing. Begin at 42 weeks or in the event of decreased fetal movements. Criteria for determining a satisfactory nonstress test are based on assessment of variability for normalcy, fetal heart rate acceleration of at least 15 beats per minute above the baseline in response to fetal movement, and any decelerations either spontaneous (more ominous) or in response to uterine activity or fetal movement (see Chapter 7).

3. Contraction stress test (CST). There are two types of contraction stress tests: oxytocin and nipple stimulation (see Chapter 7). Some clinicians prefer using the contraction stress test instead of the nonstress test because the CST directly tests the uteroplacental unit. A contraction stress test definitely should be performed in the event of a suspicious or nonreactive nonstress test *unless* there was a terminal tracing (i.e., straight line or flat variability and no fetal movement). A CST should *not* be done in the presence of an NST terminal

tracing, as the baby's life may be jeopardized. Instead, consult with your physician for evaluation for immediate delivery.

4. Amniotic fluid volume. Oligohydramnios occurs because of decreased urine production by a fetus that is chronically stressed from uteroplacental insufficiency. Amniotic fluid volume should be assessed at each visit. Oligohydramnios is recognized clinically (by abdominal palpation) by "molding" of the uterus around the fetus, being easily able to outline the fetus, and finding the fetus not ballottable. If you are unable to determine oligohydramnios clinically and an ultrasound is needed to evaluate amniotic fluid volume, then obtain a biophysical profile at the same time.

5. Maternal weight gain. Weight loss may indicate developing postmaturity syndrome (i.e., decreasing amniotic fluid volume, decreasing fetal subcutaneous fat). Postdates babies are large babies accompanied by continuing increase in fetal and maternal weight gain. Postmature babies are small babies with fetal and maternal weight loss.

6. Some clinicians also do a weekly biophysical profile, including placental grading if available, or assess estriol levels if the capability for doing biophysical profiles is not available. Other clinicians say that the use of a combination of fetal movement recordings, nonstress testing, indicated contraction stress testing, and clinical assessment of amniotic fluid volume provides sufficient information about fetal status for evaluation. If this combination indicates stress in the fetus, delivery should be accomplished rather than further testing.

In women in whom all parameters are normal, whose pregnancies carry no other obstetric or medical risk factors, whose weight gain pattern is adequate, and who continue to maintain weight, expectant management is appropriate. Any intervening obstetric or medical risk factors (e.g., preeclampsia, hypertension, diabetes, renal disease) preclude conservative management since these greatly increase the morbidity and mortality of the fetus, probably secondary to increased impairment of the placental blood flow. Consult with your physician.

You will find it necessary to offer support to the woman who does not give birth within her estimated time of delivery. Her own expectations as well as those of her partner and family can be disruptive intervening factors. The anticipation of the "big day" which does not occur, plus the increasing physical discomforts, all increase pressure on you as the clinician to terminate the pregnancy.

Some clinicians advocate induction of labor and delivery of every woman who reaches 42 weeks. This management option carries the risks of increased cesarean section secondary to failed induction as well as inducing many women who are not truly postdates, since accurate diagnosis of gestational age is difficult. Only about one-third of all pregnancies labeled postdates are actually postdates pregnancies. The cervix usually is not "ripe" and therefore inducible in postdates pregnancy. Evaluation of the inducibility of the cervix is essential when considering the management of the postdates pregnancy. If the cervix is clearly inducible at the end of 42 weeks it may be better to induce the woman than to continue to follow her with fetal evaluation tests. If your protocol mandates pitocin induction and delivery at 42 weeks, you may wish to initiate other methods of induction at 41½ weeks such as nipple stimulation, sexual intercourse if the membranes are intact, stripping of the membranes, and castor oil (2 oz).

Other clinicians advocate a less agressive approach to postdates pregnancy: expectant management and careful observation of the mother and fetus. The mother is observed for weight gain, blood pressure, and psychological status. The fetus is observed for continued growth, intactness of the fetoplacental unit, and presumptive development of the postmaturity syndrome.

Delivery is indicated when there are signs of uteroplacental insufficiency and a compromised fetus, evidenced by oligohydramnios with or without a nonreactive nonstress test with decreased fetal movements, or a positive contraction stress test. Consultation with the physician is necessary.

BIBLIOGRAPHY

Aladjem, S., and Brown, A. K. (Eds.). *Clinical Perinatology*. St. Louis: Mosby, 1974.

Anderson, G. V. (Moderator). Symposium: Ob-gyn emergencies: obstetric hemorrhage. *Contemporary OB/GYN* 2:59, 1973.

Anderson, G. V. (Moderator). Symposium: Ob-gyn emergencies: Part 2. *Contemporary OB/GYN* 2:75, 1973.

Bahr, J. E. Herpesvirus hominis type 2 in women and newborns. *MCN* 3:16, 1978.

Baker, D. A. Hepatitis B infection in obstetrics and gynecology. *Infectious Disease Letters for Obstetrics-Gynecology* 6(3):13−20 (March) 1984.

Banatvala, J. E. et al. Serological assessment of rubella during pregnancy. *Obstet. Gynecol. Surv.* 26:232, 1971.

Barss, V. A., Benacerraf, B. R., and Frigoletto, F. D. Second trimester oligohydramnios, a predictor of poor fetal outcome. *Obstet. Gynecol.* 64(5):608−610 (November) 1984.

Beasley, R. P. Hepatitis B virus as the etiologic agent in hepatocellular cancer: Epidemiologic considerations. *Hepatology* 2:21S−26S, 1982.

Benjamin, F., Bassen, F. A., and Meyer, L. M. Serum levels of folic acid, vitamin B_{12}, and iron in anemia or pregnancy. *Am. J. Obstet. Gynecol.* 96:310, 1966.

Berman, L. B. The pregnant kidney. *J.A.M.A.* 230:111, 1974.

Boehme, T. L. Hepatitis B: The nurse-midwife's role in management and prevention. *J. Nurse-Midwifery* 30(2):79−87 (March/April) 1985.

Boyce, A., Mayaux, M. J., and D. Schwartz. Classical and "true" gestational postmaturity. *Am. J. Obstet. Gynecol.* 125(7):911−914, 1976.

Burrow, G. N. The thyroid in pregnancy. *Med. Clin. North Am.* 59:1089, 1975.

Carpenter, M. W., and Couston, D. R. Criteria for screening tests for gestational diabetes. *Am. J. Obstet. Gynecol.* 144(7):768–772, December 1, 1982.

Carr, M. C. Serum iron/TIBC in the diagnosis of iron deficiency anemia during pregnancy. *Obstet. Gynecol.* 38:602, 1971.

Centers for Disease Control. Recommendations for the use of hepatitis B vaccine. *Infectious Disease Letters for Obstetrics-Gynecology.* 4(10):55–60 (October) 1982.

Centers for Disease Control. Sexually transmitted diseases treatment guidelines 1982, *Morbidity and Mortality Weekly Report — Supplement.* 31(25):33S–

Chen, W., Palav, A., and Tricomi, V. Screening for diabetes in a prenatal clinic. *Obstet. Gynecol.* 40:567, 1972.

Chesley, L. C. *Hypertensive Disorders in Pregnancy.* New York: Appleton-Century-Crofts, 1978.

Chesley, L. C. Hypertensive disorders in pregnancy. *J. Nurse-Midwifery* 30(2):99–104 (March/April) 1985.

Chesley, L. C. Plasma and red cell volumes during pregnancy. *Am. J. Obstet. Gynecol.* 112:440, 1972.

Chez, R. A., and Lind, T. The oral glucose tolerance test. *Contemporary OB/GYN* 8:71, 1976.

Clark, J. F. J. Preventing maternal death in advanced abdominal pregnancy. *Contemporary OB/GYN* 12:137, 1978.

Coodley, E. L. Heart disease in pregnancy. *Postgrad. Med.* 47(4):195, 1970.

Corlett, R. C., Jr. Hyperemesis gravidarum and pancreatitis. *Contemporary OB/GYN* 9:25, 1977.

Crenshaw, C., Jr., Darnell-Jones, D. E., and Parker, R. T. Placenta previa: A survey of twenty years experience with improved perinatal survival by expectant therapy and cesarean delivery. *Obstet. Gynecol. Surv.* 28:461, 1973.

Davidsohn, I., and Henry, J. B. (Eds.). *Todd-Stanford Clinical Diagnosis by Laboratory Methods, 14th.* Philadelphia: Saunders, 1969.

De Alvarez, R. R. The kidney in pregnancy. *Hosp. Prac.* 8(5):129, 1973.

Dienstag, J. L., Wands, J. R., and Koff, R. S. Acute hepatitis. In Petersdorf, R. G. et al. *Harrison's Principles of Internal Medicine, 10th.* New York: McGraw-Hill, 1983.

Eden, R. D. et al. Comparison of antepartum testing schemes for the management of the postdate pregnancy. *Am. J. Obstet. Gynecol.* 144(6):683–692, 1982.

Edwards, M. S. Venereal herpes: A nursing overview. *Obstet. Gynecol. Neonat. Nurs.* 7:7, 1978.

Elliott, J. P., and Flaherty, J. F. The use of breast stimulation to prevent postdate pregnancy. *Am. J. Obstet. Gynecol.* 149(6):628–632, July 15, 1984.

Engstrom, J. L. Quickening and auscultation of fetal heart tones as estimators of the gestational interval: A review. *J. Nurse-Midwifery* 30(1):25–32 (January/February) 1985.

Fleury, F. J. Clinical management of genital herpes. *Contemporary OB/GYN* 7:36, 1976.

Foster, S. Sickle cell anemia: Closing the gap between theory and therapy. *Am. J. Nurs.* 71:1952, 1971.

Freda, V. Hemolytic disease. *Clin. Obstet. Gynecol.* 16:72, 1973.

Gabbe, S. G. et al. Management and outcome of class A diabetes mellitus. *Am. J. Obstet. Gynecol.* 127(5):465–469, March 1, 1977.

Gabbe, S. G. et al. Management and outcome of pregnancy in diabetes mellitus, classes B to R. *Am. J. Obstet. Gynecol.* 129(7):723–732, December 1, 1977.

Gillmer, M. D. G. et al. Carbohydrate metabolism in pregnancy: Part I. Diurnal plasma glucose profile in normal and diabetic women. *Br. Med. J.* 3:399–404, August 16, 1975.

Gillmer, M. D. G. et al. Screening for diabetes during pregnancy. *Br J. Obstet. Gynaecol.* 87:377–382 (May) 1980.

Golditch, I. M., and Boyce, N. E., Jr. Management of abruptio placentae. *J.A.M.A.* 212:288, 1970.

Gottesman, R. L., and Refetoff, S. Diagnosis and management of thyroid diseases in pregnancy. *J. Reprod. Med.* 11:19, 1973.

Granados, J. L. Survey of the management of postterm pregnancy. *Obstet. Gynecol.* 63(5):651–653 (May) 1984.

Greenhill, J. P., and Friedman, E. A. *Biological Principles and Modern Practice of Obstetrics.* Philadelphia: Saunders, 1974.

Hardy, J. B. Answers to questions on infections in the pregnant patient. *Hosp. Med.* 6(12):44, 1970.

Hafez, E. S. E. Physiology of multiple pregnancy. *J. Reprod. Med.* 12:88, 1974.

Hendricks, C. H., and Brenner, W. E. Toxemia of pregnancy: Relationship between fetal weight, fetal survival, and the maternal state, *Am. J. Obstet. Gynecol.* 109:225, 1971.

Hobbins, J. C., and R. L. Berkowitz. Ultrasonography in the diagnosis of intrauterine growth retardation. *Clin. Obstet. Gynecol.* 20(4):957–968 (December) 1977.

Hobbins, J. C., Winsberg, F., and Berkowitz, R. L. *Ultrasonography in Obstetrics and Gynecology, 2nd.* Baltimore: Williams & Wilkins, 1983.

Holder, W. R., and Knox, J. M. Syphilis in pregnancy. *Med. Clin. North Am.* 56:1151, 1972.

Horger, E. O. Hemoglobinopathies in pregnancy, *Clin. Obstet. Gynecol.* 17:127, 1974.

Howe, C., Martin, M. C., and Pernoll, M. L. *Hemorrhage during Late Pregnancy and the Puerperium.* Series 3, Module 4, A Staff Development Program in Perinatal Nursing Care. White Plains, N. Y.: March of Dimes–Birth Defects Foundation, 1984.

Josey, W. E., Nahmias, A. J., and Naib, Z. M. The epidemiology of type 2 (genital) herpes simplex virus infection. *Obstet. Gynecol. Surv.* 27:295, 1972.

Jovanovic, L., and Peterson, C. M. New options for the pregnant diabetic. *Contemporary OB/GYN* 77–94 (March) 1983.

Jovanovic, L. et al. Feasibility of maintaining normal glucose profiles in insulin-dependent pregnant diabetic women. *Am. J. Med.* 68:105–112 (January) 1980

Kelley, M. Nurse-midwifery management of pre-eclampsia: Two case studies. *J. Nurse-Midwifery* 30(2):105–111 (March/April) 1985.

Kincaid-Smith, P. Bacteriuria and urinary infection in pregnancy. *Clin. Obstet. Gynecol.* 11:533, 1968.

Kitay, D. Z. Folic acid deficiency. *Contemporary OB/GYN* 10:30, 1977.

Kitay, D. Z. Bleeding disorders in pregnancy. *Contemporary OB/GYN* 7:87, 1976.

Knox, G. E. How infection damages the fetus. *Contemporary OB/GYN* 12:96, 1978.

Knox, G. E., Huddleston, J. F., and Flowers, C. E. Management of prolonged pregnancy: Results of a prospective randomized trial. *Am. J. Obstet. Gynecol.* 134(4):376–384, 1979.

Krugman, S. Hepatitis B virus infection and pregnancy. *Infectious Disease Letters for Obstetrics-Gynecology* 2(5):25–30 (May) 1980.

Langer, O., Sonnendecker, E. W. W., and Jacobson, M. J. Categorization of terminal fetal heart-rate patterns in antepartum cardiotocography. *Br. J. Obstet. Gynaecol.* 89:179–185 (March) 1982.

Ledger, W. J. When to hospitalize in incomplete abortion. *Hosp. Prac.* 3(7):30, 1968.

Leveno, K., J. et al. Appraisal of "rigid" blood glucose control during pregnancy in the overtly diabetic woman. *Am. J. Obstet. Gynecol.* 135(7): 853–862, December 1, 1979.

Lewis, J. L., Jr. (Moderator). Symposium: Managing the hydatidiform mole patient. *Contemporary OB/GYN* 3:117, 1974.

Lin, C. C. Intrauterine growth retardation. In Wynn, R. M. (Ed.) *Obstetrics & Gynecology Annual, Vol. 14.* Norwalk, Conn.: Appleton-Century-Crofts, 1985.

Lind, T. et al. Changes in serum uric acid concentrations during normal pregnancy, *Br. J. Obstet. Gynaecol.* 91:128, 1984.

Lind, T., and Harris, V. G. Changes in the oral glucose tolerance test during the puerperium. *Br. J. Obstet. Gynaecol.* 83:460–463 (June) 1976.

Lindheimer, M. D., and Katz, A. I. Managing the patient with renal disease. *Contemporary OB/GYN* 3:49, 1974.

Lindheimer, M. D. (Guest Editor), Medical complications of pregnancy: An invitational symposium. *J. Reprod. Med.* 11:1, 1973.

Lukens, J. N. Iron deficiency and infection. *Am. J. Dis. Child.* 129:160, 1975.

Manning, F. A. et al. Fetal biophysical profile scoring: A prospective study in 1184 high-risk patients. *Am. J. Obstet. Gynecol.* 140:289, 1981.

McCormick, M. C. The contribution of low birth weight to infant mortality and childhood morbidity. *N. Engl. J. Med.* 312(2):82–90, January 10, 1985.

McFee, J. G. Anemia in pregnancy — a reappraisal. *Obstet. Gynecol. Surv.* 28:769, 1973.

McFarland, K. F., Murtiashaw, M., and Baynes, J. W. Clinical value of glycosylated serum protein and glycosylated hemoglobin levels in the diagnosis of gestational diabetes mellitus. *Obstet. Gynecol.* 64(4):516–518 (October) 1984.

McKenzie, A. W. Skin disorders in pregnancy, *Practitioner* 206:773, 1971.

Marymont, J. H., Jr., and Herrman, K. L. Rubella in pregnancy: Review of current problems. *Postgrad. Med.* 56:167, 1974.

Merkatz, I. R. et al. A pilot community-based screening program for gestational diabetes. *Diabetes Care* 3(3):453–457 (May-June) 1980.

Messer, R. H. Pregnancy anemias. *Clin. Obstet.*

Gynecol. 17:163, 1974.

Mestman, J. H. A practical approach to thyroid function tests. *Contemporary OB/GYN* 9:28, 1977.

Mikat, D. M., and Mikat, K. W. *A Clinician's Guide to Bacteria, 3rd.* Indianapolis, Ind.: Eli Lilly and Company, 1977.

Nahmias, A. J. et al. Perinatal risk associated with maternal genital herpes simplex virus infection. *Am. J. Obstet. Gynecol.* 110:825, 1971.

Nichols, C. W. Clinical management of size/dates discrepancy. *J. Nurse-Midwifery* 30(1):15–24 (January/February) 1985.

Nichols, C. Postdate pregnancy, Part I. A literature review. *J. Nurse-Midwifery* 30(4):222 (July/August) 1985.

Nichols, C. Postdate pregnancy, Part II. Clinical implications. *J. Nurse-Midwifery* 30(5):259 (September/October) 1985.

Ockner, R. K. Acute viral hepatitis. In Wyngaarden and Smith (Eds.). *Cecil Textbook of Medicine, Vol. 1.* Philadelphia: Saunders, 1982.

Oparil, S., and Swartwout, J. R. Heart disease in pregnancy. *J. Reprod. Med.* 11:2, 1973.

O'Sullivan, J. B., and Mahan, C. M. Criteria for the oral glucose tolerance test in pregnancy. *Diabetes* 13(3):278–284 (May/June) 1964.

O'Sullivan, J. B. et al. Screening criteria for high-risk gestational diabetic patients. *Am. J. Obstet. Gynecol.* 116(7):895–900, August 1, 1973.

Page, E. W. On the pathogenesis of preeclampsia and eclampsia. *J. Obstet. Gynaecol. Br. Comm.* 79:883, 1972.

Prez, R. D. Tuberculosis. In Wyngaarden and Smith (Eds.). *Cecil Textbook of Medicine, Vol. 2.* Philadelphia: Saunders, 1982.

Pritchard, J. A., MacDonald, P. C., and Gant, N. F. *Williams Obstetrics, 17th.* Norwalk, Conn.: Appleton-Century-Crofts, 1985.

Reid, D. W., Ryan, K. J., and Benirschke, K. *Principles and Management of Human Reproduction.* Philadelphia: Saunders, 1972.

Robertson, E. G. The natural history of oedema during pregnancy. *J. Obstet. Gynaecol. Br. Comm.* 78:520, 1971.

Sadovsky, E. et al. The definition and the significance of decreased fetal movements. *Acta Obstet. Gynecol. Scand.* 62:409, 1983.

Schneierson, S. S., and Sewell, A. F. *Atlas of Diagnostic Microbiology.* North Chicago, Ill.: Abbott Laboratories, 1971.

Schreier, A. C. The nurse-midwifery management of physiological edema in pregnancy. *J. Nurse-Midwifery* 21:18, 1976.

Schwartz, R. O., and Di Pietro, D. L. B-hCG as a diagnostic aid for suspected ectopic pregnancy. *Obstet. Gynecol.* 56(2):197–203 (August) 1980.

Scott, J. R. Vaginal bleeding in the midtrimester of pregnancy. *Am. J. Obstet. Gynecol.* 113:329, 1972.

Seeds, J. W. Impaired fetal growth: Definition and clinical diagnosis. *Obstet. Gynecol.* 64(3):303–310 (September) 1984.

Seeds, J. W. Impaired fetal growth: Ultrasonic evaluation and clinical management. *Obstet. Gynecol.* 64(4):577–584 (October) 1984.

Shih, T., and Gabbe, S. G. Fetal movement: The fetus in distress. *Contemporary OB/GYN* 9:73, 1977.

Soler, N. G., and Malins, J. M. Prevalence of glucosuria in normal pregnancy. *Lancet* 1:619, 1971.

Speroff, L. et al. Pregnancy-induced hypertension. *Contemporary OB/GYN* 9:137, 1977.

Stubblefield, P. G., and Berek, J. S. Perinatal mortality in term and post-term birth. *Obstet. Gynecol.* 56(6):676–682, 1980.

Takahashi, K. et al. Uterine contractility and oxytocin sensitivity in preterm, term, and postterm pregnancy. *Am. J. Obstet. Gynecol.* 136:774–779, 1980.

Talkington, K. M. et al. Effect of ingestion of starch and some clays on iron absorption. *Am. J. Obstet. Gynecol.* 108:262, 1976.

Taylor, E. S. Risk of toxoplasmosis infection from cats. *Curr. Med. Dialog.* November, 1973, p. 871.

Thornton, Y. S., Yeh, S., and Petrie, R. H. Antepartum fetal heart rate testing and the post-term gestation. *J. Perinat. Med.* 10:196–202, 1982.

Tobin, J. O'H. Herpesvirus hominis infection in pregnancy. *Proc. Royal Soc. Med.* 68:371, 1975.

Tsai, A., Reuler, J., and Rubenstein, A. Diabetes and pregnancy. *J. Reprod. Med.* 11:23, 1973.

Tyson, J. E. (Ed.). *Symposium on Pregnancy — The Medical Clinics of North America.* Philadelphia: Saunders, 1977.

VanNagell, J., Koepke, J., and Dilts, P. V., Jr. Preventable anemia and pregnancy. *Obstet. Gynecol. Surv.* 26:551, 1971.

Vorherr, H. Placental insufficiency in relation to postterm pregnancy and fetal postmaturity. *Am. J. Obstet. Gynecol.* 123(1):67–103, 1975.

Whalley, P. J., Martin, F. G., and Peters, P. C. Significance of asymptomatic bacteriuria detected during pregnancy. *J.A.M.A.* 193:879, 1965.

Wilhelm, H. S. Congenital toxoplasmosis, *J. Am. Med. Women's Assoc.* 27:598, 1972.

Yeh, S. Y., and J. A. Read. Management of post-term pregnancy in a large obstetric population. *Obstet. Gynecol.* 60(3):282–287, 1982.

Zuspan, F. P. (Coordinator). Anemia in pregnancy: An invitational symposium. *J. Reprod. Med.* 6:94, 1971.

Zuspan, F. P. (Moderator). Symposium: Hypertension in pregnancy: The problems. *Contemporary OB/GYN* 6:120, 1975.

III   Management of the Intrapartal Period

10

Diagnosis of Labor and Management of False and Early Labor

SIGNS AND SYMPTOMS OF IMPENDING LABOR

There are a number of premonitory signs and symptoms that may alert you to a woman's approaching labor. A woman may exhibit any, all, or none of these but it is useful to keep them in mind when seeing a woman late in her pregnancy so appropriate anticipatory counseling and guidance can be given. The signs and symptoms of impending labor are lightening, cervical changes, false labor, premature rupture of membranes, bloody show, energy spurt, and gastrointestinal upsets.

Lightening

Lightening, which occurs approximately 2 weeks before labor, is the descent of the presenting part of the baby into the true pelvis.

The baby's head, if there is a cephalic presentation, usually is fixed or engaged afterwards. The woman frequently refers to lightening as "the baby has dropped." She will experience a decrease in the minor discomfort of shortness of breath she has had during the third trimester because lightening will give her more room in the upper abdomen for lung expansion. However, lightening will cause other discomforts due to the pressure of the presenting part on structures in the area of the true pelvis. Specifically, she will have:

1. Frequency of urination because the bladder feels pressure and has less room for expansion
2. An uncomfortable feeling of generalized pelvic pressure, which may make her feel awkward and produces the constant sensation that something needs to come out or that a bowel movement is needed

3. Leg cramps, which may be caused by the pressure of the presenting part on the nerves that course through the foramen obturator and lead to the legs
4. Increased venous stasis producing dependent edema because the pressure of the presenting part inhibits blood return from the lower extremities

Lightening lowers the height of the fundus to a position similar to that of the eighth month of pregnancy, and you are no longer able to ballotte the previously movable head of the baby above the symphysis pubis during abdominal palpation. Your examining fingers will now diverge rather than converge during the fourth step of Leopold's maneuvers.

Since lightening usually does not occur prior to labor except in primigravidas, it is probably the result of the increasing intensity of the Braxton Hicks contractions combined with the good abdominal muscle tone more common to primigravidas.

The nurse-midwife's knowledge of lightening is of value in being able to reassure the woman of the normality of the bodily changes she is experiencing and explain why they are occurring. Lightening also provides a good opportunity to review with the woman her plans for labor. Moreover it provides an indication of the adequacy of the pelvic inlet. Because the length of time between lightening and true labor varies with individuals, it is of little use in predicting the onset of labor except in a most generalized fashion of a few days to a couple of weeks. However, lightening tends to encourage the woman that the long-awaited end of pregnancy is within sight.

Cervical Changes

As labor approaches the cervix becomes "ripe." Contrasted with the usual closed, long, soft cervix of pregnancy it becomes still softer, like the consistency of pudding, and evidences some degree of effacement and perhaps slight dilatation. Evaluation of ripeness is relative to the individual woman; for example, a grand multipara's cervix may normally be 2 centimeters dilated as opposed to a primigravida's normally closed cervix.

It is thought that these cervical changes are brought about by the increasing intensity of the Braxton Hicks' contractions. A cervix may be ripe for a variable period of time prior to labor. Ripeness indicates a readiness of the cervix for labor. It is of value in assuring the patient that she will go into labor with the onset of labor contractions and that the time of labor is relatively close at hand, and in assessing the probable success of an indicated induction of labor.

False Labor

False labor consists of painful uterine contractions that have no measurable progressive effect on the cervix and are in actuality an exaggeration of the usually painless Braxton Hicks' contractions which have been been occurring since about 6 weeks' gestation.

False labor may occur for days or intermittently even 3 or 4 weeks before the onset of true labor. False labor is genuinely painful and a woman may lose sleep and energy coping with it. She has no way of knowing for sure whether she is in true labor since this can be determined only by vaginal examination. The intermittent recurrence of false labor and trips back and forth to your office or the hospital are exhausting and frustrating to the woman and her family. This calls for a great degree of understanding, patience, support, reassurance, and many explanations on the part of all obstetrical team members who see the woman during her trips to your office or the hospital. False labor, however, does indicate the approach of labor.

Premature Rupture of Membranes

Normally the membranes rupture at the end of the first stage of labor. Rupture before the onset of labor is called premature rupture of the membranes and occurs in about 12 percent of women. Approximately 80 percent of near-term women with premature rupture of membranes begin labor spontaneously within 24 hours (see Chapter 14).

Bloody Show

A mucus plug, created by cervical secretions from proliferation of the glands of the cervical mucosa early in pregnancy, serves the function of a protective barrier and closes the cervical canal throughout pregnancy (Fig. 10-1). Bloody show is the expulsion of this mucus plug.

Bloody show is most often seen as a tenacious, blood-tinged mucus discharge which must be carefully differentiated from frank bleeding. Women often refer to the discharge as "seeing the sign." Occasionally the entire mucus plug is expelled en masse, making inexperienced obstetrical personnel think the umbilical cord has prolapsed when the plug is expelled during labor and seen extruding from the woman's vagina.

Bloody show is a sign of imminent labor, which usually takes place within 24 to 48 hours. Bloody show as a sign of labor is of no value if a vaginal examination has been done within the past 48 hours, because a blood-tinged mucus discharge during this time may be only the effect of minor trauma to or disruption of the mucus plug during the examination.

Energy Spurt

Many women experience an energy spurt approximately 24 to 48 hours before the onset of labor. After days or weeks of feeling tired

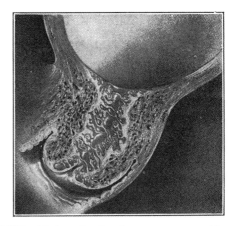

FIGURE 10-1. Cervix in pregnancy. Note the elaboration of the mucosa into a honeycomblike structure, the meshes of which are filled with a tenacious mucus (the mucus plug). (Reproduced by permission from J. A. Pritchard and P. C. MacDonald. *Williams Obstetrics, 15th.* New York: Appleton-Century-Crofts, 1976.)

(physically tired and tired of being pregnant) they get up one day to find themselves full of energy and vigor. Typically these women do things like clean the house, wash and iron curtains, scrub floors, cook and freeze food, and perform a variety of other household tasks which they either have not had the energy to do or now feel need doing before the baby's arrival. Consequently they enter labor exhausted and often have long, difficult labors.

There is no known explanation for this energy spurt other than it is nature's way of giving a woman the energy she needs for the work of labor. Women should be informed of the possibility of their having this energy spurt and advised to deliberately refrain from expending it and instead to conserve it for use during labor.

Gastrointestinal Upsets

In the absence of any causative factors for the

occurence of diarrhea, indigestion, nausea, and vomiting, it is thought they might be indicative of impending labor. No explanation for this is known, but some women do experience one to all of these signs.

DATA BASE FOR DIAGNOSIS OF LABOR

Contractions

Labor itself is an intricate interplay of physiologic and psychologic forces within the woman and the effect of these forces on the process of birth and on the baby. These forces result in the birth of the baby. The primary physiologic force during labor is that of uterine contractions. It is impossible to understand and evaluate labor progress, to understand the discomforts of labor, to devise comfort measures, or to be aware of complications without a thorough comprehension of uterine contractions and their action.

The uterine contractions of labor are unique as the only painful physiologic muscular contractions in the body. Furthermore, these contractions are involuntary as they are under intrinsic nervous control. This means that the woman has no physiologic control over the frequency and duration of these contractions nor does any extrauterine neural process.

Uterine contractions are intermittent, providing for a period of uterine relaxation between contractions. These periods of relaxation between contractions are essential for:

1. Providing rest to the uterine muscle because a sustained contraction of severe intensity could rupture the uterus
2. Providing rest to the woman, who would be unable to cope with a sustained uterine contraction of several hours duration
3. Maintaining the welfare of the baby since uterine contractions constrict the placental blood vessels and a sustained contraction

would produce fetal hypoxia, anoxia, and death

The duration of a uterine contraction varies considerably depending on where the woman is in her labor. The contractions of active labor range from 45 to 90 seconds with an average of 60 seconds. In early labor the contractions may be only 15 to 20 seconds in duration.

Timing of the frequency of contractions is done from the beginning of one contraction to the beginning of the next contraction. Note is also taken of the duration of the contraction which, when subtracted from the frequency, gives one the length of the period of relaxation. For example, a woman who begins a contraction at 5:05, 5:10, 5:15, 5:20, and 5:25, each lasting 60 seconds, is having a frequency of contractions of every 5 minutes and a duration of 60 seconds. It is obvious that the period of relaxation of 4 minutes between the end of one contraction and the beginning of the next is more than adequate for the welfare of baby, mother, and uterine muscle. An absolute critical point is reached when the contractions are more frequent than every 2 minutes and have a duration longer than 90 seconds, because there is not sufficient relaxation time. This does not happen with normal spontaneous labor but must be closely guarded against during pitocin induction or augmentation of labor.

In evaluating the frequency and intensity of uterine contractions it is important to know that each contraction has three phases: increment, acme, and decrement. The increment phase is longer than the other two phases combined. The experienced hand can feel a contraction coming on before the woman can feel it. Conversely, the woman may feel the contraction for several to many seconds after the experienced hand feels it has gone. What the woman is feeling may be the aftermath of the pain just experienced. When one considers, in addition, the extreme variations in individual pain thresholds it becomes apparent that to time contractions on the basis of the woman's vocal or behavioral manifestations of pain is most inaccurate.

This holds true also for evaluating the intensity of a contraction. A frightened woman who is unknowledgeable about what is happening to her and unprepared in the physical and breathing techniques that can help her cope with her contractions may cry out in pain and thrash about in her bed with the mildest of contractions. Conversely, the woman who has been prepared for her childbearing experience and is supported by her significant other or a professional prepared in labor support, or the woman who is a stoic, may never evince loss of control or cry out even with the most severe contractions. Intensity, therefore, can be evaluated only by the indentability of the uterine wall by one's fingers during the acme of the contraction or by the uterine lead of a fetal monitor. A good, effective labor contraction is one in which the uterine wall cannot be digitally indented or has reached a uterine pressure of more than 40 millimeters of mercury during the acme of the contraction.

The timing of contractions for frequency, duration, and intensity must be evaluated not only for each factor but also for the interplay of the three factors. Generally speaking, uterine contractions follow a pattern which starts with infrequent or irregular contractions (e.g., every 20 to 30 minutes) of short duration (15 to 20 seconds) and mild intensity; becomes more frequent, longer, and more severe as labor progresses; and are usually every 2 to 3 minutes, lasting 60 to 90 seconds, and of severe intensity by the end of the first stage of labor. However, there are infrequent variations of this pattern which also result in birth of the baby. If a woman starts her contractions with a frequency of every 5 minutes, lasting 60 seconds of moderately hard intensity, don't expect them to become irregular, of short duration, and mild intensity before becoming more frequent, longer, and harder — unless she develops

uterine dysfunction. Also, women have been known to deliver babies with 5- to 7-minute contractions lasting 30 to 40 seconds and of mild to moderate intensity.

Normal uterine contractions also follow another pattern, known as the normal gradient pattern. This term refers to synchronous activity of the uterine muscle which exhibits itself as stronger and longer in the fundal portion of the uterus, decreasing in the midportion, and minimal to nonexistent toward the cervix. This pattern is essential to dilatation of the cervix. The effect of contractions on the uterus is to differentiate it into two zones: (1) The upper, contracting zone, which thickens and expels the baby during labor, and (2) the lower zone, composed of the isthmus of the uterus (known during labor as the lower uterine segment) and the cervix. The lower zone does not contract but thins out into an expanded muscular tube through which the baby can pass. Differentiation of the uterus into 2 zones is accomplished through a mechanism of contraction in the upper zone in which the muscle does not return to its original length during relaxation even though the tension is one of relaxation, but stays relatively fixed at a shorter length. The upper zone is thus kept in constant contact with the intrauterine contents, and the uterine cavity becomes progressively smaller with each successive contraction. In order for this to occur, a decrease in volume is required in the intrauterine contents in the upper zone, which is accomplished by expansion of the musculature of the lower zone so that more of the intrauterine contents can distend its walls. The muscle fibers of the lower zone lengthen under the influence of upper-zone contractions and do not return to their shorter length during relaxation, even though the tension is one of relaxation, but remain relatively fixed at a longer length. The changes in the two zones complement each other: the upper zone thickens only to the extent that the lower zone expands and thins. If the uterus were to contract equally all over rather than in its normal gradient pattern, nothing would be accomplished. If the lower zone were to contract more than the upper zone, labor would be dysfunctional and cervical dilatation would not occur.

Effacement and Dilatation

Effacement and dilatation are the direct result of the contractions described above. They are also the result of the indirect effects of the contractions, which cause the fetal membranes or the presenting part to exert pressure against the cervix and lower uterine segment.

Effacement is the shortening of the cervical canal from its usual length of 2 to 3 centimeters to one in which the cervical canal is obliterated leaving only the external os as a circular orifice with thin edges. This shortening results from the lengthening of the muscular fibers around the internal os as they are taken up into the lower uterine segment. Effacement is facilitated by the cleftlike arrangement of the endocervix, which in effect unfolds like an accordian as it is stretched and taken up to become part of the lower uterine segment. The process of effacement is also facilitated by the expulsion of the mucus plug. Effacement is clinically evaluated in terms of percentages, with no effacement being 0 percent and complete effacement being 100 percent.

Dilatation is the enlargement of the external cervical os from an orifice of a few millimeters to an opening large enough for the baby to pass through. In addition to the primary action of the contractions, dilatation is facilitated by the hydrostatic action of the amniotic fluid under the influence of the contractions, causing the membranes to serve as a dilating wedge in the area of least resistance in the uterus. If the membranes have ruptured, the pressure of the presenting part on the cervix and the lower uterine segment has a dilating effect.

Dilatation is clinically evaluated by measuring the diameter of the cervical opening in centimeters, with 0 centimeters being a closed external cervical os and 10 centimeters being complete dilatation. The magic number of 10 centimeters is based on the fact that the suboccipital-bregmatic diameter of the fetal head, which is the widest diameter of the flexed head in the normal mechanisms of labor, is 9.5 centimeters at term.

Initial effacement and dilatation vary between a primigravida and a multigravida entering labor. A primigravida's cervix is frequently 50 to 60 percent effaced and a fingertip to 1 centimeter dilated prior to labor as the result of the Braxton Hicks' contractions before labor begins. Such early effacement and dilatation are part of the cervical changes that contribute to the "ripeness" of the cervix as a premonitory sign of labor. Progressive cervical change in a primigravida in labor is generally sequential, then simultaneous, with 50 to 100 percent effacement occurring first, followed by a progressive combination of any remaining effacement and dilatation. A primigravida with a paper-thin cervix is on the verge of active labor. The cervix of a multigravida entering labor is frequently 1 to 2 centimeters dilated (or more, depending on parity) with little to no effacement.

Development of clinical judgment in your fingers for assessing centimeters of dilatation is facilitated not only by practice on cervical effacement and dilatation models but also by running your fingers around the edge of and across every circular object with which you come into contact (e.g., assorted drinking glasses, telephone dials and receivers, circular ashtrays, flat circular knobs on machines), estimating its diameter in centimeters, and then checking its acutal measurement with a centimeter measuring tape or ruler.

Because it is difficult at times to distinguish between true and false labor contractions the only indicator which enables one to diagnose labor accurately is progressive cervical change, that is, cervical effacement *and* dilatation. All information concerning the contractions, location of pain, and the premonitory signs of labor is useful in differentiating between early labor and false labor but is adjunctive to assessment of the cervix.

Station

Station is the relationship of the lowermost part of the presenting part to an imaginary line drawn between the ischial spines of the woman's pelvis. The lowermost part of the presenting part at the level of the ischial spines (i.e., at the imaginary line) is called 0 station. Station is measured in terms of centimeters above or below the level of the ischial spines with above being designated as −1, −2, −3, −4, and −5 station, and below being designated as +1, +2, +3, +4, and +5 station. A −5 station is equivalent to a floating head and a +5 station is equivalent to a head at the vaginal orifice. See Figure 10-2.

Frequently a description of 0 station is given inaccurately as a definition of engagement. The reason for this error is that generally speaking, when the head is engaged the lowermost part of the presenting part is at the level of the ischial spines because the distance from the pelvic inlet to the ischial spines is usually 5 centimeters and the distance from the biparietal diameter of the full-term fetal head to the occiput is 4½ centimeters. However, this is not always true inasmuch as pelvic structure may vary with the individual woman and the size of the fetal head may alter this finding. For example, a preterm infant of 34 weeks gestation may well have its head engaged and be at a −1 station. It must be remembered that the definition of engagement is when the widest diameter of the presenting part (which, in a cephalic occipital presentation, is the biparietal diameter) has passed through the pelvic inlet.

Station is at times difficult to ascertain if there has been considerable molding of the

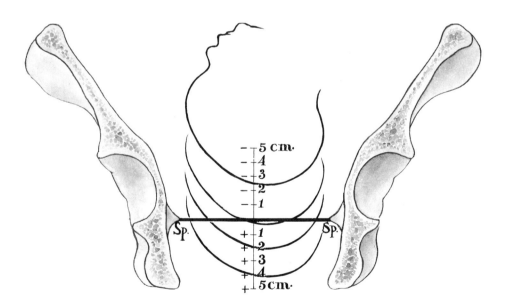

FIGURE 10-2.   Diagrammatic presentation of the station, or level of descent, of the fetal head through the pelvis. The location of the forward leading edge (lowest part of the head) is designated in centimeters above or below the plane of the interspinous line. (Reproduced by permission from J. P. Greenhill and E. A. Friedman. *Biological Principles and Modern Practice of Obstetrics.* Philadelphia: Saunders, 1974.)

fetal skull and development of caput suc-cedaneum. In a cephalic presentation, the actual lowermost part of the presenting part, which is the skull bones, may be a centimeter or so higher than the caput, which is what one's fingers are feeling. This is important to remember if one is concerned about the ade-quacy of the midpelvis and is using station as an indication that the fetal head has maneuvered this portion of the pelvis.

History, Physical and Pelvic Examination

When a woman presents herself for examin-ation thinking that she is in labor you need to evaluate her possible labor status, assess the well-being of both the mother and the baby, screen for immediate complications, and, on the basis of these findings and other factors, make a decision of whether or not the woman is in labor or needs any medical help or inter-vention.

Evaluation of labor status refers to just that information needed to determine where a woman is in the progress of her labor and to anticipate her continued progress. It has nothing to do with the well-being of either the mother or the baby. Table 10-1 outlines the history, physical examination, and pelvic examination used in assessing a woman in possible labor. The items which pertain to evaluation of labor status are indicated with an asterisk (*). The significance of each item (why the item is important information to obtain) is in the right-hand column.

If the woman is admitted to the hospital, a more extensive history than is given here is taken or reviewed from her prenatal record. This history is discussed in Chapter 11. A finding indicative of any complication requires taking a history related to that complication.

A more extensive physical examination is also done and reviewed from the patient's prenatal record if she is admitted to the hospital. This is also discussed in Chapter 11. A finding

indicative of a complication requires physical examination pertaining to that complication. For example, an elevated blood pressure, with or without the presence of edema, is an indi-cation for eliciting and evaluating deep tendon reflexes as well as taking a history for symptoms of toxemia.

Other vaginal findings may be ascertained during the course of following a woman's progress during labor. If, however, there is any reason to question the adequacy of a woman's pelvis at this time — because of a larger baby than she previously had, or a large baby in a primigravida, or a small body frame or an unengaged head in a primigravida — now is the time to do clinical pelvimetry. It is easier to perform clinical pelvimetry with the woman on an examining table than in a bed.

Determining the Status of the Membranes

Determination of whether the membranes have ruptured is essential and at times difficult. (Also see Chapter 14.) This diagnosis is made difficult by a hazy history, false-positive results on the nitrazine paper test, and the fact that the membranes may have a high leak which has sealed over as a result of the pressure of the presenting part against the cervix and lower uterine segment.

When a woman gives a history suggestive of ruptured membranes and she is not in active labor, a sterile speculum examination is in-dicated to observe the cervix for escaping amniotic fluid and, some feel, a nitrazine test. A nitrazine test is properly perfomed during the sterile speculum examination and *not* by holding a strip of nitrazine paper between gloved fingers and inserting them in the vagina. Neither is a nitrazine test done during a sterile speculum examination by clamping a strip of nitrazine paper with a ring forceps and placing it at the cervical os. Remember that the nitra-zine paper is not sterile.

The nitrazine paper test is based on the fact
(*text continues on page 220*)

Table 10-1. Data Base for Diagnosis of Labor: History, Physical Examination, and Pelvic Examination.

Item	Significance
History	
*Age	An age of under 16 and over 35 predisposes the woman to a number of complications. Under 16 increases the incidence of toxemia. Over 35 there is an increased incidence of prolonged labor due to cervical rigidity and uterine dysfunction, premature labor, placenta previa, multiple pregnancy, breech presenations, fetal congenital malformations, and maternal mortality frequently associated with increased parity.
*Gravida and para	Parity has an effect both on the duration of labor and on the incidence of complications. A cervix which has been completely dilated in a previous labor offers less resistance to being dilated again, thereby shortening the length of labor. In addition, multiparas have more pronounced fundal dominance with their contractions and more relaxed pelvic floors, which offer less resistance to the passage of the baby and decrease the length of labor. However, the duration of labor in grand multiparas may again progressively increase with greater numbers of babies, presumably resulting from changes in the uterine musculature which is often referred to as "exhaustion of the uterine muscle." It is not uncommon to see a woman having a longer labor with her eighth full-term baby than she had with her first baby. Increased parity increases the incidence of complications, with the incidence of abruptio placentae, placenta previa, uterine hemorrhage, maternal mortality, perinatal mortality, and double ovum twinning increasing in Gravida 5 and above.
*Time of onset of contractions and the frequency and duration of the contractions from onset to present	This information is necessary in order to establish the start of labor, usually timed from when the contractions became regular, and to differentiate between true and false labor contractions. False labor contractions do not increase in frequency, duration, and intensity; are irregular; and are of short duration. True labor contractions may start as irregular and of short duration but then become regular with increased frequency, duration, and intensity.
*Intensity of the contractions when lying down contrasted to when walking around	This information helps to differentiate between true and false labor contractions. True labor contractions are intensified by walking, whereas false labor contractions are rarely intensified by walking and may actually be relieved.
*Description of the location of discomfort or pain felt with contractions	This information also helps to differentiate between true and false labor contractions. False labor contractions are usually felt in the lower abdomen and groin. True labor contractions are usually felt as radiating across the uterus from the fundus to the back.
*Length of previous labor	If a previous labor has been within the past few years the length of that labor is a good indication of the potential length of this labor, allowing for the differences between a primigravid and secundigravid labor and the labor of increasing great parity.

TABLE 10-1. (Continued)

Item	Significance
*Number of years since the last baby	If there are a number of years between babies a woman may have a length of labor more similar to her first one. If 10 or more years have passed since her last baby she is predisposed to prolonged labor and the complications of placenta previa, abruptio placentae, maternal mortality, and perinatal mortality.
Delivery method of previous deliveries	To rule out previous cesarean section.
Size of largest and smallest previous babies	The size of the largest baby delivered vaginally assures the adequacy of the woman's pelvis for up to that size baby. It also provides baseline information for anticipating possible complications when compared with the estimated fetal weight of this baby and is important for decision making concerning the route of delivery in breech presentations.
	History of a baby over 9 pounds and/or abortions and preterm babies are an indication to screen the woman for diabetes.
	A woman who has a history of small babies by the same father will tend to have a smaller baby this time. This may, however, be affected by nutrition.
EDD and present weeks of gestation	This is baseline data for evaluating gestational size; if labor is at term or premature; and possible complications for the weeks of gestation.
*Absence, presence, or increase in bloody show	Bloody show is a premonitory sign of labor. An increase in bloody show is indicative of impending second stage of labor.
Absence or presence of vaginal bleeding	Bleeding is abnormal. Since vaginal examination is almost always contraindicated in the presence of bleeding, the woman must be asked if she has had any vaginal bleeding prior to doing a vaginal examination. Frank bleeding requires physician consultation and referral.
*Membranes ruptured or not	Ruptured membranes are a premonitory sign of labor. Because ruptured membranes predispose both mother and baby to high risk factors due to the increased risk of intrauterine infection, a history of ruptured membranes demands determining by examination whether or not they have indeed ruptured. Women are not always clear as to whether their membranes have ruptured or not because a slow leak can easily be confused with incontinence of urine. A history of a sudden gush of water which ran down her legs and filled her shoes and subsequently necessitated her wearing a sanitary pad, or of wetting of clothes, is a pretty good history that the membranes have ruptured.
Any prenatal problems	It is essential to screen the woman quickly for antepartal complications which may affect the intrapartal period (e.g., preeclampsia, anemia) or masquerade as signs of labor (e.g., urinary tract infection).
Physical Examination Vital signs: BP, T, P, R	An elevated or lowered blood pressure is indicative of the hypertensive disorders of pregnancy or shock, respectively. An elevated systolic but normal diastolic blood pressure may indicate anxiety.

Item	Significance
	An elevated temperature is indicative of an infectious process.
	An elevated pulse may indicate infection, shock, or anxiety.
	An elevated respiratory rate may indicate shock or anxiety.
FHT	To assess the status of the baby. A fetal heart rate below 120 or above 160 may be indicative of fetal distress and warrants immediate evaluation.
*Contraction pattern	The frequency, duration, and intensity of the contractions must be accurately assessed to determine labor status.
*Engagement	Determined by abdominal palpation, an unengaged or unfixed head on a primigravida in labor is indicative of possible cephalopelvic disproportion. Such a finding requires repeating clinical pelvimetry during the vaginal examination and evaluation in relation to the estimated fetal weight.
*Estimated fetal weight and fundal height	For evaluation in relation to the weeks of gestation. A smaller than expected estimated fetal weight (EFW) and fundal height indicates either that the woman's dates are in error or that she has a small-for-dates baby. A larger than expected EFW and fundal height indicates that the woman's dates are in error, or a large baby (indicative of diabetes), or multiple gestation, or polyhydramnios. A large baby also forewarns you of (1) the possibility of postpartum uterine atony producing hemorrhage or (2) possible shoulder dystocia. An EFW 1 or more pounds larger than her preceding babies, even though not excessive in size, also alerts you to the possibility of difficulty with delivery of the shoulders.
*Lie, presentation, position, and variety	To ascertain an abnormal lie (i.e., transverse), presentation (i.e., breech), or position (i.e., mentum, brow, military). Also to determine variety, as a posterior variety may lengthen or increase the discomfort of the first stage of labor. A woman in even very early labor must be admitted to the hospital if she has a transverse lie. A primigravida with a breech presentation is at risk and should also be admitted.
Edema of the extremities	This is one of the classic signs of preeclampsia. Ankle, pretibial, finger, and facial edema is checked for and evaluated. Ankle edema alone may simply be dependent edema resulting from the decrease in venous blood flow caused by pressure from the enlarged uterus.
Pelvic Examination *Effacement and dilatation	To determine if progressive cervical change has occurred and diagnose labor. Also to determine what stage and phase of labor the woman is in if in labor.
*Position of the cervix	The cervix is usually far back and directed posterior prior to labor. Movement of the cervix so it is directed forward in a midline position indicates readiness for, or entry into, labor.
*Station	To determine descent of the fetal head. Descent of the fetal head is one of the mechanisms of labor and is indicative of progress and pelvic adequacy.

Item	Significance
*Lie, presentation, position, and variety	To confirm abdominal findings. Sometimes it is easier to obtain these findings upon vaginal examination because the presenting part — suture lines, fontanels, and skull bones (if a cephalic presentation); a hand, or foot — can be directly felt.
*Whether or not the membranes have ruptured	To confirm or rule out a history of ruptured membranes or detect a rupture of membranes not reported for reasons stated under *History*.

* Starred items pertain to evaluation of labor status.

that its usually yellow color turns blue-green to deep blue when moistened by contact with a substance with an alkaline pH. The pH of amniotic fluid is an alkaline 7.0 to 7.5. Unfortunately, the pH of blood, of cervical mucus, and of secretions produced by certain vaginal infections are also alkaline, and if present may invalidate the test for rupture of the membranes. The chance of an invalid nitrazine test is reduced, and sterility is maintained, by obtaining a specimen during the sterile speculum examination with a sterile cotton-tipped applicator or cotton ball at the cervical os, avoiding all structures while withdrawing the specimen, and then touching it to the nitrazine paper. (The emphasis on sterility is to reduce the chance of infection in the event the membranes are ruptured, especially if there is no labor.) However, the specimen is obtained from the same area where extrusion of the mucus plug occurs, and some minute bleeding accompanies its disruption. Also it is possible that the collecting device actually rubbed against the membranes, which would render the resulting positive nitrazine test invalid. Therefore, while the nitrazine test can be a helpful adjunct, it should not be relied on for making a definitive diagnosis.

Collection of a specimen from the cervix or vaginal pool can be used for doing a fern test for detecting amniotic fluid in the secretions. This test is based on being able to observe microscopically a fernlike crystallization of the sodium chloride in amniotic fluid when the specimen is dried. However, a moderate amount of bloody show or vaginal or cervical secretions due to an infection can interfere with this test, rendering it invalid.

Digital examination for rupture of the membranes is most helpful, especially if speculum findings are inconclusive and you are not concerned with premature rupture of the membranes and the development of chorioamnionitis. If the membranes are not easily felt over the presenting part or as bulging it is helpful either to have the woman bear down or to apply fundal pressure, which may cause the membranes to bulge if they are there. Membranes in close contact with a head feel smooth and slick to the touch in contrast with the slightly irregular and comparatively more coarse feel of hair. A digital examination is *not* necessary for diagnosing ruptured membranes if findings during the speculum examination are definitive (see Chapter 14).

Diagnosis is definitive for ruptured membranes (1) when you see amniotic fluid escaping from the cervical os and pooled in the vaginal vault during speculum examination or (2) when the membranes are not felt over the presenting part at the cervical orifice. When you feel the membranes bulging against your examining fingers during vaginal examination of the cervix, other possibilities must be considered. They are (1) unruptured membranes, (2) a high leak that is occluded by pressure from the presenting part, or (3) escape of fluid trapped between the membranes with rupture of the chorion only but not the amnion.

DIFFERENTIAL DIAGNOSIS

In making a diagnosis of labor you must differentiate not only between true and false labor but also any discomforts or complications that masquerade or can be misinterpreted as labor. These most commonly include urinary tract infections and what may be called "the general miseries of the end of pregnancy," which some women have to a rather severe degree. Abruptio placentae with a posterior placenta should also be considered (see Chapter 9).

The suprapubic, flank, and back pain which may be associated with a urinary tract infection are frequently mistaken by both patient and examiner as symptomatic of labor. Added to this is the possibility of misinterpreting the frequency and urgency of urination associated with urinary tract infection as merely that experienced by the woman from pressure of the enlarged uterus on the bladder, especially if lightening has occurred. A urinary tract infection should be suspected in this situation in the absence of uterine contractions and cervical effacement and dilatation. This picture may be complicated in the presence of false labor contractions, and a diagnosis of urinary tract infection can be missed in the diagnosis of false labor.

When a urinary tract infection is suspected a careful history of any previous urinary tract infections, fever, chills, nausea and vomiting, frequency, urgency, dysuria, suprapubic pain, flank pain, lower back pain, and hematuria should be taken; a physical examination for temperature, suprapubic pain, and CVA tenderness should be made; and collection of a urine specimen for routine analysis, culture, and sensitivity is indicated as the necessary data base from which to confirm or rule out the infection. In the meantime, true labor is ruled out in the absence of cervical change and false labor is ruled out in the absence of irregular uterine contractions which are relieved by walking.

The general miseries of the end of pregnancy are frequently seen in, but not limited to, women who have been having periodic episodes of false labor. These women are terribly uncomfortable; have muscular aches and pains, particularly in the back, abdomen, and legs; walk and move with great lassitude and difficulty; haven't been eating well; are somewhat emotionally depressed because they are tired of being pregnant; are physically tired; are not sleeping well; and generally "just don't feel good." Labor is absent as is the presence of any causative disease process for these symptoms.

MANAGEMENT OF FALSE LABOR AND OF EARLY LABOR

The management of care of the woman with false labor and of the woman with the general miseries of the end of pregnancy is the same. Both require a large dose of patience, understanding, explanations, and TLC (tender, loving care). These requirements also extend into the home, and willing family members need to offer support and patience.

The woman is sent home with two sleeping pills, such as two 100-milligram tablets of sodium secobarbitol (Seconal). She is instructed to soak in a tub of warm or hot water filled enough to cover her abdomen; then, after getting out of the tub, to drink a hot drink of her preference (tea, coffee, milk, chocolate) with sugar, or a glass of wine, with which she takes one of her sleeping pills; and then to go to bed for a back rub and sleep. If she is not asleep in an hour, she may repeat the sleeping pill. The tub bath relaxes and soothes her aching muscles through the action of dilatation of the blood vessels, thus increasing blood flow and oxygenation to the area, and through the action of the psychologically soothing motion of the water. It would be dangeous for her to take a sleeping pill prior to the tub bath and to fall asleep in the nearly full tub of water. She will need help from family members to get in and out of the tub. The hot drink, made for her by a family member, is the time-honored method for facilitating sleep. The addition of sugar to the drink provides needed calories and energy to the body's cells. Sherry is often used also to promote relaxation. The back rub, given by a family member, again gives relief to aching muscles and bespeaks TLC. The sleeping pills are given the woman as an adjunct in case the other measures are not sufficient to assure a good sleep.

It is frequently difficult to differentiate between false labor and the early latent phase of labor in a woman. The management of care of such a woman, in the absence of any complications, will vary according to the setting in which she will labor and deliver. If she plans to deliver in a hospital the plan will vary according to hospital policies, hospital facilities, distance the woman lives from the hospital, availability of transportation for the woman, the coping abilities of the woman and her family, and the woman's preference. If, for example, the hospital has a unit for labor observation or early labor, admission to this unit is appropriate. If, however, the hospital does not have such a unit and also has a policy that patients are not to be admitted to the labor and delivery suite until in active labor unless the membranes are ruptured, or admitted to the hospital except with complications, then you must decide whether to keep the woman in the hospital emergency room or area where you examined her for labor or to send her home until labor is more definitively established. In such a situation a compromise is generally struck between realities and the philosophy that a woman will probably feel and cope better in the more pleasant, familiar surroundings of her home.

Since walking may stimulate true labor or relieve false labor, the woman is usually asked to walk outside or in designated areas of the hospital and return to be rechecked in 1 to 2 hours. If no change in the cervix is noted upon this repeat examination and if the woman lives nearby, has no transportation problems, and wants to go home, she is managed for false labor and sent home. If, however, the woman lives a great distance away and the diagnosis of false labor or early latent phase labor is still not yet able to be determined, the woman may be asked to walk for another couple of hours and again be rechecked before a final decision is made to send her home. Some women who live many miles from the hospital would rather walk for hours in the hospital until they are convinced that this is false labor than have the anxiety of thinking she might not return in time and deliver either at home or en route. A combination of lack of cervical progress and exhaustion finally culminate in a change of preference to go home and the woman is sent home on the regimen for false labor for a much needed rest.

Management of the woman in the early latent phase of labor again varies according to the setting in which she will labor and deliver. If she plans to deliver in a hospital, the management of care varies according to hospital policies, hospital facilities, distance the woman lives from the hospital, availability of transportation for the woman, the coping abilities of the woman and her family, and the woman's preference. If the hospital has an early labor unit, admission to it is appropriate. This enables the woman to undergo routine admission procedures and spend her early labor in a more homelike atmosphere. Comfortable chairs for her and her significant other; availability of materials and personnel to explain the progress of labor and helpful breathing and relaxation techniques; time-passing materials such as playing cards, books, television, and magazines; and freedom to walk and move around are basics in such a unit. If the hospital does not have such a unit, a woman who lives nearby and has readily accessible transportation may prefer to go home and return to the hospital when her labor is more active. A woman who lives some distance from the hospital may have friends or relatives with whom she would prefer to spend this period of early labor. Even if a hospital does not have a 4-centimeter dilatation admission requirement some women who live too far away to return home for early labor prefer to walk outside or in designated areas of the hospital, frequently going to the cafeteria or snack shop for tea or coffee with sugar before being admitted to the labor and delivery suite. Any time a patient in early labor has entered the active phase of the first stage of labor, ruptures her membranes, or develops signs and symptoms of a complication, she is admitted to the labor and delivery suite.

The bibliography is at the end of Chapter 13.

11

Initial Evaluation of the Mother and Fetus in Labor

When a woman is admitted to the labor and delivery suite in active labor a complete evaluation of her condition and the condition of her baby is conducted. This includes a history, physical and pelvic examination, and laboratory tests.

HISTORY

The history is similar, with modifications, to the history outlined in Chapter 3 with the additions outlined for history in Chapters 5 and 10. It includes the following categories with modifications given:

1. Identifying information — name, age, race, gravida, para, LMP, EDD, and weeks gestation
2. Labor history — contractions, bloody show, status of fetal membranes, any vaginal bleeding, when she ate last

3. Present pregnancy history — where received antepartal care, any antepartal complications and treatment (this segment may be summarized, if normal, as "normal antepartal course"), drugs and medications taken during pregnancy, and special tests (e.g., sonography) during pregnancy and why
4. Past obstetric history — explanation of gravida and para numbering for this woman, any complications during previous childbearing experiences (antepartal, intrapartal, postpartal), number of years since last baby, length of last labor, size of largest and smallest previous babies, any fetal deaths
5. Past medical history (see Chapter 3)
6. Family history (see Chapter 3)

If admission is for a reason other than labor — such as premature rupture of membranes, vaginal bleeding, or a medical complication —

the appropriate related history needs to be taken and the physician notified. (See "Chief Complaint" and "History of Present Illness" in Chapter 3.)

If the woman's prenatal record is available in the labor and delivery suite it is often used as the source of information for the above outlined history, with the exception of the labor history. This spares the woman from having to reiterate history she has given before, from being disturbed at a time when she is coping with the demands and stresses placed upon her by her condition and situation, and from being disrupted while concentrating on her breathing exercises during contractions. However, a few critical items of history should be double-checked, specifically the existence of any of the following: drug allergies, blood transfusions and reactions, and major obstetrical or medical complications.

PHYSICAL AND PELVIC EXAMINATION

A screening physical examination is done on all women upon their admission to the labor and delivery suite. This not only provides up-to-date baseline data but also screens for any infectious disease. If the woman's prenatal record is available in the labor and delivery suite the physical examination which was done during her initial antepartal visit is reviewed for any medical abnormalities or disease. (See Chapters 3 and 5.) The admission examination is somewhat abbreviated, as follows in outline form:

1. General observations
2. Vital signs
3. Gross observation of all the various anatomic parts and systems with specific questioning and examination of the following:
   a. head and eyes — questioning for headaches, dizziness, any visual disturbances (blurring of vision, scotomata, diplopia, spots before eyes, flashing lights); and ophthalmoscopic examination
   b. mouth and throat — examination of the lips, tongue, and oropharynx
   c. neck — examination of the lymph node groups and the thyroid gland
   d. cardiorespiratory system — questioning for breathing difficulties and any known cardiac or respiratory disease; auscultation of the heart and lungs
   e. breasts — questioning for any known breast disease; inspection of the nipples and breasts and palpation of the breasts in the supine position (see Chapter 40)
   f. gastrointestinal system — questioning for epigastric pain; observation for belching or burping and vomiting (signs of transition); and examination of the abdomen (detailed later in this chapter)
   g. urinary system — questioning for known urinary tract disease and the signs and symptoms of a urinary tract infection (see Chapter 10); examination for CVA tenderness (see Chapter 42)
   h. genitals — questioning (if prenatal record is not available) for any known venereal disease, date and results of last Pap smear and vaginal infection; pelvic examination (detailed later in this chapter)
   i. endocrine system — questioning for any known endocrine disease and to ascertain the need for diabetic screening (questioning done if there is no prenatal record available)
   j. musculoskeletal, vascular, and central nervous systems — questioning for syncope, convulsions, and any difficulties with edema, or varicosities; observation of any obvious skeletal deformities, especially those which might indicate pelvic deformity or difficulties with positioning for delivery; and examination for edema (ankle, pretibial, hands, and face), varicosities (legs and vulva), Homan's sign, and deep tendon reflexes and clonus (see Chapter 43)
   k. skin — questioning and examination

for rashes, lesions, jaundice, lice, and so on

A more comprehensive review of systems and physical examination can be performed postpartally if the woman entered the labor and delivery suite in late active labor without prenatal care. The above outline is sufficient for gross general screening and screening for major medical problems which might affect a safe intrapartum period for the woman. If the woman has been closely followed throughout her antepartal course by a consistant care provider, this repeat of history, other than the labor history, and the total gross screening physical examination are not necessary.

In addition to the above, thorough abdominal and pelvic examinations are essential for evaluation of labor status and the well-being of the fetus.

Abdominal Examination
Abdominal examination is done for the following:

Contraction pattern
Engagement
Abdominal scars (obtain explanation if any)
Lie
Presentation
Position
Variety
Fetal heart tones
Fundal height
Estimated fetal weight
Abdominal girth when indicated (see Chapter 41)

Pelvic Examination
Pelvic examination is done for the following:

Position of the cervix
Effacement
Dilatation
Molding
Caput succedaneum
Station
Lie
Presentation
Position
Variety
Synclitism/asynclitism
Status of fetal membranes
Evaluation of vaginal orifice and perineal body
Evaluation of bony pelvis, including clinical pelvimetry

(See Chapters 10 and 12 for explanation of the items included in this abdominal and pelvic examination.)

LABORATORY TESTS

The laboratory tests ordered upon admission of the woman to the labor and delivery suite may vary by policy from clinical setting to clinical setting but generally include the following:

Hematocrit — ordered *stat.* or done by the nurse-midwife (see Chapter 35).
VDRL
Urinalysis — minimum of dipstick test for protein, glucose, and acetone; in some settings a urine specimen is collected and sent to the laboratory for routine microscopic examination or done *stat.* by the nurse-midwife.

In addition, a type and crossmatch blood sample is drawn (although it may or may not be sent immediately to the lab, depending on the woman's condition) if any of the following are present:
Grand multiparity
Anemia
Overdistended uterus
Candidacy for cesarean section
Rh-negative blood
Bleeding

History of postpartum hemorrhage

The blood for the laboratory tests is drawn by the nurse-midwife (see Chapter 34). If the woman will be having an intravenous infusion, the blood specimens are obtained at the same time the IV is started (see Chapter 36).

The woman's prenatal record is reviewed for the results of the following laboratory tests and adjunctive studies done during pregnancy. Those with an asterisk are recorded in the admission note; the others are reviewed but usually recorded only if results are abnormal.

*Blood group (ABO)
*Rh factor
Indirect Coombs' test

Serology
GC cultures
Pap smear
*Last hemoglobin and hematocrit
Last urinalysis
Rubella titer
Chest roentgenography
Sickle cell screening
Tuberculin screening
Any special tests

A finding of any sign or symptom of a medical or obstetrical complication requires physician consultation.

The bibliography is at the end of Chapter 13.

12

The Normal First Stage of Labor

Labor comprises those processes that result in the expulsion of the products of conception by the mother. It begins with true labor contractions, as evidenced by progressive cervical change, and ends with the delivery of the placenta. The cause of the onset of spontaneous labor is not known, although a number of interesting theories have been advanced and it is known how to induce labor under certain conditions. (See *Williams Obstetrics* [1] for review and critique of the theories of the onset of labor.)

The first stage of labor is defined as beginning with true labor contractions, as evidenced by progressive cervical change, and ending with the cervix completely dilated (10 centimeters). It is known as the stage of cervical dilatation.

DATA BASE FOR THE FIRST STAGE OF LABOR

Components of the data base for determining

the well-being of the mother and the fetus during the first stage of labor are as follows:

1. Continuing evaluation of any significant findings from the history, physical and pelvic examinations, and laboratory work done upon admission to labor (see Chapter 11)
2. Evaluation of the progress of labor
3. Evaluation of the woman's behavior and her response to labor and her significant others
4. Continuing evaluation of the normality of the fetal presentation, position, and variety; and fetal adaptation to the pelvis
5. Evaluation of the fetal heart tones
6. Evaluation of the woman's vital signs and other physical signs and symptoms
7. Continued screening for signs and symptoms of obstetrical complications and fetal distress (see Chapter 14)

In order to evaluate any of the components of the data base, one must know what the parameters of normal are for each of the specific pieces of information obtained for each component.

The Progress of Labor

The first stage of labor is divided into two sequential phases: latent and active. The active phase is further subdivided into three sequential phases as defined and described by Friedman [2]: acceleration, maximum slope, and deceleration (Fig. 12-1). What is referred to as the transitional phase of labor (from approximately 8 centimeters to 10 centimeters) roughly corresponds to the deceleration phase. Each phase of labor is characterized not only by measurable physical changes but also by psychologic changes. The physical changes are used to evaluate progress in labor, while the psychologic changes are used to estimate where in labor a woman is and to aid in devising appropriate support and comfort measures.

The average length of time for each phase and stage of labor enumerated here and the progress within each phase and stage as detailed in this section is according to Friedman [2] and serves as a guide for normality. This does not mean however, that a woman who does not follow this labor curve is not having a normal labor, but it does signal that this woman needs to be carefully and comprehensively evaluated to assess that she and her fetus indeed are still within the realm of normal and will remain so over time. The operative word is *progress*. If there is not progress in one area (e.g., dilatation), is there progress in another area (e.g., descent, working through any psychologic obstacle)? Is the progress sufficient for current and projected maternal and fetal well-being?

Latent Phase

The latent phase covers the period of time from the beginning of labor to the point when dilatation begins to progress actively. This generally is from the onset of regular contractions to 3 to 4 centimeters dilatation or to the beginning of the active phase. Little to no descent of the presenting part occurs during the latent phase.

Contractions become established during the latent phase as they increase in frequency, duration, and intensity — from every 10 to 20 minutes lasting 15 to 20 seconds of mild intensity to a moderate intensity (averaging 40 mm Hg at their acme from a baseline uterine tonus of 10 mm Hg) and occurring approximately every 5 to 7 minutes and lasting 30 to 40 seconds.

Usually the woman during the latent phase of labor experiences a mixture of emotions: she is excited, happy, and relieved that the end of pregnancy has come and the long period of waiting has ended, but she feels a sense of anticipation and some apprehension about what is yet to come. Generally she is not too uncomfortable and copes well with her situation. For a woman who has been suffering from the general miseries of the end of pregnancy and false labor, the emotional response is at times dramatic in terms of relief, relaxation, and increased coping ability. Even though tired, she knows she is at last actually in labor and what she is now experiencing is productive.

Active Phase

The active phase covers the period of time from the start of active progression of dilatation to the completion of dilatation. This is generally from 3 to 4 centimeters, or the end of the latent phase, to 10 centimeters dilatation, or the end of the first stage of labor. Progressive descent of the presenting part occurs during the latter part of the active phase (deceleration) and during second stage.

The *acceleration phase* starts the active phase of labor and leads into the phase of maximum slope. The *phase of maximum slope* is the time when cervical dilatation is occurring most rapidly and increasing from 3 to 4 centimeters

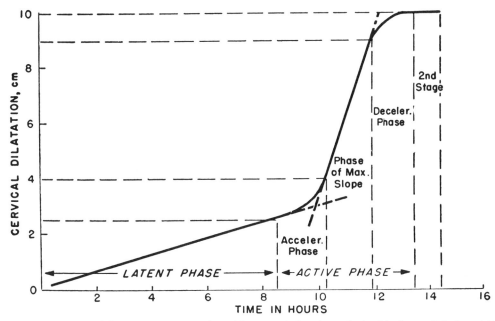

FIGURE 12-1.   Primipara labor curve. (Reproduced by permission from E. A. Friedman. Primigravid labor: A graphicostatistical analysis. *Obstet. Gynecol.* 6:569, 1955.)

to about 8 centimeters. Normally this dilatation is constant, averaging 3 centimeters per hour with a minimum rate of not less than 1.2 centimeters per hour in nulliparas. In multiparas, the average rate of dilatation during the phase of maximum slope is 5.7 centimeters per hour with a minimum rate of 1.5 centimeters per hour. The *deceleration phase* is the end of the active phase, during which there is a slowing down of the rate of dilatation from 8 to 10 centimeters while descent reaches its maximum rate. The average maximum rate of descent in nulliparas is 1.6 centimeters per hour and normally at least 1.0 centimeter per hour. In multiparas the rate of descent averages 5.4 centimeters per hour with a minimum rate of 2.1 centimeters per hour.

Contractions during the active phase become increasingly more frequent, of longer duration, and of greater intenstiy. Effective contractions are those which have a normal triple gradient pattern, reach a uterine pressure of 40 to 50 millimeters of mercury during the acme of the

contraction, and return to a resting uterine tonus of 10 millimeters of mercury. By the end of the active phase, contractions are usually coming every 2 to 3 minutes, lasting around 60 seconds, and reaching firm intensity (more than 40 mmHg) with an average of about 55 millimeters of mercury.

As labor progresses through the phase of maximum slope the woman may become increasingly apprehensive. As the contractions become harder, last longer, and occur more often it becomes apparent to her that she cannot control the fact of their happening. With this realization she becomes more serious. She wants someone with her as she is frightened of being left alone with the contractions with which she is no longer sure she can cope. She experiences a number of ill-defined doubts and fears. She can tell you she is scared but is unable to tell you what she is scared of.

During the deceleration phase the woman is ending the first stage of labor. This has long been known as the *transitional phase* as the woman nears entry into, and prepares for, the second stage of labor. A large number of signs and symptoms, including behavior changes, have been identified as indicative of this transition. Those occurring late in the transitional phase are known as the signs of impending second stage and are marked with an asterisk (*) in the following listing of the signs and symptoms of transition:

Beads of perspiration on the upper lip or brow
Shaking legs
Chattering teeth
Cramps in the buttocks, thighs, or calves of the legs
Hiccupping
Belching and burping
Thirst
Anorexia
Nausea and possible vomiting
Inability to breathe abdominally
Irritable abdomen — increased tenderness to touch over the abdomen and back
Marked restlessness
Natural amnesia between contractions — appears exhausted and is difficult to rouse
Difficulty in readily comprehending directions
Contractions every 1½ to 2 minutes, lasting 60 to 90 seconds, of severe intensity — seem almost continuous and are quite painful
Toes curl with contractions
Generalized discomfort
Doesn't want to be touched
Eager to be "put to sleep"
Bewildered, frustrated, and exasperated by the severity of the contractions
Severe low backache
Marked decrease in the sense of modesty
Unable to cope with the contractions if left alone
Irritable behavior
Pulling or stretching sensation deep in the pelvis
Rejection of those about her
Quite apprehensive
*Increase in bloody show

*Rectal pressure, feeling of having to have a bowel movement, repeated requests for a bedpan or to go to the bathroom
*Uncontrollable desire to bear down
*Membranes rupture
*Rectal and perineal bulging and flattening
*Expulsive grunt upon exhalation

Usually a combination of several of these are exhibited by the woman during transition. It is not uncommon to have a woman exhibit all or nearly all of these signs and symptoms, particularly if she is a primigravida who has not had the benefits of preparation for childbearing classes.

Continuing evaluation of the progress of labor is thus based on findings obtained during vaginal and abdominal examination of the woman and observation of her behavior. It is in addition to the data base, including evaluation of labor status, obtained when the woman first presented herself for diagnosis of labor (see Chapter 10). Specifically, evaluation of the progress of labor is based on the following items of information:

Effacement
Dilatation
Station
Contraction pattern — frequency, duration, and intensity
Behavior changes
Signs and symptoms of transition and impending second stage

There are other observations you can make that indicate the woman's progress in labor. These are based on the fact that descent of the fetus in the pelvis changes the location of findings elaborated from the fetus. The low back pain a woman experiences is caused by the pressure of the fetal head against her spine. This is not a generalized pain but rather one that can be precisely pinpointed for you by the woman. As descent occurs the location of this back pain correspondingly moves down her lower spine. Also, the location of the fetal heart tones moves lower in her abdomen as descent occurs.

Fetal Normality

Presentation, Position, and Variety

Determination of the lie, presentation, position, and variety of the fetus is essential information for the data base. These determinations require an understanding of the words used and of the anatomical landmarks of the fetal skull in relation to the maternal pelvis.

Lie is the relationship of the long axis of the fetus to the long axis of the mother. There are three possible lies: longitudinal, transverse, and oblique (Fig. 12-2).

Presentation is determined by the presenting part, which is the first portion of the fetus to enter the pelvic inlet.There are three possible presentations: cephalic, breech, and shoulder. The first two are further subdivided — cephalic: vertex, sincipital, brow, and face; breech: frank, full (or complete), and footling, which can be single or double.

The *attitude* of the fetus is its characteristic posture. This is determined by the relationship of the fetal parts to each other and the effect this has on the vertebral column. The attitude of the fetus varies according to its presentation. For example, a fetus in a vertex presentation has a well-flexed head, flexion of the extremities over the thorax and abdomen, and a convex curved back; while a fetus with a face presentation has a head which is acutely extended, flexion of the extremities on the thorax and abdomen, and a vertebral column which not only is straightened but also has some degree of arching (Fig. 12-3).

Position is the arbitrarily chosen point on the fetus for each presentation in relation to the left or right side of the mother's pelvis. These are shown in Table 12-1.

Position is commonly used to refer to the designations of left occipital anterior (LOA), right sacral transverse (RST), and so forth. This is what is expected as an answer to the question "What is the position?" Technically this is not accurate, but it serves as a shorthand form since such a designation gives not only the position and variety but also the lie and presentation. For example, the designation LOA tells you that the lie is longitudinal, the presentation is vertex, the position is the occiput in the left side of the mother's pelvis, and the variety is the occiput in the anterior portion of the pelvis.

Variety is the same arbitrarily chosen point on the fetus used in defining position in relation to the anterior, transverse, or posterior portion of the pelvis. Table 12-2 summarizes the possibilities.

Transverse and oblique lies in labor are abnormal conditions. They require referral of women who have them to the physician and most likely necessitate cesarean section. Approxi-

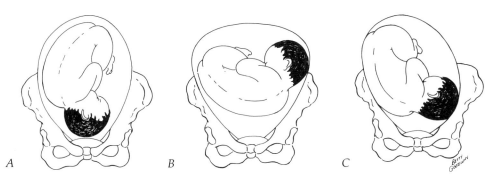

FIGURE 12-2.   Lies. A. longitudinal; B. transverse; C. oblique.

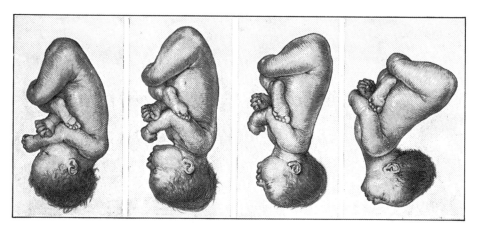

FIGURE 12-3. Attitude of the fetus in vertex, sinciput, brow, and face presentations. (Reproduced by permission from J. A. Pritchard and P. C. MacDonald. *Williams Obstetrics, 15th.* New York: Appleton-Century-Crofts, 1976.)

TABLE 12-1. Position for Each Presentation

Presentation	Position — To Right or Left of the Mother's Pelvis
Cephalic:	(Specific for each subdivision)
Vertex	Occiput
Sincipital	Sinciput (bregma, anterior fontanel)
Brow	Brow
Face	Mentum (chin)
Breech:	(Same for each subdivision)
Frank	Sacrum
Full	Sacrum
Footling	Sacrum
Shoulder	Acromion

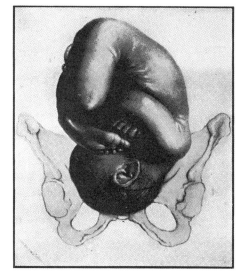

FIGURE 12-4. Left occiput transverse (LOT), anterior view. (Reproduced by permission from J. A. Pritchard and P. C. MacDonald. *Williams Obstetrics, 15th.* New York: Appleton-Century-Crofts, 1976.)

mately 0.5 percent of women enter labor with a shoulder presentation.

Of the presentations associated with a longitudinal lie, the most common is the vertex cephalic presentation. It has an incidence of approximately 95 percent. Of these, approximately two-thirds will be positioned with the occiput in the left side of the mother's pelvis (LOA, LOT, LOP) and one-third with the occiput in the right side of the mother's pelvis (ROA, ROT, ROP). Because the head usually enters the inlet with the occiput directed to the transverse portion of the mother's pelvis, the most common position at the onset of labor is left occiput transverse (LOT). Figures 12-4 and 12-5 show left occipital positions.

Approximately 3.0 to 3.5 percent of women will enter labor with a breech presentation

TABLE 12-2. Possibilities of Fetal Relationships to the Maternal Pelvis

Lie	Presentation	Position and Variety	
Longitudinal	Cephalic: vertex	ROA ROT ROP	LOA LOT LOP
	sincipital brow	These two presentations usually convert to either a vertex or face presentation	
	face	RMA RMT RMP	LMA LMT LMP
	Breech: frank, full, and footling	RSA RST RSP	LSA LST LSP
Transverse	Shoulder	RAA RAP	LAA LAP
		A transverse variety is not possible	
Oblique	Nothing is felt at the inlet. There is no presentation, position, or variety associated with this lie. An oblique lie usually is a transitory condition.		

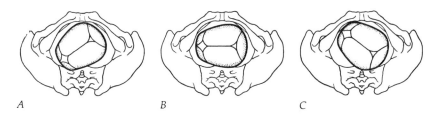

FIGURE 12-5. Left occiput varieties, view from below. A. Left occipital anterior (LOA); B. Left occipital transverse (LOT); C. Left occipital posterior (LOP). (Reproduced by permission from J. A. Pritchard and P. C. MacDonald. *Williams Obstetrics, 15th*. New York: Appleton-Century-Crofts, 1976.)

and 0.5 percent with a face presentation. The nurse-midwife collaborates with a physician in the management of women with a breech or face presentation. (See Chapter 15.)

It is thought that the reason why the vast majority of presentations are cephalic at term is the interrelationship between the decreased amount of amniotic fluid and the piriform shape of the uterus, with the roomier portion being in the fundus. Although the breech of the fetus (podalic pole) is smaller than the fetal head (cephalic pole), the combination of the breech and the flexed lower extremities is bulkier because the flexed upper extremities

TABLE 12-3. Essential Landmarks of the Fetal Skull

Anatomical part	Description
Bones:	
frontal	There are two frontal bones.
parietal	There are two parietal bones.
occipital	There is one occipital bone.
Sutures:	
frontal	The frontal suture is between the two frontal bones.
sagittal	The sagittal suture is between the two parietal bones.
coronal	There are two coronal sutures, each between the frontal and parietal bones on either side of the head.
lambdoid	There are two lambdoid sutures, each between the parietal bones and the upper margin of the occipital bone on either side of the head.
Fontanels:	
anterior	Formed by the meeting of the frontal, sagittal, and two coronal sutures. This is roughly the shape of a diamond ($\Diamond$), and four sutures can be felt leading off the anterior fontanel in four different directions as indicated by the points on the diamond.
posterior	Formed by the meeting of the sagittal and the two lambdoid sutures. This is roughly the shape of a triangle (∇), and three sutures can be felt leading off the posterior fontanel in three different directions as indicated by the points of the triangle. The occipital bone, which serves as the base of the triangle, can also be felt.

are not as close to the head as the lower extremities are to the breech. Prior to the thirty-second week of pregnancy the bulkiness of the poles of the fetus is not a factor in fetal presentation because the amniotic cavity is large in relation to the total fetal mass. The incidence of breech presentation at this time may be as high as 50 percent. After the thirty-second week the combination of fetal growth and the decrease in amniotic fluid causes the fetus to be constrained by the uterine walls. The fetus thus accommodates itself to the shape of the uterus so that the majority of the earlier breech presentations spontaneously convert to vertex presentations by term. Those which do not convert spontaneously may be responding to abnormal uterine shape, extension of the fetal vertebral column, placenta previa, hydrocephaly, or unknown influences. Hydrocephaly must be ruled out because this condition makes the cephalic pole bulkier than the podalic pole. Therefore, accommodation by the fetus will put the larger cephalic pole in the fundus and accounts for the high incidence of breech presentation when the fetus is hydrocephalic.

Vaginal examination during labor after the cervix has begun to dilate is invaluable for confirming abdominal findings as well as enabling more definitive diagnoses regarding the fetal presentation, position, and variety. This is because the fetal suture lines and fontanels, portions of the fetal face, portions of the fetal pelvis, or the fetal extremities (hands or feet) can now be felt. Since the cephalic vertex presentations are by far the most common it is vital to be well versed in the essential landmarks of the fetal skull as indicated in Table 12-3 and Figure 12-6.

Position and variety of the vertex presentation, therefore, are determined vaginally by feeling the anterior or posterior fontanel (its shape and the sutures leading off the fontanel) and identifying which fontanel is in which side and portion of the maternal pelvis. In order to identify which part of the fetal skull one is feeling, it helps to remember that the sagit-

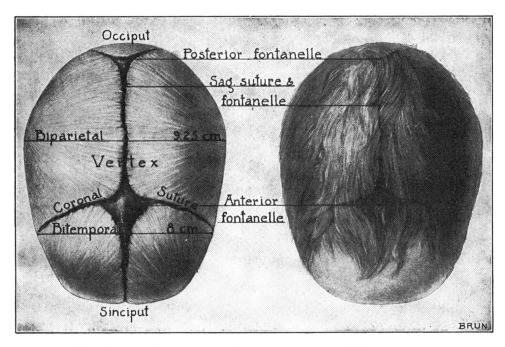

FIGURE 12-6.   Fetal head at term showing various fontanels, sutures, and diameters. (Reproduced by permission from J. A. Pritchard and P. C. MacDonald. *Williams Obstetrics, 15th*. New York: Appleton-Century-Crofts, 1976.)

tal suture is the only suture that has the anterior fontanel at one end and the posterior fontanel at the other end.

Adaptation to the Pelvis

Vaginal examination during labor also provides other information regarding the adaptation of the fetus to the pelvis. This information includes synclitism/asynclitism, molding, and caput succedaneum.

Synclitism/Asynclitism.   Synclitism and asynclitism are terms to describe the relationship of the sagittal suture of the fetal head to the symphysis pubis and the sacrum of the maternal pelvis. This relationship is determined when the anteroposterior diameter of the fetal head is in alignment with the transverse diameter of the pelvic inlet, which is the usual case for entry into the pelvic inlet and engagement. This places the sagittal suture

line of the fetal skull directly across the pelvic inlet in the same line as the transverse diameter of the inlet and the occiput of the fetal head in the transverse portion of the mother's pelvis. *Synclitism* is the term used when the sagittal suture is midway between the symphysis pubis and the sacral promontory. *Asynclitism* indicates that the sagittal suture is directed either towards the symphysis pubis or towards the sacral promontory (Fig. 12-7). Determination of whether this is anterior asynclitism or posterior asynclitism is *not* based on which maternal pelvic structure the sagittal suture is closer to but instead is based on which parietal bone is dominant. Therefore, anterior asynclitism occurs when the anterior parietal bone (the one closest to the symphysis pubis) becomes the lowermost part of the presenting part, due to deflection of the head toward the sacral promontory, causing the sagittal suture to lie closer to the sacral promontory. Posterior

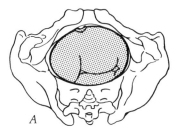 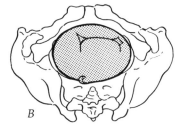

FIGURE 12-7. Asynclitism. A. anterior; B. posterior.

asynclitism occurs when the posterior parietal bone (the one closest to the sacral promontory) becomes the lowermost part of the presenting part as a result of deflection of the head toward the symphysis pubis, causing the sagittal suture to lie closer to the symphysis pubis. In normal labor the head usually enters the pelvic inlet with a moderate degree of posterior asynclitism and then changes to anterior asynclitism as it descends further into the pelvis before the mechanism of internal rotation takes place. This sequential change from posterior to anterior asynclitism facilitates the mechanism of descent; it is an accommodation by the fetus to take advantage of the roomiest portions of the true pelvis.

Molding. Molding and caput succedaneum result from pressure exerted on the fetal head by the maternal structures of the birth canal. Molding is the change in the shape of the head as a result of the soft skull bones overriding or overlapping because they are not yet firmly united and movement is possible at the sutures. The shape the head becomes depends on the presentation because this determines which parts of the skull are subjected to pressure. Due to the prevalence of occipital cephalic presentations, the usual molding is the over-riding of the parietal bones over the occipital bone which, in effect, obliterates the posterior fontanel and leaves a ridge. When there is overlapping of the parietal bones at the sagittal suture, which is not uncommon, the parietal bone that was anterior in the pelvis overlaps the "posterior" parietal bone, which was de-

pressed because of pressure from the sacral promontory. Therefore, in an ROT position that rotates to ROA, the left parietal bone overrides the right parietal bone, and vice versa for an LOT position that rotates to LOA.

Molding involves the totality of the skull with overlapping in one area being counter-balanced with movement elsewhere. This creates harmony between the base and the vertex of the skull in order to prevent destructive tension and possible rupture of the cranial membrane, the dura mater.

Caput succedaneum. Caput succedaneum is the formation of an edematous swelling over the most dependent portion of the presenting fetal head. Pressure around the presenting part by the cervical opening produces congestion and edema of the portion of the fetal head over the cervical opening. If the fetal membranes are ruptured and the fetal head instead of the membranes is functioning as the dilating wedge against the cervical opening, a greater amount of caput succedaneum will be formed. Caput succedaneum can be differentiated from *cephalhematoma* by virtue of the fact that caput succedaneum crosses suture lines as a generalized swelling whereas a cephalhematoma, which is a bleeding beneath the periosteum, may occur over more than one cranial bone but is limited to each individual bone and does not cross any sutures.

The formation of a few millimeters of caput succedaneum is not unusual or abnormal. Extensive formation of caput succedaneum which makes the identification of fetal sutures and fontanels impossible, combined with severe amounts of molding, is usually seen only when labor is prolonged and cephalopelvic disproportion must be suspected.

Fetal Heart Tones
Evaluation of the fetal heart is based on a combination of rate and pattern, with the latter being most significant when there is deviation from normal. The work of Caldeyro-Barcia and associates in South America and Hon, Paul, and associates in the United States has contributed immeasurably to fetal heart evaluation and understanding of both clinical assessment and interpretation of findings. Their work has invalidated former teachings such as waiting 30 seconds after a contraction is over to count the fetal heart tones by auscultation with a fetoscope in order to avoid error in the count caused by the "normal bradycardia" occurring with a contraction. There is no such thing as a normal bradycardia occurring with contractions (see Chapter 14.) Therefore to evaluate the fetal heart only between contractions may completely mislead the clinician and cause failure to detect early evidence of fetal distress.

Fetal heart rate must be evaluated both during and between contractions not only because the information gathered from these two times has different significance but also because the one provides the baseline from which the other deviates. Changes in the fetal heart rate that are associated with uterine contractions are known as *periodic fetal heart rate changes.* The fetal heart rate that is present between periodic fetal heart rate changes or, if there are no periodic fetal heart rate changes, the fetal heart rate that is present between contractions is known as the *baseline fetal heart rate.*

Norms. The normal range of the baseline fetal heart rate is 120 to 160 beats per minute. When there is instantaneous continuous recording of the fetal heart rate, such as is obtained by electronic fetal monitoring, it is obvious what the fetal heart rate level is over a period of time. In order for a change in this level to be considered the new level, the fetal heart rate must be at the new level for at least 10 minutes. If this change is an increase in the baseline fetal heart rate it is called a *rise.* If this change is a decrease in the baseline fetal heart rate it is called a *fall.* A baseline fetal heart rate level in the range of 161 to 180 beats per minute is termed moderate tachycardia, with marked tachycardia being a baseline fetal heart rate level above 180 beats per minute. At the other end of the range of normal, a baseline fetal heart rate level in the range of 119 to 100 beats per minute is termed moderate bradycardia, with marked bradycardia being a baseline fetal heart rate level below 100 beats per minute.

Variability (irregularity) of the baseline fetal heart rate refers to short-term fluctuations from the baseline fetal heart rate level and is classified according to the degree of this fluctuation. This can range from no variability, in which there are no fluctuations visible on the tracing from a fetal heart monitor, through an average fluctuation, consisting of 4 to 9 percent of the baseline fetal heart rate level, to a marked fluctuation, which consists of more than 15 percent of the baseline fetal heart rate level. Contrary to previous teachings, marked variability, by itself, does not indicate fetal distress. In fact, baseline fetal heart rate level variability is a far better sign of fetal well-being than an absence of variability because variability indicates that the nervous system mechanism for controlling heart rate is well developed, functioning, and not affected by either maternal medication or a deleterious fetal condition.

Periodic fetal heart rate changes, baseline fetal heart rate levels in the range of tachycardia or bradycardia, and either lack of fetal heart rate level variability or marked variability associated with periodic fetal heart rate changes are all abnormal. These are discussed in detail in Chapter 14.

Methods. Evaluation of the fetal heart is accomplished by use of one or more of several different methods: fetoscope (e.g. headscope, Lefscope), ultrasound (e.g., Doptone), external fetal monitor, and internal fetal monitor. The last two methods can also include electronic measurement of uterine activity. Each method has its place, advantages, and disadvantages depending on the situation.

FETOSCOPE AND ULTRASOUND. In order to obtain any valid information at all from use of the fetoscope it must be used at the right time. The fetal heart tones must be listened to during a contraction as well as between contractions. The best method is to start listening midway between two contractions and continue listening through the next contraction to the midpoint between it and the following contraction. The fact that averaging of the rate of the fetal heart does not give an accurate pattern of the fetal heart rate can be alleviated to some extent by shortening the amount of time the fetal heart tones are counted to obtain the average. This will more closely approximate the beat-to-beat rate obtained on monitor tracings. For example, counting the fetal heart rate for 60 seconds to ascertain the rate for one minute will not give you the same results as two 30-second countings or four 15-second countings. The common practice of counting just once for 15 or 30 seconds and multiplying times 4 or 2, respectively, to obtain the rate is unfortunate and not equivalent to counting for 60 seconds. More frequent counting of the fetal heart tones for several consecutive short periods of time during the time when the fetus is most apt to be stressed (i.e., during the contraction) gives the most reliable information for detecting abnormal or periodic fetal heart rate changes or patterns when using a fetoscope or ultrasound. To increase accuracy in counting fetal heart tones when counting for several consecutive short periods of time, it is helpful to allow a 5-second break between periods of counting (e.g., count 5 seconds, take a 5-second break; count 5 seconds, take a 5-second break; etc.). The fetal heart tones are also counted between contractions in order to establish the baseline fetal heart rate. This baseline should be determined by listening between several consecutive contractions rather than listening just once.

Evaluation of the fetal heart by use of a fetoscope is limited when compared to electronic fetal monitoring, but it is more than adequate and safe, when properly used, for the fetus of an obstetrically and medically normal woman. In fact, it may be an even safer method than all others for the fetus of a normal woman since there are potential hazards involved with the most comprehensive method of fetal heart evaluation, which is internal fetal monitoring, and the long-term effects of ultrasound are not yet known.

Use of ultrasound methods (e.g., Doptone) is equivalent to use of a fetoscope. The main usefulness of ultrasound monitoring is in being able to detect the existence of fetal heart tones difficult or impossible to hear with a fetoscope and render them accessible to counting and evaluation.

EXTERNAL FETAL MONITOR. Use of the external fetal monitor has a number of drawbacks. The monitor, which has two straps encircling the woman and firmly affixed to her abdomen, is uncomfortable to the patient. It also has the effect of restricting her movement and changes of position; these activities may change the tension on the straps and dislodge the transducers, thus giving inaccurate data. The transducers and straps need frequent adjustments. In addition, maternal activity and any surface brushing of the transducers (e.g., manual adjustments or accidental touching of the transducers, sheets rubbing across the transducers) as well as internal noises of the mother (e.g., bowel sounds) create static noise, which interferes with obtaining a clear recording of either the fetal heart tones or uterine activity. Furthermore, the location of the straps and transducers combined with limited maternal activity inhibits the initiation of a number of support and comfort measures for the woman related to the abdomen and lower back (e.g., effleurage, position changes, back rubbing). The best recordings are obtained if the woman remains quietly on her back. This may adversely affect the fetus as well as the comfort of the mother. The supine position may interfere with placental blood flow due to supine hypotensive syndrome caused by the weight of the uterus and its contents on the maternal inferior vena cava. In effect, then, this method may create fetal distress which did not exist prior to this intervention and interference with normal processes. On the other hand, external fetal monitoring has the advantage of not requiring that the fetal membranes be ruptured in order to initiate this method of evaluation. Therefore, it is useful for short-term evaluation such as with contraction stress tests (CST) or to confirm or rule out suspicious findings detected by fetoscope if the membranes have not ruptured.

INTERNAL FETAL MONITOR. The internal fetal monitor provides the most reliable, comprehensive data of all the methods of fetal heart evaluation. Its other advantage is that once the fetal electrode is attached and the intrauterine catheter is in place, the woman is able to move about freely in bed without disruption of either, and her activity does not cause artifacts in the recording of the fetal heart and uterine activity patterns. It is not, however, without its disadvantages. Use of the internal fetal monitor requires ruptured membranes because the fetal electrode is attached directly to the fetus and the intrauterine catheter is placed within the uterine cavity. There must also be 1 to 2 centimeters of cervical dilatation and the presenting part of the fetus needs to be down to at least a −2 station.

Rupture of the fetal membranes carries with it its own potential hazards to the fetus because the amniotic fluid, when contained within the membranes, protects the fetal head and umbilical cord from undue and uneven pressure. Without this protection there is more extensive molding of the head, which may exhibit itself by periodic heart rate pattern changes identifiable as early deceleration resulting from head compression, as well as more extensive formation of caput succedaneum. Studies have shown that uneven head compression, which may occur without the protective membranes, causes abnormal changes in fetal electroencephalogram findings and may cause brain damage due to trauma. Without the protection of the fetal membranes containing the amniotic fluid, the umbilical cord may be compressed between the uterus and the fetus during contractions, particularly if the cord has looped itself around the fetal trunk or neck. Periodic heart rate pattern changes identifiable as variable deceleration result from cord compression. The earlier the rupture of the membranes, the greater the hazards. Spontaneous rupture of the membranes normally occurs at the end of the first stage of labor, thereby protecting the fetus from uneven and undue pressure during the process of dilatation.

Other complications that may arise from internal monitoring include uterine rupture or abruption of the placenta during the process of inserting the intrauterine catheter, scalp abscess resulting from infection at the point of attachment of the fetal scalp electrode, or, rarely, fetal death caused by puncture of the scalp of a fetus who has a bleeding disorder. The incidence of scalp abscess is reduced when attention is paid to sterile technique during the attachment process and during subsequent vaginal examinations.

The fetal monitors have the advantage of giving a visual correlation of the fetal heart rate pattern with the uterine contractions. This is important. One should not be fooled into thinking that periodic fetal heart rate changes can be accurately identified and documented with only the fetal heart rate pattern. If you pick up a possibly abnormal fetal heart rate change with a fetoscope and are confirming or ruling out this possibility with electronic fetal monitoring, or if electronic fetal monitoring is indicated from the beginning due to an obstetical or medical problem, then you must have both a fetal heart rate pattern and a contraction pattern. It is the correlation of these two patterns that enables you to accurately identify any abnormal periodic heart rate changes (e.g., late decelerations). This assessment *cannot* be done accurately with electronic monitoring of the fetal heart and a hand on the abdomen to detect contractions. Both the fetal heart *and* the contractions must be electronically monitored and visually recorded.

Use of the fetal monitors for women with medical or obstetrical complications that may compromise the baby is an invaluable aid in effecting a viable outcome for the fetus. Electronic fetal monitoring alone is insufficient when the fetal heart rate pattern indicates possible distress. The measurement of *fetal scalp pH* is an important adjunct to management and will decrease unnecessary cesarean birth based on electronic fetal monitoring alone. A fetal scalp pH of 7.20 to 7.25 is of serious concern, and the test should be repeated in half an hour. A second pH of 7.20 is considered the critical level for immediate cesarean section. The entire field of perinatology combined with the resources available in the labor intensive care unit and the neonatal intensive care unit has had a dramatic effect on salvaging babies who in earlier years probably would have died or been brain damaged.

The vast majority of births, however, are normal and uncomplicated. For them this advanced technology is neither required in order to effect the safe delivery of a healthy baby nor is it desirable. Use of the fetal monitors is intrusive both in its procedure and in its effect on an orientation of family-centered care, quiet work and joy, nonintrusive facilitation of natural processes within the realm of normal, and focus on the woman (as opposed to machines). Finally, the reliability of any information obtained by use of fetal monitors is subject to the state of maintenance and repair of the machines. It is wise not to forget the ever-available and valid use of the experienced clinician's own hands, ears, and judgment in evaluation.

Maternal Physiologic Changes

There are a number of normal maternal physiologic changes that take place during labor. It is important to know those which may be ascertained clinically in order to accurately interpret certain signs, symptoms, and physical and laboratory findings as normal or abnormal during the first stage of labor (Table 12-4). They may also be significant factors to consider in management of the care of the woman.

MANAGEMENT PLAN FOR THE NORMAL FIRST STAGE OF LABOR

Management of the first stage of labor includes the diagnosis of labor, management of false labor, management of early labor, and the initial evaluation of the mother and fetus as discussed in Chapters 10 and 11. Thereafter, nurse-midwifery management of care during the first stage of labor includes responsibility for the following, all of which may be going on simultaneously:

1. Continuing evaluation of maternal well-being.
2. Continuing evaluation of fetal well-being.
3. Continuing evaluation of the progress of labor.
4. Bodily care of the woman.
5. Supportive care of the woman and her significant other/family.
6. Continuing screening for maternal or fetal complications (this content may be found in Chapter 14).
7. The thirteen basic management decisions.

The thirteen basic management decisions

TABLE 12-4. Significance of Maternal Physiologic Changes Occurring during Labor

Physiologic Change	Significance
Blood pressure:	
Rises during contractions with the systolic rising an average of 15 (10−20) mm. Hg and the diastolic rising an average of 5−10 mm. Hg.	To ascertain the true blood pressure, be sure to check it well between contractions.
Between contractions the blood pressure returns to its prelabor levels.	
A shift of the woman from supine to lateral eliminates the change in blood pressure during a contraction.	
Pain, fear, and apprehension may further raise the blood pressure.	If a woman is extremely fearful or apprehensive, consider the possibility that an elevated blood pressure is being caused by this rather than by preeclampsia. Check other parameters to rule out preeclampsia. Give supportive care and medications which will relax the woman before making a final diagnosis if preeclampsia is not readily evident.
Metabolism:	
During labor both aerobic and anaerobic carbohydrate metabolism steadily rise. These increases are due largely to anxiety and to skeletal muscle activity.	
The increased metabolic activity is reflected by an increase in body temperature, pulse, respirations, cardiac output, and fluid loss.	The increase in body temperature, pulse, and respirations is discussed separately in the following paragraphs.
	The increase in cardiac output and fluid loss affects renal considerations and necessitates concern for and preventative action against the development of dehydration.
Temperature:	
Slightly elevated throughout labor; highest during and immediately after delivery.	A slightly elevated temperature may be normal. If the labor is prolonged, however, an elevated temperature may be indicative of dehydration and other parameters should be checked. Also, if the membranes ruptured prematurely an elevated temperature may be indicative of infection and cannot be considered normal in these circumstances.
To be considered normal, this elevation should not exceed 1 to 2°F (0.5 to 1°C). It reflects the increase in metabolism that occurs during labor.	
Pulse (cardiac rate):	
Marked change during contractions with an increase during the increment, a decrease during the acme to a rate lower than that between contractions, and	

TABLE 12-4. (Continued)

Physiologic Change	Significance
an increase during the decrement to the rate usual for the woman between contractions.	
The marked decrease during the acme of the uterine contraction does not occur if the woman is in a lateral rather than a supine position.	
The pulse rate between contractions is slightly higher than during the immediate prelabor period. This reflects the increase in metabolism that occurs during labor.	A slightly elevated pulse may be normal. Check other parameters to rule out an infectious process.
Respirations:	
A slight increase in respiratory rate is normal during labor and reflects the increase in metabolism that is occurring.	It is difficult to obtain accurate findings regarding respirations as they are affected in both rate and rhythm by excitement, pain, apprehension, and the utilization of breathing techniques.
Prolonged hyperventilation is abnormal and may result in alkalosis.	The woman should be observed for and be aided in control of her breathing to avoid prolonged hyperventilation, which is evidenced by her feeling tingling in her extremities and feeling dizzy.
Renal changes:	
Polyuria is frequent during labor. It may be the result of a further increased cardiac output during labor and probable increase in glomerular filtration rate and renal plasma flow. This is less pronounced in the supine position, which has the effect of decreasing urine flow during pregnancy.	The bladder must be frequently evaluated (every 2 hours) for distention and emptied to prevent (1) obstruction of labor by a full bladder that prevents descent of the presenting part and (2) trauma to the bladder from prolonged undue pressure, which will cause hypotonia of the bladder and urinary retention during the immediate postpartal period.
Slight proteinuria (trace, 1+) is common in a third to half of women in labor.	More frequent in women who are primiparas, or have anemia, or are in prolonged labor.
Proteinuria 2+ and above is definitely abnormal.	Indicative of preeclampsia.
Gastrointestinal changes:	
Gastric motility and absorption of solid food are severely reduced. This, combined with a further decrease in the secretion of gastric juice during labor, brings digestion to a virtual standstill and yields a significantly prolonged gastric emptying time. Liquids are not affected and leave the stomach in the usual amount of time. Food ingested during the immediate prelabor period or the prodromal or latent phase of labor will most likely remain in the stomach throughout labor.	If general anesthesia becomes necessary, when the woman last ate solid food is of concern because of the dangers of regurgitation and aspiration. It is also a matter of discomfort and general misery during transition. Women, therefore, are instructed not to eat a big meal when they think they are going into labor but rather to restrict themselves to liquids to which sugar (for energy) is added.
	Intake during labor should be limited to liquids.

Physiologic Change	Significance
Nausea and vomiting are not uncommon during the transition phase marking the end of the first stage of labor.	Oral medications are rendered ineffective during labor.
	Gastrointestinal changes are probably a response to one or a combination of the following factors: uterine contractions pain fear and apprehension medications complications
Hematologic changes:	
Hemoglobin increases an average of 1.2 gm/100 ml during labor, returning to prelabor levels the first postpartum day in the absence of abnormal blood loss.	Don't be falsely reassured that a woman is not anemic if the results are borderline and thus be lulled into not thinking of the increased risks of the anemic woman during the intrapartal period.
Blood coagulation time decreases while there is a further increase in plasma fibrinogen during labor.	These changes decrease the risk of postpartum hemorrhage in the normal woman.
The white blood cell count progressively increases throughout the first stage of labor by about 5000 to an average total WBC count of 15,000 at the time of complete dilatation. There is no further increase after this.	Increased white cell count is not necessarily indicative of an infectious process when at this level. If much above this level check other parameters for an infectious process.
Blood sugar decreases during labor, dropping markedly in prolonged and difficult labors, most likely as a result of the increase in activity of the uterine and skeletal muscles.	Use of laboratory tests to screen a woman for diabetes during the intrapartum period would yield most inaccurate and unreliable results.

are the decisions that are routinely made about each woman in labor and individualized for that woman. Some decisions are predetermined by virtue of the setting where labor and delivery are taking place. Other management decisions may need to be made depending on the woman, her condition, her situation, and the setting. However, the following thirteen decisions are the most common management decisions made in a hospital after the decision is made to admit the woman to the labor and delivery suite:

1. Whether or not to give the woman an enema
2. Whether or not the woman is to have a perineal shave and, if so, what variety of shave
3. Whether or not the woman is to have an IV
4. Whether or not there are any position or ambulation limitations and, if so, what these are
5. Whether or not the woman may have food or fluids by mouth and, if so, precisely what is allowed
6. Whether or not to give the woman medication and, if so, what, how much, and when
7. The frequency with which the woman's vital signs (blood pressure, pulse, and temperature) are to be checked

8. The frequency with which the fetal heart tones are to be checked and how this will be done
9. The frequency with which vaginal examinations are done
10. Identification of the woman's significant others and their roles
11. Whether to artificially rupture the membranes and, if so, when
12. Determination of when there is a need for physician consultation or collaboration
13. Whether to move the woman to the delivery room, and if so, when

Many of these decisions are made over again several times during the course of labor as the woman's condition changes and labor progresses. Each must be considered in relation to the individual woman at that time. However, in so doing there are specific factors to consider in making each decision. These management decisions are found scattered across the various categories of management responsibilities enumerated at the beginning of this section and will be discussed as they relate to these responsibilities and the woman's progress through the first stage of labor.

Admission

When the woman is admitted to the labor and delivery suite she undergoes an admission procedure. This procedure varies from hospital to hospital but generally includes the following:

1. Change from street clothing to a hospital gown
2. Tagging and marking of the woman's personal belongings
3. Identification band for the woman
4. Filling out of chart forms and signing of necessary permission forms
5. Carrying out the admission orders
6. Initial evaluation of the woman and fetus

in labor — history, physical and pelvic examinations, and laboratory tests (see Chapter 11)

The admission orders include not only the routine laboratory tests as listed in Chapter 11 but also your decisions regarding an enema, perineal shave, food and fluids by mouth, an IV, ambulation, medication, and electronic fetal monitoring.

Enema
The purpose of an enema is threefold: (1) to stimulate uterine contractions, (2) to assure a clean field without fecal material at the time of delivery, and (3) to eliminate a possible deterrent to accurate and comfortable examination. For years textbooks have said that an enema creates more room in the pelvis for the baby and prevents interference with fetal descent due to large amounts of fecal material. The fact is, however, that only a severe impaction might decrease pelvic roominess or have an effect on fetal descent. Otherwise the fecal material is simply squeezed out and is not a hindrance to the passage of the fetus through the pelvis.

Whether or not an enema can stimulate labor is a controversial issue. Personal clinical experience and observation of the results dictates each clinician's response to and use of enemas for stimulation of labor. Even those who don't have much faith in enemas will use them for stimulation of labor in hopes of their effectiveness if they are caught in a dilemma and don't want to intervene with more potent and potentially dangerous methods of stimulating labor.

The purposes of an enema must be weighed against the following factors in making a decision about an enema:

1. Discomfort to the woman.
2. The woman's agreement to the procedure and lack of strong negative reaction to it. If a woman has strong negative feelings about

getting an enema but is given it anyway, she may retain it. Retention of the enema defeats all the reasons for giving it, especially the one about having a clean delivery field since the enema will be expelled at the time of delivery.

3. Need for stimulation of uterine contractions, for example, because of a desultory latent phase or hypotonic uterine dysfunction.

4. Present labor status. If a woman is in the late first stage of labor or having rapidly progressive labor, especially a multipara, expulsion of an enema may be accompanied by expulsion of the baby.

5. Station — location of the presenting part. If the presenting part is unengaged or above the ischial spines, there is a risk of prolapse of the umbilical cord accompanying expulsion of the enema. The risk is less if the membranes are intact but it still is a risk.

6. Whether or not the membranes are ruptured. If the membranes are ruptured there is an increased risk of possible intrauterine infection. Extreme care should be taken in cleansing the perineal area following expulsion of the enema.

7. The presence of any complications that would contraindicate an enema, such as vaginal bleeding with suspected abruptio placentae or placenta previa (avoid bringing either of these conditions to a life-threatening crisis), premature labor (avoid stimulating labor), breech presentation (danger of a prolapsed cord), severe pre-eclampsia (need for the woman to be as quiet and undisturbed as possible).

It becomes evident that routine enemas for all women do not constitute good management since these factors would not be given consideration in such a situation. The ideal situation for ordering an enema is (1) when it is indicated, (2) when the woman has agreed to its necessity, (3) when the presenting part is an engaged fetal head, (4) when the membranes are intact, and (5) when there are no complications contraindicating the enema. This, however, is not always the situation. Most nurse-midwives feel that there must be a real indication for an enema — either an extremely full bowel or the need for stimulation of uterine contractions — to warrant the discomfort to the woman.

The nurse-midwife's rule of thumb is applicable in making a decision about an enema: "If I, as a nurse-midwife, cannot handle the possible results of this action, then I won't do it." Therefore, many nurse-midwives will not order or give an enema to a woman when the presenting fetal head is unengaged, especially if the membranes are ruptured, because of the danger of possible prolapse of the umbilical cord. However, there are times when the clinician is in a dilemma. A calculated risk may then be taken, that is, the risk is known and deliberately taken because without this action there may be an even greater problem — for example, a situation in which there is the need to stimulate the labor of a woman at term with several hours of premature rupture of membranes, a high presenting part, and no labor, who is contraindicated for pitocin induction or augmentation. The risks of the enema can be reduced by having her expel it in a bedpan while lying in bed and by giving her perineal cleansing care following expulsion. When a nurse-midwife takes a calculated risk she or he does so in consultation with both the woman and the physician.

If the decision is made to give an enema to a woman the next decision to make is what kind and how much of an enema. Soapsuds enemas, because they are irritating, are thought to be more effective for stimulating labor than just warm tap water. A small tapwater or Fleets enema will suffice if cleansing of the lower bowel is all that is wanted. The old "3H" enema (high, hot, and a hell of a lot) should be avoided. The water should be body temperature for comfort, the tube inserted the usual distance for giving an enema, and the fluid given gently and slowly with the tubing pinched off during any contractions. The amount can vary, with 500 to 1000 cc used for stimulating contractions, depending on the woman's toleration, and smaller amounts used for cleansing enemas. Someone should be with or near the woman while she is expelling the enema in case of strong expulsive contractions, rupture of membranes, prolapse of the umbilical cord, or birth of the baby during expulsion. Unless contraindicated it is easiest for the woman to expel the enema in a toilet. The fetal heart tones should be checked after the enema is expelled.

Perineal Shave

The primary purpose of a perineal shave has long been said to be the prevention of infection. Full preparation (prep) of the perineum, involving the shaving of the mons pubis, vulva, perineal body, and anal region is no longer considered necessary. Full preps were done in the thought that they not only prevented infection but also provided for cleanliness and easier viewing of the perineum. They were also an embarrassing, uncomfortable, and often insulting procedure and created a most irritating time during the period of hair regrowth.

To prevent infection, hair must be kept out of episiotomy wounds and perineal lacerations. Shaving the perineal body is thought by some clinicians to be generally all that is necessary for this purpose. Longer hairs from the vulval area which extend to the area of the perineal body can be clipped. Some clinicians, however, prefer that the vulva also be shaved to prevent wound contamination. The decision may be based on the individual woman's hair pattern. Shaving the vulva from the level of the clitoris down and also shaving the perineal body is called a poodle prep or partial prep. A mini prep usually involves shaving of the perineal body only. Whatever terminology is used, it should be clear within the setting exactly what is wanted.

So far as the other reasons for a full prep are concerned, cleanliness is a matter of washing and drying, and viewing the perineum is a matter of looking. In fact, there is very little pubic hair around the vaginal introitus and across the perineal body. Many clinicians believe in no prep at all, especially if delivery over an intact perineum is planned.

Foods and Fluids by Mouth

A woman in labor, even in early labor, should not eat solid food. If she does it will most likely remain in her stomach throughout labor or be vomited during transition. This is because of the severe decreases in secretion of gastric juice, gastric motility, and gastric absorption during labor. These decreases do not affect liquids, which leave the stomach in the usual amount of time. Liquids, therefore, may be ingested during labor.

Oral intake during labor, therefore, should be limited to fluids. The best liquids for women to have are clear liquids to which sugar (for energy) has been added, such as tea or coffee. If these are not available, hard candies provide flavor and energy, and water provides fluid. Excessive fluids are not desirable because they may produce nausea and discomfort. Large quantities of chilled, sweetened fruit juices are gas producing and possibly cause nausea and vomiting. Most women want only to moisten their dry mouths and parched throats and should be given the means for immediate and continuing relief.

Even fluids need to be restricted if general inhalation anesthesia is anticipated.

Intravenous Infusion

The purposes of an intravenous infusion are twofold: (1) as a lifeline for medications, fluid, or blood in the event of an obstetric disaster and (2) as a means of maintaining maternal hydration. An intravenous infusion is mandatory if one of the following conditions is present:

1. Gravida 5 or greater

2. An overdistended uterus for any reason, including:
   a. multiple gestation
   b. polyhydramnios
   c. an excessively large baby (estimated at 9 pounds or more)
3. A pitocin induction or augmentation
4. History or presence of any other condition that predisposes an immediate postpartal hemorrhage
5. Maternal dehydration or exhaustion
6. Any obstetric or medical condition which is life threatening, such as abruptio placentae, placenta previa, ruptured uterus, preeclampsia or eclampsia

The decision of whether or not to start an intravenous infusion on a woman other than one for whom it is mandatory becomes, in practice, largely a matter of what the individual clinician believes in and is comfortable with in consultation with the woman. Some clinicians believe "it is better to be safe than sorry" and want all of their clients to have an IV. Other clinicians believe it is unnecessary to subject all women to the pain, bother, and restrictions of an IV and want none of their clients to have an IV unless there is an indication for it. These clinicians, however, reserve the right to start an IV in the event the woman's condition changes so that either maternal hydration cannot be maintained with oral fluids (e.g., too much nausea and vomiting for desire and retention of oral fluids) or complications are now an anticipated possibility.

The usual intravenous solution for a woman in labor consists of 1000 cc D_5W or D_5RL given at 125 cc per hour. This may vary if the woman is mildly dehydrated, in which case approximately 300 cc may be run in and then the IV slowed to 125 cc per hour. IVs on women in labor should always be started with an intravenous intracatheter (see Chapter 36). An intravenous intracatheter is used because, as opposed to a butterfly needle or a straight needle, it permits the woman more free movement of her arm without trauma to the involved blood vessel and has the best chance of staying in the vein should she become physically active during labor.

Position and Ambulation
A woman in labor should assume a position that is comfortable for her, provided that there are no contraindications to it. Positions may include supine (with the head of the bed at any angle of inclination, or flat), lateral recumbent, knee-chest, all-fours, sitting, standing, walking, and squatting. The only contraindications relate to the status of the membranes in relation to fetal lie and size and to the need for specific positions.

If the membranes have ruptured and the fetal presenting part is a transverse lie, an ill-fitting breech presentation or a small fetus (less than 2000 grams), each of which poses a risk of a prolapsed cord, then the positions should be limited to those which will not increase the risk of prolapsed cord. These positions are the supine position with the head of the bed (including the pillows) elevated no higher than 20 to 30 degrees, the lateral recumbent position, and the knee-chest position.

The lateral recumbent position (Fig. 12-8) has several beneficial effects, which are as follows:

1. Better coordination and greater efficiency of uterine contractions because they are of stronger intensity and decreased frequency than when the woman is in a supine position.
2. Facilitation of kidney function (urine flow is decreased in the supine position).
3. Facilitation of fetal rotation in posterior positions.
4. Relief of uterine pressure on, and compression of, the major maternal blood vessels (the inferior vena cava and the aorta) which may result when the woman is supine.

These beneficial effects can be used to good advantage in the following situations and constitute the conditions in which the woman should assume the lateral recumbent position:

1. Maternal supine hypotensive syndrome
2. Fetal distress (to reduce uterine activity, relieve pressure on the umbilical cord, or eliminate hypoxia resulting from maternal supine hypotensive syndrome)
3. ROP or LOP fetal positions if long arc rotation is slow; if ROP the woman should be on her right side, if LOP the woman should be on her left side
4. Severe preeclampsia (for best urine flow)
5. Mild uterine hypertonicity or ineffectual uterine contractions

A woman in labor should be allowed to ambulate when and for as long as she desires, provided there are no contraindications. Walking in early labor may stimulate labor. Many women experience relief and cope with their labor better when they can walk. The woman's freedom to walk, sit in a chair, use the toilet, and so forth is certainly more conducive to a comfortable and progressive labor oriented to normal processes than is the sickness orientation of being confined to bed.

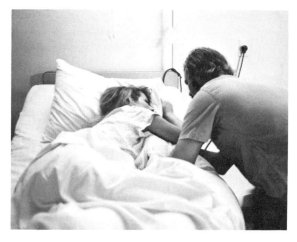

FIGURE 12-8. Father/husband supporting woman in active labor. The woman is in left lateral recumbent position.

There are, however, times when the woman should not be out of bed or ambulating. These are as follows:

1. When the membranes are ruptured and the fetus is either small (under 2000 grams) or in a footling or ill-fitting breech presentation or transverse lie. In such events there is a risk of cord prolapse which is increased if the woman is upright.
2. When the woman has been medicated with any drug which might make her lightheaded, dizzy, or unsteady on her feet.
3. During rapidly progressive labor, late first stage labor in multiparas, or second stage labor in primigravidas, unless this is a planned squatting or standing birth.
4. Any obstetric or medical complications requiring that the woman remain in bed, (e.g., abruptio placentae, placenta previa, severe preeclampsia).

Medication

Commonly Used Drugs and Practices. Medication during labor may have one or all of the following purposes: pain relief, decrease of anxiety and apprehension, sedation, and control of vomiting. Drugs commonly used during labor may fulfill one or more of these purposes. The drugs most commonly used by nurse-midwives and the purposes they serve are listed in Table 12-5. Drugs used less commonly during labor by nurse-midwives include alphaprodine (Nisentil, a narcotic analgesic), propiomazine hydrochloride (Largon, an ataractic), pentobarbital (Nembutal, a barbiturate sedative), and ethchlorvynol (Placidyl, a nonbarbiturate sedative).

The decisions to be made regarding medication during labor are:

1. Whether to give a medication
2. Which medication to give
3. Dosage of the medication to be given
4. Route to use in giving the medication, if there is a choice

5. When to give how much of what medication by what route

This final decision summarizes the other decisions and emphasizes the importance of the timing in giving the medication in relation to the status and progress of labor.

The nurse-midwife is not limited to a single dose of a single medication. She or he may mix drugs (adding them together), divide doses, and repeat doses, usually with a total maximum for each drug for labor as stated in the nurse-midwife's standing orders; these decisions can be made without consulting a physician. It should be remembered that the ataractics (tranquilizers) potentiate the action of the narcotic analgesics.

The most common practices of nurse-midwives in relation to the most commonly used drugs are summarized in Table 12-6. Nurse-midwives using Nisentil usually administer 30 milligrams subcutaneously during active labor or 10 to 15 milligrams intravenously postpartum, or both. Nisentil is more rapid acting and of shorter duration than Demerol.

Factors Affecting Medication Decisions. What the nurse-midwife decides to do regarding medications will be based on his or her consideration of the following factors.

WOMAN'S DESIRE FOR MEDICATION. Some women want as much medication as they can get. Usually such women do not understand why you can't give them enough to take the

TABLE 12-5. Medications Commonly Given during Labor

Trade name (generic name)	Classification	Pain relief	Decrease anxiety and apprehension	Sedation	Antiemetic
Demerol (meperidine)	Narcotic analgesic	X		X (mild)	
Phenergan (promethazine)	Ataractic		X	X (moderate)	X (moderate)
Vistaril (hydroxyzine)	Ataractic		X	X (moderate)	
Seconal (secobarbital)	Barbiturate sedative		X (mild)	X	X (mild)

TABLE 12-6. Common Practices in Medication Administration during labor

Trade name	Single dose and route	General timing
Demerol	50 mg. IM 12.5−25 mg. IV	Active labor Active labor
Phenergan	25−50 mg. IM or IV	Early or active labor, or both
Vistaril	50 mg. IM	Early or active labor, or both
Seconal	100 mg. p.o. 100 mg. IM	False labor Early labor

pain away, even after you explain several times. Generally such women are having a difficult time coping with their labor, are quite frightened, and have had little to no education or preparation regarding childbirth.

On the other hand are the women who have read extensively, attended preparation for childbirth classes, practiced breathing and muscle techniques for labor, and want to experience as much of the labor as they can without medication. Some of them are adamantly opposed to any medication.

Prepared childbirth means the woman's knowledgeable, active participation in the natural, normal processes of childbearing — it does *not* mean childbirth without medication. Natural childbirth devotees who have lost sight of the meaning of prepared childbirth and have distorted it into meaning childbirth without medication may suffer tremendous and damaging feelings of failure and guilt if they "succumb" to their own expressed need for medication during labor. Such women need help in revising their definitions and expectations of themselves and in acceptance of their own behavior. Medication that takes the edge off the pain but leaves the woman fully aware and still able to participate actively in her experience is not only well within the realm of success but also desirable for a woman who needs it, because it may be just what enables her to stay in control of herself and to continue coping with the demands of her condition and situation.

The art of medication during labor comprises achieving this balance of the woman's desire, need, and facilitation of her coping abilities within the parameters of safety. In order to do this you must know the woman's viewpoints and preferences regarding medication during labor. Ideally this has been discussed prior to labor as part of providing continuity of care; however, this is not always the situation. You must be careful not to assume or impose your own values and beliefs regarding medication. Ask the woman what she wants and then strive for the art within the limits of safety and her desire.

LABOR STATUS. The timing of when the medication is given is vitally important. The following principles should be observed:

1. The progress of labor is evaluated carefully and the giving of medication timed so it will *not* be at its peak action at the time the baby is born. Otherwise the baby might be sleepy and have some respiratory depression. This principle does not apply to very small doses of medication (e.g., 25 mg. of Demerol) as long as this dose is not the last of an accumulation of doses but is rather a single and only dose for the total of labor, as might occur if the woman arrives in the labor and delivery suite far advanced in labor.

2. A narcotic analgesic should not be given until the woman is in active labor. If given before the contractions are well established, as in the latent phase of labor, the drug will most likely render the contractions ineffectual by diminishing their frequency, duration, and intensity. In effect, while the woman is extremely comfortable, you have lengthened the total labor by several hours, for which she would probably not thank you if she knew. If the membranes are ruptured this could constitute a dangerous lengthening of labor. After the woman is in well-established active labor a narcotic analgesic will not affect the contraction pattern.

3. The ataractics do not affect uterine contractions and will not slow down or delay the progress of labor. In fact, because of their calming effect on the woman, progress of labor is often facilitated as the woman relaxes and begins to work with rather than against her labor.

4. The sedatives are for use:
   a. when the woman is in false labor.
   b. when the woman is in early labor and is exhausted and needs a rest.

c. as part of the treatment for hypertonic uterine dysfunction, to stop the present labor with its abnormal gradient contraction pattern.

FETAL SIZE. Because of developmental immaturity and a high risk of respiratory distress in a preterm (premature) or small-for-gestational-age fetus, all medications are withheld from the woman during labor in order not to depress the baby. Unlike full-term babies, small or premature babies cannot handle any amount of drugs crossing the placental barrier.

FETAL CONDITION. If there is any evidence of fetal distress, regardless of fetal age or size, all medications are withheld from the woman in order not to further stress the fetus who no longer is able to handle drugs crossing the placental barrier.

For any fetus at risk — such as those of diabetic mothers, severely preeclamptic mothers, or those who are postterm — judicious, very small dosages might be tried and the fetus carefully monitored for the drug's effect. Further medication is based on this trial and the status of the condition that is placing the fetus at risk. In such cases internal fetal monitors will probably be used, permitting comprehensive monitoring of the fetal response.

MATERNAL SIZE. The amount of medication is limited by the fact that the fetus cannot tolerate the levels it would take to totally alleviate the woman's pain. Thus, if the woman is large, additional medication cannot be given in accord with her increased body size. On the other hand, you still need to consider the body size of the small, petite woman in determining the amount of medication within the limits imposed by the fetus.

WOMAN'S RESPONSE TO SUPPORT IN LABOR. Support for women in labor is discussed in detail later in this chapter. It has been said that effective supportive care in labor is worth 100 to 200 milligrams of Demerol. If the woman is responding well there is a corresponding decrease in the amount of medication needed.

This is typical of women who have undergone preparation for childbearing. It can also be true for the unprepared patients, depending on a number of variables such as the patient's pain threshold, how early in labor you establish contact with her, how much educational and breathing preparation you can give her during early labor, the presence and help of her significant other, her previous experience and what she has heard from others regarding labor, and the situational circumstances determining the amount of continuing constant supportive care which can be given her. There are women and circumstances, however, in which the woman is unable to cooperate with and respond well to the support; these women will need more medication, within the limits of safety.

NEED FOR MEDICATION. The woman's need for medication encompasses and summarizes her desire or preference regarding medication, her labor status, and her response to support in labor. In addition to and underlying these factors is the amount of real pain she is feeling. This varies for each woman, depending on her pain threshold and on the amount of anxiety and tension she has and their effect on intensifying the amount of pain.

It is not uncommon to see women in early normal labor complaining of great pain as evidenced by thrashing about, doubling up, and much vocal expression. Yet you palpate only mild, brief contractions. A dramatic change in behavior can be wrought with attention geared to what the woman is feeling physically and experiencing psychologically in relation to this. Most likely she is frightened. Supportive care alone or in conjunction with a little ataractic often changes her into a smiling, coping woman rapidly progressing into active labor. She has no need for a narcotic analgesic at this time.

On the other hand, in medicating a woman, you should always be anticipating when she is really going to need it most — which is during transition — and plan accordingly. A woman's pain in labor, as she is experiencing it, should never be scoffed at regardless of your findings — she is feeling it and needs to have this respected. Again, the art of medicating involves a total plan of supportive care, including medication, over the totality of labor as designed for each woman within the limits of safety.

Continuing Evaluation of Maternal Well-being

Continuing evaluation of maternal well-being includes continuing evaluation of the following:

1. Vital signs:
   a. blood pressure
   b. temperature
   c. pulse
   d. respirations
2. Bladder distention
3. Urine:
   a. protein
   b. ketones
4. Hydration:
   a. fluids
   b. nausea/vomiting
5. General condition:
   a. fatigue and physical depletion
   b. behavior and response to labor
   c. pain and coping ability

An inherent part of this continuing evaluation is determination of when there is a need for physician consultation in the event your evaluation reveals deviation from normal.

Vital Signs
The parameters of normal and their significance for all the maternal vital signs were detailed earlier in this chapter regarding the data base for the first stage of labor (Table 12-4). All of the vital signs are checked every time the woman is seen for diagnosis of labor and again upon admission to the labor and delivery suite. Thereafter, the frequency of checking vital signs may vary with the hospital since each usually has a policy regarding this to

assure a minimum standard. Any greater or lesser frequency desired or indicated than that stated by policy requires a specific order. The following schedule for checking vital signs reflects generally accepted norms of frequency for a normal woman during the active phase of the first stage of labor:

1. Blood pressure — every hour
2. Temperature, pulse, and respirations:
   a. every 2 hours (or every 4 hours) when the temperature is normal and the membranes are intact
   b. every hour (or every 2 hours) after the membranes have ruptured

Bladder
The woman's bladder should be evaluated for distention at least every 2 hours during the active phase of the first stage of labor. The bladder needs this attention because it is a pelvic organ. With the descent of the fetal presenting part into the true pelvis, the bladder is compressed so that distention occurs with only approximately 100 cc of urine in the bladder. This distention is visible above the symphysis pubis. If the bladder is not carefully attended to and emptied, but instead allowed to become more and more distended, the following may result:

1. Obstructed labor — an over-distended bladder can impede the progress of labor by preventing fetal descent.
2. Difficulty in management of an immediate postpartal hemorrhage resulting from uterine atony — an overdistended bladder displaces the postpartal uterus, thereby inhibiting its ability to contract and effect uterine hemostasis.
3. Difficulty in management of shoulder dystocia — an overdistended bladder interferes with descent of the shoulders and decreases the amount of room in the true pelvis.
4. Discomfort to the woman — a distended bladder increases the discomfort or pain

in the lower abdomen that women frequently experience during labor.

5. Bladder hypotonicity, urine stasis, and infection during the postpartal period, resulting from trauma from pressure exerted on the distended bladder during labor.

Assessment of the bladder is done routinely every 2 hours to be sure distention does not go undetected. However, every time the woman's abdomen is bared for abdominal examination or taking of the fetal heart tones, the contour of her abdomen should be noted for bladder distention. A distended bladder appears as a bulge above the symphysis pubis and, in severe cases, may extend as high as the umbilicus. When the fetus is in a posterior position the contour of the woman's abdomen may look as though she has a full bladder; distention must then be ruled out.

In the event of bladder distention all measures must be taken to facilitate the woman's efforts to void. The best method is for her to walk to the toilet if there are no contraindications to her ambulating. If she is unable to be out of bed and if having her listen to the sound of running water, blowing on her thumb, dabbling her fingers in water, running warm water over her perineum, putting oil of peppermint in the bedpan, applying light suprapubic pressure, and having her practice perineal relaxation do not result in her voiding, then the nurse-midwife must decide for or against catheterization. This decision is based on weighing the risk of infection with catheterization against the risk of postpartal infection plus the other possible problems and sequelae if the woman is not catheterized. This latter risk is evaluated on the basis of the severity of the distention, her labor status, and her progress in labor.

Urine
When a woman does void during labor, the urine should be examined by dipstick for protein and ketones. This is subsequent to the initial specimen collected at the time of admission for routine microscopic examination.

The results of examination of the urine for protein should be evaluated in relation to the type of urine specimen it was and the contaminants it might have in it. This is important because the urine is being examined for protein as a routine screening for one of the signs of preeclampsia. If there is protein in the specimen it is vital to know whether or not this is proteinuria. If the specimen was a voided specimen and the woman has a copious amount of bloody show, the specimen will be contaminated with blood. The results are thereby rendered worthless because the positive protein results may be due to the contamination of blood protein. If, however, the specimen was obtained during catheterization the results may be considered valid. The results from carefully collected clean-catch specimens under favorable conditions (i.e., without contamination from vaginal discharges) may also be considered valid.

Examination of the urine for ketones is for the purpose of screening the patient for maternal exhaustion and distress inclusive of dehydration, electrolyte imbalance, and nutritional deficiency during labor. Since most of the other signs and symptoms of maternal exhaustion and distress are difficult to differentiate from normal physiologic changes and physical manifestations during labor, the presence or absence of ketonuria is essential for establishing a differential diagnosis and instituting corrective treatment. (See Chapter 14.) It is most important to use dipstick testing of the urine for ketones to evaluate the well-being of a laboring woman who does not have an intravenous infusion, in order to evaluate the adequacy of her oral intake of liquids for maintenance of hydration. Good oral fluid intake is not usually possible in prolonged labor or when there has been uterine inertia. Ketonuria would indicate the need for an IV.

Hydration
The maintenance of hydration throughout labor is essential for the well-being of the woman.

The time span of labor does not lend itself to evaluation of hydration on the basis of such things as skin turgor. On the other hand, signs of dehydration such as dry or cracked lips, a dry mouth, or a parched throat may not be due to dehydration at all in a woman in labor but may instead be due to the type of breathing she is doing with her contractions. Evaluation, thus, is based on the previously stated screening for ketonuria and on a knowledge of the woman's fluid intake (by whatever route) and loss. Concentration of the urine should also be noted.

Not only the woman's fluid intake (as discussed earlier in this chapter under "Admission") but also any loss of fluids affects the maintenance of hydration. Excessive nausea or vomiting in a woman without an IV will decrease her desire for or ability to cooperate with oral fluid intake. Excessive vomiting in a woman with an IV must be counterbalanced by an increase in her IV fluids. While a strict intake and output record need not be kept on a normal laboring patient, her labor record should reflect her fluid intake, urinary output, and the amount of any emesis.

General Condition
Evaluation of the well-being of the woman necessarily includes evaluation of several areas that interrelate and overlap: her state of fatigue and physical depletion, her behavior and responses to labor, and her perception of pain and ability to cope with labor.

Her state of fatigue and physical depletion is affected by her state of fatigue upon entering labor, maintenance of hydration during labor, length of labor, and her ability to cope with the demands placed upon her by her condition and situation. These may form a vicious cycle of interplay: a lack of ability to cope may increase fatigue and fatigue may decrease her ability to cope; or the longer the labor, the greater the fatigue, but fatigue may also cause labor to be longer. An occasional woman enters labor truly exhausted and dehydrated from days of the general miseries of the end of pregnancy or from false labor. She should be evaluated for a management plan of helping her rest during early labor with 100 milligrams of secobarbital (Seconal) intramuscularly while hydrating her with intravenous fluids.

A woman's behavior normally changes throughout labor as described earlier in this chapter. These changes can be used in evaluating her behavior and response to labor. Her behavior is also affected by her degree of self-confidence, her anxiety and fear, and the amount of pain she is experiencing. In another cycle of interplay, these in turn affect her coping ability, and her ability to cope affects her self-confidence, anxieties, and fears. Intervention during labor is most effective in women who have had preparation for childbearing during pregnancy. With or without this preparation, evaluation of behavior during labor will aid in determining a number of the support and comfort measures needed, including the need for medication.

Continuing Evaluation of Fetal Well-Being

Assessment of fetal well-being includes continuing evaluation of the following:

1. Normality of the fetal lie, presentation, attitude, position, and variety
2. Fetal adaptation to the pelvis
3. The fetal heart rate and pattern

Evaluation of the fetal lie, presentation, attitude, position, and variety is done first by abdominal palpation (see "Abdominal Palpation and Leopold's Maneuvers" in Chapter 41) and confirmed by vaginal examination as discussed in detail earlier in this chapter. The first part of this chapter also discusses the information needed to evaluate fetal adaptation to the pelvis: synclitism/asynclitism, molding of the fetal skull, the formation of caput succedaneum, and the parameters of normal for each.

THE NORMAL FIRST STAGE OF LABOR 257

All the information in these two categories of evaluating fetal well-being is obtained whenever the woman is evaluated for diagnosis of labor, upon admission to the labor and delivery suite, and any other time a vaginal examination is done during labor, whether for purposes of updating this information or to evaluate the progress of labor by cervical change and fetal descent.

One of the management decisions is the frequency with which the fetal heart tones are to be checked and how this will be done. The possibilities include intermittent auscultation of the fetal heart; intermittent external fetal monitor strips; continuous external fetal monitoring; and continuous internal fetal monitoring. This management decision should be based on indicated need. If the woman is healthy and has had an uncomplicated pregnancy, there is no need for electronic fetal monitoring. It should also be remembered that external electronic fetal monitoring uses ultrasound (see Chapter 7 for discussion of ultrasound).

The frequency of evaluation of the fetal heart rate and pattern using auscultation with a fetoscope or ultrasonic method (e.g., Doptone) is every 30 minutes during active labor. In addition, the fetal heart is checked at other times during the course of a normal labor, including the following:

1. When the membranes rupture
2. After expulsion of an enema
3. Whenever there is any sudden change in the contraction or labor pattern
4. After giving the woman medication and again at its peak action time
5. Whenever there is any indication that an obstetric or medical complication is developing

In order to establish what the baseline fetal heart rate is and whether this rate changes during or immediately following contractions when counting the fetal heart beats (i.e., without beat-to-beat electronic recording of them),

the following method should be used. Start listening midway between two contractions. Count the fetal heart beats for 5 seconds, break for 5 seconds, count again for 5 seconds, and continue this pattern of listening through the contraction to midway between it and the following contraction. Note the amount of irregularity as well as the rate. Palpate the contractions of the uterus while listening to the fetal heart in order to correlate any change in the fetal heart rate with when the change occurs in relation to the increment, acme, and decrement of the uterine contraction. This is done to determine if there are periodic fetal heart rate changes and if electronic fetal monitoring is indicated.

The parameters of normal for the baseline fetal heart rate, irregularity, and periodic fetal heart rate changes are discussed earlier in this chapter. See also "Location of Fetal Heart Tones" in Chapter 41 for locating the point of maximum intensity in accord with the position of the fetus and for the recording of findings.

In using a fetoscope it helps to be able to hear the fetal heart if you remember that the fetoscope is constructed to take advantage of bone conduction of sound. For this reason, keep your fingers off the piece extending from the listening bell pressed into the woman's abdomen and the metal band pressed against your forehead (stem). Fingers on this piece disrupt the conduction of sound. Most people automatically put their fingers on the stem in order to steady the fetoscope. The fetoscope can instead be steadied without interfering with the conduction of sound by simply pressing the piece that fits over the head against the top or the back of the head.

The proper amount of pressure with which to press the listening bell of the fetoscope into the woman's abdomen varies with each woman, depending on fetal position and maternal size. Generally speaking one should start in a location with light pressure and then press more firmly until the fetal heart tones are heard well. It is possible to press too lightly or too strongly and to obliterate the sound of the fetal heart tones either way. The pressing can be done, without placing your fingers on the stem, by simply pressing with your forehead against the stem.

Continuing Evaluation of The Progress of Labor

The following items of information are used in the continuing evaluation of the progress of labor:

1. Effacement
2. Dilatation
3. Station
4. Contraction pattern:
   a. frequency
   b. duration
   c. intensity
5. Maternal behavior changes
6. Signs and symptoms of transition and impending second stage
7. Position of low back pain
8. Position of location of maximum intensity of fetal heart tones

The first four of the above items are discussed in Chapter 10 and their parameters of normal for the phases of the first stage of labor are given earlier in this chapter. The first part of this chapter also discusses the last four of the items listed above for continuing evaluation of the progress of labor.

The findings obtained from examination and/or observation of these eight items are evaluated in relation to the following information which was obtained from the woman when initially evaluated for labor (see Chapter 10):

Age
Gravida and para
Time of onset of true labor
Length of previous labor
Number of years since last baby

Size of largest previous baby
EDD and present week of gestation

and in relation to the following information obtained in continuing evaluation of the fetus:

Estimated fetal weight
Presentation, position, and variety
Synclitism/asynclitism
Molding
Caput succedaneum

and in relation to the following information obtained in continuing evaluation of the woman:

Bladder status
General condition including her state of hydration, fatigue, and physical depletion

and, finally, in relation to whether or not the woman has had any medication, and if so, what, how much, by what route, and when.

Management Decisions

Management decisions relating to the continuing evaluation of progress in the first stage of labor include the following:

1. The frequency of vaginal examinations
2. Whether or not to artificially rupture the membranes
3. Management of an anterior cervical lip
4. Whether to move the woman to the delivery room and, if so, when
5. Whether there is need to consult with the physician

Frequency of Vaginal Examinations. The frequency with which vaginal examinations are done is dependent on the woman's condition and on the clinician's ability to use other parameters for evaluating progress in labor. It is not always necessary to do a vaginal examination in order to evaluate the progress of labor.

The practice of hourly vaginal examinations only subjects the woman to unnecessary discomfort, intrusion, and increased risk of infection. Astute observation of the woman (possible only if the observer stays in the room) — her behavior, contraction pattern, the signs and symptoms of transition, and changing location of back pain and fetal heart tones — suffice to give the nurse-midwife a good idea of whether or not the woman's labor is progressive. This does not negate performance of a vaginal examination if there is either a question of progress or if you are not sure of your observations and interpretation of them.

If the membranes have ruptured prematurely, vaginal examinations are restricted to none except by permission of the person responsible for the obstetric management of the woman. This restriction is imposed because of the increased risk of introducing contaminants and the development of intrauterine infection without the protective barrier of the membranes. (See Chapter 14.) For the normal intrapartal woman there are four times when a vaginal examination is indicated:

1. Upon admission, to establish an informational baseline
2. Before deciding upon the kind, amount, and route of medication to give when need for medication is determined
3. To verify complete dilatation in order to either encourage or discourage maternal pushing effort
4. After spontaneous rupture of the membranes if a prolapsed cord is suspected or is a possibility

Other than these four times, vaginal examinations serve no function in normally progressive labor other than to reassure the insecure clinician.

Artificial Rupture of the Membranes. Whether or not to artificially rupture the membranes

(perform an amniotomy) depends on the indications for amniotomy weighed against possible undesirable effects of doing so and potential hazards if conditions do not meet certain criteria. These three categories of decision making factors are as follows:

1. Indications for artificial rupture of the membranes include the following:
    a. to attach an internal fetal monitor electrode
    b. baby about to be born with the membranes intact at the time of delivery
    c. need to stimulate labor, for example, in hypotonic uterine dysfunction
    d. to facilitate fetal descent and reduce the possibility that the force of the pushing contractions will lead to sudden and vigorous rupture of the membranes that will cause the cord to prolapse
2. Possible undesirable effects of artificial rupture of the membranes:
    a. cord compression
    b. uneven head compression with more extensive molding and caput succedaneum possibly causing brain damage, especially if ruptured early in labor
3. Hazards and conditions:
    a. potential prolapse of the umbilical cord if ruptured with the fetal head unengaged, a compound presentation, an ill-fitting breech presentation, or a small baby (less than 2000 grams)
    b. potential intrauterine infection if the membranes are ruptured before labor is established and prolonged rupture of the membranes results

Because of the potential hazards, the standing orders and protocols of most nurse-midwives limit the nurse-midwife to artificial rupture of the membranes only if the following criteria are met:

1. Active labor — contraction pattern well

established and cervix dilated 4 to 5 centimeters

2. Cephalic vertex presentation with the head engaged

This also means that if the nurse-midwife decides that the membranes need to be needled to facilitate descent of a floating fetal head, she or he will need to consult and collaborate with a physician since the physician will need to perform this type of amniotomy.

In the past it was not uncommon to rupture the membranes at 4 to 5 centimeters "in order to speed up labor" in a normal labor for no reason other than to shorten the whole process for the mother and the attendants. Now that possible undesirable effects to the fetus have been identified with early rupture of the membranes, most nurse-midwives will not perform an amniotomy on a normal patient until late in labor, and then only if there is an indication, even if criteria are met much earlier in labor.

The technique of performing an amniotomy is based on the following principles:

1. Do the amniotomy between contractions so that:
   a. the force behind the rupture is reduced
   b. the membranes are not stretched tightly against the fetal head and you have a little room in which to safely grasp the membranes in order to tear them.
2. Use an instrument which will be effective quickly and easily, such as an Allis clamp or various hooks put out by companies for this purpose. An instrument that simply glides and slips along the membranes frustrates the clinician and prolongs the discomfort of a vaginal examination for the woman.
3. After rupturing the membranes, leave your fingers in the vagina through the next contraction in order to:
   a. evaluate the effect of the amniotomy on the cervix and on the fetus — dilatation, descent, and rotation

b. assure that there was no prolapse of the umbilical cord

4. Have the fetal heart tones evaluated during and after artificial rupture of the membranes to evaluate the immediate effect of the amniotomy on the well-being of the fetus.

Management of an Anterior Cervical Lip. Sometimes progress at the end of the first stage of labor is impeded by the development of an anterior lip of cervix. In other words, the cervix may be completely dilated with the exception of this anterior lip, which may be becoming increasingly edematous. Occasionally, an anterior lip of cervix starts developing earlier in the first stage of labor and may be felt when cervical dilatation is only 6 centimeters. If it becomes extremely edematous it is a matter of concern not only because of impeding the progress of labor but also because of an increasing potential for damage to the cervix as it is caught between the fetal head and the symphysis pubis. The extreme of this is separation of the anterior lip from the cervix if ignored.

Early development of an edematous anterior cervical lip is infrequent. Watchful waiting and noninterference are usually sufficient until dilatation reaches the point where the anterior lip is all that remains and it can be managed as described below. If the anterior cervical lip becomes so extremely edematous before the end of dilatation as to be of serious concern and further waiting is questionable practice, the edema can be reduced by positioning the woman on the delivery room table, doing a speculum examination, and puncturing the edematous lip of the cervix multiple times with a needle.

Management of an anterior lip when there is otherwise complete or nearly complete dilatation is as follows:

1. Doing a vaginal examination, place your fingers on the anterior lip at its junction with the fetal head.

2. During a contraction, run your fingers back and forth the distance of the junction of the anterior cervical lip with the fetal head and push it backwards until it slips over the fetal head and above the inferior border of the symphysis pubis.
3. Hold it there and maintain its position while waiting for the next contraction.
4. Continue to hold it in position while asking the woman to push down during the next contraction.
5. Allow your fingers, but not the cervix, to be pushed downwards and out as the fetal head fills the space and presses against the inferior border of the symphysis pubis.
6. Do not remove your fingers from the vagina until you are sure that the cervical lip will remain in its new position both during and between contractions.

The second stage of labor has now begun. You will need to examine the cervix for lacerations after delivery of the placenta.

Moving the woman to the delivery room. Bed deliveries for uncomplicated deliveries in the hospital are much more acceptable now than they were 10 years ago. Many hospitals have instituted birth rooms, in-hospital alternative birth centers, or combination labor and delivery rooms. One outcome of this development is that women do not have to move from bed to table at the critical moment of giving birth. Since there often is now an option, the management decision must be made as to whether to move the woman to the delivery room. This decision, however, may be predetermined by hospital policy which specifies criteria as to who can deliver in a birth room or a combination labor and delivery room and who must be delivered in the delivery room. These criteria are generally based on any developing complications or on procedures which need to be done (e.g., forceps delivery, epidural anesthesia).

Some hospitals, though, still require that the woman be moved to the delivery room for birth. Deciding exactly when is the best time to do so is a refined art.

The ideal timing is such that the woman is moved in an unrushed fashion; there is time for her to move from her bed to the delivery room table between contractions; preparations (getting legs into stirrups or being positioned for dorsal delivery, perineal cleansing, draping) are done at a steady, quiet, nonfrantic pace; there is time for procedures that have been selected as part of the management plan (e.g., pudendal block); and immediate delivery follows completion of all preparations, thereby keeping at a minimum the amount of time the woman's legs are in stirrups. All this is ideally accomplished without having to tell the woman to pant in order to prevent her from pushing and having the baby before all is ready.

Experience in refining observations and a sixth sense are required in order to achieve this ideal. However, there are a few cardinal generalities that are valid enough of the time to be useful:

1. Primigravidas are moved to the delivery room after complete dilatation, and, depending on the amount of descent, after some time of pushing or until the time-honored maxim of "fifty cents is the price of admission to the delivery room" is achieved. The fifty cents indicates the size of a half-dollar as the amount of fetal head visible at the vaginal introitus *between* contractions. If a pudendal block is planned, the patient should be moved when the fifty cents' worth of caput is visible *with* a contraction.
2. Multiparas are moved to the delivery room before complete dilatation, at approximately 8 centimeters during transition. If you wait longer you are inviting the baby's being born in uncontrolled fashion in bed en route to the delivery room.
3. Progress of labor must be taken into account in making this decision. A rapidly progressive labor or a more desultory type of

labor invalidates the above two statements, and the timing of moving the woman to the delivery room needs to be adjusted accordingly. The rapidity of second stage labor is affected by the degree of relaxation, stretch, and give in the vagina and perineum as well as by the parity.

Remember, it is far better to have a nice, calm, controlled delivery in bed — even an "unsterile" one — en route to the delivery room than to have a wild scene of madly rushing personnel dashing around while yelling at the woman not to push in order to pour some solution frantically over her perineum and don gloves so the delivery can be called sterile. Still better would be to have realized the mistiming and simply left the bed with the woman in it in her labor room and set up for a delivery there with solution and gloves if this is what is required in the setting.

Consultation with a Physician. The need for consultation with a physician is determined by the nurse-midwife as she or he evaluates the normality of the woman, fetus, and progress of labor; screens for medical and obstetrical abnormality; and anticipates possible potential problems. The parameters of normal were covered earlier in this chapter. Screening for and disposition of complications, including when to consult with the physician, are covered in Chapter 14.

Bodily and Supportive Care of the Woman

Purpose of Supportive Care

One of the hallmarks of a nurse-midwife is the constant care she or he gives the woman throughout labor. This does not mean remote control management of the woman but, rather, an active and participating presence in the room both to manage the care of the woman obstetrically and to provide or facilitate the provision of indicated supportive care. Women's horror stories of being left alone in fear and in pain without knowing what was going on, with only an hourly check of the blood pressure and fetal heart tone and a "mashing" of her abdomen for comfort and company, are anathema to the nurse-midwife. This sort of trauma experienced by a woman in labor may have a negative psychologic affect upon her for the rest of her life and upon her relationship with the child, whom she may see as the causative factor for her trauma.

In order to provide supportive care one must know how to do so. Otherwise the caretaker becomes frustrated in not knowing how to help the woman in labor and uncomfortable with the woman's suffering, with the end result that the caretaker removes herself or himself from the situation by leaving the room. From this scenario come the horror stories and the trauma experienced by women. Supportive care during labor miraculously changes this entire scenario. The dramatic effects relate not only to the woman's psyche but also to the physiologic effects on the fetus, who benefits from less medication and a naturally shorter labor. It has been said that effective supportive care is worth 100 to 200 milligrams of Demerol, 2 to 3 hours of labor, and uncountable psychologic benefits.

Lesser and Keane [3] identified five needs of a woman in labor as follows:

1. Bodily or physical care
2. Sustaining human presence
3. Relief from pain
4. Acceptance of attitudes and behavior
5. Information and reassurance of a safe outcome for herself and her baby

The following listing of support and comfort measures include specific actions for meeting these five needs. By implementing these you become at least one sustaining human presence for the woman. The basis for deciding which support and comfort measures to implement, and when and where, lies in your observations of the woman, the mutual accord between you and her as to what might be helpful, and where she states her discomfort or pain is. Inherent throughout is the acceptance of the woman's attitudes and behavior with the philosophic belief that whatever she is doing is the best she is capable of at that moment. Supportive care requires patience and understanding on your part and perseverance in your efforts to help her. She so desperately needs positive input — not negative reactions — in order to continue coping with her condition and situation and to have a sense of satisfaction afterwards.

The support and comfort measures that emphasize explanations and teaching — meeting the woman's need for information — are means of breaking the fear-tension-pain syndrome described by Dick-Read [4]. This vicious cycle occurs when fear causes both mental and muscular tension, which in turn causes pain, which in turn increases fear, and so forth. Dick-Read advocated breaking this cycle with education to reduce fear, combined with exercises geared towards further facilitating muscular relaxation. Subsequent natural psychoprophylactic methods of childbearing vary in the emphasis of their preparatory muscular and breathing exercises but all educate the woman as to the processes occurring within her body and the means to facilitate her coping with them, thereby reducing fear.

The following listing of support and comfort measures describes in some detail the "what-to-dos." Of equal importance is determining *how* to do the what-to-dos in terms of purpose, approach, implementation, and expectations of results. Five of these considerations are:

1. The support and comfort measures that are listed constitute an armamentarium from which to choose. Not all women need all of these measures. Some women will respond to none of them. Some women will find some measures helpful and others irritating. Which are considered helpful and which are considered irritating will vary from woman to woman. You can but try each that may be indicated and seek validation from the woman as to its helpfulness. Ask. Do not go strictly on the woman's behavior, especially if nonresponsive, as you can misinterpret her behavior. Ask if a certain measure is helping or not and if she wants you to continue it. Use your knowledge of labor processes, combine this with the woman's need-for-help, learn from each experience with a laboring woman, and think up support and comfort measures other than those listed here. Do not be limited by books and articles; use your intelligence, ingenuity, and compassion.

2. Define your purpose, that is, what you are trying to accomplish with your support and comfort measures and care of a woman. One such statement of purpose would be to facilitate the efforts of the woman to cope effectively with, and function capably in response to, the demands being placed upon her by her condition and situation.

3. How you talk with a woman in labor may determine your effectiveness with her. It does no good to give her instructions or coach her with her breathing if she can't hear you. The advent of a contraction is also the advent of her directing her total mental concentration toward her response to that contraction. For the unprepared woman in particular this concentration and response may be one of fear and bodily tension and pain. You will need to "break through" or "break into" this mind set. To do so requires your speaking with a degree of authority and firmness with enough vocal timbre and projection to be heard. Whispering, unless directly into her ear (which most women find irritating), is useless. Soft-spoken instructions from a distance (i.e., across the room, from the foot of the bed) are also a waste of breath. This does not mean, however, that you should shout or yell at the woman. This is equally useless, only heightening the

woman's sense of aloneness and pain, and is nonhelpful and intolerable behavior towards a woman in labor.

4. The key to success in supportive care is your own involvement (Fig. 12-9). Involvement means facilitating others in their support as well as doing things yourself. There will be times when you are as exhausted, or more so, than the woman after the delivery because you will have breathed, rubbed, and pushed with her throughout her labor in addition to all your other responsibilities. Supportive care demands your presence if you are the one giving it. You cannot simply make an hourly visit and then conduct supportive care from afar with a string of orders. This does not mean, however, that you are the only one capable of giving supportive care. Far from it. Use others — nursing staff and significant others. Involve them so that each feels the importance of his or her contribution in the totality of the management of the care of the woman through childbirth.

5. Be realistic in your expectations of what you can accomplish with your support and comfort measures. It is unrealistic to think you can take away all the woman's discomfort and pain and make her a fully capable, blissfully happy mother-to-be throughout her labor. While it is true that some women, especially prepared women, do well in coping effectively with their labor, are well in control of themselves and measures that relieve their discomfort, and respond with relief and gratitude to everything you do, there are other women, usually unprepared, who will scream, thrash, and writhe their way painfully and miserably through labor and seemingly get no relief from anything you do, no matter what you do. Don't feel you have failed. If you talk with such a woman about her experience the next day she probably will tell you that your perseverance, which gave her a sustaining human presence, meant everything to her.

Allow for individual attitudes and behavior. In some cultures women are supposed to scream during labor in order to atone for their sins. The more and louder and longer the screaming, the more sins are atoned for. Other women try to be stoics when what they really need is to be encouraged to yell at the peak of hard contractions. Each woman comes into labor with her own set of expectations, fears, preparation, pain threshold, personality and behavioral makeup, and way of experiencing what is happening to her. You must adapt to her, not her to you, and quickly learn her individuality in order to facilitate her coping efforts as you manage her care for an optimally safe outcome for herself and her baby.

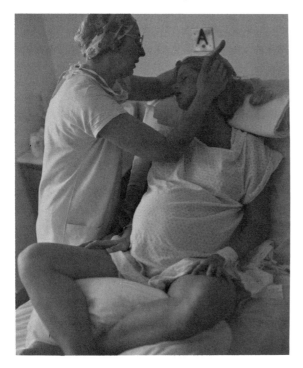

FIGURE 12-9.   Nurse-midwife supporting woman in labor.

Support and Comfort Measures
Positioning.   Positioning   involves   placing

pillows, rolled blankets or towels, or a combination of these in strategic spots to promote relaxation, reduce muscle tension, and eliminate pressure points. This can be done in any position the woman assumes.

A pillow under her head should always be the bare minimum provided a laboring woman. If there are no pillows, make one. This is done simply and quickly by taking two full sheets or two blankets, letting them "fall out" and stuffing them into a pillow case. This pillow is more comfortable if the sheets or blankets are shaken out first rather than placed in their folded state inside the pillow case. It takes only a few more seconds to do and the results are worth it.

For the explicit purpose of promoting generalized relaxation, the woman is encouraged to assume a side or elevated supine position if in bed. Figures 7-3 and 12-10 demonstrate the position of the pillows and rolled blankets and towels for those two positions.

Relaxation exercises. There are three relaxation exercises:

1. *Progressive relaxation.* This type of relaxation needs to be practiced during the antepartal period so that a woman can quickly will herself to muscular relaxation and, if needed, the catching of catnaps between contractions. It is an exercise in which the woman concentrates on deliberately tightening a single muscle group (e.g., hand, arm, leg, face) as tight as possible and then letting it go as limp as possible. This is done sequentially and progressively from one end of the body to the other, ending in total body relaxation and rest or sleep.

2. *Controlled relaxation.* This type of relaxation also needs to be practiced during the antepartal period in order to make effective use of it during labor (Fig. 7-6). The idea behind it is having one muscle group contracted while keeping other muscle groups relaxed. This is akin to labor, in which the uterus is tightly contracted, and the desire is *not* to tense the remainder of the muscle groups in response. It is practiced by tightening one muscle group while relaxing its counterpart. For example, in order of increasing difficulty:

   Right arm tightened, left arm relaxed (and vice versa)

   Left leg tightened, right leg relaxed (and vice versa)

   Right arm and right leg tightened, left arm and left leg relaxed (and vice versa)

   Left arm and right leg tightened, right arm and left leg relaxed (and vice versa)

3. *Deep breath and sigh after each contraction.* This relaxation can be taught in the immediate active labor situation if it is not already known. It consists simply of the woman's taking a deep breath and letting it all out in "a big heavy sigh" after the contraction is over. This serves a double function. It not only promotes relaxation but also acts as a cleansing breath to counteract any possible hyperventilation from more rapid breathing during the contraction or to break a pattern of rapid breathing

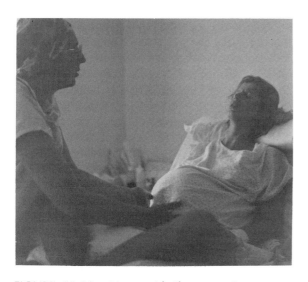

FIGURE 12-10. Nurse-midwife supporting woman in labor in elevated supine position.

at this time. Relaxation is further promoted if you give the woman a mental image of how you want her to look and feel after her sigh. For example: "Let yourself sink into the bed and go loose like a rag doll" (or a wet dishrag or a limp noodle).

Breathing Exercises.   If you have not taught the woman you are working with during labor, you must be knowledgeable about and able to adapt and facilitate her efforts in whatever breathing methodology she has learned and practiced and believes in. During labor is no time to teach her your way of doing it nor to even hint that her way is anything but the best. For her, her way *is* the best. If you are unfamiliar with her way, ask her to teach you how you can best help her.

If a woman enters active labor with no preparation in childbearing and no practice in breathing exercises, you are limited in what you will be able to teach her. If she is in active labor already you probably will not be able to teach her the breathing of Lamaze preparation and the Lamaze philosophy of active "working with" participation and concentration; this method requires training and practice. You might be able to teach her a basic pant-pant-blow rhythm to be sped up or down with your guidance for the purpose of distraction. This gives her something to concentrate on other than the contraction and its pain.

You might be able to teach her abdominal breathing; the advantage to this is that the woman feels relief when she is doing it. Abdominal breathing is effective for two reasons: (1) half is psychologic because it provides distraction by giving her something else to concentrate on and (2) half is physiologic because it lifts the abdominal wall up off the contracting uterus, thereby reducing pressure and giving subsequent reduction of pain. However, during transition the woman is no longer able to do abdominal breathing, and pant-pant-blow breathing or a superficial chest breathing will need to be taught and used at that time.

Which of the above you teach may depend on what the individual woman responds to and is able to do. At times you may be happy just to get the woman to breathe. Some very frightened, unprepared women may simply hold their breath and not push throughout a contraction. This causes a certain degree of tissue hypoxia, which increases pain. Your instruction may be limited in such situations to nothing more than repeated authoritative urgings: "Breathe!"

Regardless of method, one essential form of breathing is panting. If learned during the antepartal period a more controlled form of panting can be used. However, panting in the form of a rapid, shallow, throat breathing, illustrated by you and described as "panting like a dog" can be learned instantly while in labor. It is used whenever you want to prevent the woman from pushing. It does no good to tell a woman "Don't push," no matter how loudly and forcibly said, without showing her how not to push. It is impossible for anyone to pant and push at the same time. Panting is, however, a very exhausting type of breathing. Therefore, it should be used only when indicated, as in the following situations:

1. If the woman is pushing prior to complete dilatation of the cervix. Constant pushing of the presenting part against an undilated cervix serves only to make the cervix edematous which, if severe enough, may impede labor or, at the very least, increases the chance of cervical laceration and hemorrhage as the congested cervix becomes friable.

2. In order to deliver the head of the baby between contractions. You may instruct a woman to pant through her contraction and then push without a contraction so the head will ease out without the combined force behind it of both the contraction and the push.

3. If you discover a cord tightly around the baby's neck after the head is born and you decide to clamp and cut the cord immedi-

ately. You don't want the mother to push until you have completed this action.

The other essential form of breathing, that used for the maternal pushing effort, is described in Chapter 49.

In all teaching of breathing, you will get the idea across to the woman most quickly and effectively if you demonstrate it to her and then do it with her. If the woman is not learning a breathing exercise until in active labor and so has not previously practiced it, it may be necessary for you to breathe with her during every contraction. Prepared or unprepared, a woman needs reminding, encouragement, and positive reinforcement with *each* contraction. She will not remember what you say from contraction to contraction and will quickly exhaust herself if she has to rely upon herself for coaching. You may sound like a broken record to yourself but for her each contraction is a new experience to be coped with and gotten through.

Prevention of Exhaustion and Provision for Rest. Prevention of exhaustion and provision for rest between contractions is another support and comfort measure. Prevention of useless exhaustion is done in four ways, the latter three also providing for rest between contractions:

1. Utilization of the proper breathing at the proper time is basic to preventing useless exhaustion. As stated previously, panting is an exhausting type of breathing to be used only when it is mandatory that the woman not push. Controlled types of breathing, whether Lamaze or abdominal, are also tiring if used in early, latent-phase labor before they are really needed. Natural, normal breathing should be encouraged during this time.

2. Organization of necessary procedures to be done. Plan procedures so that as many as possible are done sequentially in the shortest possible time span (or number of intervals between contractions). It is exhausting to the woman when there is always something to be done after every contraction.

3. Control of the environment is done in accord with what is most restful to the individual woman (which may vary from your idea of what is restful). This includes control of lighting, air, external noises, room arrangement, and so forth as well as who is in the room doing and saying what.

4. Control of who is in the room doing and saying what affects exhaustion and provision for rest. (The woman's significant others and their involvement are discussed later in this chapter. The present discussion relates to personnel, both professional and nonprofessional.) All too frequently there is talking among the people in the room (often over and across the woman in her bed) on subjects totally unrelated to her labor and not involving her. There may be such involvement in the conversation that the woman's entry into her next contraction goes unnoticed and her needs-for-help ignored. This not only constitutes extreme rudeness and reflects a lack of respect but also illustrates a total misplacing of focus, which should be on the woman. The room of a woman in active labor is no place for constant chatter either among personnel or of a social nature with the woman or her significant others. The old maxim "Silence is golden" is most apropos between contractions unless the woman evinces need for a social exchange (extremely unlikely during active labor) or there is need to communicate instructions or explanations. During a contraction a quiet, firm voice of encouragement gives instruction and praise. Afterwards, silence. This makes the room quiet, devoid of distractions, and conducive to rest. The focus should be upon the woman and all aspects that will facilitate her efforts to cope and work with her labor.

Assurance of Privacy and Prevention of Exposure. Assurance of privacy and prevention of exposure are of particular importance in a teaching hospital. Professional faculty and staff in a teaching hospital often think that because a patient is in their hospital they can assume the patient's willing submission to the learning needs of a large variety of professional students. Often this is not the case. Most patients are in teaching hospitals (generally university medical centers) either because of their medical condition or because of their finances and with no comprehension of the bewildering array of students seemingly affronting pieces of their mind and body.

Privacy refers not only to maintaining the integration of their wholeness as a human being but also to respect for the patients themselves and their bodies, which is their right as individuals. Imagine the shock to a woman in the delivery room lifting up to push, only to confront five to fifteen pairs of eyes all zeroed in on her perineum without her prior knowledge or informed permission. What a difference it would have made to have discussed this with her beforehand and to have requested her permission for an extraordinary number of observers. Furthermore, a smaller number of observers should be introduced personally so that first contact is person-to-person rather than eyes-to-body. Discretion should always be exercised. If the patient is assured by your actions that there will be no surprises, relaxation is promoted.

Privacy and prevention of exposure also pertain to respect for the woman's sense of modesty. The extent of what has traditionally been considered modesty varies widely today. Women who are knowledgeable about and feel good about their bodies generally do not feel the need to be carefully draped to prevent exposure of external genitals. To them this connotes a traditional attitude of shame regarding these areas — an attitude with which they completely disagree — and they are as apt to

be insulted if you drape them as the traditionally modest woman is apt to be acutely embarrassed if you don't drape her. It is best to ask the woman her preferences concerning draping.

Explanation of the Process and Progress of Labor. Women who have been prepared for childbearing are knowledgeable about the processes of labor and want and need to be kept informed as to precisely where they are in their progress through these processes. Women who have not been prepared for childbearing usually want to know what is going on inside their bodies. If you are with an unprepared woman during the latent phase of labor, you will have the time and the woman's undivided attention, if she is interested, to explain briefly the processes of labor and what she will be experiencing in relation to them (Fig. 12-11). The labor plates in the *Birth Atlas* [5] published by Maternity Center Association are the most useful teaching aid for this purpose. If the unprepared woman is already into active labor, then explanations are limited to the briefest of explanations about the essence of labor progress, such as cervical effacement and dilatation. A quick and graphic way of explaining cervical effacement and dilatation is to use your hands showing 0 percent, 50 percent, and 100 percent effacement; and 1 centimeter, 5 centimeters, and 10 centimeters dilatation and stating that it takes longer to get from 0 to 5 centimeters than it does to get from 5 to 10 centimeters dilatation. The explanation of effacement is most useful when differentiating between true and false labor and explaining why you want the woman to walk for a while. It is unessential to explain effacement to a woman in active labor. Explanation of dilatation is useful at both times.

Outside of the philosophic belief about the rights of individuals to know what is occurring with their bodies, explanations regarding the process and progress of labor are done in an effort to intervene in the aforementioned fear-

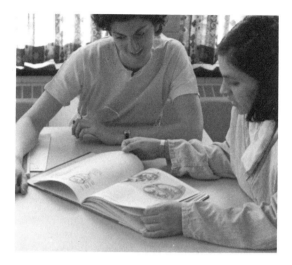

FIGURE 12-11. Nurse-midwife and woman in early labor reviewing the processes of labor. (Photograph by Patricia Urbanus, CNM).

tension-pain cycle. Explanation reduces fear of the unknown and alleviation of fear decreases the pain resulting from tension caused by fear.

Explanation of Procedures and Imposed Limitations. Each procedure should be explained and the patient's agreement obtained prior to doing the procedure. In order to cope effectively with it the woman needs to perceive the procedure as one that she needs and one that will be helpful to her. The woman also needs to understand the helpfulness or necessity of imposed limits (e.g., no food, no ambulation if the membranes are ruptured and the presenting part is breech or unengaged or ill-fitting), again, in order to cope effectively and to function capably within the situation.

Keeping Clean and Dry. Cleanliness and dryness promote comfort and relaxation and decrease the risk of infection. A possible combination of bloody show, perspiration, amniotic fluid, solutions for vaginal examination, and feces creates a feeling of messiness, discomfort, and general misery. A shower can change a

woman's entire outlook and feeling to one of well-being if there are no contraindications to ambulation and there are available facilities. If a shower is not possible,a sponge bath or a bed bath is also refreshing.

Subsequent attention to perineal care and keeping dry continues the feeling of well-being. This is maintained by changing the gown if the one she has on becomes damp with perspiration; changing sheets if they become wet from solutions, discharges, or perspiration; giving perineal care to remove any solutions or discharges, using careful front-to-back technique; and frequently changing the absorbent pad beneath her buttocks. Emphasis on cleanliness of the perineum and anything that comes close to the perineum, as well as scrupulous attention to handwashing by both the woman and all in contact with her, decreases the chance for intrauterine infection developing from contamination at the vaginal introitus.

Tub Bath. A tub bath can be the most relaxing and facilitative support and comfort measure to the woman. The tub needs to be deep enough for the water to cover her abdomen. This provides a form of hydrotherapy and bouyancy which is soothing and helps her cope with the contractions.

Mouth Care. A woman in labor will develop bad breath, a dry mouth, dry or cracked lips, a parched throat, and coated teeth, especially if in labor for a number of hours without oral fluids and without mouth care. If all these develop the woman is uncomfortable and it is unpleasant to those attending her. Some of this can be avoided if the woman is able to ingest liquids during her labor. Some of it develops by virtue of mouth breathing, slight dehydration, lack of moisture in the mouth, or passage of time without mouth care. Mouth care consists of the following:

1. Brushing teeth — women should be en-

couraged to bring their toothbrush and toothpaste with them to the hospital for use during labor.

2. Mouthwash — diluted or undiluted according to patient preference.
3. Glycerin swabs for the lips.
4. Vaseline for the lips.
5. Sips of water or clear liquids with sugar added for hydration and moistening of the mouth and throat.
6. Hard candies for moistening the mouth and throat — women should be encouraged to bring these with them to the hospital.
7. Moist washcloth — this is invaluable if the woman's oral fluid intake is restricted. Wet a washcloth with cold water and squeeze out the water just the right amount so that when the woman chews and sucks on it she will get enough moisture to moisten her mouth but not enough to swallow. As crude as this may sound, the vast majority of women in this situation find it one of the most helpful comfort measures.

Contrary to popular labor room practice, ice chips are *not* recommended because they have the opposite effect from that desired. Instead of providing moisture and relief, they actually have a drying effect. Use of ice chips simply increases the discomfort of a dry mouth and dry lips and causes an insatiable craving and need for more. Sips of water are far more satisfying and thirst quenching, and also contribute to hydration.

Usefulness of a Washcloth. If you were ever faced with the selection of one item to help you provide support and comfort to a woman in labor, a washcloth is the item to choose. A washcloth can be used in multitudinous ways. A few examples are:

1. To refresh by cleansing/washing.
2. To wipe away facial perspiration — wet the cloth with cold water; if there is no cold water, wet it and then cool it with air

breezes like those created when used as a fan. (See "Fanning" below.)

3. To serve as a moist warm or hot pack.
4. To serve as a cold compress.
5. To moisten dry lips and a dry mouth as described previously under "Mouth Care."
6. To use as a fan (there are more efficient and effective ways of fanning a patient — see "Fanning").
7. To use as a "security blanket" — some women clutch it in a manner akin to Linus and his blanket.

Fanning. Even in labor rooms with the best of temperature control, women generate a lot of heat with their energy output. They will perspire and complain at times of being warm. In labor rooms that are not air-conditioned in the summer the stickiness becomes miserable. If there are no fans you need to create means of fanning the patient. The following are three possibilities:

1. Use of a washcloth as a fan was mentioned previously. This is performed by holding the washcloth by two adjacent corners with your two hands and then flipping it around and around on itself, first going one way and then the other. It will flip more easily if it is damp. However, this requires a lot of your energy to create only a little amount of breeze in a very circumscribed area.
2. Better yet is the use of a glove package. This provides a fairly stiff expanse of paper which can be used as a fan with one hand. It has the advantage of mobility and can be directed at any part of the woman's body.
3. The best method for cooling the woman's upper body is to simply grasp the lower front hem of her gown, make sure it is loose from underneath the woman at the lower sides, and flap it. This creates a breeze over her entire body from the perineum up across her abdomen, breasts,

and head. Hospital gowns are ideal for this.

Back Rub.   Two types of back rubs are useful in providing support and comfort to a woman in labor. One is the usual generalized, overall back rub which is used to promote relaxation. The second is called the OB back rub. Both have the effect of expressing care for the woman and assuring a sustaining human presence for as long as the back rub is given. Lotion or powder should be used to reduce friction and prevent skin irritation.

The OB back rub consists of applying pressure to a specific spot on the woman's lower spine (Fig. 12-12). The woman can tell you precisely where this spot is because it is a localized pain caused by the pressure of the fetal head against her spine. This pain is exaggerated if the fetus is in an occipital posterior position, thereby often making low back pain the woman's primary complaint. You will need to recheck with the woman frequently about the proper location of the pressure you are applying as the pain will move downward as the mechanism of labor of descent of the fetal head occurs. The application of external pressure on the spine counteracts the internal pressure on the spine by the fetal head and thus reduces the pain.

The OB back rub is done by placing the palm of your hand against the spot identified by the woman and then applying pressure. You can massage the spot and adjacent area at the same time by circularly moving your palm on that spot without lifting your palm or moving it off of the identified spot. The woman can also guide you as to the proper amount of pressure. Too much pressure is painful; too little pressure is ineffective. Bracing the elbow of the arm of your pressure-applying hand against your body or against the bed will enable you to achieve greater pressure if needed. It also will enable you to continue the back rub over a longer period of time because your muscles do not tire as easily if your arm is

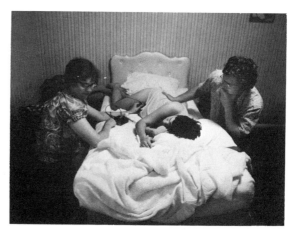

FIGURE 12-12.   Father/husband giving woman an OB back rub.

braced. The OB back rub generally is done just during contractions; this is usually when the woman experiences the greatest discomfort or pain in her lower back. Check with the woman before beginning an OB back rub. Some women don't have this pain, and your energy could be better spent where she is feeling a need for help.

It is difficult to do the OB back rub if the woman is in a supine position; it is hard for you to reach the right area and you have to lift up to apply pressure. At times some degree of relief can be obtained by folding a small towel and placing it at the specific spot so she lies on it. It will provide counterpressure.

Heat/Cold to the Lower Back.   Heat applied to the woman's lower back in the area where the fetal head presses against the spine will decrease the pain. The heat increases circulation to the area, thereby combatting tissue anoxia caused by the pressure. Care must be taken not to burn the woman not only by the temperature of the application but also by putting heat on an area to which creams or ointments have already been applied.

Some clinicians have found that the application of cold decreases the pain when heat does not. Supposedly the relief results from a numbing effect probably due to superficial vasoconstriction.

Abdominal Rub. The abdominal rub is a *light* rubbing (massage) of the entire abdomen usually done in a circular fashion and often concentrating twice as much rubbing in the lower abdominal area if the woman is feeling pain there. It differs from effleurage in its technique, in its rationale, and in who does it. It is done by an attendant (e.g., significant other, nurse, nurse-midwife) using one hand while the other hand is doing something else, such as feeling the contraction, doing the OB back rub, or holding the woman's hand.

The abdominal rub is particularly effective with women whose previous babies were born at home with a granny midwife in attendance. When such a woman is asked what the midwife did that helped her the invariable response is that the midwife rubbed her stomach. For you to do the same becomes very comforting and familiar in a strange environment, and it expresses caring to the woman. It also increases circulation to the area, thereby dilating blood vessels which have become constricted from contractions and caused tissue anoxia. The increased blood flow combats the tissue hypoxia and provides a physiological basis for a decrease in pain.

Effleurage. Effleurage is a technique used in the Lamaze and other psychoprophylactic methods of childbearing. By definition, effleurage means "feather touch," which describes the amount of pressure to be used in doing it. It is usually done by the laboring woman, using both hands and following a definite pattern over primarily her lower abdomen (symphysis pubis to just above her umbilicus) as illustrated in Figure 12-13. Using all her fingers on both hands, with the fingers loosely separated, the woman covers the entire lower abdominal area with the two circular patterns: up and outward from her umbilicus, down

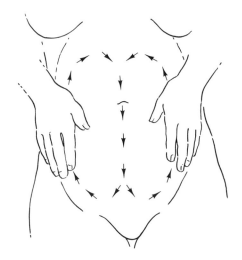

FIGURE 12-13.   Effleurage pattern.

and around, or in a reverse pattern. Its effectiveness is both psychologic and physiologic — psychologic in that it is one more thing to concentrate on, along with her breathing, other than discomfort, and physiologic in that the action also increases circulation to the area, combatting tissue hypoxia and thus decreasing pain.

Heat to the Lower Abdomen.   The application of heat to the woman's lower abdomen decreases pain by virtue of the resulting increased circulation that reduces tissue anoxia caused by contraction and tension. There is a problem with the application of heat to the lower abdomen. In order to get enough heat to be effective you need to use a hot pack of bath towels. When these are wet, even when wrung out, they are often too heavy for the woman to tolerate. They are, however, just the right relief measure for some women.

Empty Bladder.   This subject was discussed earlier in this chapter. In addition to the effect of a full bladder on the progress of labor and possible later effects on bladder hypotonicity, urine stasis, and bladder infection, there is the very real fact that a full bladder accentuates, and in part creates, a woman's lower abdominal pain. This pain can be greatly relieved if the woman's bladder is emptied.

Medication. Medication was discussed as one of the management decisions earlier in this chapter. It should be recognized that the judicious use of medication also constitutes a support and comfort measure.

Cold Compresses. Some clinicians have found that if all else seems ineffective cold compresses to the axilla and groin bring relief and calm some women.

Support during Vaginal Examinations. This subject is discussed in Chapter 44. You may not have time, or need, to go through all the components of support discussed there. At the very least, however, the following should be observed:

1. An empty bladder — desirable also for the other reasons discussed in this chapter
2. Explanation of why you are doing the examination
3. Positioning of the woman's arms beside her body
4. Help with relaxation breathing throughout the examination
5. Encouragement and aid in relaxation throughout the examination
6. Super-gentle verbal and physical approach
7. Warning and explanation if what you are about to do will hurt her
8. Information giving and explanation of findings

Alleviation of Leg Cramps. Leg cramps during labor usually are so acute they capture the woman's total attention and demand immediate relief. Cramps probably are caused by pressure of the presenting part on the nerves to the extremities as they cross through the obturator foramen in the pelvis.

The woman's legs must never be massaged because of the risk of unwittingly dislodging unknown thrombi developed during months of trouble with venous return and possible varicosities. Besides, there is a way of obtaining immediate relief for leg cramps without running this risk. That is to straighten the woman's leg and dorsiflex her foot. Alternating relaxation with dorsiflexion of her foot increases the rapidity of the effectiveness. The dorsiflexion should be forcibly exaggerated to effect relief.

Use of Physical Touch. This means the touching of the woman by you (e.g., on her leg, head, arm) for no other purpose than to touch her. Most people who touch mean to convey caring, comfort, and understanding in an effort to soothe, calm, dispel loneliness, and so forth. However, touching is effective only if you are comfortable in touching others *and* if the woman is comfortable with being touched. Don't force yourself to touch in the labor situation if it is uncomfortable for you. Your discomfort will be sensed by the woman and the action rendered ineffective. If you are "a toucher" then you must be acutely sensitive to the woman's response to your touch. If she withdraws or acts repelled, confirm her desire not to be touched and respect her wishes. Don't force touch upon her. Even women who do not like to be touched do find your hand better to grasp than the cold metal of siderails in a hospital labor room, so this must be checked out separately. Touching can be extremely effective when both the toucher and the touched are comfortable with it.

On the other hand, some women in labor are extreme touchers. Their use of touch is not the same as just described; it is more like a cry for help. Usually done by extremely frightened younger girls, this kind of contact includes throwing their arms around your neck and forcibly hanging on to you during a contraction. It is imperative that you do not reject the girl in this situation, even if you are a nontoucher. Hold her. Then, between contractions, ascertain the problems and location of pain and either find a significant other for her to hang on to or tell her you have to be free bodily to do other things to help her but that she can hang on to one of your hands.

Significant Others. This most important of all support and comfort measures was deliberately left for last because you need to know the other support and comfort measures in order to guide the significant others in providing them for the woman.

The first step is to identify the woman's significant other(s) whom she wants with her during the childbirth process — father of the baby, parent, grandparent, sibling, friend, children, other relative. In many hospital settings the woman has to identify one person who is so designated and accepted as the person who will be with her in the labor room, because many hospital labor rooms cannot philosophically or physically accommodate more than one significant other at a time. The second step is to determine whether the significant other chosen by the woman wishes to be with her during labor.

In a hospital setting the significant others may feel strange, frightened, intimidated, and insecure. They should be made to feel welcome and wanted in the labor room by the staff and viewed as important participants in the ongoing events. These persons should not be relegated to an outer corner of the room but should be given territorial space at the side of the woman. Unprepared significant others usually are glad to do anything you suggest and show them how to do. Prepared significant others have probably planned beforehand with the woman what they will do. Inquire about their plans so you will facilitate rather than frustrate them.

And what do the significant others do? They do anything within their capability that is agreeable to the woman, themselves, and you. The woman will respond to the prepared significant other with whom she has practiced and on whom she relies for coaching. Unprepared husbands, mothers, and grandmothers

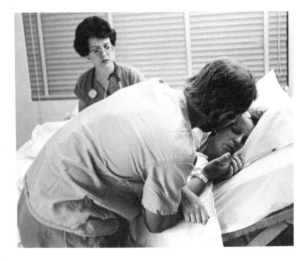

FIGURE 12-14.   Father/husband supporting woman with nurse-midwife facilitating efforts of both.

learn quickly and do well in coaching breathing. The significant other can be involved in such activities as the uses of a wet washcloth, hand holding, fanning, and abdominal rubbing. Men make the best back rubbers, especially for the OB back rub.

The fact that it is procedure time does not mean that the significant other has to leave the room. The decision about staying in the room and supporting the woman during a vaginal examination is up to the woman and the significant other. Husbands in particular frequently resent being sent out of the room at this time. On the other hand, some women or husbands prefer that he not be there. Determine the wishes of the woman and her significant other.

The most important thing in working with women and their significant others is to facilitate their relationship. Do not try to make yourself the most important person in the woman's eyes but rather foster the importance of the significant other (Fig. 12-14). You are a vital, but transient, person in the woman's life. The relationship between the woman and her significant other involves a continuing commitment in daily life.

REFERENCES

1. Pritchard, J. A., MacDonald, P. C., and Gant, N. F. *Williams Obstetrics, 17th.* Norwalk, Conn.: Appleton-Century-Crofts, 1985, pp. 295–303.
2. Friedman, E. A. *Labor: Clinical Evaluation and Management, 2nd.* New York: Meredith, 1978.
3. Lesser, M. S., and Keane, V. R. *Nurse-Patient Relationships in a Hospital Maternity Service.* St. Louis: Mosby, 1956.
4. Dick-Read, G. *Childbirth without Fear, 2nd.* New York: Harper & Row, 1959.
5. Dickinson, R. L., Belskie, A., and Hoffman, M. *Birth Atlas, 6th.* New York: Maternity Center Association, 1968.

Bibliography is at end of Chapter 13.

13

The Normal Second Stage of Labor

The second stage of labor begins with complete dilatation of the cervix and ends with the birth of the baby. It is known as the stage of expulsion.

DATA BASE OF THE SECOND STAGE OF LABOR

Components of the data base for determining the well-being of the mother and fetus during the second stage of labor are a continuation of the data base and its evaluation for the first stage of labor. These include:

1. Continuing evaluation of any significant findings from the history, physical and pelvic examinations, and laboratory work done upon admission to labor or developing during the first stage of labor. (See Chapter 11 and the first part of Chapter 12.)

2. Continuing evaluation of the progress of labor.
3. Continuing evaluation of the fetus.
4. Continuing evaluation of the woman.
5. Continuing screening for signs and symptoms of obstetrical complications and fetal distress. (This content may be found in Chapter 14.)

Again, the parameters of normal must be known in order to evaluate the specific pieces of information obtained for each component of the data base.

The Progress of Labor

Descent of the fetal presenting part, which began during the first stage of labor and reached its maximum speed toward the end of the first stage of labor, continues its rapid pace through the second stage of labor until reaching the perineal floor. The average maximum rate of descent is 1.6 centimeters per hour in nulliparas and 5.4 centimeters per hour in multiparas. Engagement should have occurred in nulliparas no later than during the active phase of the first stage of labor. Lack of engagement at the onset of the second stage of labor in multiparas is abnormal.

Contractions during the second stage are frequent, strong, and slightly longer — that is, approximately every 2 minutes, lasting 60 to 90 seconds — of strong intensity, and becoming expulsive in nature. After the painful contractions she experienced during transition the woman usually feels relief to be in second stage and able to push if she so desires. For most women, pushing gives utmost satisfaction inasmuch as it is a feeling of active involvement and accomplishment and their effort is rapidly bringing about the climax of their labor. A sense of anticipation again pervades this period. These women do not find the contractions very painful; instead they find the combination of the contraction and the work of pushing exhausting. On the other hand, some women feel acute pain with each push and fight the contractions and any effort to get them to push. Usually such a person is quite frightened; frequently her resistance diminishes as she is reassured and helped to push effectively and as some degree of natural anesthesia occurs because of the pressure of the baby's head against the pelvic musculature and other tissue.

As in the first stage of labor, the woman's behavior and physical manifestations can also reflect progress during the second stage. An irresistible desire to push usually signals the arrival of the second stage of labor. This is not always true, however, particularly if the fetal head has not descended well into the pelvis. In such instances the woman may not feel the urge to push because the reflex mechanism which will make her feel like pushing does not occur until the fetal head presses against the pelvic floor. For such a woman to feel like pushing after she has entered second stage

informs you that some degree of descent has taken place. Descent can also be detected by progressively lower location of the fetal heart tones and a progressively lower point of back pain. Confirmation, when necessary, is by vaginal examination.

On the other hand some women feel like pushing before second stage. This occurs when the fetal head is very low in the pelvis. The reflex mechanism is initiated too early and makes the woman feel in constant need of having a bowel movement. Consequently she frequently asks for a bedpan. This is a difficult situation for her because she must not push prior to complete dilatation of the cervix. Such action will cause edema and friability of the cervix and possible subsequent cervical lacerations, which, in turn, can be the cause of hemorrhage.

In the natural course of labor there is often a lull, or quiet period, between first and second stage. The hard contractions of transition are now past and the cervix is fully dilated. The woman's body seems to "take a breath" before starting expulsive efforts. The contractions space out and are not so intense. The woman rests and may even nap. This quiet period may last as long as an hour and is longer in primigravidas than in multigravidas. Gradually momentum builds as the fetal head descends through the pelvis; the contractions become more forceful and the woman begins to voluntarily bear down with expiratory, grunty, short pushes. The woman's grunts may be gutteral and her face contorted with effort (Fig. 13-1).

Rectal bulging, perineal bulging, and progressive visibility of the fetal head at the vaginal introitus are indicative of approaching delivery (see Fig. 13-2). Another almost infallible signal of imminent delivery is the patient's verbal expression, "My baby's coming!" In 99.99 percent of instances in which this occurs the baby is indeed coming, often in spite of a vaginal examination with findings to the contrary a few minutes earlier. The average length of the second stage, according to Friedman [1], is 1 hour for primigravidas and 15 minutes for multiparas. Generally, a second stage that lasts longer than 2 hours for a primigravida or 1 hour for a multipara is considered abnormal by those who agree with Friedman.

The Mechanisms of Labor

Engagement and descent are two of the mechanisms of labor. The mechanisms of labor are the positional movements that the fetus undergoes to accommodate itself to the maternal pelvis. This is necessary inasmuch as the larger diameters of the fetus must be in alignment with the larger diameters of the maternal pelvis in order for the full-term fetus to negotiate its way through the pelvis to be born.

Understanding of the mechanisms of labor involves a knowledge of the essential diameters of the fetal head. The diameters are as follows (see Fig. 13-3):

Biparietal (9.25 centimeters) — the distance between the two parietal eminences; the largest transverse diameter of the fetal head

Suboccipitobregmatic (9.5 centimeters) — the distance from the junction of the neck and the occiput to the bregma (anterior fontanel)

Suboccipitofrontal (10.5 centimeters) — the distance from the junction of the neck and the occiput to the brow

Occipitofrontal (11.5 centimeters) — the distance from the occiput to the bridge of the nose

Trachelobregmatic (9.5 centimeters) — the distance from the junction of the neck and lower jaw to the bregma

Occipitomental (13.5 centimeters) — the distance from the posterior fontanel to the mentum (chin); the largest diameter of the fetal head

In order to evaluate progress of the fetus through the pelvis, screen for developing complications, and manage the actual delivery appropriately, it is important to be well versed in

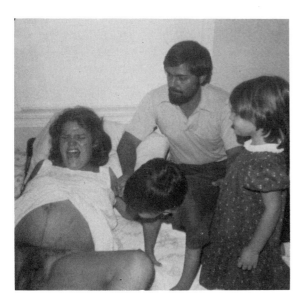

FIGURE 13-1. Children who have been prepared for the sounds and sights of labor and delivery are not disturbed by them and instead focus on being able to see more and more of the baby's head as it appears at the introitus.

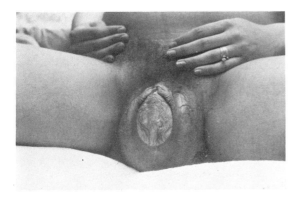

FIGURE 13-2. Perineal bulging. Note the relaxation and control of the woman.

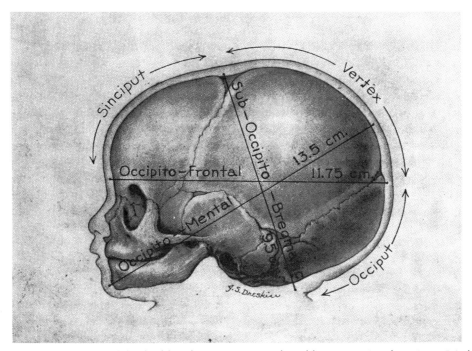

FIGURE 13-3. Diameters of the fetal head at term. (Reproduced by permission from J. A. Pritchard and P. C. MacDonald, *Williams Obstetrics, 15th.* New York: Appleton-Century-Crofts, 1976.)

the mechanisms of labor for each fetal presentation, position, and variety. The mechanisms of labor for all varieties of the cephalic vertex presentation are covered in this chapter. Mechanisms of labor for all other presentations are presented in sections pertaining to abnormalities or emergencies.

There are eight basic positional movements which take place when the fetus is in a cephalic vertex presentation. These are as follows:

Engagement
Descent throughout
Flexion
Internal rotation ____° to the _____ position
Birth of the head by _____
Restitution 45° to the _____ position
External rotation 45° to the _____ position
Birth of the shoulders and body by lateral
    flexion via the curve of Carus

Although the mechanisms of labor are listed separately, some overlap or occur simultaneously.

Engagement takes place when the biparietal diameter of the fetal head has passed through the pelvic inlet. See the first part of Chapter 12 for an explanation of the contribution of asynclitism to descent of the fetal head into the true pelvis.

Descent occurs throughout the mechanisms of labor and is therefore both requisite to and simultaneous with the other mechanisms. Descent is the result of a number of forces, including contractions (which straighten the fetal spine, bring the fundus into direct contact with the breech, and exert pressure of the fundus on the breech) and the maternal pushing effort with contraction of her abdominal muscles.

Flexion is essential to further descent. This mechanism substitutes the smaller suboccipitobregmatic diameter for the larger fetal head diameters that exist when it is either not completely flexed, or in a military attitude, or in some degree of extension. Flexion occurs when the fetal head meets resistance; this resistance increases with descent. It is first met from the cervix, then the sidewalls of the pelvis, and finally the pelvic floor. Some degree of flexion, therefore, may occur prior to engagement.

Internal rotation brings the anteroposterior diameter of the fetal head into alignment with the anteroposterior diameter of the maternal pelvis. This is most commonly accomplished by rotation of the occiput to the anterior portion of the maternal pelvis, beneath the symphysis pubis. If internal rotation has not occurred by the time the fetal head has reached the pelvic floor it takes place shortly thereafter. Internal rotation is essential for vaginal birth to occur except for abnormally small babies. To understand why, one need only look at the dimensions and planes of the pelvis. The inlet has a larger transverse diameter than anteroposterior diameter, while the midplane and outlet have larger anteroposterior diameters than transverse diameters. Internal rotation is effected by the V-shape of the pelvic floor musculature and the decreased dimensions of the pelvic cavity due to the ischial spines. The amount of internal rotation is determined by the distance the occiput has to travel from its original position upon entering the pelvis to the occiput anterior or occiput posterior position. The distance is described as the degrees in a circle, as indeed it is a portion of the arc of a circle which is being traversed (Fig. 13-4).

When the occiput rotates from an LOP, ROP, LOT, or ROT position the shoulders also rotate with the head until the LOA or ROA position has been reached. As the occiput rotates the final 45° into the occiput anterior position the shoulders do not continue their rotation with the head but, instead, enter the pelvic inlet in one of the oblique diameters (the left oblique diameter for an LOA and the right oblique diameter for an ROA). The entire mechanism,

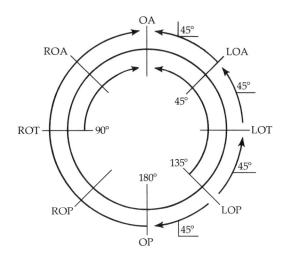

FIGURE 13-4. Degrees of internal rotation.

therefore, has the effect of twisting the neck 45°.

Birth of the head is by *extension* for occiput-anterior deliveries. This mechanism is different when the occiput rotates to an occiput-posterior position, as is explained later in this chapter. Extension must occur when the occiput is anterior because of the resistant force of the pelvic floor forming the curve of Carus, which directs the head upward to the vulval outlet. The suboccipital region, or nucha, impinges under the symphysis pubis and acts as a pivotal point. The fetal head is now positioned so that further pressure from the contracting uterus and maternal pushing serves to further extend the head as the vulvovaginal orifice opens (see Fig. 13-5). Thus the head is born by extension as the occiput, sagittal suture, anterior fontanel, brow, orbits, nose, mouth, and chin sequentially sweep over the perineum. The suboccipito-frontal diameter is thus the largest diameter to pass through the vulvovaginal orifice.

Restitution is the rotation of the head 45° either to the left or right, depending on the direction from which it rotated into the occiput anterior position. In effect, restitution untwists the neck and brings the head so it is again at a right angle with the shoulders. The sagittal

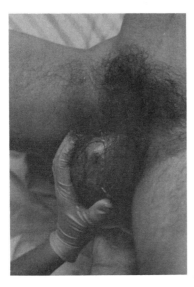

FIGURE 13-5. Perineal distention with head extension.

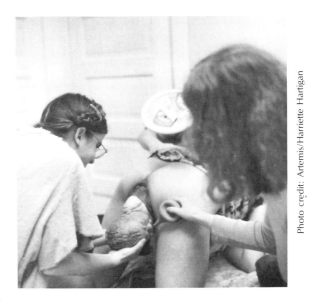

FIGURE 13-6. Birth of the posterior shoulder by lateral flexion. The woman is in the knee-chest position. Note the distended, intact perineum.

suture is now in one of the oblique diameters of the pelvis and the bisacromial diameter of the fetus is in the other oblique diameter of the pelvis.

External rotation occurs as the shoulders rotate 45°, bringing the bisacromial diameter into alignment with the anteroposterior diameter of the pelvic outlet. This causes the head to rotate externally another 45° into the LOT or ROT position, depending on the direction of restitution.

Birth of the shoulders and body is by lateral flexion via the curve of Carus. The anterior shoulder comes into view at the vulvovaginal orifice, where it impinges under the symphysis pubis, while the posterior shoulder distends the perineum and is born by lateral flexion (see Fig. 13-6). After the shoulders are delivered the remainder of the body follows the curve of Carus and is readily born.

The *curve of Carus* is the pelvic curve at its lower end as determined by pelvic structure. The products of conception must follow this curve for birth. The pelvic cavity actually resembles a curved cylinder so that the direction

of either the baby or the placenta coming through it is first downward from the axis of the inlet to just above the tip of the sacrum and then forward, upward, and outward to the vulvovaginal orifice.

Occiput Anterior

Variations of these positional movements are based on the position and variety and must be delineated for each. The mechanisms of labor for a fetus in the LOA, LOT, LOP, ROA, ROT, and ROP positions that deliver in an occiput anterior position are as follows (see Fig. 13-7):

1. Engagement takes place for LOT and ROT positions with the sagittal suture of the fetus in the transverse diameter of the pelvic inlet and the biparietal diameter of the fetus in the anteroposterior diameter of the pelvic inlet. For LOA, ROA, LOP, and ROP positions, engagement of the fetal head takes place with the sagittal suture in one of the oblique diameters of

Photo credit: Artemis/Harriette Hartigan

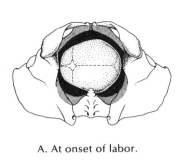

A. At onset of labor.

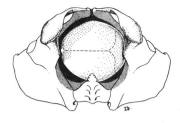

B. Descent and flexion.

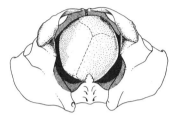

C. Internal rotation: LOT to LOA.

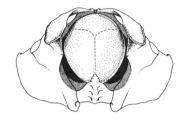

D. Internal rotation: LOA to OA.

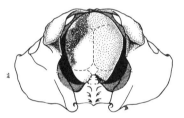

E. Extension beginning.

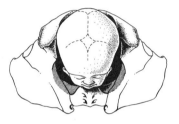

F. Extension complete.

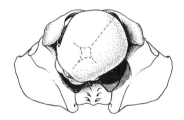

G. Restitution: OA to LOA.

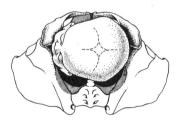

H. External rotation: LOA to LOT.

FIGURE 13-7.   LOT → OA mechanisms of labor. (Reproduced by permission from H. Oxorn and W. H. Foote. *Human Labor and Birth, 3rd.* New York: Appleton-Century-Crofts, 1976.)

the pelvis. This would be the right oblique diameter for LOA and ROP positions and the left oblique diameter for ROA and LOP positions. The biparietal diameter would thus be in the oblique diameter of the pelvis, opposite from the one the sagittal suture is in. The sagittal suture is used as the fetal landmark determining in which oblique diameter the fetal head is entering the pelvis.

2. Descent occurs throughout.
3. Flexion substitutes the suboccipitobregmatic diameter for the diameter which entered the pelvic inlet.
4. Internal rotation takes place
   45° (for LOA and ROA positions)
   90° (for LOT and ROT positions)
   135° (for LOP and ROP positions — long arc rotation)
   to an occiput-anterior position in the anteroposterior diameter of the mother's pelvis.
5. Birth of the head by extension.
6. Restitution 45° to the LOA or ROA position: L (left) for those which started the mechanisms of labor with the occiput in the left side of the pelvis and R (right) for those which started the mechanisms of labor with the occiput in the right side of the pelvis.
7. External rotation 45° to the LOT or ROT position: L (left) or R (right) determined by the direction of restitution. This brings the bisacromial diameter of the shoulders into the anteroposterior diameter of the maternal pelvis.
8. Birth of the shoulders and body by lateral flexion via the curve of Carus.

Persistent Posterior

Persistent posterior occurs when a right or left occiput posterior position undergoes internal rotation through a short arc of 45° to a direct occiput posterior position in the anteroposterior diameter of the maternal pelvis instead of a long arc rotation of 135° to a direct occiput anterior position as described earlier. Short arc rotation is much less common, occurring approximately 6 to 10 percent of the time and most frequently in conjunction with an anthropoid or android type of pelvis.

Persistent posterior is considered a variation of normal. Its effect on the length of labor is debatable and such that if there is an effect it is only slight and does not warrant delay in consulting with a physician in the event of prolongation beyond the parameters of normal during any phase or stage of labor.

Diagnosis of a posterior position is by abdominal examination and confirmed by vaginal examination. Observation of the contour of the abdomen may be the first clue of a posterior position. A depression the shape of a saucer is commonly seen at or just below the umbilicus. This depression is due to the fact that there is not a smooth anterior curve but rather a gap between the cephalic and podalic poles of the fetus, since the shoulder is posterior rather than anterior. If the head is not engaged there is a bulge between the symphysis pubis and the saucer-shaped depression. The total contour thus resembles a full bladder, which must be ruled out.

The mechanisms of labor for a fetus in the LOP or ROP positions that delivers in an occiput posterior position are the same as for those that rotate to an occiput anterior position except as noted and explained (see Fig. 13-8):

1. Engagement takes place in the right oblique diameter for the ROP position and in the left oblique diameter for the LOP position.
2. Descent occurs throughout.
3. Flexion.
4. Internal rotation takes place 45° to an occiput posterior position in the anteroposterior diameter of the mother's pelvis.
5. Birth of the head by the double mechanism of flexion and then extension. The sinciput impinges beneath the symphysis pubis and becomes the pivotal point for delivery of the head. The head stays in flexion as the occiput distends the perineum and is born to the nape of the neck. The remainder

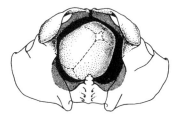

A. ROP: onset of labor.

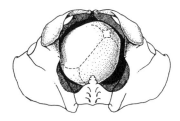

B. Descent and flexion.

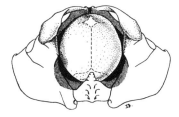

C. Internal rotation: ROP to OP.

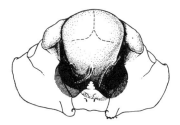

D. Birth by flexion.

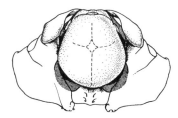

E. Head falls back in extension.

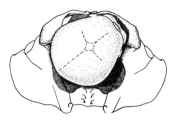

F. Restitution: OP to ROP.

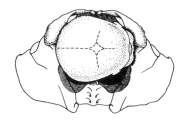

G. External rotation: ROP to ROT.

FIGURE 13-8. ROP → OP mechanisms of labor. (Reproduced by permission from H. Oxorn and W. H. Foote. *Human Labor and Birth, 3rd.* New York: Appleton-Century-Crofts, 1976.)

of the head is then born by extension starting with the anterior fontanel and ending with the chin as the head falls back towards the rectum with the face looking upward.

6. Restitution 45° to the LOP or ROP position depending on whether internal rotation was from the LOP or ROP position.

7. External rotation 45° to the LOT or ROT position.

8. Birth of the shoulders and body by lateral flexion via the curve of Carus.

Fetal Normality

Evaluation of the fetus during the second stage of labor includes evaluation of the amount of caput succedaneum and molding, as discussed previously for the first stage of labor; evaluation of the normalcy of progress being made in the mechanisms of labor; and continuing evaluation of the fetal heart tones, as discussed earlier for the first stage of labor.

Periodic fetal heart rate changes of the early deceleration type may occur as delivery nears (see Fig. 13-9). Early deceleration, caused by compression of the head, is a uniform-shaped pattern reflecting the uniform shape of the contraction. Head compression occurs at this time because of the pressure exerted on the fetal head by the pelvic floor and perineum during contractions and further exaggerated by the woman's pushing effort. Usually the fetal heart rate does not fall below 100 beats per minute during the deceleration period, and the baseline fetal heart rate is usually within normal range in an early deceleration pattern. There are no changes in the fetal acid-base balance with head compression. Early deceleration is not considered an indication of acute fetal distress but needs to be differentiated carefully from a late deceleration pattern; the latter is an ominous pattern which is due to uteroplacental insufficiency. A baseline bradycardia may occur when the fetal head descends rapidly into the pelvis and needs to be carefully evaluated (see Chapter 14).

Maternal Physiologic Changes

The normal maternal physiologic changes discussed in the data base for the first stage of labor (Table 12-4) continue through the second stage of labor. Any variations from what was said before are noted.

Blood Pressure.
Blood pressure may rise another 15 to 25 millimeters of mercury with contractions during the second stage. Maternal pushing effort also affects the blood pressure, causing variation from an increase to a decrease and ending at a level slightly above normal. It is important, therefore, to evaluate the blood pressure well between contractions. A slight rise in blood pressure levels at an average of 10 millimeters of mercury between contractions when a woman has been pushing is normal.

Metabolism.
The steady rise in metabolism continues through

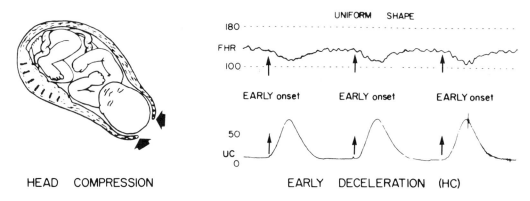

FIGURE 13-9. Early deceleration in fetal heart rate pattern. (Reproduced by permission from E. H. Hon. *An Introduction to Fetal Heart Rate Monitoring.* Los Angeles: University of Southern California, 1973.)

the second stage with the maternal pushing effort adding further skeletal muscle activity to contribute to this increase.

Pulse.
The pulse rate varies during each maternal pushing effort. Overall, it is elevated throughout the second stage with a definite tachycardia reaching a peak at the time of delivery.

Temperature.
The highest elevation of temperature is at the time of delivery and immediately thereafter. A normal increase is 1 to 2 degrees Fahrenheit (0.5 to 1 degree Celsius).

Respirations.
Respirations are the same as discussed for the first stage of labor.

Gastrointestinal Changes.
The severe reduction in gastric motility and absorption continues through the second stage. Usually the nausea and vomiting of transition subside during the second stage but they may persist for some women. Vomiting, when it occurs, is normally sporadic. Persistent, constant vomiting at any time during labor may be abnormal and indicative of obstetric complications such as uterine rupture or toxemia.

Renal Changes.
These changes are the same as discussed for the first stage of labor.

Hematologic Changes.
Hematologic changes are the same as discussed for the first stage of labor.

MANAGEMENT PLAN FOR THE SECOND STAGE OF LABOR

Management of the second stage of labor is a continuation of the responsibilities included in the management of the first stage of labor as follows:

1. Continuing evaluation of maternal well-being.
2. Continuing evaluation of fetal well-being.
3. Continuing evaluation of the progress of labor.
4. Bodily care of the woman.
5. Supportive care of the woman including her significant others and family.
6. Continuing screening for maternal and fetal complications. (This content may be found in Chapter 14.)

These additional responsibilities are included in the management of the second stage of labor:

7. Preparation for delivery.
8. Management of the delivery.
9. Management decisions for the second stage of labor.

Second stage management decisions include the following:

1. The frequency with which the woman's vital signs (blood pressure, pulse, and temperature) are to be checked.
2. The frequency with which the fetal heart tones are to be checked.
3. Whether or not to encourage the maternal pushing effort.
4. Location of the delivery.
5. Whether to move the woman to the delivery room, and if so, when.
6. Position of the woman for the delivery.
7. Whether or not to catheterize the woman immediately prior to delivery.
8. Whether or not to support the perineum, and if so, how.
9. Whether or not to cut an episiotomy.
10. If the decision is to cut an episiotomy, what type.
11. Type of analgesia/anesthesia.
12. Whether or not to deliver the baby's head with a contraction or between contractions.
13. Whether or not to use a Ritgen maneuver.

14. When to clamp and cut the umbilical cord.
15. Determination of when there is a need for physician consultation or collaboration.

The decisions may vary in accord with the woman, her desires, her condition, and her situation. Each decision is made in relation to the unique individuality and circumstances of the woman at that given moment. There are, however, specific factors to be considered in making each decision and these are presented in the discussion of each management decision. These decisions are scattered across the various categories of management responsibilities and are discussed as they relate to these responsibilities and the woman's progress through the second stage of labor.

Continuing Evaluation of Maternal Well-being

Continuing evaluation of maternal well-being during the second stage of labor includes the items used in first stage evaluation. The following list shows additional items specific to the second stage of labor marked with an asterisk.

1. Vital signs:
   a. blood pressure
   b. temperature
   c. pulse
   d. respirations
2. Bladder
3. Urine
   a. protein
   b. ketones
4. Hydration
   a. fluids
   b. nausea or vomiting
   *c. perspiration
5. General condition
   a. fatigue and physical depletion
   b. behavior and response to labor
   c. pain and coping ability
*6. maternal pushing effort

*7. need for analgesia or anesthesia
8. Perineal integrity

Vital Signs
The parameters of normal and their significance were given in the preceding chapter on the normal data base for the second stage of labor. The frequency with which vital signs are checked is increased during the second stage of labor. This frequency may vary somewhat from setting to setting or from clinician to clinician but the following schedule reflects generally accepted standards for a normal woman during the second stage of labor:

Blood pressure — every 15 minutes
Temperature, pulse, and respirations — every hour (whether or not the membranes have ruptured no longer affects this frequency)

It is important to remember in interpreting the blood pressure that the blood pressure *between* contractions, when it should be taken, is now normally increased by an average of 10 millimeters of mercury if the woman has been pushing.

Bladder
Management of the woman's bladder during the second stage of labor and the rationale for this management are the same as discussed for the first stage of labor.

In addition, a decision has to be made about catheterizing the woman immediately prior to delivery. The phrase "immediately prior to delivery" means as part of the sequence of events in preparing for the delivery, so this would be toward the end of the second stage of labor. If catheterization is to be done it is usually done after the woman is prepped (scrubbed) and draped and before any other procedure such as pudendal block or cutting of an episiotomy. This timing is chosen so that the catheter can be inserted before the fetal head gets any lower in the pelvis, since further descent makes the catheterization more difficult.

The following factors are considered in

making the decision whether or not to catheterize the woman at this time:

1. Whether or not the bladder needs emptying:
   a. is it distended?
   b. has the woman voided within the last 2 hours?
   c. what has been her fluid intake since her last voiding?
2. The increased risk of a bladder infection with catheterization.
3. Whether or not a possible potential complication is being anticipated:
   a. immediate postpartum hemorrhage
   b. shoulder dystocia
   (Management of both of these complications includes having an empty bladder. Precious time can be gained if an empty bladder is already assured.)

Generally speaking, if the bladder is obviously distended the decision is to catheterize the woman in order to avoid further trauma to the bladder, decrease the discomfort in her lower abdomen, and circumvent a problem with the bladder in the event of the aforementioned complications. If the bladder is not obviously distended, the decision is based on your calculation of the probability of the woman's having one of the two complications. A low probability does not warrant catheterization. High probability does warrant catheterization if the woman has not recently voided, even if a distended bladder is not obvious. The woman should end this phase of labor with an empty bladder. This accomplishment requires careful monitoring of the bladder during first and second stage labor (see Chapter 12) and use of all measures to get the woman to void naturally (see Chapters 12 and 24). It is uncommon for a woman cared for by a nurse-midwife to need catheterization.

If catheterization is performed and the fetal head is into the true pelvis, the direction of the catheter is different from usual. The urethra is displaced to conform with the contour of the fetal head, which is displacing it. Therefore, immediately upon entry of the catheter into the urethra, it is necessary to direct the catheter upward and over the fetal head while going inward. Otherwise, by going straight in as usual the catheter simply won't go in and you will only have succeeded in traumatizing the urethra. Sometimes it is helpful to splint the urethra vaginally by placing a finger below it as the catheter is being inserted. Going up and over the fetal head also means that more than usual of the catheter will be inserted before reaching the bladder. (These same pointers should be remembered if it is necessary to catheterize a woman during the first stage of labor and the fetal head is into the true pelvis.)

Urine, Hydration, and General Condition
Management of these three areas during the second stage of labor and the rationale for their management is the same as for the first stage of labor.

Hydration, however, is further affected during the second stage of labor by fluid loss through the skin in the form of perspiration. The woman may perspire profusely from the effort of pushing, especially if the environment is not air-conditioned and it is summer in a geographic area that is both hot and humid.

The general condition of the woman during the second stage is going to depend on her general condition resulting from the first stage of labor. If she enters the second stage of labor exhausted, she is going to have difficulty in mustering the energy required for pushing, especially if a primigravida. This is because the average length of a primigravid second stage is longer than that of a multipara. This problem is often overcome, however, if the woman believes that delivery is near. This thought, thus, needs to be fostered. This is not difficult as it is a truism, especially in comparison with the length of the first stage of labor. Most women respond well to evidence of progress. There can be no greater encouragement than for them to see for themselves the bulging of their rectum and perineum and the color of their baby's hair (if a cephalic presen-

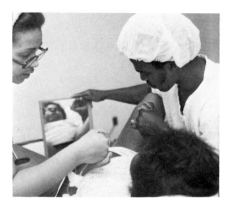

FIGURE 13-10. Father/husband and nurse-midwife supporting a woman during second stage. A mirror has been placed between her legs so she can visualize the progress made from her pushing efforts.

tation) and to touch the baby's head. A padded mirror propped on her bed between the woman's legs so she can see the effect of her pushing effort is invaluable for this purpose (Fig. 13-10).

Maternal Pushing Effort

The maternal pushing effort must be evaluated for effectiveness. Proof of effectiveness is the progressive descent and sequence of the mechanisms of labor by the fetus. This is generally evidenced by the sequential bulging of the rectum, then the perineum, and finally visualization of an ever-increasing amount of the fetal presenting part at the enlarging vaginal orifice. In the absence of progress it is essential to reevaluate pelvic adequacy and rule out arrest in the mechanisms of labor by careful vaginal examination. If neither of these difficulties exists the problem is probably either ineffectual pushing or a psychologic obstacle. Recognition that a psychologic obstacle can affect the progress of labor is an old/new observation. It is more apt to be seen in out-of-hospital settings where the woman's emotions are less controlled by external environmental forces. Dramatic change in the progress of labor can be effected by working through whatever psychological block the woman has.

Management of the second stage of labor in relation to the maternal pushing effort is largely a matter of individual clinician belief. It ranges from those who believe in vigorously encouraging the maternal pushing effort as soon as the woman is completely dilated to those who believe that the word *pushing* should never be used and the woman should bear down only as she feels like it. Management by the bulk of nurse-midwives lies somewhere between these two extremes in a rather common-sense approach.

Those clinicians who advocate vigorous encouragement of the maternal pushing effort as soon as the woman is completely dilated probably do so out of concern that to do otherwise may prolong the second stage of labor and increase the possibility of a traumatic forceps delivery. Their fear is allayed if they quickly see evidence of progress. This attitude is more prevalent in hospitals with rigid policies dictating time limitations on the duration of second stage. Excessive encouragement to push reflects a general impatience, which is fostered by the need to be assured that the fetus has made it through the mechanisms of labor all right without any complications arising from arrest at any point.

Proponents of the other extreme point to Beynon's study [2] as proving the above fears groundless. They also point out that having the woman push only when she wishes is a much more natural approach that eliminates what they consider to be frenzied harrassment of the woman to push and disruption of a possibly heretofore calm, relaxed situation of breathing and working with the contractions.

Several anatomic, physiologic, and psychologic considerations enter this controversy:

1. The natural maternal pushing effort is in response to a reflex mechanism which is not initiated until the fetal head is pressing against and distending the pelvic floor.
2. The reflex mechanism is thereafter triggered with each contraction; the maternal

response of pushing is activated shortly after the onset of the contraction, after it has started to build toward its acme.

3. It is possible to teach a woman to push effectively in the absence of the reflex mechanism, for example if she has spinal anesthesia or when the fetal head has not yet descended to the pelvic floor.

4. It is possible for the natural maternal pushing effort to be ineffectual. This is more likely in the frightened woman with no preparation for childbirth.

5. There are times when a woman needs to push as a result of developing complications or from the effects of anesthesia.

6. The breathing used in the natural pushing effort is that of a series of short pushes, each approximately five seconds long, often during the expiratory phase of respiration. This reduces the possibility of fetal hypoxia and acidosis which may result from repeated breath-holding after inspiration and prolonged bearing down.

7. Slow distention of the perineal musculature is less apt to result in lacerations or the need for an episiotomy than when the tissue layers have been stretched rapidly.

8. The incidence of uterine prolapse and cystocele may be lessened because of less strain on the cardinal ligaments if only the natural bearing down of the woman is allowed instead of subjecting the ligaments to undue strain caused by forced pushing.

9. Birth trauma to the fetal head may be lessened because of gradual, even pressure against the head and easing of that pressure rather than sudden prolonged spurts of pressure and abrupt release of pressure.

10. The ability of the woman to "open up" facilitates the progress of second stage. Helping her to open up includes the following:

    a. positioning — especially squatting

    b. open mouth, open throat, and guttural sounds

    c. deliberate perineal musculature relaxation

    d. visualization and imaging techniques learned during preparation for childbirth

Taking all of this into consideration, it seems reasonable to use an approach that combines the best of the two methods. In this approach, the "natural" method is used unless or until there is evidence of a need for the woman to push deliberately. In such an event the woman is taught, if she was not already taught in preparation for childbirth and parenthood classes, how to push. (See Chapter 49). The woman also is taught how to push effectively if her natural efforts at pushing are ineffectual.

Need for Analgesia/Anesthesia

Analgesia during the second stage of labor usually is the continuation in action of analgesia given the woman during the first stage of labor. This was discussed in Chapter 12.

Some clinicians find the use of a methoxyflurane (Penthrane) mask helpful at times, particularly with women who did not have any preparation for childbirth. Penthrane is a halogenated anesthetic which may be given at concentrations that result in analgesia rather than anesthesia. Given for obstetric analgesia it is self-administered by the woman by way of a hand-held inhalator such as the Cyprane or the Duke inhalator. Penthrane has largely replaced the use of trichloroethylene (Trilene) because it is less risky in its potential side effects. Penthrane inhalation used with contractions only during the second stage of labor will not cause respiratory depression of either the fetus or the woman. In order to avoid getting into levels of concentration greater than analgesia it is important that the woman does not continue inhaling the anesthetic after the contraction begins to go away or between contractions. However, since there is a slight time lag between the start of inhalation and the onset of analgesia, the woman needs to breathe the Penthrane deeply and quickly as soon as she feels the contraction beginning. This should carry her through the acme of the contraction, at which time she should no longer inhale the anesthetic. More than this usage may adversely affect the contractions by causing a temporary decrease in their frequency, duration, and intensity. Penthrane is not routinely used by nurse-midwives for labor analgesia. It is useful when a narcotic analgesic is not possible or when the woman is unprepared for childbirth and has an expectation of a gas mask. It is also helpful for use during cervical inspection and repair but may add to the postpartum blood loss by contributing to uterine atony.

Anesthesia is for the delivery itself. Nurse-midwives may perform either a pudendal block or a local infiltration of the perineal body, or a combination of both, to provide anesthesia when necessary for normal spontaneous vaginal deliveries. Correctly performed, both are safe procedures with minimal to no effect on the baby and constitute the safest known methods (for both mother and baby) of regional and local obstetric anesthesia.

If an episiotomy is planned, then pudendal block is the method of choice for the following reasons:

1. It anesthetizes a larger area so anesthesia is provided if there are lacerations in an area other than the perineal body (e.g., periurethral lacerations) or if it is necessary to extend the episiotomy. A pudendal block anesthetizes the perineum and vulva including the clitoris, labia majora, labia minora, perineal body, and rectal area. A local infiltration anesthetizes only that tissue infiltrated with an anesthetic agent.
2. There is no tissue distortion with a pudendal block because the trunk of a major nerve is anesthetized, thereby anesthetizing all its branches and the tissue it innervates. Local infiltration distends the tissues into which the anesthetic agent is injected,

thereby distorting their size and making proper approximation of tissue layers more difficult.

3. Pudendal block also anesthetizes the lower vaginal tract thereby alleviating any discomfort or pain a woman may have from the tissue stretching taking place from distention by the fetal head. The sensation of stretching may be actually more frightening from fear of "ripping open" than painful for some women, especially those who did not have any preparation for childbirth education. This alone may constitute a reason for performing a pudendal block. If an episiotomy is being cut it then spares the unprepared woman from being frightened by the sudden sensation of her "bottom splitting open" at the time the cut is made. A pudendal block is also sometimes used for the sole purpose of relaxing the perineal musculature, especially if the woman is tightening up from pain and fear. An episiotomy may or may not subsequently be necessary.

Selection of a local infiltration as the anesthesia of choice is discussed in Chapter 52, as are the different techniques used for performing a local infiltration both prior to delivery for cutting an episiotomy and after delivery for repair of an episiotomy or lacerations. The technique, relevant anatomy, and necessary equipment and materials for performing a pudendal block are discussed in Chapter 51.

Perineal Integrity

Evaluation of perineal integrity is for the purpose of determining if delivery can possibly occur over an intact perineum or if an episiotomy is indicated. This decision is continually re-evaluated until the baby is born.

There are a number of techniques which facilitate delivery over an intact perineum. Each has its advocates and detractors. The first division of thinking is between "hands on" and "hands off." The hands-off proponents feel that hands on interferes with the natural timing and stretching by the mother, especially in squatting and standing positions. They believe that touching stimulates muscle contraction and is distracting to the woman. Some birthing women in other positions have vocalized distress over being touched on the perineum, feeling that the area is already supersensitive and hyperstimulated. These women find perineal massage or any stretching technique irritating.

The hands-on advocates believe that a number of techniques facilitate the stretching of the perineum. They vary amongst themselves as to which single or combined techniques are the best. The techniques include:

1. Prenatal digital stretching of the vaginal outlet by the woman or her partner.
2. "Ironing out" the perineum by sweeping your fingers back and forth from side to side in the vagina just ahead of the fetal head. The pressure applied to iron out, or stretch, the muscles also stimulates the pushing reflex.
3. Warm compresses to the perineum. These increase circulation to the area thereby promoting muscle relaxation.
4. Perineal massage. This is usually done with warmed oil. The warm oil increases circulation to the area and avoids friction from the massage. The massage is to promote perineal relaxation. Concern has been expressed about the use of the oil. Care should be taken that the oil not enter the vagina or be used for ironing out the perineum so there is no chance of its getting in the baby's mouth or respiratory tract.
5. Perineal support at the time of birth. Some clinicians do this by directly bracing the perineal body with their hand. Other clinicians place their thumb and middle finger across from each other in the left and right groin and press inward to provide a little extra give across the perineal body (see Fig. 13-11).
6. Fetal head control by asserting pressure

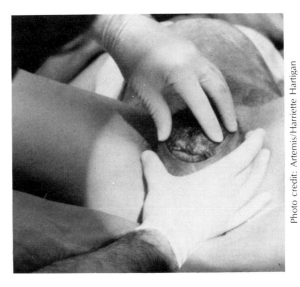

Photo credit: Artemis/Harriette Hartigan

FIGURE 13-11. Combination of fetal head control and perineal support at the time of crowning.

against the fetal head to keep it well flexed and then allowing gradual extension as the perineum stretches (Fig. 13-11). This is absolutely essential in lithotomy and most dorsal positions in order to prevent tears. Some clinicians believe that if fetal head control is done properly then there is no need to touch the perineum. Other clinicians combine fetal head control and perineal hands-on techniques. Still other clinicians combine only fetal head control and perineal support.

Maternal self-control is key to whatever method of delivering over an intact perineum you use. A woman who is out of contol is more apt to tear or need an episiotomy.

Need for, and Type of, Episiotomy

Initial evaluation of the perineum should be done prior to the time of delivery. The perineum is evaluated for its length, thickness, and distensibility. This evaluation aids in determining whether or not an episiotomy is indicated and, if so, what kind of episiotomy. An extremely thick perineum may be found in athletes, is the result of muscular overdevelopment, and is apt to be rigid and resistant to distension, thereby necessitating an episiotomy. A short perineum may indicate performing a mediolateral episiotomy rather than a median (midline) episiotomy, if an episiotomy is necessary, in order to avoid injury to the rectal sphincter and wall.

Your findings are evaluated in relation to the following considerations when making a decision about cutting an episiotomy:

1. *The woman's preference.* Most woman who state a preference usually request that an episiotomy not be done. They generally respond well to a plan of not cutting an episiotomy unless absolutely necessary in your judgment (i.e., last minute episiotomy to prevent an inevitable tear or for a high probability of shoulder dystocia). If episiotomy does become necessary, you should inform the woman and discuss it with her to the best of your capability in the situation. Using the rationale of prophylactic gynecology is not considered valid in this plan.

2. *Your beliefs about episiotomy as prophylactic gynecology.* Proponents of an episiotomy as prophylactic gynecology state that an episiotomy saves the muscles from being stretched and that proper reapproximation of the tissues and building up of the perineal musculature during the repair will result in a better structure with better muscle tone. The detractors of this theory state that there are no studies which support this belief and that, regardless, there is no need to put the woman through all this trauma in order for her to have a good structure with good muscle tone. Instead, muscle tone is not only regained but improved by doing perineal tightening exercises (Kegel exercises). In response, the proponents point out that there is no guarantee that the woman will do the exercises even if taught and that an episiotomy and repair are assured hap-

penings. The detractors feel that this is an unvalidated assumption and that the women they care for will exercise if properly motivated to do so.

Both sides of the argument are concerned with the relationship of childbearing to gynecological problems later in life, such as uterine prolapse, cystocele, and stress incontinence, which are affected by lax tone in the muscles and ligaments of the pelvic floor that support the pelvic organs.

3. *The size of the baby.* Cutting a good-sized episiotomy may be indicated for delivery of the preterm or SGA (small-for-gestational-age) baby, depending on the relaxation of the perineum. Also, depending on the length and distensibility of the perineum and the control of the woman, a baby estimated to be 4000 grams or 9 pounds or more may cause need for an episiotomy either to prevent laceration or in anticipation of a possible shoulder dystocia.

4. *Self-control of the woman.* A woman who is in good control of herself, that is, able to respond to directions as to when to push and when to breathe in order to slowly ease the baby's head out, is a far better candidate for no episiotomy and for delivering over an intact perineum. An uncontrolled woman is nearly guaranteed to lacerate, and repair of an episiotomy in this situation is much to be preferred.

5. *Anticipation of a shoulder dystocia.* Precious time is saved and your efforts facilitated if you already have an episiotomy in the event of a shoulder dystocia. Expectation of a shoulder dystocia is grounds for cutting an episiotomy.

6. *Fetal malpresentations and malpositions.* A malpresentation or malposition in an average-sized baby means that (1) the widest diameter of the fetal head coming through the pelvic outlet and vaginal orifice is larger than usual, thereby creating a higher probability of laceration and (2) you or the physician may need room for

manipulations in order to effect a safe delivery.

Final evaluation of the perineum is made immediately prior to the birth of the head as it is distending the perineum and dilating the vaginal orifice. If the decision has been made to deliver over an intact perineum, the perineum must be watched carefully for signs of impending tearing. An earlier decision not to cut an episiotomy may be reversed at this last minute in the presence of one additional consideration:

7. *An inevitable laceration of the perineal body.* This is evidenced by narrow white lines resembling stretch marks and visible just beneath the perineal skin. These appear just prior to laceration and probably represent beginning tearing of the underlying tissues. A quick episiotomy prior to the moment of crowning is possible and can substitute for an inevitable tear. The result is a better anatomical and artistic repair than repair of a jagged laceration.

If the decision is made to cut an episiotomy, then the next decision is to decide what type of episiotomy will be cut: midline (median) or mediolateral. The following are factors to be considered in making this decision:

1. *How much room is needed in relation to the length of the perineal body.* If the distance between the posterior fourchette and the rectal sphincter is unusually short, a mediolateral episiotomy is indicated in order to avoid extension by laceration into the rectal sphincter and rectum.
2. *How much room is needed as determined by the reason for the episiotomy.* If the episiotomy is being cut because you have determined a need for additional room, such as in the management of a shoulder dystocia, a mediolateral episiotomy is indicated. If the episiotomy is being cut for either prophylactic gynecological factors or prevention of a perineal laceration, then the room

you can get from cutting a mediolateral episiotomy is not needed and a midline episiotomy will suffice.

3. *A midline episiotomy is easier to repair than a mediolateral episiotomy.* This is because a mediolateral episiotomy is cut on a slant in relation to the perpendicular midline of the perineum. This means that the size of the bites for each half of a single stitch on either side of the incisional line will be deliberately unequal, that there is an increased risk of entering the rectum during the repair due to greater retraction of the medial aspect of the incision, that manipulation of the necessary equipment and materials is more awkward, and that approximation of tissues yielding good functional and artistic results is more difficult.
4. *A midline episiotomy is less painful than a mediolateral episiotomy during the healing process.* This is because there are fewer nerve branches involved in the locale of a midline episiotomy and its repair. It is also because the arrangement of the muscles that have been cut across and into with a mediolateral episiotomy causes points of stretch that pull on the incisional repair line, thereby causing pain. This is in contrast with a midline episiotomy that is cut into the central tendinous point of the perineum and only separates the two sides of pairs of muscles rather than cutting across the muscles themselves.

How to cut the episiotomy you have decided upon is discussed in Chapter 60. Relevant anatomy also is discussed. When cutting an episiotomy it is vital to remember that with the cut there is a sudden release of a previously restraining force against the progress of the head. Depending on when you cut it (i.e., during a contraction or not, while the woman is pushing or not, how distended the vaginal orifice is), it is possible for the fetal head to suddenly "pop" — a totally uncontrolled delivery of the head. Since this can be damaging to both the baby and the woman, you need to control the baby's head as you cut. This is done with the vaginal hand which is already delineating the area to be cut and protecting the baby's head.

Continuing Evaluation of Fetal Well-Being

Continuing evaluation of fetal well-being during the second stage of labor is a continuation of the evaluation of the well-being of the fetus during the first stage of labor. It consisted of evaluating the following:

1. Normalcy of the fetal lie, presentation, attitude, and variety.
2. Fetal adaptation to the pelvis (synclitism or asynclitism, molding of the fetal skull, the formation of caput succedaneum).
3. The fetal heart rate and pattern.

Evaluation of fetal well-being during the second stage of labor in addition includes:

4. Evaluation of the normalcy of progress being made in the mechanisms of labor.

Numbers 1, 2, and 4 are determined during a vaginal examination. The first two were discussed in Chapter 12, relating to the first stage of labor. Evaluation of the normalcy of progress being made in the mechanisms of labor is done by evaluating the progress of the fetus through the pelvis (engagement and descent) and the cardinal turning movements of the fetus (flexion and internal rotation) as identified by the changing position (variety) of the fetal head prior to delivery. This evaluation was discussed in the first part of Chapter 12 relative to the normal data base for the first stage of labor.

Evaluation of the fetal heart rate and pattern is also the same as that discussed for the first stage of labor with the exception of an increased frequency for checking and evaluating the fetal heart when using a fetoscope or ultrasonic method during the second stage of labor. Clinicians vary in what they consider this frequency should be but most agree that it should be at least every 15 minutes. The variance in opinion is not that the fetal heart evaluation should be any less frequent but, rather, more frequent. Some clinicians believe the fetal heart should be evaluated every 5 minutes during the second stage of labor. Others believe it should be checked at the end of and after each contraction during which the woman pushes.

It is important to remember in interpreting the fetal heart rate and pattern toward the end of the second stage that an early deceleration pattern of a periodic fetal heart rate change is not considered an indication of acute fetal distress. Instead it is a not unexpected happening because an early deceleration pattern is caused by head compression. Increased pressure on the head occurs as the second stage progresses and delivery nears. The pressure is a result of the resistance of the pelvic floor and perineum during contractions. This may be further intensified by the addition of the maternal pushing effort.

Continuing Evaluation of The Progress of Labor

Continuing evaluation of the progress of the second stage of labor is based on the following:

1. Contraction pattern
2. Length of second stage
3. Descent/station
4. Progress through the mechanisms of labor other than descent and engagement

The norms for these items were discussed earlier in this chapter.

Management decisions relating to the continuing evaluation of the progress of labor include the following:

1. Whether to move the woman to the delivery room and, if so, when

2. Whether or not there is a need to consult with the physician

The timing for moving primigravidas and multiparas to the delivery room was discussed in Chapter 12 under management of the first stage of labor. The decision concerning physician consultation is made by the nurse-midwife as she (1) continues to evaluate the normality of the progress of labor, the well-being of the fetus, and the well-being of the mother, (2) continues to screen for abnormalities and complications, and (3) anticipates potential problems on the basis of her or his interpretation of findings resulting from this data base evaluation. Screening for the collaborative management of complications during labor, including when to consult with the physician, is discussed in Chapter 14.

Evaluation of progress through the mechanisms of labor is essential to detecting deep transverse arrest and concomitant second stage hypotonic uterine dysfunction (see Chapter 14). Generally, the fetus is not in danger if hypotonic uterine dysfunction occurs and *is not ignored.*

The fetus is in danger in the situation in which there are strong, expulsive contractions and maternal pushing effort but failure to progress because of some form of fetopelvic disproportion, including deep transverse arrest. The fetus is then subjected to a literal battering. It is mandatory that the progress of labor as determined by progressive descent be carefully assessed.

Detection of progressive descent was discussed in preceding chapters and includes the following:

1. Progressively lower location on the woman's spine of the point of back pain due to pressure from the fetal head
2. Progressively lower location in the woman's abdomen of the maximum point of intensity of the fetal heart tones
3. Increasing desire of the woman to push, which indicates descent of the fetal head

to the pelvic floor and subsequent initiation of the reflex mechanism for pushing
4. Vaginal examination findings indicative of descent by virtue of a change in station, which is evidence of progress through the pelvis
5. Rectal and perineal bulging
6. Appearance of the presenting part at the vaginal orifice
7. The woman's assertion that her baby is coming, confirmed by either observation or examination

Engagement should have occurred during the active phase of the first stage of labor in the nullipara and by the onset of the second stage of labor in the multipara. Failure of engagement to have occurred by entry into the second stage of labor is a signal of a potential problem.

Bodily and supportive care of the woman

Bodily and supportive care during the second stage of labor are continuations of the care begun during the first stage of labor, modified to meet the woman's changing needs as she progresses through labor. All support and comfort measures are subject to the manner in which each woman experiences and accepts them; their effectiveness is ascertained with this in mind. There are a few additional measures and considerations specific to the second stage of labor — those pertaining to breathing, pushing, and the woman's significant others.

Breathing.
A controlled form of breathing, such as that used during the active phase of the first stage of labor, should be used through the contractions if the woman does not yet feel like pushing. This type of breathing starts with a cleansing breath, then goes into a slow chest breathing that increases in speed as the contraction reaches its acme, then slows down as the contraction tapers off, and ends with another cleansing breath.

A woman may need help with her breathing and in making effective use of either her natural pushing desire or a deliberate pushing effort. The breathing used for her pushing is discussed in detail in Chapter 49.

The woman needs to be instructed to pant if she feels like pushing but you don't want her to push. Panting may be a quick inhalation followed by a forcible exhalation and repeated immediately. It may also be a rapid, shallow throat breathing as described, along with when to use it during both the first and second stages of labor, in Chapter 12. The woman's ability to pant and not push can be critical and should be taught when she enters the second stage of labor as a form of anticipatory instruction if it has not been taught before.

Pushing.
A woman who feels like or needs to push can be helped in a number of ways in order to make her effort as effective as possible. Her significant other can also be involved in helping her push in a way that will make that person feel important, contributing, and participating in the experience (Fig. 13-12). These techniques are described in detail in Chapter 49.

Significant others
Ideally, the matter of whom the woman wants present at the time of birth has been discussed and planned for some time in advance. If the delivery will be in a hospital delivery room the number of significant others usually is limited

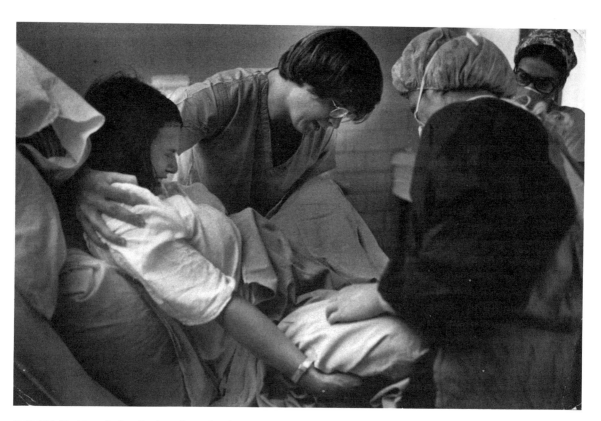

FIGURE 13-12.   Father/husband involved in second stage pushing effort.

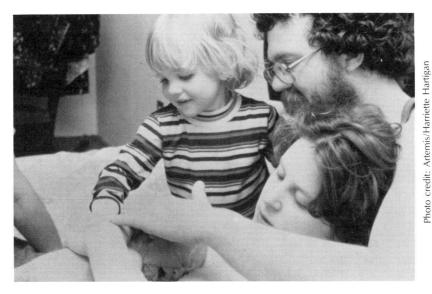

Photo credit: Artemis/Harriette Hartigan

FIGURE 13-13. Sibling presence at birth.

to one. Depending on the size of the labor room, more than one significant other might be permitted. The policies regarding the presence of significant others at the time of delivery vary with hospital settings. The major current controversy in the more enlightened hospitals is the presence of siblings at the time of birth (Fig. 13-13). See Chapter 20 regarding the presence of significant others, including siblings, at a childbirth center or home births. Restrictive policies have been one of the reasons for couples' seeking childbirth alternatives to the hospital setting.

If the delivery is going to be in the delivery room, the significant other again needs to be welcomed and made to feel wanted and needed, as in the labor room. Give the person territorial space beside the woman, provide a stool to sit on, and emphasize his or her importance in being there. If the significant other has to change clothes in order to be in the delivery room, allow plenty of time so that the person doesn't miss the delivery. Include the significant other in your explanations of the ongoing activities.

The significant other's activities during the second stage of labor again depend on the person's capabilities and wishes and how much participation is agreeable to the woman, the person, and you. For example, activities might include a continuation of what they were doing during the first stage of labor (e.g., back rubbing, coaching breathing, timing contractions, fanning). The significant other might also help the woman in the technique of pushing, encourage her, wipe her face, share the anticipation and then the moment of birth with her, and cut the umbilical cord.

Preparation for delivery

It is the nurse-midwife's responsibility to assure that all is in readiness for the delivery when managing the labor and delivery of the woman. Management decisions included in preparation for delivery in the hospital involve the location of the delivery and the position of the woman for delivery. Since subsequent preparations are somewhat dependent upon these two decisions, these decisions will be discussed first.

Location of the Delivery
The location of the delivery should have been planned long before the time of labor. Whether or not they can have what they want in terms of having their significant others with them, dorsal or other position for delivery, no routine episiotomy, no separation of themselves from their baby, and so forth, will determine for some parturients the location of the delivery in or out of the hospital. The alternatives for delivery within a hospital are the delivery room, the labor room, or a birthing room. Newer hospitals often are designed now for combination labor and delivery rooms or birthing rooms for normal women.

The planned location of the delivery may change due to unforeseen circumstances. For example, the delivery may be planned for the delivery room but if all the delivery rooms are occupied at the time your patient is ready to deliver, the locale may change to the labor room. Development of complications may also dictate a change of locale. For example, in this instance, the delivery may have been planned for the labor room but there has been evidence of fetal distress as labor nears the end. There is need for a low forceps delivery and the availability of immediate newborn resuscitation equipment. Hence the locale changes to the delivery room.

Position of the Woman for Delivery
Position of the woman for delivery refers to whether she will deliver in the lithotomy, dorsal, left lateral, squatting, standing, or knee-chest position. Any of the positions can be used in the labor room or in a birthing room and many women prefer a squatting, standing, knee-chest, left lateral or dorsal position for delivery. The usual positions in a hospital delivery room are lithotomy or dorsal. The dorsal position is most apt to be used by women with normal deliveries when cared for by nurse-midwives in a hospital delivery room. Nurse-midwives believe that in neither of these positions does the woman have to be flat on her back; rather, they encourage a semisitting or "back up" and "legs down" modification of these positions (Fig. 13-14). In deciding which of these two positions to utilize for the delivery of a woman without complications in a delivery room the following should be considered:

1. The woman's preference. Although the dorsal position is a more natural position for the woman, some women prefer the lithotomy position as being more comfortable because their legs are supported. Many women, usually those who are not knowledgeable about what is happening to themselves, have no preference.
2. The condition of the woman's legs. A woman with severe varicosities should be delivered in dorsal rather than lithotomy position. This position avoids pressure on the legs and in the popliteal space which is exerted by both the full-leg and knee-break stirrups and causes circulatory interference. The risk of thrombophlebitis would be quite high with the woman in stirrups.
3. The control and cooperation of the woman. A dorsal delivery is more effective when the woman is cooperative and in control of herself. The lithotomy position does give the clinician an element of control in the event the woman is out of control.
4. Any existing or anticipated complications. In the event of any existing complications (e.g., malpresentations, multiple gestation) or anticipated complications (e.g., shoulder dystocia), the woman should be in a lithotomy position because the clinician needs all possible visualization and room in which to function with ready, direct access to the woman.

General Preparations
What the general preparations consist of depends, in part, on the location of the delivery. The following description of preparations are for a delivery in the delivery room because

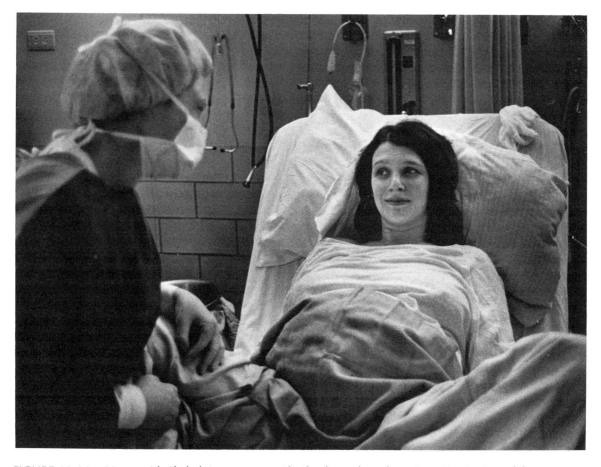

FIGURE 13-14.   Nurse-midwife helping woman with "back up, legs down" positioning in a delivery room.

this setting is the most formal and involves the most detail. Certain principles from this description can be extrapolated for preparations for delivery in other settings. Examples are warmth for the baby, a sterile or clean area for delivery which also protects the underlying furnishings from fluids, and organization of necessary equipment and supplies. The pacing of the preparations depend on the timing of their performance in relation to the woman's progress of labor. The ideal pacing is one of steady progression with neither frantic haste nor long waiting for the actual delivery after all is in readiness.

An effective learning tool for nurse-midwifery students in thinking through the responsibilities and the multiple preparations for delivery is to play a mental game in which you envision yourself making the decisions, performing some preparatory acts, and directing others in the performance of other preparatory acts in a given situation. Once you have the basics drilled you can alter the game by changing variables in the situation (e.g., primigravida versus multipara, different settings, precipitous second stage) and "live" through what you would do from beginning to end, in sequence, in each situation. The value of these mental games lies in the fact that when faced with the actual situation you have already thought through your actions and will thus both face and manage the situation with greater equanimity and more seasoned judgment.

The following are basic steps in preparing for a delivery in the delivery room:

1. Notify the nursing staff that the woman you are caring for is nearing delivery by informing them of your findings and estimation of how soon you are going to want to move her to the delivery room. Notification should be approximately upon entry into transition for a multipara and into second stage labor for a primigravida.

2. Make sure that the significant others have already changed clothes into acceptable attire for the delivery room, or that they do so now.

3. Make sure that the newborn resuscitation equipment and supplies have been checked, that is, are present and in working condition.

4. Request that blankets be warmed for the baby if there is not a blanket warmer in the setting.

5. Make sure that the source of heat for the baby is functioning, e.g., radiant heater, incubator.

6. Make the decision of when to move the woman to the delivery room.

7. Notify the nursing staff, if not in the room, of your decision.

8. Assist with movement of the woman from the labor room to the delivery room.

9. Depending on the availability of nursing staff, assist with movement of the woman safely onto the delivery room table and removal of the labor room bed or transport cart from the room.

10. See to it that the significant others are capped and masked prior to entry into the delivery room and that they are safely seated on stools beside the woman and out of the way of the nursing personnel, general activities going on in the room, and sterile fields (Fig. 13-15).

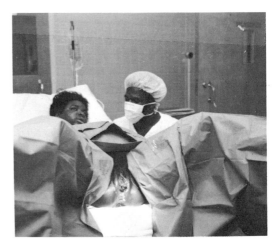

FIGURE 13-15. Woman and father/husband ready for delivery in a delivery room.

11. Inform the woman and her significant others that you are leaving the room to scrub but that you will be right outside the door. Tell them that you will keep an eye on her as will the nurses in the room and that the next time they see you it will be in a cap and mask.

12. Inform the nursing staff of the following:
    a. that you are leaving to scrub
    b. the position of the woman for delivery (lithotomy or dorsal), as this makes a difference in what is or is not done with the stirrups and the end of the delivery table
    c. what size gloves you wear
    d. whether or not you want a pudendal set, Iowa trumpet, and/or needle and syringe for local infiltration, and what local anesthetic
    e. anything else you are going to want that is necessary for the circulating nurse to get or do while she is doing her other tasks

    Nurse-midwives who were former labor and delivery room nurses remember what it was like to try to jump six different directions at the same time and resent having to try while wishing that the person giving the orders was better organized. Experienced delivery room circulating nurses have developed a routine that efficiently accomplishes a myriad of essential tasks in a short amount of time while also continuing support and instruction of the woman. By your telling them what you will need before you need it, they can incorporate your requests smoothly into their routine and have everything ready and waiting for you by the time you're back in the room from scrubbing. If you wait until you are scrubbed and in the room to tell them your glove size and ask for other needed items, you not only disrupt an effective routine but frustrate both the nurse who can't get it all at once and yourself as you end up waiting — which, depending on the circumstances, may or may not matter.

13. Don a cap and mask if this was not done before. While it is considered better technique to have on a cap and mask when entering the delivery room at any time, it is not generally considered a serious breach in technique to have been in the delivery room without wearing a cap and mask if none of the sterile packs are open or sterile fields uncovered, as is usually the situation at the time of moving the woman into the delivery room.

14. Scrub. This is a surgical scrub. If you did a surgical scrub upon entry to the labor and delivery suite (a good idea), then the length of your scrub now can be cut in half. Remember to put on your cap and mask before starting your scrub. Otherwise, upon realizing that you have not yet done so, you have to break scrub, put on your cap and mask, and then start your scrub over again.

It is essential while scrubbing to keep an eye on what is going on in the delivery room, specifically watching for signs of imminent delivery. Most delivery rooms are adjacent to the scrub sinks, which enables easy visual checking while scrubbing. Needless to say, a controlled delivery of the fetal head is eminently more important than a complete, or any, scrubbing of your hands. Scrub time is also good thinking time to review, even if quickly, your management plan for delivery of this individual woman and baby.

15. When you reenter the delivery room from scrubbing, the woman will be positioned for delivery, the sterile delivery table of supplies and instruments uncovered, chart forms started, and so forth. You should be familiar with the delivery room, where equipment and supplies are, the routines of the circulating nurse, and how to function within the room so if need be you know how to operate the delivery room table, fix stirrups, adjust lights and mirror, and so on.

16. Dry your hands and arms, using surgical technique.

17. Gown, using sterile technique.

18. Glove, using sterile technique.

19. The person who does the perineal prep varies. In some settings it is the circulating nurse; in other settings it is the person helping the woman deliver her baby (you). (See Chapter 50 for the procedure.)

If the woman is in lithotomy position it is at the time of doing the perineal prep that the table is broken. *Once the table is broken it is imperative that you keep at least one eye on the woman's perineum at all times no matter what else you are doing.* This is a vital safety feature for the about-to-be-born baby.

20. Draping of the woman is in accord with the drapes provided and institutional procedure. After the woman is draped, if she is in stirrups, you can more easily keep your eye on the perineum if you bring the instrument table up beside you with the end slanted under her leg.

21. If the woman so desires, request that the overhead mirror be adjusted so the woman and her significant others can watch the delivery of the baby. It helps in adjusting the mirror for you to hold your hand right in front of the vaginal orifice and ask if they can see your hand. This is because a hand may be more recognizable to them. After the mirror is adjusted you can point out landmarks, the area to watch, and what they can expect to see.

22. Request either sterile normal saline or benzalkonium (Zephiran) to be put in either a separate sterile splash basin or in a kidney basin if there is one on the instrument table. This is for wetting your gloves for vaginal examinations and rinsing off your gloves of powder, blood, and so on.

23. Organize your instrument table. The instrument table is set up in an organized fashion but needs further organizing by you. It is helpful to separate what you will need to manage the delivery of the baby from the other instruments and supplies on the table; i.e., two clamps and a pair of scissors for clamping and cutting the umbilical cord, and the bulb syringe for oropharyngeal and nasal suctioning of the baby. Then if you need any of these items in a hurry you will have them available rather than trying to find them and losing precious time. It also helps to separate out the scissors for cutting an episiotomy, even if one is not planned, in case you reverse this decision at the last minute.

   The remainder of the table can be reorganized as events progress and you need different items; for example, reorganize the table for repair work when ready to do this by separating the needleholder, suture scissors, pickup forceps, suture, and local infiltration apparatus from the other instruments and supplies.

24. Do a vaginal examination to:
    a. reconfirm the presentation and position of the baby
    b. ascertain the station, if needed
    c. again evaluate the distensibility of the woman's perineum

25. If indicated, perform either a pudendal block or a local infiltration. See Chapters 51 and 52 for how to do these.

26. If indicated, cut the appropriate type of episiotomy. See Chapter 60 for how to do this.

Throughout all these preparations for delivery you will have continued to keep the woman and her significant others informed of and involved in the ongoing activities, coached her in her breathing and pushing effort, and responded to any questions or concerns they might have. You will also have assumed management of the delivery room. By this is meant the fact that you are responsible not only for what is occurring at the perineum, the delivery, the mother, the baby, and the significant others but also for everything that is going on in the delivery room, as it all affects directly or indirectly these central people. In this capacity you must not only be aware of everything transpiring in the room but also either be in accord with what is happening or redirect any activity with which you do not agree. You are the one looked to for direction and instructions. You are in control of the situation for the safety of mother and baby and the best possible experience for them within their framework.

Management of the delivery

Management of the delivery includes the hand maneuvers used to assist the baby's birth, the immediate care of the newborn, and the following management decisions:

1. Whether to deliver the baby's head with a contraction or between contractions

2. Whether or not to use a Ritgen maneuver
3. When to clamp and cut the umbilical cord

Hand Maneuvers

The hand maneuvers for delivery of the baby in an occiput anterior (OA) position with the mother in a lithotomy position and with the mother in a dorsal position are detailed in the Skills section of this book (Chapters 53 and 54). The hand maneuvers for differing presentations and positions of the baby are detailed in the discussion of managing the delivery and the mechanisms of labor for each (i.e., breech, face) in Chapter 15. The hand maneuvers for a persistent occiput posterior (OP) position are the same as for an occiput anterior except for control of the head. The direction of pressure to help maintain the head in flexion and then to allow gradual extension when the head is occiput posterior is exactly opposite from the direction of the pressure exerted for the same purpose when the head is occiput anterior.

The hand maneuvers you use for delivering a baby in every position must be drilled thoroughly prior to use so they become second nature to you. Those used infrequently should be reviewed periodically and drilled so when you need them you know them.

Delivery of the Baby's Head

Whether to deliver the baby's head with a contraction or between contractions or to use a Ritgen maneuver may not be your deliberate decision. A woman who is out of control and pushing with all her might despite all efforts to get her to stop will determine how the head is born.

Between Contractions. The idea behind delivering the baby's head between contractions is that the combination of the contraction and the maternal pushing effort actually constitutes exertion of a double force at the moment of birth. This makes the birth of the head more rapid and the release of restraining pressure more abrupt, both of which increase the risk of intracranial damage to the baby and lacerations to the woman. If the woman is in control of herself it is possible for her to follow your instructions and to pant through a contraction and then gently push in between contractions, an action that will ease the baby's head out with the least amount of trauma to the baby and to the woman.

Ritgen Maneuver. The Ritgen maneuver, or modified Ritgen maneuver, is a technique by which the clinician controls the delivery of the baby's head (see Fig. 13-16). It is performed as follows:

1. One hand remains on the occiput as described in the hand maneuvers for delivery in Chapters 53 and 54, for control of the baby's head.
2. The other hand is covered with a towel to protect it from contamination.
3. The draped hand then exerts inward pressure posterior to the woman's rectum until the baby's chin is located and in the grasp of the fingers.
4. Forward and outward pressure is then exerted on the underneath side of the chin and the head is controlled between this hand and the hand exerting pressure on the occiput.

Most nurse-midwives do not routinely use the Ritgen maneuver. They believe the baby's head can be controlled in other ways (see Chapters 53 and 54) that are better for the baby and mother because they allow for gradual natural processes, are less interfering, and are less uncomfortable than the Ritgen maneuver. The concern for discomfort is based on the fact that the anus is extremely distended with the bulging of the rectal wall into it. The Ritgen maneuver increases this anal stretching and most likely subjects it and the rectal wall to direct pressure and the rough surface of the

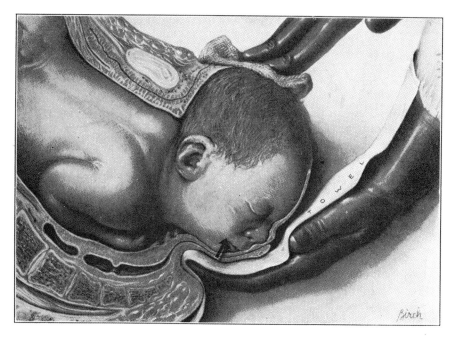

FIGURE 13-16. Ritgen maneuver. The arrow indicates the direction of moderate pressure applied to the fetal chin by the posterior hand. (Reproduced by permission from J. A. Pritchard and P. C. MacDonald. *Williams Obstetrics, 15th.* New York: Appleton-Century-Crofts, 1976.)

towel. It is also associated with an increased incidence of periurethral lacerations.

However, it is useful to know how to do the Ritgen maneuver because it does enable you to "get hold of" the baby's head earlier and to deliver the baby's head faster in a controlled fashion if there is an urgent need for immediate delivery. It is possible to institute the Ritgen maneuver when the head is distending the vulva about half as much as it will when crowning, at which time it encircles the largest diameter of the head at the moment before birth. A combination of an episiotomy and a Ritgen maneuver will shorten the end of the second stage of labor and bring it quickly to an end, if needed.

Clamping and Cutting the Umbilical Cord
Clamping the umbilical cord is done by placing two instrument clamps on the cord with enough room between them to allow for easy cutting of the cord. After applying the first clamp, experienced clinicians routinely strip the cord the distance to the location of application of the second clamp. This prevents the spurting of blood from a distended umbilical vessel at the time of cutting. When a clamp has been applied, care must be taken so that the weight of the clamp is supported and not allowed to exert pull or tension at the site of insertion into the baby. Many clinicians do this by hooking the ring of the finger hold of the instrument over a finger of the hand that is holding or supporting the baby. This leaves the other hand free for cutting. There is no pain for either the baby or the woman at the site of the cutting of the umbilical cord.

The timing of cutting the umbilical cord is a long-standing controversy between those advocating delayed clamping of the cord and those who don't think it makes any significant difference when the cord is clamped. In fact, neither early nor late clamping and cutting of the umbilical cord has any effect on the rate of infant mortality in term gestations. Entering into this debate is the further controversial issue of whether or not to deliberately hold the baby at or below the level of the vaginal introitus, thereby holding the baby at or below the level of the placenta. Lowering the infant, combined with delayed cord clamping, will result in a placental transfusion of approximately 80 milliliters of blood. Whether this placental transfusion is desirable, especially for preterm newborns, is also controversial. It is clear, however, that placental transfusion is *not* desirable if there is a known blood incompatibility between the mother and the baby.

Leboyer [3], in his plea for decreasing the violence of childbirth to the baby, advocates delayed clamping of the cord for an entirely different reason. He believes that the baby's transition to breathing air can be made more easily without trauma and without danger of anoxia. This is accomplished with patience and by allowing the newly born baby to have two sources of oxygen during this transition: (1) from the lungs and (2) from the placenta through the umbilical cord. Then when the gradual transition from dependence on the placenta to dependence on the lungs is completed, as evidenced by cessation of cord pulsations, the umbilical cord is clamped and cut. This process is completed by approximately 4 to 5 minutes after birth.

Immediate Care of the Newborn
Immediate assessment and resuscitation of the newborn are detailed in Chapter 22. However, it does not hurt to reemphasize vital points of care during the first minute of life as this is the climax of the second stage of labor. From the point at the end of the delivery of the baby (with the baby either in a football hold in your arm and hand or on the mother's abdomen), the usual steps of care are as follows:

1. Establish a clear airway. In normal births

this usually involves:
   a. holding or positioning the baby so that the head is lower than the body and is turned somewhat to the side for purposes of drainage
   b. wiping off the baby's face and head and wiping fluid from the nose and mouth
   c. suctioning the nasal and oral passages with a soft rubber bulb syringe
2. Keep the baby warm. This is initiated by wiping off and drying the baby so body heat is not lost. Subsequent actions vary but may include:
   a. bodily contact with the mother
   b. radiant heater
   c. warmed blankets
3. Show the baby to the mother and her significant others or place the baby on the mother's abdomen if not already there (Fig. 13-17).
4. Clamp and cut the umbilical cord. See preceding discussion.
5. Assign the 1-minute Apgar score (preferably done by nursing staff).

If the baby is taken to a warmed crib, incubator, or Kreiselman, the bulb syringe is

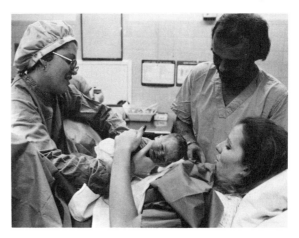

FIGURE 13-17. Nurse-midwife placing baby on mother's abdomen immediately after birth. Note the baby's open eyes.

also taken as well as the cord clamp and scissors for the final clamping and cutting of the cord. During this minute of life while doing the above, you have also grossly examined the baby for any visible deformities or congenital defects.

While you are applying the cord clamp approximately 1 to 2 centimeters from the baby's skin edge, cutting off the excess cord, and completing your gross examination, remember to *keep one eye on the mother's perineum to note any sudden hemorrhaging or signs of placental separation.*

An alternative to the management and immediate care of the newborn presented in this chapter is to use all or part, in modification, of the Leboyer approach to childbirth and the immediate care of the baby. This is detailed in the management of the third stage of labor, Chapter 16.

REFERENCES

1. Friedman, E. A. *Labor: Clinical Evaluation and Management, 2nd.* New York: Meredith, 1978.
2. Beynon, C. L. The normal second stage of labor: A plea for reform in its conduct. *J. Obstet. Gynaecol. Brit. Empire* 64:815, 1957.
3. Leboyer, F. *Birth without Violence.* New York: Knopf, 1976.

BIBLIOGRAPHY FOR CHAPTERS 10, 11, 12, AND 13

Anderson, E. Rationale for use of ketostick, labstick in obstetric labor: Detection of ketosis. Unpublished paper, 1974.

Berger, G. S., and Maynard, L. How routine should FHR monitoring be? *Contemporary OB/GYN* 12:35, 1978.

Beynon, C. L. The normal second stage of labour: A plea for reform in its conduct, *J. Obstet. Gynaecol. Brit. Empire* 64:815, 1957.

Bing, E. *Six Practical Lessons for an Easier Childbirth.* New York: Grosset & Dunlap, 1967.

Bonica, J. J. *Principles and Practice of Obstetric Analgesia & Anesthesia.* Vol. 1. Philadelphia: Davis, 1967.

Bowe, N. L. Intact perineum: A slow delivery of the head does not adversely affect the outcome of the newborn. *J. Nurse-Midwifery* 26(2):5−11 (March/April) 1981.

Brown, C. Therapeutic effects of bathing during labor. *J. Nurse-Midwifery* 27(1):13−16 (January/February) 1982.

Caldeyro-Barcia, R., et al. Effect of position changes on the intensity and frequency of uterine contractions during labor. *Am. J. Obstet. Gynecol.* 80:284, 1960.

Caldeyro-Barcia, R. Some consequences of obstetrical interference. *Birth Family J.* 2:34, 1975.

Caldeyro-Barcia, R. The influence of position during the second stage of labor. *ICEA Conference Proceedings,* 1978.

Chagnon, L. J., and Heldenbrand, C. L. Nurses undertake direct and indirect fetal monitoring at a community hospital. *J. Obstet. Gynecol. Neonat. Nurs.* 3:41, 1974.

Cogan, R., and Edmunds, E. P. The unkindest cut? *Contemporary OB/GYN* 9:55, 1977.

Danforth, D. N. (Ed.). *Obstetrics and Gynecology, 4th.* Philadelphia: Harper & Row, 1982.

Dickinson, R. L., Belskie, A., and Hoffman, M. *Birth Atlas, 6th.* New York: Maternity Center Association, 1968.

Dick-Read, G. *Childbirth without Fear, 2nd.* New York: Harper & Row, 1959.

Eckstein, K., and Marx, G. F. Aortocaval compression and uterine displacement. *Anesthesiology* 40:92, 1974.

Fischer, S. R. Factors associated with the occurrence of perineal lacerations. *J. Nurse-Midwifery* 24(1):18−26, 1979.

Friedman, E. A. An objective method of evaluating labor. *Hosp. Prac.* July, 1970.

Friedman, E. A. *Labor: Clinical Evaluation and Management, 2nd.* New York: Meredith, 1978.

Friedman, E. A. Labor in multiparas: A graphicostatistical analysis. *Obstet. Gynecol.* 8:691, 1956.

Friedman, E. A. Primigravid labor: A graphicostatistical analysis, *Obstet. Gynecol.* 6:567, 1955.

Friedman, E. A. The functional divisions of labor. *Am. J. Obstet. Gynecol.* 109:274, 1971.

Gaskin, I. M. *Spiritual Midwifery,* Rev. Ed. Summertown, Tenn.: The Book Publishing Company, 1977.

Gimbel, J., and Nocon, J. J. The physiological basis for the Leboyer approach to childbirth. *J. Obstet. Gynecol. Neonat. Nurs.* 6:11, 1977.

Greenhill, J. P., and Friedman, E. A. *Biological Principles and Modern Practice of Obstetrics*. Philadelphia: Saunders, 1974.

Hamlin, R. H. J. *Stepping Stones to Labour Ward Diagnosis*. Adelaide, Australia: Rigby Limited, 1959.

Haverkamp, A. et al. The evaluation of continuous fetal heart monitoring in high-risk pregnancy. *Am. J. Obstet. Gynecol.* 125(3):310–320, June 1, 1976.

Hellman, L. M., and Pritchard, J. A. *Williams Obstetrics, 15th*. New York: Appleton-Century-Crofts, 1976.

Hendricks, C. H. The hemodynamics of a uterine contraction, *Am. J. Obstet. Gynecol.* 76:969, 1958.

Highley, B. L., and Mercer, R. T. Safeguarding the laboring woman's sense of control. *Am. J. Maternal Child Nurse.* 3:39, 1978.

Hon, E. H. *An Introduction to Fetal Heart Monitoring, 2nd*. North Haven, Conn.: Corometrics Medical Systems, 1975.

Hon, E. H., and Paul, R. H. *A Primer of Fetal Heart Rate Patterns*. North Haven, Conn.: Corometrics Medical Systems, 1970.

Intrapartum Module. Nurse-Midwifery Education Program, University of Mississippi Medical Center, Jackson, Mississippi (Baton Rouge draft), 1976.

Kier, J. *Woman's Guide to a Stress-Free Pregnancy and Creative Childbirth*. Houston, Texas: Butterfly Books, 1985.

Kitzinger, S., and Simkin, P. *Episiotomy and the Second Stage of Labor*. Seattle, Wash.: Pennypress, 1984.

Leboyer, F. *Birth without Violence*. New York: Knopf, 1976.

Lesser, M. S., and Keane, V. R. *Nurse-Patient Relationships in a Hospital Maternity Service*. St. Louis: Mosby, 1956.

Lynaugh, K. H. The effects of early elective amniotomy on the length of labor and the condition of the fetus. *J. Nurse-Midwifery* 25(4):3–9 (July/August) 1980.

MacLaughlin, S. M., and Taubenheim, A. M. A comparison of prepared and unprepared first-time fathers' needs during the childbirth experience. *J. Nurse-Midwifery* 28(2):9–16 (March/April) 1983.

Merkatz, I. R. et al. An association between low maternal serum a-fetoprotein and fetal chromosomal abnormalities. *Am. J. Obstet. Gynecol.* 148(7):886–894, April 1, 1984.

Miller, J., Williams, H. B., and Macarthur, J. L. Hemoglobin changes in labor and the puerperium. *Am. J. Obstet. Gynecol.* 78:303, 1959.

Morton, R., and Chesley, L. C. Intrapartum proteinuria. *Obstet. Gynecol.* 7:373, 1956.

Myles, M. F. *Textbook for Midwives, 8th*. London: Livingstone, 1975.

Noble, E. *Childbirth with Insight*. Boston: Houghton Mifflin, 1983.

Noble, E. Controversies in maternal effort during labor and delivery. *J. Nurse-Midwifery.* 26(2):13–22 (March/April) 1981.

Oxorn, H., and Foote, W. R. *Human Labor & Birth, 3rd*. New York: Appleton-Century-Crofts, 1975.

Parer, J. T., and Dulock, H. L. (Eds.) *Intrapartum Evaluation of the Fetus*. Supplemental issue, *J. Obstet. Gynecol. Neonat. Nurs.* 5(5), (September/October) 1978.

Paul, R. H., and Petrie, R. H. *Fetal Intensive Care*. Wallingford, Conn.: Corometrics Medical Systems, 1981.

Peterson, G. *Birthing Normally: A Personal Growth Approach to Childbirth, 2nd*. Berkeley, Calif.: Mindbody Press, 1984.

Pritchard, J. A., MacDonald, P. C. and Gant, N. F. *Williams Obstetrics, 17th*. Norwalk, Conn.: Appleton-Century-Crofts, 1985.

Reid, D. E., Ryan, K. J., and Benirschke, K. *Principles and Management of Human Reproduction*. Philadelphia: Saunders, 1972.

Roberts, J. Alternative positions for childbirth. Part 1. First stage of labor. *J. Nurse-Midwifery* 25(4): 11–18 (July/August) 1980.

Roberts, J. Alternative positions for childbirth. Part 2. Second stage of labor. *J. Nurse-Midwifery* 25(5): 13. (September/October) 1980.

Roberts, J. E., and Kriz, D. M. Delivery positions and perineal outcome. *J. Nurse-Midwifery* 29(3): 186–190 (May/June) 1984.

Schrag, K. Maintenance of pelvic floor integrity during childbirth. *J. Nurse-Midwifery* 24(6):26–31 (November/December) 1979.

Schwarz, R. H. (Moderator). Symposium: Managing premature rupture of membranes. *Contemporary OB/GYN* 8:140, 1976.

Shearer, M. H. Some deterrents to objective evaluation of fetal monitors. *Birth Family J.* 2:58, 1975.

Taylor, E. S. *Beck's Obstetrical Practice, 9th*. Baltimore: Williams & Wilkins, 1971.

Taylor, E. S. *Beck's Obstetrical Practice and Fetal Medicine, 10th*. Baltimore: Williams & Wilkins, 1977.

Taylor, P. M., Bright, N. H., and Birchard, E. L. Effect of early versus delayed clamping of the umbilical cord on the clinical condition of the newborn infant. *Am. J. Obstet. Gynecol.* 86:893, 1963.

Thoms, H., Roth, L. G., and Linton, D. *Understanding Natural Childbirth.* New York: McGraw-Hill, 1950.

Wiedenbach, E. *Clinical Nursing — A Helping Art.* New York: Springer, 1964.

Wiedenbach, E. *Family-Centered Maternity Nursing, 2nd.* New York: G. P. Putnam's Sons, 1967.

Williams, H. V. (idem: Burst). Unpublished presentation: Workshop on Labor and Delivery Care.

American College of Obstetrics and Gynecology Conference on Obstetric, Gynecologic and Neonatal Nursing, 1965.

Wynn, R. M. (Translator of original article by Ferdinand August Max Franz von Ritgen, 1855). XXIII. Concerning his method for protection of the perineum. *Am. J. Obstet. Gynecol.* 93:421, 1965.

Yeates, D. A., and Roberts, J. E. A comparison of two bearing-down techniques during the second stage of labor. *J. Nurse-Midwifery* 29(1):3–11 (January/February) 1984.

Ziegel, E., and VanBlarcom, C. C. *Obstetric Nursing, 6th.* New York: Macmillan, 1972.

14

Screening for and Collaborative Management of Selected Variations of Normal, Abnormality, and Complications During the First and Second Stages of Labor

Coauthored by
Therese A. Dondero, C.N.M.
Director, Midwifery Service
North Central Bronx Hospital
Bronx, New York

This chapter includes conditions and complications which actually may occur before or without labor (e.g., premature rupture of membranes, umbilical cord prolapse). The more common complications of labor are discussed in this chapter. No effort has been made to differentiate them by stage of labor because most of them can occur in either the first or second stage.

The nurse-midwife must be familiar with these complications in order to recognize their development or existence as early as possible. The nurse-midwife then enters into a collaborative relationship with the consulting physician for the management of care of patients with these conditions. In addition to contributing to the medical management of care the nurse-midwife also contributes patient advocacy, provides continuity of care, protects the normal labor process insofar as possible, and promotes family-centered care and alter-native safe labor birth options (including delivery by the nurse-midwife) appropriate to the situation.

This chapter reflects the fact that there are usually progressive levels of intervention in the recognition and evolution of the complicated clinical situation. The nurse-midwife should evaluate the need for each intervention, the safety of nonintervention, the disruption in the normal process an intervention will cause, and the risk-benefit ratio of intervention and nonintervention. Some of the complications discussed in this chapter alter the normal physiological condition of the mother and the environment for the fetus. Because of this altered condition and environment the normal reserve of the mother and the fetus is compromised, thereby dictating the need for earlier and more agressive intervention than is indicated for a normal progressive labor.

Other complications, rarely seen in obstetric

practice and having the characteristics of being either so catastrophic that there is no question of urgent need for a physician (e.g., amniotic fluid embolism) or rather esoteric causes of other complications for which physician consultation will have already been sought, are not included. Examples of this latter category include Bandl's retraction ring, or pathologic uterine constriction rings, and causes and results of cervical dystocia including cervical rigidity, conglutination of the cervix, cervical stenosis, and annular detachment of the cervix, all of which would cause failure or lack of progress in labor and earlier consultation for dysfunctional labor. The nurse-midwifery student who is interested in these more esoteric complications is encouraged to pursue this interest in medical obstetric textbooks and journals.

PREVIOUS CESAREAN SECTION

The management of care of women who have had one or more previous cesarean sections has undergone a revolution in the past several years. From an earlier "once a section, always a section" philosophy, cautious attempts at vaginal birth after cesarean section (VBAC) in highly selected women came into practice in the early 1970s. Today all women with previous low transverse cesarean sections should be encouraged to labor rather than have a planned repeat cesarean section.

The risk to a woman having a vaginal birth who has had a previous cesarean section is related to the type of uterine incision and in some instances to the gestational age at which the section was performed. The crucial piece of information is whether or not the incision was transverse and in the lower uterine segment. Any incision that extends into the uterine muscle mass of the uterine corpus or fundus increases the risk of uterine rupture. Since the lower uterine segment is poorly developed in early gestation, a cesarean section done before

28 weeks without labor necessarily involves the corpus muscle mass, even with a low transverse incision. Safety of a subsequent vaginal delivery in such a situation is thus questionable, especially if there had been no labor. With labor the lower uterine segment develops even in second trimester.

The risk to a woman of having a repeat cesarean section is the increased morbidity and mortality associated with cesarean section. This risk is statistically outweighed for those women with classical scars (described below) but not for women with low transverse scars:

There are two types of cesarean sections:(1) the classical section, which involves a vertical uterine incision, and (2) a low transverse (horizontal) uterine incision. There are variations of these two basic incisions referred to as the inverted-T incision and the low vertical incision, which is a classical incision that does not extend into the fundus. The risk of subsequent uterine rupture is directly related to the type of uterine scar. For women who have had a previous low transverse uterine incision the risk of uterine rupture is between 0.25 percent and 0.6 percent. For women with a previous classical, inverted-T, or low vertical incision, the risk of uterine rupture both before the onset of labor and during labor is much higher (approximately 2 percent prior to labor and 5 percent during labor).

Rupture of a low transverse uterine incision, if it occurs, is not generally catastrophic or life threatening to either the mother or the baby. Such a rupture is usually no more than a dehiscence of the old scar and an incidental finding during uterine exploration following a vaginal birth or during an elected repeat cesarean section. To be life threatening, dehiscence of a uterine scar needs either to extend into the rich blood supply found in the uterine corpus and fundus or to disrupt the placenta, which is normally located in the uterine fundus. Because of these possibilities VBAC is not attempted for women with classical, inverted-T, or low vertical scars. VBAC, however, is a safe procedure for those with previous low transverse uterine incisions. Further, the significance of the following as they relate to uterine rupture is minimal:

1. Number of previous cesarean sections
2. Interval of time since the last cesarean section
3. Any intervening vaginal deliveries

Management options for labor and delivery are discussed during the prenatal period. This discussion starts upon observation, during the initial visit, that the woman has undergone a previous cesarean section. The data base obtained during the initial visit includes:

1. History
   a. type of cesarean section
   b. reason for cesarean section
   c. length of labor
   d. weeks gestation at time of cesarean section
2. Physical examination
   a. abdominal scar (describe)
3. Pelvic examination
   a. clinical pelvimetry
   b. nonparous cervix and vaginal introitus if all previous babies have been delivered by cesarean section

You should obtain the record of the previous labor and surgery. A copy of the labor record is quite revealing and helpful in the subsequent labor.

If the previous incision was low transverse, the management options are (1) a scheduled, elective repeat cesarean section, (2) an elective repeat cesarean section after the onset of labor, or (3) a vaginal delivery. If the previous uterine incision was classical, inverted-T, or low vertical, then a repeat section without labor is the management. The options available to the woman should be reviewed with her, along with a discussion of the risks and benefits of a repeat cesarean section versus a VBAC. Docu-

mentation that this discussion has taken place should be recorded in the chart.

If a woman chooses to have a scheduled elective repeat cesarean section without waiting for the onset of labor it may be necessary to confirm fetal maturity by early ultrasound or late amniocentesis for fetal lung maturity, or both, in order to avoid iatrogenic prematurity. These interventions are avoided if the woman enters spontaneous labor prior to the repeat section.

If a woman chooses to have a vaginal birth she will have some special needs for support in her decision. Referral to a special VBAC course or support group may help her overcome any negative feelings and fears she has from her previous experience. Support throughout the antepartal course is especially important when there are family members who might be skeptical about the woman's decision. Body image, fear of failure, and self-image as a woman should be explored antepartally by the nurse-midwife.

The nurse-midwife should be cautious in labeling a woman a poor candidate for vaginal delivery on the basis of a previous diagnosis of cephalopelvic disproportion (CPD). Many diagnoses of cephalopelvic disproportion have been made which do not reflect actual CPD but, rather, an unknown reason for failure to progress in labor. Approximately 30 to 40 percent of women with a previous cesarean section for CPD (or failure to progress) will deliver vaginally in a subsequent pregnancy, and deliver babies larger than the one for which CPD was the diagnosis.

Discussion with your consulting physician regarding a woman with a previous cesarean section should include your findings, your discussion with the woman, and her decision about delivery. Depending on policy, your physician consultant may or may not have to be present for labor or delivery of this woman. Delivery should be in the hospital.

A candidate for VBAC should be allowed to labor normally. She may have a psychological milestone to overcome at the point in labor at which she experienced the difficulties which led to the previous cesarean section. Also, from this point she will subsequently progress like a primigravida if she has never delivered vaginally. Thus it is important to note the point in the previous labor at which arrest or difficulty occurred as this is the point in the present labor where progress might be slow or nonexistent. Support and exploration of fear of failure is essential when that point in labor is reached.

Management of care of the VBAC woman in labor and for delivery is the same as for any woman in labor (see Chapters 10, 11, 12, and 13). There are some clinicians who believe the woman should have an intravenous line and fluids, should have all food and fluids withheld, and should be internally monitored in the event she is the rare person who will have a catastrophic uterine rupture requiring an immediate emergency repeat cesarean section. Other clinicians believe these precautions are not necessary. There is also disagreement about the use of pitocin for induction or augmentation of labor. Some clinicians emphasize the potential danger of pitocin contractions, while others believe that if labor is not contraindicated, pitocin is not contraindicated. Most clinicians do not advocate the use of epidurals because the signs and symptoms of uterine rupture may be masked or confused. All interventions should be evaluated as any interventions are evaluated for safety and interference with normal labor progress and mechanisms. The woman should be more closely monitored for the signs and symptoms of uterine rupture (see page 338).

In management of the third stage of labor it is useful to remember that there is an increased incidence that the placenta may be implanted over the uterine scar. This leads to an increased incidence of placenta accreta. For this reason, in the event of a retained placenta you may wish to ask your consulting physician to attempt the manual removal of the placenta rather than do it yourself.

The performance of manual exploration of the uterine cavity immediately after birth to rule out scar dehiscence is another area of controversy. The individual situation and events during labor should be considered and discussion as to the absolute necessity of this procedure explored with your consulting physician. The management of scar dehiscence following vaginal birth, if asymptomatic, is to do nothing as the defect will heal itself by six weeks postpartum.

PRETERM LABOR

Preterm, or premature, labor is labor commencing any time after the 20th week of gestation and up to the 37th week of gestation by dates.

Preterm birth is the leading cause of perinatal morbidity and mortality. Premature birth occurs in 6 percent to 10 percent of all pregnancies in the United States. It accounts for 75 percent of all perinatal deaths and up to 50 percent of the neurologic handicaps found in infancy. The incidence of premature birth varies among different populations, with the lowest incidence in the socioeconomically more advantaged sector and the highest incidence occurring in the medically indigent population. This higher frequency of preterm labor among low-socioeconomic women is probably due to poor nutrition and inadequate prenatal care.

Any woman who has delivered prematurely in a past pregnancy has a 25 to 50 percent risk of recurrence of premature birth. It is sometimes difficult to distinguish, from the history of birth weight and supposed months of gestation, whether a previous infant was preterm or growth-retarded. Therefore, an attempt should be made to obtain the medical records for any woman who has had a previous infant weighing less than 2500 grams or who has delivered prior to 36 weeks gestation.

Management of preterm labor is predicated on first identifying the woman at risk for this complication. Predisposing factors include:

1. Lower socioeconomic status
2. Poor nutritional status (low prepregnancy weight, weight gain less than 10 pounds by the 20th week of gestation, weight loss, inadequate protein and calorie intake: see Chapter 8)
3. Previous history of a premature labor or birth
4. Multiple gestation
5. Cigarette smoking
6. Use of street drugs
7. Alcohol abuse
8. Urinary tract infections
9. Hemoglobinopathies
10. Sudden, severe stress
11. Second trimester induced abortions
12. Premature rupture of the membranes
13. Uterine anomalies
14. High maternal fever: 38.4°C (101°F) or greater
15. Abdominal surgery
16. Incompetent cervix
17. Inadequate prenatal care

There is some thought that vaginitis causes some degree of uterine activity that may predispose the untreated woman to premature labor.

Screening, therefore, consists of identification both of the predisposing factors for preterm labor during routine prenatal care and of the signs and symptoms of preterm labor. The signs and symptoms of preterm labor are as follows:

1. Painful menstrual-like cramps — may be confused with round ligament pain
2. Dull low backache — different from the usual low backache a pregnant woman may have
3. Suprapubic pain or pressure — may be confused with urinary tract infection
4. Sensation of pelvic pressure or heaviness
5. Change in character or amount of vaginal discharge (thicker, thinner, watery, bloody, brown, colorless)
6. Diarrhea

7. Unpalpated contractions felt more often than every 10 minutes for 1 hour or more and not relieved by lying down
8. Premature rupture of the membranes

The signs and symptoms of preterm labor should be included as a routine part of prenatal patient education around 20 to 24 weeks of gestation.

A woman with a history of one previous premature labor or birth and no signs and symptoms of preterm labor in this gestation should have the following done in relation to the other predisposing factors, in addition to routine screening for complications:

1. Monthly screening for asymptomatic bacteriuria
2. Treatment of any vaginal and cervical infections
3. Diet history and appropriate nutritional counseling
4. Reinforcement of routine instructions about the signs and symptoms of preterm labor
5. Counseling, if necessary, regarding cigarette, drug, and alcohol use
6. Encouragement to communicate if she is having personal stresses in order to obtain appropriate help with stress reduction

If a woman has a history of two or more previous premature labors or births, or has a multiple gestation, and shows no signs and symptoms of preterm labor, then in addition to the above the following should be done:

1. Vaginal examination every 2 weeks for cervical changes in position, consistency, effacement, and dilatation, and station of the presenting part
2. Change and/or reduction in workload if job involves heavy lifting, pushing, or pulling, long hours, or rotating shifts
3. Use of condoms during sexual intercourse to prevent prostaglandin in the semen from causing uterine irritability

A woman with signs and symptoms of preterm labor, with or without any predisposing factors, should be seen immediately. You should notify your consulting physician and make the following assessment:

1. History
   a. signs and symptoms of preterm labor
   b. signs and symptoms of urinary tract infection
   c. signs and symptoms of vaginitis or cervicitis
   d. signs and symptoms of viral or bacterial infection
   e. signs and symptoms of premature rupture of membranes
2. Physical examination
   a. vital signs (especially temperature and pulse)
   b. evaluation of gestational age
   c. evaluation of contractions*
   d. evaluation of fetal heart rate*
   e. abdominal palpation for presentation, position, multiple gestation, estimated fetal weight, and assessment of abdominal pain
   f. costovertebral angle tenderness
   g. assessment of low back pain and suprapubic pain

* How evaluation of the contractions and fetal heart rate is done may vary from place to place by institutional policy but it should be remembered that external electronic fetal monitoring involves encircling straps which may cause uterine irritability and increase contractility.

3. Pelvic examination
   a. speculum examination for evaluation of any existing vaginitis or cervicitis, premature rupture of membranes, bloody show, meconium
   b. digital examination for evaluation of any existing cervical changes and of the station of the presenting part (not done if premature rupture of membranes is diagnosed upon speculum examination)
4. Laboratory tests
   a. *stat.* microscopic urinalysis
   b. urine culture and sensitivity
   c. wet mount of any vaginal discharge
   d. complete blood count (CBC) and differential (if has signs and symptoms of infection)
   e. fern test
   f. nitrazine test

An accurate diagnosis of preterm labor is critical to determine the appropriate treatment. Contractions alone are not enough to diagnose preterm labor. A diagnosis of preterm labor is made between 20 and 37 weeks gestation by dates when there are (1) uterine contractions (frequency of at least every 10 minutes) and ruptured membranes or (2) uterine contractions (frequency of at least every 10 minutes) and intact membranes and progressive cervical change over several hours of observation.

Women with signs and symptoms possibly indicative of preterm labor should be collaboratively managed with your consulting physician in the hospital. Management of care includes bed rest (left lateral position), hydration, and treatment of any infection until uterine activity no longer meets the definition of preterm labor and there is no evidence of progressive cervical change or ruptured membranes. If these criteria are achieved, the woman is then sent home with the following instructions:

1. Limit activity — curtail working hours in a nonstrenuous and nonstressful job, or take a leave of absence from a strenuous or stressful job; do no heavy housework.
2. Arrange for support systems for household and child care responsibilities.
3. Engage in no sexual activity until reevaluation in 1 week. Resumption of sexual activity depends on uterine activity and the presence of any predisposing factors to preterm labor. If sexual activity is sub-

sequently resumed, condoms should be used. If resumption of sexual activity causes an increase or recurrence of uterine contractions, the couple should be advised to abstain from sexual intercourse or other sexual activity that leads to orgasm in the woman.

4. Return for routine prenatal care and reevaluation for preterm labor in 1 week. Continuation of routine prenatal care is every other week until 36 weeks and then weekly. In the event of a recurrence of the signs and symptoms of preterm labor, immediate reevaluation should be done and weekly visits initiated.

5. Continue to follow previous instructions on nutrition, signs and symptoms of preterm labor, stress reduction, and use of cigarettes, drugs, and alcohol.

Women who meet the definition of preterm labor who are less than 4 centimeters dilated and less than 34 weeks gestation are candidates for tocolysis. Tocolysis is the use of medication which will inhibit uterine contractions. Varous tocolytic agents are available to attempt to stop uterine contractions (e.g., ritodrine, magnesium sulfate, terbutaline). If these agents are to be successful, accurate early diagnosis of premature labor must be made. Close collaboration with your consulting physician is needed to develop a comprehensive plan of care for a woman should premature labor occur.

The first line of action, however, takes place during the observation period when assessing the woman for preterm labor. During this time a woman may respond positively to simple bed rest and hydration. If she does not respond positively to bed rest and hydration or if she is in obvious progressive labor upon admission to the hospital, your consulting physician may decide to initiate tocolysis. The woman should first be carefully screened for contraindications to tocolysis. Contraindications include:

1. Vaginal bleeding

2. Pregnancy-induced hypertension
3. Dead fetus or major fetal malformation incompatible with survival
4. Intrauterine infection
5. Cardiac disease
6. Hyperthyroidism
7. Diabetes
8. Pulmonary hypertension
9. Preexisting maternal medical conditions that would be seriously affected by the known pharmacologic properties of a betamimetic drug (e.g., hypovolemia, cardiac arrhythmias associated with tachycardia or digitalis intoxication, uncontrolled hypertension, pheochromocytoma, and bronchial asthma already treated by betamimetics or steroids)
10. Known hypersensitivity to any component of the product
11. Elderly multiparas (because of potential for myocardial insufficiency)

In addition to screening for contraindications, the nurse-midwife obtains necessary baseline laboratory data (CBC and complete chemistries: kidney and liver function tests, glucose levels). During the initiation of the intravenously administered tocolytic agent, the nurse-midwife monitors the woman for maternal tachycardia, cardiac arrhymias, hypotension, chest pain or tightness, and other possible side effects (tremors, palpitations, nervousness, restlessness). A record of intake and output is started.

The danger with tocolytic drugs is pulmonary edema and myocardial infarction. Maternal tachycardia above 130 beats per minute is considered a first warning of myocardial complications, and an EKG should be obtained if this occurs. The dosage is reduced if unacceptable side effects result, until a tolerable level is found. The infusion is stopped if labor progresses despite treatment at the maximum tolerated dose.

If the tocolytic agent is tolerated, the infusion is continued 12 to 24 hours after the contractions stop. During this time the fetal heart rate, uterine contractions, and the maternal blood pressure and pulse rate are monitored and recorded hourly. Intake and output are recorded every 4 hours. Ongoing laboratory tests include a hematocrit every 4 hours and electrolytes and blood glucose every day because of the metabolic effects of the drugs. Successful intravenous therapy may be followed by oral maintenance doses of the tocolytic agent, begun while the woman is still receiving the intravenous tocolytic. The intravenous medication is reduced as the oral tocolytic is administered. The oral preparation is continued until 34 weeks gestation — or until premature labor again ensues, whereupon intravenous tocolysis is begun.

Treatment of premature labor depends upon gestational age, underlying maternal disease, and the status of the membranes. The risk-benefit ratio must be carefully weighed in considering the use of tocolytic agents. These drugs are extremely toxic and may produce dangerous side effects in the mother. Undoubtedly the fetus experiences the same side effects as the mother. Also, there is some question of the effectiveness of the tocolytic drugs, as the literature contains conflicting reports. The question then becomes one of environment: is the fetus better off in the uterus or outside the uterus? Thus, should labor be allowed to proceed or should a potentially unsafe and possibly ineffective effort be made to stop it?

Women receiving tocolytics for preterm labor require intensive support to help them overcome the physical side effects of the drugs. Continuous monitoring and support by the nurse-midwife to help alleviate the anxiety produced by these side effects contributes to the success of the tocolysis.

When labor is successfully inhibited with tocolysis, monitoring at home and during prenatal visits may be done by the nurse-midwife. Continued education and observation are required to see this woman to term, if possible.

With all women at risk for premature labor,

care must be taken not to produce extreme anxiety as this in and of itself has been implicated as a causative factor. Certainly, for a woman who has delivered prematurely in the past, the subsequent pregnancy will be fraught with anxiety. Your screening and instructions to the woman, if done appropriately, will decrease this anxiety. You should attempt to make her feel that she has some degree of control over, and contribution to, the situation. This is done through trusting her suspicions and her reports about her observations of any important changes. Availability of telephone contact with you to allay fears or review her uneasiness about what she is feeling will help her to feel that she is a valued participant in her care.

Nurse-midwifery management of preterm labor is conducted in collaboration with the consulting physician. This collaborative management includes the following:

1. Reaching a decision regarding the route of delivery. This decision is based on the presentation and gestational age.
2. Giving no analgesic, ataractic, or sedative medication prior to delivery.
3. Maintaining careful monitoring of the fetus during labor. A preterm baby has less reserve to tolerate the stresses of labor.
4. Carefully weighing the usefulness of internal electronic fetal monitoring against the dangers involved in application of the scalp clip. The preterm fetus has wider fontanels and a different skull bone density and consistency. The decision is based on real need for internal electronic fetal monitoring and on gestational age.
5. Administering pudendal block or local infiltration anesthesia (or both) if cutting an episiotomy. Epidural anesthesia by a physician is all right.
6. Making an episiotomy if you determine the need for one. The need for an episiotomy depends on the estimated fetal weight and the relaxation of the perineum.

7. Arranging for the pediatrician to be notified and present at delivery.
8. Making provisions for keeping the baby warm and for transporting the baby if necessary and if the delivery does not take place in a Level III hospital.

PREMATURE RUPTURE OF THE MEMBRANES

Premature rupture of the membranes (PROM) may be technically defined as rupture of the membranes prior to the onset of labor, regardless of gestational age. In practice and in research, however, premature rupture of the membranes is defined in accord with the number of hours that elapse from the time of rupture until the onset of labor. This interval is called the latent period and may last 1 to 6 or 12 or more hours. The absence of a uniformly accepted method of establishing the diagnosis of premature rupture of the membranes makes comparison of studies difficult and results in the lack of a standard operational definition. The incidence of premature rupture of the membranes is 2.7 percent to 17 percent, depending on the length of the latent period used in making the diagnosis.

The incidence of premature rupture of the membranes is higher when there is polyhydramnios, fetal malpresentation, or multiple gestation. Possible complications resulting from premature rupture of the membranes include premature labor, intrauterine infection, and prolapsed umbilical cord.

Since the risk of intrauterine infection (chorioamnionitis) is increased with rupture of the membranes, it is important for you to make an accurate diagnosis without increasing the risk of infection. Leakage of amniotic fluid has to be differentiated from urinary incontinence, vaginal or cervical discharge, semen, or (rarely) rupture of the chorion. The diagnosis is made by the following:

1. History
   a. amount of fluid loss — rupture of the membranes may initially cause a large gush of fluid followed by a continuous discharge. In some instances of ruptured membranes, however, the only symptoms noted by the woman may be a small, continuous discharge (clear, cloudy, yellow, or green) and a feeling of moistness on her panties.
   b. inability to control leakage with Kegel exercises — differentiates from urinary incontinence.
   c. time of rupture.
   d. color of fluid — amniotic fluid can be clear or cloudy; if meconium stained it will be yellow or green.
   e. odor of fluid — amniotic fluid has a distinct musty odor which differentiates it from urine.
   f. last sexual intercourse — expulsion of semen from the vagina can sometimes be mistaken as amniotic fluid.
2. Physical examination
   a. abdominal palpation to ascertain amniotic fluid volume. When there is a frank rupture of the membranes it is possible to detect the decrease in fluid because there is increased molding of the uterus and abdominal wall around the fetus and decreased ballottability compared to examination findings before rupture of the membranes. Leaking membranes do not give these same changes in abdominal findings.
3. Sterile speculum examination
   a. inspection of the external genitalia for signs of fluid.
   b. visualization of the cervix for a flow of fluid from the os.
   c. visualization of pooling of amniotic fluid in the vaginal vault.
   d. if fluid is not seen, have the woman bear down (valsalva maneuver), or exert gentle fundal pressure, or gently elevate the presenting part abdominally to allow

fluid to pass by the presenting part in the event of a high leak so observation of the leaking fluid can be made.

    e. observation of any fluid for the presence of lanugo or vernix caseosa if the pregnancy is further than 32 weeks gestation.

4. Laboratory tests

    a. positive fern test — ferning, also called arborization, on a microscope slide is due to the presence of sodium chloride and protein in amniotic fluid. (During the sterile speculum examination, use a sterile cotton swab to obtain a specimen of the fluid either from the posterior vaginal fornix or directly from the fluid exuding from the cervical os. Smear the specimen on a microsope slide and allow to dry thoroughly. Inspect under a microscope for a fern pattern.)

    b. positive nitrazine paper test — this mustard-gold pH-sensitive paper will turn dark blue in the presence of alkaline material. The normal pH of the vagina during pregnancy is 4.5 to 5.5; the pH of amniotic fluid is 7.0 to 7.5. (Place a piece of nitrazine paper against the blade of the speculum after withdrawing the speculum from the vagina.)

The fern test is more reliable than the nitrazine paper test. This is because a number of materials besides amniotic fluid have an alkaline pH, including cervical mucus, blood, urine, and glove powder. Thus, if a specimen is taken directly from the cervical os and then smeared on nitrazine paper, a false-positive color change may result.

The earlier an examination is performed after the rupture occurs, the easier it is to diagnose ruptured membranes. When more than 6 to 12 hours pass, many of the diagnostic observations become unreliable because of lack of fluid. Observation of fluid coming from the cervical os is diagnostic of ruptured membranes. In the absence of direct visualization of fluid from the os, a history strongly suggestive of rupture, with a positive fern test, is diagnostic.

The other action the nurse-midwife takes during the initial evaluation of the woman for diagnosis of ruptured membranes is to do a cervical culture for group B beta-hemolytic streptococci. Even though a preliminary report will not be available for 24 hours (48 hours for a final report), this action will provide the pediatrician with the earliest possible data for management of the newborn. Some laboratories with special laboratory techniques are able to give cervical culture results in 6 to 8 hours. If the results are positive for group B beta-hemolytic streptococci and the woman is not yet in labor or has not yet delivered, this information will influence management of care to effect delivery as rapidly as possible. Some clinicians will also start antibiotics.

The incidence of chorioamnionitis increases in direct relationship to the number of pelvic examinations performed. Therefore, the fewer examinations performed the less risk there is of chorioamnionitis developing. For example, the palpation of forewaters does not preclude the existence of ruptured membranes with a high leak. A digital examination, therefore, during the initial examination only exposes the woman to an unnecessary increase in risk of infection. Your plan of management should include the knowledge that 80 to 85 percent of women of all gestations with premature rupture of the membranes will be in labor within 24 hours. Another 10 percent will be in labor within 72 hours. This leaves 5 percent whose latent period will be longer than 72 hours. The infection rate in the first 24 hours for pregnancies 37–42 weeks gestation has been reported variously from 1.6 percent to 29 percent depending on race, socioeconomic factors, receipt of prenatal care, and gestational age. In term pregnancies, there is an increase in the incidence of intrapartal fever if the latent period from rupture of membranes to onset of labor is more than 24 hours. If this latent period is in excess of 72 hours, there is a significant increase in perinatal mortality. In pregnancies less than 37 weeks gestation, however, the rates vary according to gestational age and the risks associated with prematurity are much greater than the risk of infection due to premature rupture of the membranes.

The ongoing debate over management options emanates from this information. One management option is to accomplish delivery within 24 hours of rupture of the membranes, since this is the time of greatest risk. The cesarean section rate for women at term who are induced in order to effect delivery in 24 hours is between 30 and 50 percent. Since most women at term will go into spontaneous labor within the first 24 hours after rupture of the membranes, another management option is to await the onset of spontaneous labor while observing the woman closely for signs and symptoms of chorioamnionitis.

In either management option, the performance of an initial digital examination to determine cervical dilatation is unnecessary since knowledge of the cervical findings is superfluous to the management. If the plan is for an induction in order to effect delivery within the first 24 hours, digital examination can be done at the time of induction. Determination of the presenting part is a useful piece of information to obtain by vaginal examination *if* this information cannot be acquired by abdominal palpation. In the presence of a breech presentation, digital examination for prolapsed umbilical cord is probably of greater importance than the risk of infection. If the fetal heart rate pattern is abnormal, a vaginal examination to rule out cord prolapse is warranted.

When the management plan is to deliver the woman within 24 hours of rupture of the membranes, a 12-hour leeway is usually given for the woman to enter spontaneous labor before pitocin induction is started. During this 12 hours other methods of inducing labor are used, such as castor oil (2 ounces), nipple stimulation, rupture of forewaters, or all of these. Sexual intercourse is contraindicated because of the premature rupture of membranes. Notify your physician consultant of the situation.

In either management option the management of labor care is the same as any other labor, with the following additions:

1. Assess temperature and pulse every 2 hours.
2. Count the fetal heart rate every hour as long as it remains normal. Tachycardia is indicative of intrauterine infection. Closer monitoring of the fetal heart is done during pitocin induction, either by taking the fetal heart rate after *each* contraction and listening through a contraction every 15 minutes or by continuous electronic fetal heart monitoring.
3. Avoid unnecessary vaginal examinations.
4. When doing a vaginal examination note:
   a. whether the vaginal walls are unusually warm (hot) to touch.
   b. the odor of the discharge or fluid on your gloves.
   c. the color of the discharge or fluid on your gloves.

Scrupulous attention to hydration is important in order to have a clear picture of any developing infection, since there is often a temperature elevation with dehydration.

When the management option is to await the onset of spontaneous labor regardless of the number of hours that have elapsed since rupture of the membranes, expectant management of care of the woman at home may be appropriate. A woman being managed at home should have access to transportation and needs to have someone with her for support, to do the cleaning, and to run errands outside the house. She should also be at term and have no compounding medical or obstetrical risk factors, including malpresentation or unengaged cephalic presentation.

Regardless of the management option, monitoring for signs and symptoms of chorioamnionitis is imperative. A presumptive diagnosis of chorioamnionitis is made when there is premature rupture of membranes and the woman has a temperature of 38°C (100.4°F) or greater with no obvious cause for the temperature. Foul-smelling purulent amniotic fluid gives a definitive diagnosis of chorioamniotis.

Maternal temperature and pulse are taken every 4 hours (night included). Although the definition of febrile morbidity is a temperature elevation to 38°C (100.4°F), a woman with a slowly rising temperature should be carefully observed and active management initiated which is geared toward getting her delivered before she reaches true febrile morbidity.

Fetal heart tones should also be taken every 4 hours when the woman is in the hospital. Fetal tachycardia (160 beats per minute or greater) is a relatively good indication of possible chorioamnionitis. Nonstress tests are done every 2 days to weekly (varies with clinicians).

The woman should be evaluated daily for uterine tenderness; she can do this herself. Uterine tenderness prior to delivery, however, is a difficult sign to rely upon since it is so variable and unpredictable and mimicks uterine contractions.

A white blood cell count with differential should be done daily or every other day. An elevated maternal white blood cell count, especially when accompanied by a shift to the left in bands, indicates an infectious process. An elevated white blood cell count is a late sign of chorioamnionitis, because it is possible to have an early infectious process without an elevation in white blood cells.

A cervical culture for group B beta-hemolytic streptococci is done during the initial sterile speculum examination to diagnose ruptured membranes, and weekly thereafter. The finding of a positive cervical culture requires immediate induction and delivery, regardless of gestational age, as beta-hemolytic streptococcal infection is lethal in the newborn.

It must be emphasized again that vaginal examinations are not done, as the risk of chorio-amnionitis drastically multiplies with vaginal examination. For this same reason the woman should be advised to observe pelvic precautions — no vaginal therapeutics, no douches, no sexual intercourse. Some clinicians also advise against tub baths as an added measure of precaution.

When a preterm pregnancy (less than 37 weeks gestation) is complicated by premature rupture of membranes, the risk of sepsis is outweighed by the risks of prematurity. The primary cause of perinatal morbidity and mortality in this gestational age group is directly related to prematurity and not to sepsis. In preterm premature rupture of the membranes, especially if it occurs at less than 26 weeks of gestation, fetal lung hypoplasia and limb deformities may occur secondary to oligo-hydramnios.

The current recommendation for women with preterm premature rupture of the membranes is to await the onset of spontaneous labor while observing for signs and symptoms of chorioamnionitis. These women are usually admitted to the hospital and restricted to bed rest. In the event that there is no further leakage of amniotic fluid, there is a vertex presentation, and there are no signs or symptoms of chorio-amnionitis, the woman may be followed at home. She should be placed on pelvic precautions and bed rest, instructed in the principles of good hygiene, and instructed about her return visits for the necessary screening tests for chorioamnionitis. She will need at least a weekly return to the hospital for nonstress tests and cervical culture for beta streptococci, and in addition she will need to be seen for routine prenatal care. Arrangements can be made to have her blood drawn at home for the more frequent blood tests. A cervical culture for group B beta hemolytic streptococci is repeated every week because the latent period for the onset of labor in the preterm pregnancy with premature rupture of the membranes exceeds the latent period in the term pregnancy.

Preterm rupture of the membranes can be anxiety producing for the woman and her family. Fears accompanying the anticipated birth of a premature infant as well as the added risk of chorioamnionitis should be explored with the woman. The plan of management involving a prolonged period of bed rest and hospitalization should be discussed with the woman and her family. Their understanding and cooperation are important to the continuation of the pregnancy.

The performance of a digital vaginal examination increases the risk of infection, and is not necessary for those women with preterm rupture of the membranes since these women will be managed expectantly until labor ensues or there are signs or symptoms of chorioamnionitis. If the woman develops signs or symptoms of chorioamnionitis or has a positive cervical culture for group B beta-hemolytic streptococci, immediate consultation with your physician is indicated for induction of labor and delivery. The choice of delivery method (vaginal or cesarean section) is dependent upon the gestational age, presentation, and, if present, the severity of the chorioamnionitis.

At the time of delivery appropriate cultures should be obtained. These include cultures of the uterus, both maternal and fetal sides of the placenta, umbilical cord, and gastric aspirate from the newborn. Some pediatricians also culture the baby's skin or ears or both. The presence of the pediatrician at delivery is dependent on the length of time the membranes have been ruptured, the absence or presence of infection, and the protocol of the department of pediatrics in your institution. The perinatal mortality rate for all gestational ages when there is premature rupture of the membranes is 2.6 to 11 percent.

AMNIONITIS AND CHORIOAMNIONITIS

Amnionitis is inflammation of the amniotic sac and amnion. Chorioamnionitis is inflammation of the chorion in addition to the amnion and amniotic sac. These conditions almost always coexist.

Amnionitis and chorioamnionitis most often result when there has been prolonged rupture of the membranes (over 24 hours), with or without prolonged labor, with repeated vaginal examinations or manipulative vaginal or intrauterine procedures. Amnionitis and chorioamnionitis may also infrequently occur in women with intact membranes, for unknown reasons.

Both the mother and the baby will be infected, each with further resulting complications. The mother's uterine contractility is adversely affected in that it does not contract as well or respond to oxytocin. The infected woman has the potential for being very sick both intrapartally and postpartally (see Chapter 25). The infant may develop life-threatening intrauterine pneumonia and acidosis.

Signs and symptoms of amnionitis and chorioamnionitis are as follows:

1. Maternal fever
2. Maternal tachycardia
3. Fetal tachycardia
4. Tender uterus
5. Vaginal walls unusually warm (hot) to touch
6. Foul-smelling, purulent amniotic fluid
7. Elevated white blood cell count

After delivery the following additional information indicative of infection is available: steamy translucence of the umbilical cord and fetal membranes, and the presence of polymorphonuclear leukocytes in smears of gastric aspirate from the baby and of the chorionic surface of the amnion. The infant most likely will have an Apgar score below 7 and may have hypothermia.

Intrapartal management of the woman with amnionitis or chorioamnionitis has two goals: (1) to effect delivery as quickly as possible within a time limit of 6 to 8 hours and (2) to treat the infection. These goals are achieved through collaboration with your consulting physician. Labor management of a term pregnancy complicated with chorioamnionitis includes the following:

1. Setting a time limit for delivery. Failure to meet or come within reasonable attainment of this goal indicates need for cesarean section. Cesarean section is also indicated in the presence of worsening maternal or fetal condition.
2. Pitocin induction or augmentation to shorten the latent phase of labor.
3. Rupture of forewaters if present.
4. Internal electronic fetal monitoring.
5. Scalp pH in the presence of moderate to heavy meconium staining, with or without any kind of deceleration.
6. Hydration with intravenous D_5Ringer's lactate.
7. Monitoring of vital signs every hour
8. Notification of the pediatrician

If delivery is expected within 1 or 2 hours, intravenous antibiotic therapy for the mother may be delayed until immediately after delivery. This delay is elected because the antibiotics given the mother will interfere with the pediatrician's ability to identify the causative infecting agent in the newborn. Otherwise, if a worsening maternal condition warrants treatment, intravenous antibiotic therapy should be commenced during labor. Ampicillin is the usual antibiotic used. Dosage varies according to protocol.

Birth may be accomplished in bed in a delivery room which is fully equipped for neonatal resuscitation and regulation of hypothermia. The pediatrician should be present for the delivery, and appropriate cultures of the baby (gastric aspirate, skin, ears) and a cord pH should be obtained. Cultures should also be taken from the uterus, both maternal and fetal sides of the placenta, and the umbilical cord. Intravenous antibiotic therapy is continued for the mother until her symptoms of infection subside, after which she is given oral antibiotics.

UMBILICAL CORD PROLAPSE

Prolapse of the umbilical cord is a disaster requiring prompt and knowledgeable diagnosis and action while awaiting the arrival of the physician for final resolution of the problem by cesarean section.

There are two types of umbilical cord prolapse: (1) frank and (2) occult. In frank cord prolapse the cord slips through the cervix. In occult cord prolapse the cord slips down alongside the presenting part but does not protrude through the cervix. The danger in either type of cord prolapse is fetal hypoxia secondary to compression of the cord between the presenting part and the pelvis. Frank prolapse of the cord can occur without threatening life when there is a transverse lie or footling breech, because there is no compression of the cord. The route of delivery, however, is the same (cesarean section).

The precipitating causes of cord prolapse include the following:

1. Ruptured membranes and a breech presentation, compound presentation, transverse lie, or small fetus (less than 2000 grams)
2. Administration of an enema if the membranes are ruptured and the presenting part is an unengaged head, a compound presentation, an unengaged breech or footling breech, or a shoulder
3. Amniotomy if there is an unengaged head, a compound presentation, a noncephalic presentation, or a small fetus whose presenting part (either cephalic or breech) does not fill the pelvis
4. Careless vaginal examination in the presence of tense, bulging membranes and an unengaged head, a compound presentation, or noncephalic presentation

5. Spontaneous rupture of the membranes with an unengaged head, compound presentation, or noncephalic presentation

Any time the membranes rupture, your first action should be to check the fetal heart and then to perform a vaginal examination to feel for a prolapsed cord. A thorough vaginal examination includes not only feeling around the presenting part, the cervical edge at the juncture of the presenting part and the external cervical os, and in the vagina for a frank cord but also completely checking each of the vaginal fornices and feeling around and through the thinned-out lower uterine segment to palpate for an occult cord. Sometimes a cord is felt in the vagina. At other times you are summoned by auxiliary personnel or significant others because "something came out between her legs." Vaginal examination will differentiate a cord from a mucus plug, a prolapsed foot, or a prolapsed arm.

The following actions are taken in the presence of a prolapsed cord:

1. Place your entire hand into the woman's vagina and hold the presenting part up off the umbilical cord at the pelvic *inlet*.
2. Do not under any circumstances attempt to replace the cord — it won't work, excessive manipulation may cause cord spasm, and you may accidentally cause further cord compression.
3. Inform the woman of what has happened and elicit her cooperation.
4. Summon help. Warn the woman and, if necessary, yell to get attention if the call light is out of reach.
5. Have the physician given a *stat.* call.
6. Direct others to get the woman into a position where gravity will aid in the mechanics of keeping the baby away from the pelvic inlet and pressing on the cord: knee-chest or Trendelenburg position.
7. If the cord is protruding from the vagina, direct others to wrap it loosely in a towel which is wet with normal saline.

8. Direct others to make preparations for an emergency cesarean section.
9. Under no circumstances remove your hand from the woman's vagina or from the presenting part until the baby is delivered (probably by cesarean section).

Your first action is the one that will save the baby's life. Thereafter, you are inextricably joined to the mother until the baby is delivered and you can safely remove your hand from the woman's vagina. This will call for some gymnastics on your part when the woman assumes different positions, is moved to the operating room, and is prepared for surgery.

An alternate method can be used with an *unengaged* presenting part. This method is to insert a Foley catheter, fill the bladder with 500 cc of sterile water, and clamp the catheter while your hand is in the vagina displacing the fetal head off the umbilical cord. The full bladder then displaces the presenting part and alleviates the cord compression. This technique can also be used when the presenting part is engaged if the woman is a multipara. It will be necessary, however, for you to displace the presenting part out of the pelvis with your hand before filling the bladder. Pressure on the presenting part should be evenly distributed during this maneuver. Once the bladder is filled you should again check the woman vaginally to determine that the presenting part is indeed displaced. The fetal heart should be continually electronically monitored. If bradycardia recurs, reinsert your hand into the vagina to assure that the fetal head is off the cord.

ABNORMAL FETAL HEART RATES AND PATTERNS

The normal fetal heart rate levels and amount of variability were discussed under data base of the first stage of labor in Chapter 12. As stated there and further discussed in this section, a baseline fetal heart rate in the range of tachycardia or bradycardia, periodic heart rate changes (acceleration patterns, deceleration patterns), and either lack of heart rate variability or marked variability associated with periodic heart rate changes are abnormal. All abnormal fetal heart rates and patterns require immediate notification of the physician. Detection and identification of these abnormalities are essential.

Abnormal Fetal Heart Rates

Tachycardia

Moderate tachycardia is a baseline fetal heart rate level in the range of 161 to 180 beats per minute. Marked tachycardia is a baseline fetal heart rate level above 180 beats per minute.

Tachycardia alone may indicate the following:

1. Immaturity, especially of the autonomic nervous system in a preterm fetus
2. Maternal fever, especially that resulting from intrauterine infection (amnionitis and chorioamnionitis)
3. Mild fetal hypoxia — progressive rises in the baseline fetal heart rate to levels of tachycardia may be an early indicator of fetal distress
4. Drug effect, for example, from ritodrine or hydralazine (Apresoline) administered to the mother

Tachycardia combined with either late decelerations or prolonged variable decelerations, with or without meconium, is indicative of fetal distress. This is especially true if there is also a lack of variability. Tachycardia, meconium, and maternal fever are a particularly serious combination.

Bradycardia

Moderate bradycardia is a baseline fetal heart rate level in the range of 100 to 119 beats per minute. Marked bradycardia is a baseline fetal heart rate level below 100 beats per minute.

Bradycardia with variability is generally *not* clinically significant as an indicator of *fetal distress*. If fetal bradycardia occurs, however, you should assess for signs and symptoms of fetal distress, presence of a prolapsed cord, duration of severe bradycardia, and expected length of time to delivery. It is not uncommon to get a baseline bradycardia when the fetal head descends rapidly into the pelvis. The concern is that bradycardia that occurs at the end of labor not be interpreted as a reason for emergency operative delivery. Bradycardia that persists over a period of time during the pregnancy may be indicative of maternal drug effect, maternal hypoglycemia, or fetal congenital heart lesions. In these situations operative delivery may not always be indicated.

Minimal or Absent Variability (Irregularity)

Average variability in the fetal heart rate indicates that the autonomic nervous system controlling the fetal heart rate is mature and healthy. Less than average variability, that is, minimal or absent variability, indicates depression of the autonomic nervous system due to immaturity, congenital anomalies, medication given the mother, or conditions causing fetal anoxia and acidosis.

Minimal or absent variability may be an early indicator of fetal distress. When minimal or absent variability is combined with late deceleration, serious acute fetal distress is indicated. When minimal or absent variability coexists with both late deceleration and tachycardia, fetal distress of extreme magnitude is indicated.

Marked Variability

Marked variability, by itself, does not indicate fetal distress. Marked variability associated with periodic fetal heart rate changes, however, is not normal. While experts disagree on the significance of marked variability, it has been noted that a pattern of marked variability preceding minimal or absent variability is ominous.

Deceleration patterns

Deceleration patterns are periodic fetal heart rate changes which are associated with uterine contractions. There are three deceleration patterns — early, late, and variable — which derive their names from when they begin in relation to when the corresponding uterine contraction begins. Each reflects a specific causative reason for the deceleration pattern.

Early Deceleration
Characteristics of an early deceleration pattern are as follows:

1. The shape of the fetal heart rate pattern reflects the shape of the pattern of the uterine contraction. The shape of the pattern of a uterine contraction usually is uniform in its progression through the increment, acme, and decrement phases of the contraction. Since it is this shape that is being reflected, the pattern of early deceleration is called a pattern of *uniform* shape.
2. The onset of early deceleration corresponds with the onset of the related uterine contraction.
3. The total period of deceleration from beginning to end is usually less than 90 seconds and ends when the contraction ends.
4. The early deceleration pattern occurs with each contraction with only slight variation in the pattern from contraction to contraction.
5. The baseline fetal heart rate from which deceleration occurs is usually within normal range — 120 to 160 beats per minute.
6. The lowest level of the fetal heart rate deceleration usually is not lower than 100 beats per minute.

A pattern of early deceleration (see Fig. 13-5) is thought to be due to head compression. This is the same as a Type I Dip in the literature. Early deceleration is a common pattern shortly before delivery as the head receives pressure from the perineal floor with momentary compression occurring with contractions during which the woman pushes. Early deceleration is not considered to be a pattern to be concerned about as long as it is carefully differentiated from a late deceleration pattern.

Late Deceleration
Characteristics of a late deceleration pattern (Fig. 14-1) are as follows:

1. The shape of the fetal heart rate pattern reflects the shape of the pattern of the uterine contraction. It is, therefore, a pattern of *uniform* shape.
2. The onset of late deceleration occurs late during the related uterine contraction (the onset roughly corresponds to the acme or decrement phase of the contraction).
3. The total period of deceleration from beginning to end is usually less than 90 seconds in duration. Since it starts late in the contraction, the deceleration will extend beyond the end of the contraction.
4. A late deceleration pattern may or may not occur with each contraction.
5. The fall in a late deceleration may be within the normal fetal heart rate range and may be as shallow as within ten beats of the baseline. The fall may also extend beyond the normal fetal heart rate range. The severity of the situation cannot be measured by the depth of the fall. A shallow deceleration is just as critical as a deep deceleration and is, in fact, dangerous because it is more apt to be missed.

A pattern of late deceleration is thought to be due to uteroplacental insufficiency. Late deceleration is the same as a Type II Dip in the

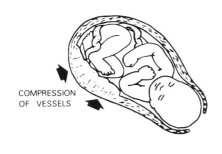

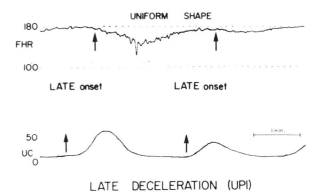

UTEROPLACENTAL INSUFFICIENCY   LATE   DECELERATION (UPI)

FIGURE 14-1.   Late deceleration of fetal heart rate pattern. (Reproduced by permission from E. H. Hon. *An Introduction to Fetal Heart Rate Monitoring.* Los Angeles: University of Southern California, 1973.)

literature. Uteroplacental insufficiency is a life-threatening condition. When a woman has late decelerations, the following should be immediately implemented:

1. Notify your consulting physician.
2. If pitocin is running, shut off the pitocin (keep the IV open with the piggyback intravenous fluid).
3. Position the woman all the way over on her left side.
4. Administer oxygen to the mother by face mask at 6 liters per minute.
5. Collect equipment and prepare the woman for a fetal scalp pH measurement.
6. If the woman has had epidural anesthesia, check her blood pressure for hypotension and, if present, elevate her legs (but not her body, i.e., do not place her in Trendelenburg position) and increase her intravenous fluids.

Causes of acute uteroplacental insufficiency include the following:

1. Hypertonic uterine contractions such as might be caused during an oxytocin induction or stimulation
2. A markedly infarcted placenta
3. Maternal supine hypotension syndrome

4. Placenta previa
5. Abruptio placentae
6. Hypertensive disorders of pregnancy
7. Intrauterine growth retardation
8. Any other condition that might interfere with placental circulation

Variable Deceleration

Characteristics of a variable deceleration pattern (Fig. 14-2) are as follows:

1. The shape of the fetal heart rate pattern does *not* reflect the shape of the pattern of the uterine contraction. In addition to varying from the shape of the pattern of the uterine contraction, variable deceleration patterns vary in their own shape from occurrence to occurrence, in duration, and in relation to the onset of the uterine contraction. Thus, its pattern is one of *variable* shape.
2. The onset of variable deceleration occurs at different times in relation to the onset and duration of the corresponding uterine contraction. For example, the onset of one variable deceleration may correspond with the onset of its related uterine contraction and the onset of the next variable deceleration may correspond with the acme of its related contraction.

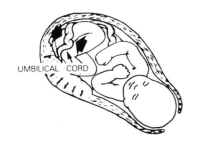

UMBILICAL CORD

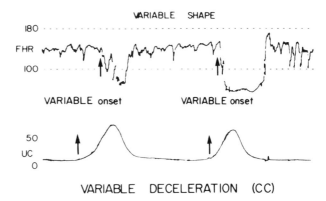

UMBILICAL CORD COMPRESSION   VARIABLE DECELERATION (CC)

FIGURE 14-2.   Variable deceleration of fetal heart rate pattern. (Reproduced by permission from E. H. Hon. *An Introduction to Fetal Heart Rate Monitoring.* Los Angeles: University of Southern California, 1973.)

3. The total period of deceleration from beginning to end varies from a few seconds to minutes.
4. The variable deceleration pattern may vary considerably in shape from contraction to contraction.
5. The baseline fetal heart rate from which deceleration occurs is usually in the low normal or normal range.
6. The fall in fetal heart rate during deceleration is usually below 100 beats per minute and may be as low as 50 to 60 beats per minute or even lower.

Variable deceleration is the same as combined Type I and Type II Dips, or as Type III Dips, in the literature. A pattern of variable decelerations is thought to be due to compression of the umbilical cord. Causes of compression of the umbilical cord include frank and occult prolapse of the cord, true knots in the cord, and positioning of the cord around the fetal neck or body. In breech presentations, variable decelerations may occur as the breech descends through the pelvis (usually in second stage) causing compression of the cord between the baby's abdomen and the mother's pelvis. Variable decelerations which have a quick recovery with a temporary compensatory elevation in fetal heart rate as it returns to baseline usually indicate a nuchal cord. This pattern can be seen anytime during descent.

Variable decelerations which are shallow with a quick return to baseline and good variability usually do not indicate fetal acidosis. However, if occurrence is frequent, notify your consulting physician. This pattern is seen most commonly in second stage, especially with an occiput posterior position.

Variable decelerations which have a slow recovery to baseline or an absence of variability, regardless of depth of fall, may indicate a more seriously compromised fetus. Your consulting physician should be immediately notified.

If a fetus has variable decelerations, regardless of type of recovery, the following should be done:

1. Change maternal position.
2. Administer oxygen to the mother by face mask at 6 liters per minute.
3. Perform a vaginal examination to:
   a. rule out a prolapsed cord if this is a possibility.
   b. ascertain whether there has been rapid descent of the head with pressure from an incompletely dilated cervix (e.g., pushing with a rim or anterior lip).
   c. determine presentation and position. Variable decelerations are often seen in

occiput posterior positions or face presentations.

4. Call your consulting physician.

Immediate management of a woman with variable decelerations depends on the experience and knowledge of the nurse-midwife interpreting the fetal monitor strip, evaluating the risk status of the pregnancy, and making the clinical judgments regarding these factors and the observations made on the fetal monitor. Less experienced nurse-midwives and students should implement the above four actions as their immediate management.

Acceleration Patterns

Acceleration patterns are transient periodic increases in the fetal heart rate. These transient accelerations are thought to be secondary to stimulation of the fetus from uterine contractions. Accelerations may represent an intact cardiovascular system in the fetus. Accelerations are often seen in breech presentations, in response to stimulation of the fetus during vaginal examinations, or as a fetal response to sound. Two acceleration patterns have thus far been identified: uniform accelerations and variable accelerations.

Uniform Acceleration
The pattern of uniform acceleration generally reflects the pattern of the related uterine contraction. A strong uterine contraction provokes a larger acceleration, while a mild contraction provokes a lesser acceleration. Uniform accelerations begin shortly after the onset of their associated contractions.

The clinical significance of uniform accelerations is not clearly understood. It is thought that they might be a reflection of stress on the fetus. Acceleration patterns have to be carefully delineated from deceleration patterns. A deceleration pattern can sometimes be misinterpreted as acceleration of the fetal heart rate

with a return to baseline. Therefore, you should determine what the baseline fetal heart rate is before diagnosing an acceleration pattern.

Variable Acceleration
The pattern of variable acceleration does not reflect the general pattern of the related uterine contraction as it is more angular in form, and its onset varies in relation to the onset of the corresponding uterine contraction.

Variable acceleration is thought to be caused by fetal movement or stimulation of the fetus (e.g., scalp electrode, vaginal examination), and not to be an indicator of any deleterious fetal condition. It is considered a possible indication of fetal well-being in an uncompromised fetus.

Sinusoidal Pattern

A sinusoidal pattern is one in which there is an undulating, repetitive, uniform pattern equally distributed at least five beats above and below the baseline and bearing no relationship to either the contraction pattern or to fetal movement. The undulation occurs at a rate of 2 to 6 cycles per minute (see Fig. 14-3).

A sinusoidal pattern is seen anytime there is fetal anemia due to disruptive factors such as abruptio placentae, placenta previa, and erythroblastosis. A persistent sinusoidal pattern may occur in cases of severe fetal distress. This is usually a serious pattern and requires immediate physician consultation.

Fetal Distress

Fetal distress can be defined as a situation in which the well-being of the fetus is compromised. This may be a chronic condition starting at some point during the antepartal period or an acute condition occurring during labor, or it may be a combination of both.

Chronic fetal stress is usually secondary to uteroplacental insufficiency during the ante-

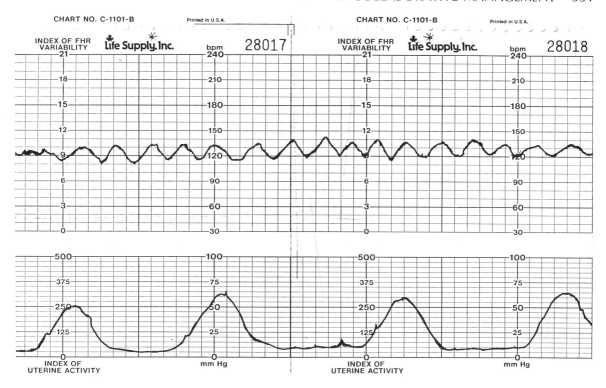

FIGURE 14-3.   Sinusoidal fetal heart rate pattern. (Courtesy of Nancy McCluggage, C.N.M., M.A.)

partal period. Clinical situations which may cause chronic fetal stress due to uteroplacental insufficiency include intrauterine growth retardation and postmaturity syndrome. Acute fetal distress may be precipitated by the onset of early labor contractions when there has been chronic antepartal fetal stress. The fetal heart rate pattern most often seen in this situation is one of late decelerations, with or without variability.

Acute fetal distress can also be due to compression of the umbilical cord (i.e., cord prolapse, nuchal cord, true knot in cord). The fetal heart rate pattern that accompanies cord compression is that of variable decelerations. Variable decelerations are also often seen in vertex presentations in the occiput posterior position during second stage or with rapid descent of the fetal head through the pelvis.

Management of acute fetal distress depends on several factors:

1. Presence of maternal complications which increase the risk for uteroplacental insufficiency (e.g., preeclampsia, hypertension, diabetes)
2. Presence of obstetrical fetal complications (i.e., postdates, intrauterine growth retardation)
3. Presence or absence of meconium
4. Stage of labor in which the abnormal fetal heart rate patterns occur

If there are underlying maternal (e.g., nutritional) or obstetrical fetal (e.g., IUGR) risk factors, the normal reserve of the fetus is compromised and the ability to respond to the added stress of uterine contractions is reduced.

There is need in such a situation for immediate notification of your consulting physician and further evaluation.

When fetal distress occurs during second stage, especially when the fetus is in an occiput posterior position, your management depends upon whether the amniotic fluid is meconium stained and the anticipated time to delivery. If you think the second stage will be over within a half hour, there is clear amniotic fluid, variability remains good, and the decelerations do not become more frequent and of longer duration, you can anticipate a good fetal outcome. If the amniotic fluid is meconium stained or you anticipate the second stage to be longer than a half hour, or there is a worsening in the fetal heart rate pattern or a loss of variability, your consulting physician should be notified and preparations made for securing a fetal scalp blood sample.

While meconium stained amniotic fluid alone is not a sign of fetal distress, conversely, the absence of meconium does not guarantee that fetal distress does not exist. The presence of meconium with any sign of acute fetal distress (i.e., any late deceleration; variable decelerations accompanied by fetal tachycardia or loss of variability; minimal or absent variability, especially when combined with late decelerations, variable decelerations, or tachycardia; or a sinusoidal pattern) is a serious development requiring prompt action as follows:

1. Notify the physician.
2. If the mother is receiving an pitocin induction or stimulation, turn off the intravenous fluids containing the pitocin. Keep the IV open with other IV fluids not containing pitocin. This will decrease uterine activity and alleviate the resulting uteroplacental insufficiency.
3. Turn the mother on either side if she is not already on her side. This serves three purposes:
   a. redistributes uterine contents so that if cord compression is the problem it may be alleviated by shifting the baby off the cord.
   b. alleviates the pressure of the uterus and its contents on the mother's great vessels (inferior vena cava and aorta), thereby alleviating supine hypotensive syndrome and its resulting uteroplacental insufficiency and fetal hypoxia if that is the cause of the acute fetal distress.
   c. reduces uterine hypertonicity and activity because the contractions are better coordinated and more efficient (with decreased frequency and increased intensity) in the lateral recumbent position.
4. Administer oxygen to the mother at a minimum rate of 6 liters per minute with a well-fitting face mask. This serves to alleviate fetal hypoxia in the presence of uteroplacental insufficiency by providing more oxygen for whatever amount of transfer is taking place. Oxygen administration is not effective when the problem is cord compression.
5. Make preparations for a fetal scalp blood sample.

If the acute fetal distress is progressively worsening or is severe, delivery by cesarean section should be anticipated and preparations begun.

CEPHALOPELVIC DISPROPORTION

Cephalopelvic disproportion (CPD), or fetopelvic disproportion, is a disproportion between the size of the fetus and the size of the pelvis in which a particular pelvis is not large enough to accommodate passage of a particular fetus through it to birth by vaginal delivery. This determination is relative. A pelvis which is adequate for passage of a 5-pound baby may not be large enough for passage of a 7-pound baby, or a pelvis large enough for a 7-pound baby may not be large enough for an 8-pound baby. Therefore, the adequacy of the pelvis must be evaluated in relation to the fetus which is to pass through it.

Evaluation of the bony pelvis and the types of pelves are discussed in Chapter 47. Included are the findings which indicate pelvic adequacy as well as the normal average length of the diameters of the pelvis. No single finding determines adequacy or inadequacy. Rather, the total pelvis (its measurements, architecture, shape, and various dimensions) should be taken into account in relation to the fetus (its size, presentation, position, variety, and normality).

The following may indicate the possibility of cephalopelvic disproportion:

1. Excessively large fetus
2. The woman's general body type and specific characteristics:
    a. shoulders wider than hips, regardless of height
    b. short, square stature
    c. short, broad hands and feet (shoe size is informative)
3. History of pelvic fracture
4. Spinal deformity, for example, scoliosis or kyphosis (note posture)
5. Unilateral or bilateral lameness (observe for limp and for marked lordosis)
6. Other orthopedic deformities, for example, rickets, fractured pelvis, pinned hip
7. Dysfunctional labor, such as uterine dysfunction
8. Malpresentation or malposition

The nurse-midwife initially evaluates a woman's pelvis during her first antepartal visit and again upon entry into labor. Any question the nurse-midwife has of the possibility of cephalopelvic disproportion is noted on the woman's chart for reevaluation upon entry into labor. Clinical pelvimetry should again be performed at the time of admission for labor to detect a truly contracted pelvis and also to anticipate where delay in descent and rotation

might occur. Therapeutic measures, such as maternal position, can then be applied early enough to facilitate the mechanisms of labor.

It is quite unusual to find a pelvis so severely contracted that labor is absolutely contraindicated. The only true test for cephalopelvic disproportion is labor. If the pelvis is obviously contracted to the point of inadequacy except for an extremely small fetus, the physician is consulted for planning a possible cesarean section.

All women who have an arrest of labor should be evaluated for cephalopelvic disproportion. This evaluation includes the following:

1. Abdominal palpation to determine fetal lie, presentation, position, flexion, engagement and station of the presenting part, and estimated fetal weight. (A common clinical phenomenon occurs in estimating the fetal weight in an arrested labor: the longer the arrest, the larger the baby becomes when the clinician is estimating the fetal weight. Usually, your initial estimation before the arrest is the most accurate since it carries the least situational bias.)
2. Assessment of uterine contractions for frequency, duration, intensity, and changes in uterine activity from that which was previously noted. A dysfunctional labor pattern is often seen in a labor complicated by CPD (see pages 335−337).
3. Pelvic examination to evaluate position of the presenting part, engagement, station, degree of flexion, synclitism/asynclitism, formation and degree of caput, molding, and progress or lack thereof in cervical dilatation and descent of the presenting part.
4. Evaluation of the pelvis by clinical pelvimetry should be repeated at this time to determine where in the pelvis the disproportion is occurring.

Cephalopelvic disproportion may be exhibited by a dysfunctional labor pattern, poorly flexed head, or an arrest of internal rotation and descent (i.e., deep transverse arrest). Cephalopelvic disproportion may or may not be accompanied by the formation of caput and molding. Suspected cephalopelvic disproportion should be discussed with your consulting physician.

Management options include maternal position changes, administration of an enema, artificial rupture of the membranes, ambulation of the woman, resting and hydration of the woman if there is maternal exhaustion, administering pitocin for the express purpose of increasing uterine activity which in turn may facilitate progress, or a combination of these measures. By improving the flexion of the fetal head or changing the position of the head, a smaller skull diameter presents which may then allow the head to pass through the pelvis.

Whenever you encounter the possibility of cephalopelvic disporportion, a time limit should be set prior to initiating the above therapeutic measures since dysfunctional labor due to cephalopelvic disproportion may result in the following tragedies:

1. Fetal damage, for example, brain damage
2. Fetal or neonatal death
3. Intrauterine infection
4. Uterine rupture
5. Maternal death

Timely collaboration with your consulting physician and timely intervention, including cesarean section if the other therapeutic measures don't work or in the presence of a worsening maternal or fetal condition, should avert these tragedies.

DEEP TRANSVERSE ARREST

Deep transverse arrest is associated with platypelloid and android pelvic types because of flat posterior pelvic configuration throughout the depth of these pelves. Additionally, platypelloid pelves are also flat in the forepelvis and android pelves have convergent side walls and prominent ischial spines. These factors inhibit the mechanism of labor of internal rotation which brings the sagittal suture from being in the transverse diameter to being in the anteroposterior diameter of the mother's pelvis. Careful clinical pelvimetry during the initial examination enables you to anticipate a potential problem.

A deep transverse arrest should be considered when there is a prolonged second stage. Signs and symptoms include:

1. Sagittal suture of the fetus in the transverse diameter of the mother's pelvis
2. Development of second stage hypotonic uterine dysfunction
3. Extensive molding of the fetal head
4. Formation of considerable caput succedaneum

The signs and symptoms given above are late indicators of deep transverse arrest. If you have identified the potential for deep transverse arrest from your initial clinical pelvimetry you need to be particularly facilitative of second stage maternal efforts. Facilitation includes positions which promote pushing (e.g., squatting, kneeling) and entry into second stage in a well-hydrated state. In order to prevent exhaustion from pushing, encourage the woman to push only with the peak of the contraction and when she feels like pushing.

It is also important to evaluate the woman's progress accurately. Extensive molding and caput formation may be misleading when evaluating station and descent. Ascertain engagement abdominally with Leopold's fourth maneuver. By vaginal examination evaluate the degree of molding and caput, locate the parietal bones by palpating past the caput, and note whether the biparietal diameter has passed through the pelvic inlet. Also estimate the amount (depth) of caput by palpating past it to skull bone and ascertain the station of the actual lowermost part of the presenting part.

Nurse-midwifery management of a woman who has obstructed labor secondary to a deep transverse arrest includes collaboration with your consulting physician. Management options include improving uterine activity to facilitate internal rotation of the fetal head. This may be accomplished by correcting maternal exhaustion if present, maternal position change to left lateral to improve contractions or to an upright position to improve maternal pushing efforts, administration of pitocin to stimulate the uterus, or a combination of these.

Improved contractions and maternal pushing efforts can sometimes overcome deep transverse arrest. When deep transverse arrest cannot be overcome, delivery is by forceps, vacuum extraction, or cesarean section as evaluated and done by your consulting physician.

UTERINE DYSFUNCTION

Uterine dysfunction is a diagnosis made by observing a prolongation of any phase or stage of labor beyond expected length. It is identified by a lack of progress in cervical effacement or dilatation or in descent of the presenting part.

Uterine activity can be measured in two ways:

1. Biophysically — this is done by using an internal pressure catheter to measure the frequency and pressure of each contraction at each phase and stage of labor.
2. By abdominal palpation and vaginal examination — This is done by palpation of the contractions and determination during vaginal examination of the progress of labor as defined by progressive effacement, dilatation, and descent of the presenting part.

Since it is still unclear what constitutes "adequate" intrauterine pressure to effect labor progress in the majority of women, measurement of effacement, dilatation, and descent is still the most accurate way to recognize uterine dysfunction.

Uterine dysfunction may reflect a biochemical problem in the woman caused, for example, by stress which results in alterations of endorphins and catecholamine production which affects uterine activity. Uterine dysfunction may also reflect the presence of another complication, in effect being a symptom of it. This underlying complication is always one of disproportion between the fetus and the soft or bony components of the birth canal, i.e., cephalopelvic disproportion (e.g., pelvic contracture, hydrocephaly), fetal malpresentations and malpositions (e.g., shoulder, face), or soft-tissue dystocias such as myomata or vaginal or uterine septa.

There are two types of uterine dysfunction: hypotonic and hypertonic. They are differentiated from each other by signs and symptoms, underlying contraction physiology, the time they occur in labor, and the effect on the mother and the fetus. The two things they have in common are that the contractions are ineffective, and cervical dilatation and fetal descent are arrested.

Hypotonic Uterine Dysfunction

In hypotonic uterine dysfunction, contractions have a normal gradient pattern (greatest in the fundus and decreasing to weakest in the lower uterine segment and cervix) but a very poor tone or intensity (less than 15 millimeters of mercury of pressure) which is too little pressure to dilate the cervix. In this situation the woman feels great because she has no pain and is able to rest. However, labor is prolonged, which increases the risk of maternal distress, hemorrhage, and, if the membranes are ruptured, intrauterine infection. The fetus usually experiences no distress unless the condition is allowed to go on over a long period of time and intrauterine infection develops.

The signs and symptoms of hypotonic uterine dysfunction are as follows:

1. *History* — contractions not painful; labor progressed well into the active phase of the first stage of labor or the second stage and then quit
2. *Physical examination* — contractions infrequent, of short duration, and mild intensity
3. *Pelvic examination* — lack of progress in cervical dilatation or fetal descent (station) in accord with expected norms because the contractions are ineffective

When the time limits described in Table 14-1 are reached, you should make a complete assessment of the woman and fetus and present the results, along with the data base you have collected during the preceding hours, to your consulting physician for the development of a collaborative management plan. If a problem is suspected or evident prior to these time limits, however, you should consult the physician immediately. A complete assessment consists of the following:

1. assessment of contractions — frequency, length, interval, intensity, and changes from what was previously observed
2. assessment for maternal exhaustion (see pages 337–338)
3. assessment of fetal well-being
4. assessment of maternal environment — note any stress factors
5. assessment of presentation, position, engagement, and station
6. assessment for cephalopelvic disproportion — molding, caput formation, flexion, synclitism/asynlitism, and pelvic adequacy
7. assessment of progress of labor — effacement, dilatation, and descent of the presenting part

TABLE 14-1. Time Limits of Normality for Determining When to Consult Physician concerning Hypotonic Uterine Dysfunction

	Primigravida	Multipara
Latent phase (first stage)	20 hours	14 hours
Active phase (first stage)	Less than 1.2 cm./hour	Less than 1.5 cm./hour
Second stage	2 hours	1 hour

There are various management options for a woman whose labor is complicated by hypotonic uterine dysfunction. The use of these options depends upon whether the parameters of normal have been met. These parameters, which should be evaluated before implementing a mangement plan, include the following:

1. Absence of fetal distress
2. Clear amniotic fluid
3. Membranes intact or ruptured membranes of a short duration and absence of signs and symptoms of chorioamnionitis (see pages 323–324)
4. Absence of signs and symptoms of maternal exhaustion
5. Adequate pelvis

If any of the above parameters are abnormal, consultation with the physician should take place earlier in the labor process regardless of the time limits described in Table 14-1.

The management options are as follows and can be used singly or in combination:

1. Modification of the environment to decrease maternal stress.
2. Correction of maternal exhaustion and dehydration through rest and fluid intake.
3. Discussion with the woman to detect any underlying fears or concerns either for herself or as they relate to the baby or

delivery. Epidural anesthesia will sometimes produce positive results if the woman's fear of pain of the birth process cannot be overcome by education, support, and communication.

4. Ambulation. This may include a shower.
5. Enema. If effective, improved uterine activity should occur within an hour or so.
6. Rupture of membranes. If effective, improved uterine activity should occur within 2 hours.
7. Nipple stimulation.
8. Pitocin stimulation if the above management is unsuccessful in accomplishing progress in labor.

In making a management plan out of the above options, you should establish an estimated time period for anticipated correction of the uterine dysfunction and communicate the plan to your consulting physician. If any of the clinical parameters are abnormal (e.g., presence of fetal distress, meconium, prolonged rupture of membranes, maternal exhaustion, malposition) immediate collaboration with your consulting physician for a more aggressive management approach is appropriate.

Hypertonic Uterine Dysfunction

In hypertonic uterine dysfunction, contractions have a distorted gradient pattern with the midportion of the uterus contracting with more force than the fundus and with portions of hypertonicity throughout the uterus. In this situation, the mother becomes literally exhausted, with a probable outcome of maternal distress and an increased risk of infection. Fetal distress may quickly develop from uteroplacental insufficiency caused by the hypertonicity of the uterus and may result in increased perinatal and infant morbidity and mortality. There is some thought that hypertonic uterine dysfunction may be a form of false labor but this has not yet been clearly delineated.

The signs and symptoms of hypertonic uterine dysfunction are as follows:

1. *History* — usually occurs in primigravidas; contractions feel excessively painful for the period of labor and the severity of the contractions by palpation; occurs early in labor during the latent phase
2. *Physical examination* — contractions are frequent and irregular in tonicity
3. *Pelvic examination* — lack of progress in cervical effacement and dilatation and in fetal descent (station) in accord with expected norms because the contractions are ineffective and the labor never really commences

The nurse-midwife collaborates with the consulting physician when the condition is first suspected. Management usually begins with stopping this discoordinate labor and inducing rest with a combination of morphine and a barbiturate. Most women will awaken in normal, coordinated labor.

MATERNAL EXHAUSTION (MATERNAL DISTRESS; KETOACIDOSIS)

Maternal exhaustion (maternal distress) should be guarded against because deterioration in the woman's condition is dangerous both to her and to her unborn baby. Checking her urine for ketones, maintaining hydration from the start of labor, and being prompt about seeking physician help if labor is not progressing within established norms should prevent the development of maternal exhaustion. In other words, in good management severe maternal distress should not occur.

The signs and symptoms of maternal exhaustion/distress are as follows:

1. *History* — feels weak, apathetic, and sick; anxious; labor is prolonged; complains of

the signs of dehydration (dry lips, dry mouth, parched throat)

2. *Physical examination* — looks distressed and is restless; rising pulse; elevated temperature; circumoral pallor; vomiting
3. *Laboratory tests* — observe urine for concentration and examine it for ketones

The nurse-midwife should have already collaborated with the consulting physician regarding abnormal length of any phase or stage of labor. Management should include correction of the fluid and electrolyte imbalance.

UTERINE RUPTURE

Uterine rupture, fortunately, is a rare event. Etiological factors in uterine rupture encompass a number of injuries to or defects of the uterus occurring either before or during the present pregnancy. The most common causes are previous surgery to the fundus or corpus of the uterus, such as a classical cesarean section; previous removal of intrauterine myomata that invaded the myometrium; and pitocin induction or augmentation of labor, especially for women with high parity. Spontaneous rupture can also occur as a result of abnormal presentations, especially in the thinned-out lower uterine segment of a grand multipara. The life of the mother (approximately 5 percent mortality) and the baby (approximately 50 percent mortality) may be dependent on the speed with which the disaster is recognized and action taken. Therefore, everyone responsible for patient care should be familiar with the signs and symptoms of uterine rupture and the immediate emergency steps to take.

Signs and symptoms of uterine rupture may be either dramatic or quiet. In dramatic rupture of the uterus the woman experiences a sharp, shooting pain in her lower abdomen at the height of a severe contraction. She feels that something has given way inside of her and may cry out that "something tore." This is followed by cessation of the uterine contractions.

The woman now has a feeling of great relief from her previous intense pain. Vaginal bleeding may be observed either as a slight amount or as a hemorrhage. Findings upon abdominal palpation are changed from previous findings as follows:

1. The presenting part is now movable above the pelvic inlet.
2. A round, firm (contracted) uterus is felt beside the fetus (the fetus is felt outside of the uterus).
3. The fetal parts are more easily palpated than before.
4. The fetal movements may become violent and then reduce to no fetal movements and no fetal heart tones — or there may be continuing heart tones.

The woman may exhibit the signs and symptoms of shock — elevated pulse (rapid and thready); decreased blood pressure; pallor; cold, clammy skin; apprehension, feeling of impending doom or death; air hunger (shortness of breath); restlessness; and visual disturbances.

In a quiet uterine rupture in which the uterus ruptures silently (without the dramatic clinical picture) the woman may or may not have some vomiting; other manifestations include increased tenderness over the abdomen, severe suprapubic pain, hypotonic uterine contractions, lack of further progress in labor, and a feeling of faintness. Eventually she will evidence a rising and rapid pulse rate, pallor, hematuria, vaginal bleeding, and some pain. The contractions may continue but they have no effect on the cervix. The fetal heart tones may be lost.

The physician is notified immediately. Other actions are:

1. Start two intravenous infusion routes with 16-gauge intracatheters: one for electrolyte solutions (e.g., lactated Ringer's solution) and the other for the blood transfusion (keep open with normal saline until the blood is obtained).

2. Notify the blood bank of your need for a *stat.* blood transfusion. Estimate the number of units needed as well as the probable need for fresh frozen plasma.
3. Administer oxygen.
4. Make all preparations for immediate abdominal surgery (laparotomy and most likely hysterectomy).
5. In desperate situations institute aortic compression and add oxytocin to the IV solution.

BLOOD TRANSFUSION REACTION

The nurse-midwife may become involved with blood transfusions as a result of obstetric complications such as postpartal hemorrhage, placenta previa, or abruptio placentae. The following steps should be taken when administering blood in order to minimize the risk of a blood transfusion reaction:

1. When initially drawing a specimen for blood typing and crossmatch, make sure the specimen is properly labeled with the correct name and chart number.
2. When you receive a unit of blood, check the name and unit number with the name and unit number of the woman to whom it is to be given. They should be the same.
3. Compare the patient's blood type with that on the unit of blood to be administered. They should be the same except in an extreme emergency, when it may be necessary to administer O-negative blood to a woman who is Rh positive.
4. Compare the unit number with the number on the vial of blood which is taped to the bag of blood. Both numbers should be the same.
5. Avoid giving blood that is ice-cold unless the situation is life threatening. The resulting chills may be mistaken as a sign of a blood transfusion reaction.

It is essential to review the signs and symptoms of blood transfusion reactions. In this presentation, all the possible signs and symptoms of all the possible complications are identified, since it is the nurse-midwife's responsibility to recognize that a reaction is taking place and to so inform the physician. It is the physician's responsibility to diagnose which complication it is and determine the appropriate management.

Subjective signs and symptoms of a blood transfusion reaction include the following:

Lumbar and leg pain
A feeling of fullness in the head
Vertigo
Headache
A feeling of chest constriction
Cold
Vague muscle weakness extending from extremities into trunk
Nausea
Apprehension
Muscle cramps
Paresthesia of hands, feet, and tongue — also of fingers and around the mouth

Objective signs and symptoms of a blood transfusion reaction include the following:

Fever
Chills
Shortness of breath
Tachycardia
Hypotension
Decreased urine output
Skin rash (urticaria)
Edema
Diarrhea
Slow, irregular pulse
Convulsions
Respiratory stridor, rales
Spasms of the hands and feet
Hyperactive reflexes
Neck vein distention

The woman may also have bronchospasm, shock, and paralysis of the respiratory muscles and myocardium, leading to cardiac arrest.

All of these signs and symptoms are due to a variety of possible complications arising from receipt of a blood transfusion, as follows: air embolism, anaphylactic shock, circulatory overload, febrile reactions, hemolytic reactions, hyperkalemia, hypocalcemia, hypothermia, and septic shock.

In the presence of a blood transfusion reaction the appropriate actions to take are as follows:

1. Stop the transfusion.
2. Flush the IV tubing and keep the IV route open with normal saline.
3. Notify the physician for diagnosis of which complication has occurred and for its management.
4. Notify the blood bank and save the unit of blood which caused the reaction for further analysis. Most blood banks have clearly outlined procedures to take when there is a transfusion reaction. They may also want to obtain blood and urine samples from the patient.

BIBLIOGRAPHY

American College of Obstetricians and Gynecologists. Guidelines for vaginal delivery after a cesarean childbirth. Committee on Obstetrics: Maternal and Fetal Medicine, ACOG committee statement, January 7, 1982.

Anderson, E. Rationale for use of ketostick, labstick in obstetric labor: Detection of ketosis. Unpublished paper, 1974.

Binkin, N. J., Koplan, J. P., and Cates, W., Jr. Preventing neonatal herpes: The value of weekly viral cultures in pregnant women with recurrent genital herpes. JAMA 251(21):2816–2821, June 1, 1984.

Boehm, F. H. FHR variability: Key to fetal well-being. Contemporary OB/GYN 9:47, 1977.

Bottoms, S. F., Rosen, M. G., and Sokol, R. J. The increase in the cesarean birth rate. N. Engl. J. Med. 302(10):559–563, March 6, 1980.

Chez, R. A. (Moderator). Symposium: Therapeutic approaches to premature labor. Contemporary OB/GYN 8:58, 1976.

Child, J., Collins, D., and Collins, J. Blood transfusions. Am. J. Nurs. 72:1602, 1972.

Creasy, R. K., and Herron, M. A. Prevention of preterm birth. Semin. Perinatol. 5(3):295–302 (July) 1981.

Davis, L. The use of castor oil to stimulate labor in patients with premature rupture of membranes. J. Nurse-Midwifery 29(6):366–370 (November/December) 1984.

Demianczuk, N. N., Hunter, D. J. S., and Taylor, D. W. Trial of labor after previous cesarean section: Prognostic indicators of outcome. Am. J. Obstet. Gynecol. 142(6):640–642, March 15, 1982.

Eggers, T. R., Doyle, L. W., and Pepperell, R. J. Premature rupture of membranes. Med. J. Aust. 209(7):93–95, 1979.

Elliott, H. R., Abdulla, U., and Hayes, P. J. Pulmonary oedema associated with ritodrine infusion and betamethasone administration in premature labour. Br. Med. J. 799–800, September 16, 1978.

Flaksman, R. J., Vollman, J. H., and Benfield, G. Iatrogenic prematurity due to elective termination of the uncomplicated pregnancy: A major perinatal health care problem. Am. J. Obstet. Gynecol. 132(8):885–888, December 15, 1978.

Friedman, E. A. An objective method of evaluating labor. Hosp. Prac. (July) 1970.

Friedman, E. A. Labor: Clinical Evaluation and Management, 2nd. New York: Meredith, 1978.

Friedman, E. A. Labor in multiparas: A graphicostatistical analysis. Obstet. Gynecol. 8:691, 1956.

Friedman, E. A. Primigravid labor: A graphicostatistical analysis. Obstet. Gynecol. 6:567, 1955.

Friedman, E. A. The functional divisions of labor. Am. J. Obstet. Gynecol. 109:274, 1971.

Friedman, E. A., and Sachtleben, M. R. High risk labor. J. Reprod. Med. 7:52, 1971.

Gibbs, C. E. Can your repeat-section patient deliver vaginally? Contemporary OB-GYN. 101–104 (February) 1983.

Gibbs, C. E. Planned vaginal delivery following cesarean section. Clin. Obstet. Gynecol. 23(2): (June) 1980.

Greenhill, J. P., and Friedman, E. A. Biological Principles and Modern Practice of Obstetrics. Philadelphia: Saunders, 1974.

Gunn, G. C., Mishell, D. R., Jr., and Morton, D. G. Premature rupture of the fetal membranes. Am. J. Obstet. Gynecol. 106:268–279, February 1, 1970.

Hameed, C. et al. Silent chorioamnionitis as a cause

of preterm labor refractory to tocolytic therapy. *Am. J. Obstet. Gynecol.* 149(7):726–730, August 1, 1984.

Hamlin, R. H. J. *Stepping Stones to Labour Ward Diagnosis.* Adelaide, Australia: Rigby, Ltd., 1959.

Herron, M. A., and Dulock, H. L. *Preterm Labor.* Series 2, Module 5. A Staff Development Program in Perinatal Nursing Care. White Plains, N. Y.: March of Dimes — Birth Defects Foundation, 1982.

Herron, M. A., Katz, M., and Creasy, R. K. Evaluation of a preterm birth prevention program: Preliminary report. *Obstet. Gynecol.* 59(4):452–456 (April) 1982.

Hon, E. H. *An Introduction to Fetal Heart Rate Monitoring*, 2nd. North Haven, Conn.: Corometrics Medical Systems, 1975.

Hon, E. H., and Petrie, R. H. Clinical value of fetal heart rate monitoring. *Clin. Obstet. Gynecol.* 18:1, 1975.

Iams, J. D. et al. Management of preterm prematurely ruptured membranes: A prospective randomized comparison of observation versus use of steroids and timed delivery. *Am. J. Obstet. Gynecol.* 151(1): 32–38, January 1, 1985.

Johnson, J. W. C. et al. Premature rupture of the membranes and prolonged latency. *Obstet. Gynecol.* 57(5):547–556 (May) 1981.

Kappy, K. A. et al. Premature rupture of the membranes: A conservative approach. *Am. J. Obstet. Gynecol.* 134(6):655–661, July 15, 1979.

Laursen, N. H. Inhibition of premature labor: A multicenter comparison of ritodrine and ethanol. *Am. J. Obstet. Gynecol.* 127:837, 1977.

Lavin, J. P. et al. Vaginal delivery in patients with a prior cesarean section. *Obstet. Gynecol.* 59(2): 135–148 (February) 1982.

Martin, J. N. et al. Vaginal delivery following previous cesarean birth. *Am. J. Obstet. Gynecol.* 146(3): 255–263, June 1, 1983.

Mead, P. B. Management of the patient with premature rupture of the membranes. *Symposium on High-Risk Pregnancy.* 1980.

Meier, P., and Porreco, R. Trial of labor following cesarean section: A two-year experience. *Am. J. Obstet. Gynecol.* 144(6), November 15, 1982.

Merrill, B., and Gibbs, C. E. Planned vaginal delivery following cesarean section. *Obstet. Gynecol.* 52(1): 50–52 (July) 1978.

Monif, G. R.G. The Derick protocol for the management of premature rupture of the fetal membranes. Part 2. *Infectious Disease Letters for Obstetrics-Gynecology.* 6(7):39–43 (July) 1984.

Morley, G. W. Once a cesarean, always a cesarean?, *JAMA* 178(12):1128–1131, December 23, 1961.

Murphy, H. Delivery following caesarean section: Ten years experience at the Rotunda Hospital, Dublin, *J. Irish Med. Assoc.* 69(20):533–534, December 18, 1976.

O'Sullivan, M. J. Ruptured uterus: Still a challenge. *Contemporary OB/GYN* 18:145–148 (July) 1981.

Pauerstein, C. J. Once a section, always a trial of labor? *Obstet. Gynecol.* 28(2):273–276 (August) 1966.

Paul, R. H., and Petrie, R. H. *Fetal Intensive Care.* Wallingford, Conn.: Corometrics Medical Systems, 1981.

Pritchard, J. A., MacDonald, P. C., and Gant, N. F. *Williams Obstetrics, 15th.* Norwalk, Conn.: Appleton-Century-Crofts, 1985.

Reid, D. E., Ryan, K. J., and Benirschke, K. *Principles and Management of Human Reproduction.* Philadelphia: Saunders, 1972.

Ritodrine in the Management of Preterm Labor: A Symposium. Cincinnati, Ohio: Merrell-National Laboratories (September) 1980.

Saldana, L. R., Schulman, H., and Reuss, L. Management of pregnancy after cesarean section. *Am. J. Obstet. Gynecol.* 135(5), November 1, 1979.

Schreiber, J. and Benedetti, T. Conservative management of preterm premature rupture of the fetal membranes in a low socioeconomic population. *Am. J. Obstet. Gynecol.* 136:92, 1980.

Seitchik, J., and Rao, V. R. R. Cesarean delivery in nulliparous women for failed oxytocin-augmented labor: Route of delivery in subsequent pregnancy. *Am. J. Obstet. Gynecol.* 143(4):393–397, June 15, 1982.

Skinner, S. J. M. et al. Collagen content of human amniotic membranes: Effect of gestation length and premature rupture. *Obstet. Gynecol.* 57:487, 1981.

Steer, C. M. *Maloy's Evaluation of the Pelvis in Obstetrics, 3rd.* New York: Plenum, 1975.

Taylor, J., and Garite, T. J. Premature rupture of membranes before fetal viability. *Obstet. Gynecol.* 64:615, 1984.

Young, D., and Mahan, C. *Unnecessary Cesareans: Ways to Avoid Them.* Minneapolis, Minn.: International Childbirth Education Association, 1980.

15

Management of Selected Obstetric Complications and Deviations from Normal

The nurse-midwife must kown how to manage certain obstetric complications and deviations from normal until they are resolved or until the physician arrives. Inevitably in her or his career the nurse-midwife will be confronted with complications or deviations from normal which will demand that action be immediately instigated. These are as follows:

1. Shoulder dystocia
2. Face presentation
3. Breech presentations
4. Multiple gestation
5. Third stage hemorrhage
6. Immediate postpartal hemorrhage
7. Low apgar score newborn

Management of the first four conditions is given in this chapter; management of third stage hemorrhage, immediate postpartum hemorrhage, and resuscitation of the low-Apgar newborn are in Chapters 17, 19, and 22 respectively.

Occasionally the nurse-midwife is confronted with these complications or deviations from normal because a patient arrives in second stage with no prenatal care or record, or because of an emergency. Theoretically, and ideally, all of these complications and deviations from normal should have been diagnosed or anticipated before delivery and before their actual occurrence. Situational circumstances, however, dictate that this will not always be the case. Rarely is a nurse-midwife confronted with any of these because of failure to have properly diagnosed or anticipated the problem.

MANAGEMENT OF SHOULDER DYSTOCIA

Shoulder dystocia, by definition, is difficulty in the birth (or delivery) of the shoulders. In practice, this refers to cephalic presentations in which the shoulders have become impacted. Shoulder dystocia occurs when one (usually the anterior) or both (rarely) shoulders impact above the pelvic brim. The typical situation is one in which the anterior shoulder becomes arrested above the symphysis pubis while the posterior shoulder gets past the sacral promontory and enters the true pelvis. The problem is fostered if the shoulders attempt to enter the true pelvis with the bisacromial diameter in the anteroposterior diameter of the pelvic inlet instead of in either the right or left oblique diameter of the pelvic inlet, which is the method of pelvic entry during the normal mechanisms of labor. The oblique diameter (12.75 centimeters) is larger than the anteroposterior diameter (10.6 centimeters for the obstetric conjugate) of the pelvic inlet.

Differential diagnosis needs to be made between shoulder dystocia and bed dystocia. Bed dystocia occurs when the woman is in a semi-Fowler's or similar propped-up position in bed, especially a soft bed that sags under her buttocks, and the baby is being born downward into the bed. In such a situation there is no room for delivery of the shoulders. This is not, however, shoulder dystocia. The problem is readily rectified by slipping something under the woman's hips which will elevate them and by reducing the upright angle of her position.

The incidence of shoulder dystocia is not accurately known because criteria for diagnosis of mild shoulder dystocia as an entity have not been developed and statistics for severe shoulder dystocia vary in the literature. There is agreement that the incidence increases considerably (although there is no agreement on how much this increase is) with increased fetal size as measured by the newborn's weight. This makes sense since the average measurement of shoulder girth increases with increased fetal weight.

The incidence of morbidity and mortality resulting from shoulder dystocia and its management (or mismanagement) is high. Fetal and newborn complications include death (intrapartal death between delivery of the head and delivery of the shoulders, resulting from anoxia; or neonatal death resulting from injuries sustained during delivery of the shoulders), brain damage, brachial plexus (Erb's) palsy, and fractured clavicle(s). Maternal complications include extensive perineal and vaginal lacerations, emotional trauma in response to a traumatic delivery, and emotional trauma and grief if the baby is either damaged or dead.

The best preparation for management of shoulder dystocia is to have anticipated it. The possibility of shoulder dystocia should be anticipated anytime any of the following conditions exist:

1. Maternal diabetes
2. Obstetric history of large babies
3. Family history of large siblings
4. Maternal obesity
5. Large fetus
6. An estimated fetal weight 1 pound or more greater than the woman's largest previous baby

The last condition is one in which you can have the worst shoulder dystocia. Frequently it is not anticipated, especially if the woman's first baby was 5 or 6 pounds and this baby is estimated at the average 7 to 7½ pounds. The chance of a shoulder dystocia is so great in this situation that proper management includes an episiotomy prior to delivery, regardless of parity.

The clinical picture of shoulder dystocia has been vividly described by Morris as follows:

The delivery of the head with or without forceps may have been quite easy, but more commonly there has been a little difficulty in completing the extension of the head. The hairy scalp slides out with reluctance. When the forehead has appeared it is necessary to press back the perineum to deliver the face. Fat cheeks eventually emerge. A double chin has to be hooked over the posterior vulval commissure, to which it remains tightly opposed. Restitution seldom occurs spontaneously, for the head seems incapable of movement as a result of friction with the girdle of contact of the vulva. On the other hand, gentle manipulation of the head sometimes results in a sudden 90 degree restitution as the head adjusts itself *without descent* [italics added] to the anteroposterior position of the shoulders.

Time passes. The child's head becomes suffused. It endeavors unsuccessfully to breathe. Abdominal efforts by the mother or by her attendants produce no advance; gentle head traction is equally unavailing.

Usually equanimity forsakes the attendants. They push, they pull. Alarm increases. Eventually

By greater strength of muscle
Or by some infernal juggle

the difficulty appears to be overcome, and the shoulders and trunk of a goodly child are delivered. The pallor of its body contrasts with the plum-colored cyanosis of the face, and the small quantity of freshly expelled meconium about the buttocks. It dawns upon the attendants that their anxiety was not ill-founded, the baby lies limp and voiceless, and too often remains so despite all efforts at resuscitation. [1]

The retraction of the head against the perineum, and seemingly back into the vagina if it were possible, is called the *turtle sign*. Morris's description is frightening, as are the potential results of severe shoulder dystocia. The danger of shoulder dystocia is in large part attributable to persons' not knowing how to manage the emergency properly. It is important that the nurse-midwife know how to manage this situation because, even with anticipation, diagnosis cannot be made until after the fetal head is born. This gives little time to resolve the problem before the baby is either damaged or dead. If the following protocol is learned, drilled, and reviewed en route to each labor and delivery situation, the nurse-midwife need not fear shoulder dystocia because he or she will know precisely what to do.

The following steps should be taken, in sequence, to manage this emergency situation of shoulder dystocia. The first five steps occur concurrently.

1. *Stay calm.* You know what to do and will effectively manage this situation.
2. *Request that the physician be given a stat. call.* If you anticipated the possibility of a shoulder dystocia, you should have previously alerted the physician of your potential need for him or her. Most likely you will have delivered the baby by the time the physician arrives. If you don't need the physician's help in delivering the baby, you still want the physician to be present because the chance is now great for a low-Apgar baby who will need resuscitation and for the mother to have an immediate postpartal hemorrhage.
3. *Request readiness of a full-scale newborn resuscitation effort.*
4. *Anticipate an immediate postpartum hemorrhage.* Most of the causes of shoulder dystocia also overdistend the uterus and predispose the woman to immediate postpartum hemorrhage. See Chapter 19 for management.
5. *Check the position of the shoulders. Rotate them into one of the oblique diameters of the pelvis* if they are in either the transverse or anteroposterior diameter of the mother's pelvis.

   Instruct the mother not to push. Rotation is accomplished by placing all of the fingers of one of your hands on one side of the baby's chest (e.g., right side) and all of the fingers of your other hand on the baby's back on the opposite side (left side) and then pressing with the amount of force necessary to move the baby. It is important that your entire hand be used rather than just two fingers of each hand because you most likely won't have the necessary strength in two fingers to move the baby. Using all of your fingers on both sides gives you the maximum strength.

It also gives you a wider area on which to exert pressure, thereby decreasing the risk of injury which is possible when all the force is concentrated on a smaller area.

Under no circumstances make the mistake of thinking that moving the head will move the shoulders. All you will do is twist the baby's neck; this may result in injury of the brachial or cervical nerve plexus or fracture of the cervical vertebrae.

6. *Request the application of suprapubic pressure while you exert your usual downward and outward pressure on the side of the baby's head.* (See Chapters 53 and 54.) This pressure should be firm but not excessive. Excessive force or traction on the baby's head may result in nerve palsy.

Suprapubic pressure is most effective if the person applying it stands on a footstool in order to get greater force behind the downward push. This person places both hands palm down, one on top of the other, in the abdominal midline just above the symphysis pubis and then pushes straight downward into the lower abdomen. *Under no circumstances allow fundal pressure to be erroneously given.* Fundal pressure will only further impact the shoulders, waste time, possibly cause injury to the fetus, and possibly rupture the uterus with disastrous sequelae to both the mother and baby. The baby will have delivered after this step if the condition was a mild shoulder dystocia. If the baby has not delivered —

7. *Cut or enlarge the episiotomy.* If an episiotomy was not already cut, cut one now and make it a *deep* mediolateral episitomy. You will get more room without getting into the bowel with a mediolateral episiotomy than you will by cutting a midline equivalent of a third- or fourth-degree laceration. With the life of the baby at stake this is no time to feel the least bit hesitant about cutting long and

deep. While cutting, request a catheter for the next step.

8. *Catheterize the woman to empty her bladder* if you don't know if she entered delivery with an empty bladder. To save precious time it would be better to routinely assure that a woman's bladder is empty at the start of delivery if there is any anticipation of a possible shoulder dystocia.

9. *Place the woman in an exaggerated lithotomy position* because this gives more room for manipulations. If the woman is in lithotomy position, position her so that her buttocks overhang the edge of the table. If the woman is in dorsal position, place an inverted bedpan underneath her buttocks and have her bring her legs up, back, and out, hanging on to them with her hands on her knees or behind her thighs (as she did when pushing) if there are no extra hands to help support her legs.

10. *Do a vaginal examination to rule out causes of labor dystocia* (after the head is born) other than impacted shoulders (shoulder dystocia). This requires the insertion of your entire examining hand as far as you can insert it. Other causes of labor dystocia to be ruled out at this time are:

a. short umbilical cord (relative or absolute)
b. enlargement of the thorax or abdomen of the fetus such as might be caused by tumors, monsters, or severe edema
c. locked twins
d. conjoined twins
e. Bandl's retraction ring

If the dystocia is diagnosed as resulting from shoulder dystocia —

11. *Attempt again to deliver the baby by again requesting the application of suprapubic pressure* while you exert firm, but not excessive, downward and outward pressure on the side of the baby's head (see

Step 5). The baby will have delivered after this step if the condition was a moderate shoulder dystocia. If the baby has not delivered —

12. (Steps 12 and 13 are reversible.) *Do the corkscrew maneuver, utilizing the screw principle of Woods* (Fig. 15-1). To do this maneuver, place your hands in the same manner as you did for rotation of the shoulders in Step 5. Rotate the baby 180°, thereby substituting the posterior shoulder for the anterior shoulder. Always rotate the body of the baby so that the back is rotated anteriorly (back up). This means that the rotation is alternately 180° clockwise and then 180° counterclockwise (or vice versa) until the baby is screwed out, but without being twisted upon itself. It also means that as you begin the maneuver your hand on the baby's back will be on the anterior shoulder pushing forward and down and your hand on the baby's chest will be pushing backward toward the posterior shoulder and up.

In order to make the best use of your natural forces you will need to switch the placement of your hands after the baby has rotated 90° before continuing on through the last 90°. For example, if the baby is positioned with its back to the mother's right in an ROT position, then the initial placement of your hands will be with your right hand pressing against the baby's chest for the posterior shoulder and with your left hand pressing against the baby's back for the anterior shoulder. After 90° rotation, which places the bisacromial diameter in the transverse diameter of the mother's pelvis, reposition your hands by exchanging their positions. This means that your left hand will now be pressing upward against the chest on the right side of the baby; and your right hand will now be pressing downward against the back on the left side of the baby for the final 90° rotation of the baby's body. The baby's body has now been rotated 180° in a clockwise direction and the posterior shoulder substituted for the anterior shoulder.

If the baby is still undeliverable, rotate the baby another 180°, again substituting the present posterior shoulder for the anterior shoulder. The direction of this rotation will now be counterclockwise, in effect rotating the baby back the way it originally came from in the preceding rotation only further down and out of the pelvis. This is accomplished by placing your hands so that your left hand will be pressing against the baby's chest for the posterior shoulder and your right hand will be pressing against the baby's back for the anterior shoulder for the first 90° of the rotation. You then switch your hands so that your left hand is now pressing downward against the right side of the baby's back and your right hand is

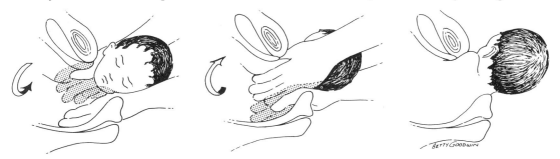

FIGURE 15-1. Corkscrew maneuver.

now pressing upward against the left side of the baby's chest for the final 90° rotation of the baby's body. Continue rotating the baby's body at least three to four times. If the baby still has not delivered —

13. *Deliver the posterior arm.* This is done by placing your entire hand deep into the vagina behind (on the back side of) the posterior shoulder. Splint the arm with your fingers and sweep it up and across the baby's abdomen and chest until the hand can be grasped with your other hand and the entire arm delivered. In doing this maneuver, resist any temptation to hook your fingers under the baby's axilla or into the armpit. This will not help you deliver the posterior shoulder as readily as the maneuver described here and most likely will cause nerve plexus injury.

14. *Attempt to deliver the baby now by the combination of suprapubic pressure and downward and outward pressure on the side of the baby's head* (see Step 6). If the baby has not delivered —

15. *Rotate the baby's body 180° again* (as described in Step 12). This will substitute the now delivered posterior shoulder for the anterior shoulder.

    If the baby did not deliver after either Step 6 or Step 11 it will have delivered after Step 12, 13 and 14, or 15 if the condition was a severe shoulder dystocia. In an exceptionally rare situation, probably not seen in the entire career of the majority of nurse-midwives, the baby will not have delivered and you then proceed to the next step —

16. *Break the baby's clavicle,* one or both as needed. Break the anterior clavicle first; this may be enough to collapse the anterior shoulder and dislodge it from behind the symphysis pubis. Breaking the clavicle is done by placing the thumbs of both hands along the clavicle and applying pressure on the middle of the clavicle where the ends of your two thumbs meet.

The danger in breaking the clavicle is the possibility of puncturing the underlying lung with the broken ends of the bone and causing pneumothorax. This, however, may save the life of the baby and therefore is preferable.

An alternate method for management of shoulder dystocia for a woman in bed has been used with success for mild shoulder dystocia, or "snug shoulders." This approach is to first turn the woman completely over on her side with her back at a right angle towards you. If delivery does not readily occur in this position then the woman is helped into a knee-chest position and an attempt is made to deliver the posterior shoulder, which is now uppermost. There is a major problem with this method and that is that it generally won't work in the event of a true, severe shoulder dystocia of the type described by Morris. It is difficult to ascertain at the beginning of a shoulder dystocia situation just how severe the problem is. Therefore, you may go through this procedure into the knee-chest position only to have to reposition the woman in the exaggerated lithotomy position in order to do the steps listed for management of shoulder dystocia. Precious time will have been wasted. Since the methodology presented for management of shoulder dystocia (Steps 1 through 16) will work for all degrees of shoulder dystocia severity, it should be the methodology used in all cases. Women who are delivering in bed simply have to carry out the additional step of moving into lithotomy position with their buttocks just over the edge of the bed.

DELIVERY OF THE INFANT WITH A FACE PRESENTATION

Many babies with face presentations begin labor either in a brow presentation or with a hyperextended head and convert to a face presentation during descent. The diagnosis of a face presentation is as follows:

1. Abdominal palpation (Leopold's third and fourth maneuvers) — the occipital bone is prominent and easily palpable; the head may feel larger than you would anticipate as compared to a well-flexed head.
2. Pelvic examination — you may be unable to clearly identify both fontanels or may feel only the anterior fontanel in an hyperextended presentation. In a brow presentation, you will feel the brow, possibly the anterior fontanel, but no other common identifying landmarks. In a face presentation, you will be able to feel the baby's eyes, nose, mouth, and chin, although initially the presenting part may feel soft and not smooth ("lumpy"), similar to a breech presentation. On further examination and palpation, the landmarks of the face become evident. The baby may even suck your finger as you approach the mouth.

Once you have diagnosed a face presentation, do not apply an internal electrode as this device will damage the infant's face or may be inadvertently applied to an eyelid.

In order to appropriately manage the delivery of a child who has a face presentation, you need to know the mechanisms of labor for this malpresentation, especially the mechanisms that vary from normal and the implications these have for the outcome. The mechanisms of labor for a face presentation are as follows:

1. Extension. The identifying feature of a face presentation is the chin (mentum) due to the fact that the head is extended rather than flexed. It is not known why in approximately 0.5 percent of all deliveries some form of interference occurs which causes the head to deflex. This means, for example, that a fetus that was an LOP or ROP converts respectively, to a RMA or LMA at the start of labor and enters the pelvis face first.
2. Engagement. Engagement takes place when the trachelobregmatic (submentobregmatic) diameter has passed through the pelvic inlet. Approximately 70 percent of all face presentations engage as either mentum anterior or mentum transverse varieties. The remaining 30 percent engage as a posterior variety. The axis of the face (midchin to midbrow, bisecting the nose) is used as the fetal diameter in relation to the mother's pelvis which determines in which oblique diameter of the pelvis engagement takes place.
3. Descent occurs throughout.
4. Internal rotation (Fig. 15-2).
   a. rotating the chin anteriorly:
      45° for RMA and LMA to MA
      90° for RMT and LMT to MA
      135° for RMP and LMP to MA
   b. rotating the chin posteriorly:
      45° for RMP and LMP to MP
   If the chin does rotate posteriorly into a mentum posterior position, the mechanisms of labor cease at this point because the baby cannot deliver vaginally from this position (Fig. 15-3). This is because the length of the neck of the fetus is only about half as long as the length of the sacrum. Therefore it is not possible for the chin to escape from the vaginal floor over the perineum, thereby allowing the remainder of the head to be born by flexion. This condition must be recognized immediately before impaction of the head takes place with its extremely poor prognosis for the fetus. Delivery is by cesarean section by the physician.
5. Birth of the head is by a double mechanism of (1) extension and (2) flexion, in this sequence. Extension in maintained until the chin is born by escaping beneath the symphysis pubis. The submento area beneath the chin impinges beneath the symphysis pubis and becomes the pivotal point for the delivery of the rest of the head by flexion. The remaining head is born sequentially starting with the mouth, then the nose, eyes, brow, anterior fontanel, and posterior fontanel, and ending with the occiput as the head flexes.

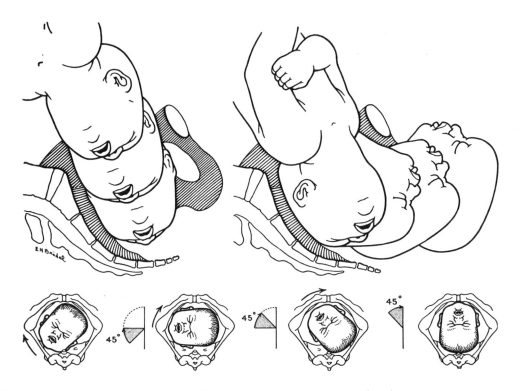

FIGURE 15-2. Mechanisms of labor for right mentoposterior position with subsequent rotation to mentum anterior and delivery. (Reproduced by permission from J. A. Pritchard and P. C. MacDonald. *Williams Obstetrics, 15th.* New York: Appleton-Century-Crofts, 1976.)

6. Restitution. Restitution takes place 45° in the direction from whence the head rotated during internal rotation. For example, if internal rotation was from an RMT to an MA, then restitution is 45° to an RMA (or LOP) position.

7. External rotation. External rotation takes place another 45° in the same direction as restitution, for example, to the RMT (or LOT) position.

8. Birth of the shoulders and body by lateral flexion via the curve of Carus.

Nurse-midwifery management of a face presentation includes the following:

1. Recognition that the position is a face presentation and notification of the physician of this malpresentation.

2. Reevaluation of the adequacy of the pelvis and consultation with the physician if there is a question of possible cephalopelvic disproprotion to rule out this condition.

3. Close monitoring of the mechanism of labor or internal rotation and immediately informing the physician if rotation is to a direct mentum posterior position.

4. For delivery of the head:

a. application of pressure on the fetal brow may be necessary to maintain extension until the chin is born. This is done by pressing on the posterior end of the perineal body as the vulvovaginal orifice distends. You need to protect your gloved

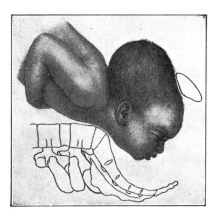

FIGURE 15-3. Face presentation, chin directly posterior, showing impossibility of spontaneous delivery unless rotation occurs. (Reproduced by permission from J. A. Pritchard and P. C. MacDonald. *Williams Obstetrics, 15th.* New York: Appleton-Century-Crofts, 1976.)

hand from contamination from the rectum during this maneuver by covering it with a towel.

    b. exertion of head control thereby allowing the gradual flexion and birth of the remainder of the head. Most face presentations deliver spontaneously with little need for extensive hand maneuvers.

5. Requesting that the pediatrician attend the delivery. If there is extensive edema of the neck (trachea), nose, and mouth, respiratory function may be compromised.

6. Reassuring parents, family, and significant others that the position of the head and neck of the baby (neck extended, head fallen backwards) and the extensive swelling of the features of the face normally disappear in a few days and show noticeable improvement in a day or so.

DELIVERY OF INFANTS WITH BREECH PRESENTATIONS

The involvement of nurse-midwives in the management of breech deliveries varies from practice setting to practice setting. Generally speaking, nurse-midwives are more apt to manage breech deliveries in a private practice setting than are nurse-midwives in a medical center, where each woman with a breech presentation is an object of competition among obstetrics residents for teaching and learning purposes. Regardless of setting, the nurse-midwife must know how to manage the delivery of a baby with a breech presentation because chances are that she will someday be confronted with delivering a breech in an unexpected or emergency situation.

An emergency breech delivery should not be caused by a lack of diagnosis by a nurse-midwife caring for the woman during the antepartal period or during labor. Expected and planned for delivery of a breech presentation by a nurse-midwife should always involve close collaboration with, and immediate availability of, the physician. This is essential because of the potential problems in breech delivery — difficulty in delivery of the after-coming head and need for extensive newborn resuscitation measures.

The nurse-midwife facilitates the mechanisms of labor of a breech presentation, follows the principle of nonintervention as long as progress is visible, and does manual extraction manipulations as indicated. Inasmuch as there is a direct relationship between the mechanisms of labor and the hand maneuvers for delivery of a breech, these are presented side by side in Table 15-1. To aid in this presentation a specific position will be utilized.

In the breech delivery in Table 15-1, the position of the fetus upon entry of the buttocks into the pelvis is LSA (left sacrum anterior). The denominator (arbitrarily chosen portion of the fetus) for determining position is the sacrum. The fetal diameter used to determine the relationship of the baby to the diameter of the mother's pelvis is the bitrochanteric diameter at the upper ends of the femurs as measured at the level of the hip joint (acetabulum). It helps to visualize *the mechanisms of labor* if you remember that they *are in sequence*

TABLE 15-1.   Correlation of Mechanisms of Labor and Hand Maneuvers for Delivery of a Breech Presentation

Mechanism of labor	Hand maneuvers
1. Descent occurs throughout. 2. Engagement of the hips takes place in an LSA position with the sacrum in the left anterior portion of the mother's pelvis and the bitrochanteric diameter in the left oblique diameter of the mother's pelvis. 3. Internal rotation of the buttocks 45 degrees from an LSA to an LST. This brings the anterior hip, which descended more rapidly than the posterior hip and initiated internal rotation when it encountered resistance from the pelvic floor, 45° forward (anterior) to underneath the pubic arch. The bitrochanteric diameter is now in the anteroposterior diameter of the mother's pelvis.	1., 2., and 3. Normally you will not need to intervene. In the event that the breech does not descend, cephalopelvic disproportion and hydrocephalus must be ruled out by the physician. It is possible, however, that failure to descend may be due to a splinting effect caused when it is a frank breech and the extension of the legs across the baby's abdomen prevents fetal maneuverability and arrests progress. In such an event, use of the Pinard maneuver will break up the breech and enable you to bring down the feet and legs, thereby changing a frank breech presentation to a footling breech presentation. This is done as follows (Fig. 15-4): a. With your vaginal hand (left hand if the baby is in a left sacrum position, right hand if the baby is in a right sacrum position) follow the posterior side of a thigh up from the buttocks to the popliteal fossa behind the knee. Your thumb will be on the anterior side of the thigh. b. Move the leg laterally away from the midline and the baby's body while pressing in the popliteal fossa. This will cause the leg to flex at the knee, thereby bringing the foot, which was at the level of the baby's face and out of reach, down to where you can grasp it. c. Bring the leg down by drawing it across the baby's abdomen in its natural range of motion and down for its delivery. d. Repeat for the other thigh, leg, and foot.

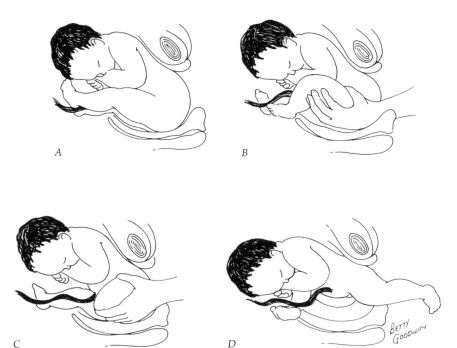

A   *B*

C   *D*

FIGURE 15-4.   Pinard maneuver. A. frank breech; B. leg abducted and flexed at knee by pressing in popliteal fossa; C. foot and leg are brought down and delivered; D. procedure is repeated for other leg and foot.

TABLE 15-1. (Continued)

Mechanism of labor	Hand maneuvers
4. Birth of the buttocks by lateral flexion. When born spontaneously, the posterior hip is born first while the anterior hip impinged beneath the symphysis pubis serves as the pivoting point for the lateral flexion necessary for the posterior hip to follow the curve of Carus to birth. The baby's body then straightens out as the anterior hip is born. The legs and feet usually follow the birth of the breech and are also born spontaneously.	4. The hand maneuver at this time is a deliberate lack of doing anything, i.e., keep your hands off the baby. The one exception to keeping your hands off the baby is if the baby is in a frank breech presentation and the extended legs prevent the necessary lateral flexion for birth of the buttocks. In such an event, Pinard maneuver is used for delivery of the feet and legs and then the buttocks. They may not if it is a frank breech presentation. In such an event, the Pinard maneuver will cause delivery of the legs and feet. Because 70 per cent of breech deliveries are frank breech presentations it is important to know how to do Pinard's maneuver inasmuch as it is the solution for three possible times of arrest during descent and delivery of the buttocks. However, prior to use during actual delivery of the buttocks, legs, and feet (i.e., during descent), cephalopelvic disproportion must be clearly ruled out.
5. (a) External rotation of the buttocks 45° from an LST to an LSA and (b) engagement of the shoulders with the bisacromial diameter in the left oblique diameter of the mother's pelvis (the same as for engagement of the buttocks). These two mechanisms occur simultaneously, with the external rotation of the buttocks being visible evidence of the entry of the shoulders into the true pelvis as the body untwists and aligns itself with the descending shoulders. Descent of the shoulders after their engagement is rapid.	5. The hands-off portion of management is maintained. The rationale for this management is as follows: a. There is no need for facilitating the progress of the mechanisms of labor until the baby is born up to the umbilicus. After that, the remainder of the baby needs to be born in 3 to 5 minutes to avoid any anoxia with resulting possible brain damage. b. Traction exerted on the baby prior to birth up to the umbilicus may cause (1) the arms to fly up in a reflex action, thereby extending them above, over, or behind the head and causing later difficulties in the delivery and/or (2) the head to deflex, which may cause dangerous problems with birth of the head. c. Natural progress using the bulk of the breech maintains cervical dilatation and lessens the possibility that the cervix may clamp around the baby's head or neck. It is a good time for requesting and obtaining a warm, dry towel for use next. When the baby is born up to the umbilicus you do two things: a. Pull down a good-sized loop of umbilical cord to avoid stress on its insertion in the umbilicus during the rest of the delivery. b. Place the warm towel around the baby from just below the umbilicus down. This serves two functions: (1) helps keep the baby warm (2) gives you a nonslippery hold on the baby, which is essential both for safety and for being able to exert the traction now needed.

TABLE 15-1.   (Continued)

Mechanism of labor	Hand maneuvers
6. Internal rotation of the shoulders 45°, bringing the bisacromial diameter of the fetus from the left oblique diameter to the anteroposterior diameter of the mother's pelvis. This is evidenced externally because the delivered body also rotates and the sacrum returns to an LST position from an LSA position.	6. After you have completed the above with birth of the umbilicus, you exert downward and outward traction while facilitating internal rotation of the shoulders with rotation of the body so the sacrum again rotates from an LSA to an LST. To do this safely without injury to internal organs or structures (e.g., kidneys, adrenal glands) resulting from the pressure you apply in order to exert traction, the placement of your hands on bone is vitally important and done as follows: a. Grasp the baby on its hips with your thumbs on either sacroiliac region and your fingers on the corresponding iliac crests (see Fig. 15-5). b. Continue this traction until you can visualize not only the lower half of the scapula of the anterior shoulder but also its corresponding axilla.

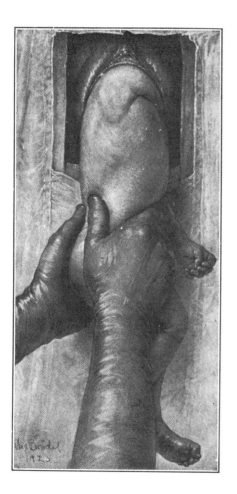

FIGURE 15-5.   Delivery of the anterior shoulder in a breech presentation by downward traction. Note the placement of the hands on the baby's hips. (Reproduced by permission from J. A. Pritchard and P. C. MacDonald. *Williams Obstetrics, 15th.* New York: Appleton-Century-Crofts, 1976.)

TABLE 15-1.   (Continued)

Mechanism of labor	Hand maneuvers
7. Birth of the shoulders by lateral flexion. When born spontaneously, the anterior shoulder impinges beneath the symphysis pubis and serves as the pivotal point for the lateral flexion necessary for delivery of the posterior shoulder via the curve of Carus. Birth of the anterior shoulder then follows as the body straightens out.	7. It doesn't matter which shoulder is delivered first. The following methodology is in accord with the mechanisms of labor. a. Grasp the feet of the baby in one hand with your index finger between the legs and your middle finger and thumb each encircling a leg (see Fig. 15-6). b. Holding the baby by its feet, exert upward traction for the entire body. Be careful that this is at an angle designed to keep the back from turning upwards so that the head will enter the pelvis in the transverse diameter.

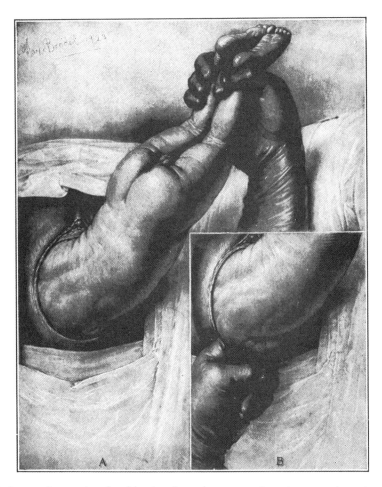

FIGURE 15-6.   Delivery of posterior shoulder in a breech presentation. A. upward traction to effect delivery of posterior shoulder; B. freeing posterior arm. (Reproduced by permission from J. A. Pritchard and P. C. MacDonald. Williams Obstetrics, 15th. New York: Appleton-Century-Crofts, 1976.)

TABLE 15-1.   (Continued)

Mechanism of labor	Hand maneuvers
	c. This draws the posterior shoulder over the perineum to birth, followed by the arm and hand of the same side.
	d. If necessary, such as when the arm has become extended, deliver the arm first. This is done as follows:
	(1) Insert the fingers of your vaginal hand (in this instance of the baby's sacrum being to the left, you would be holding the baby's feet with your left hand and your right hand would be the vaginal hand) and follow the humerus of the posterior arm until the elbow is reached
	(2) Use these fingers now as a splint for the arm and sweep it across the baby's chest downwards to delivery.
	e. Now exert downward traction on the baby for delivery of the anterior shoulder, arm, and hand. To exert this downward traction, again place your hands on the baby's hips as you did in Step 6 (see Fig. 15-5).
	f. Again, if necessary, such as when the arm has become extended, deliver the arm first as described in Step 7d.
	g. If there is a nuchal arm (the arm is extended from the shoulder but flexed at the elbow so that the lower arm is wedged behind the head), attempts to deliver it the same way as for extended arms as in Steps 7d and 7f will not work. Delivery of a nuchal arm is as follows:
	(1) Grasp the baby by placing your hands on the baby's hips as you did for Step 6.
	(2) Rotate the baby's body 90° to 180° in the direction that the baby's hand behind its head is pointing until the arm is dislodged from behind the head. This is accomplished by the friction of the body rotating against the vaginal outlet in a direction that forces the elbow towards the face and places the arm in a position from which it can now be delivered.
	(3) Deliver the arm as for an extended arm as described in Step 7d.
	(4) If both arms are nuchal arms, then repeat this process for the other arm, rotating the baby in the direction indicated, after delivery of the first arm.
	h. If all else fails (a rare circumstance), break the arm by hooking a finger over the arm and pulling on it. Such trauma is indicated when weighed against the baby's life. Such a fracture usually heals well without deformity.
8. Engagement of the head takes place with the sagittal suture in either the transverse or right oblique diameter of the mother's pelvis and the occiput in the left side of the pelvis. The head enters the pelvis as the shoulders near the outlet and may engage prior to or after internal rotation of the shoulders, thus explaining why engagement is in either the transverse or oblique diameter of the pelvis.	8. Suprapubic pressure should be applied to maintain the normal flexion of the baby's head. You request that this be done, because your hands are well occupied with delivery of the shoulders. Suprapubic pressure is continued until the head is born.

TABLE 15-1.   (Continued)

Mechanism of labor	Hand maneuvers
9. Internal rotation of the head 45° or 90°, bringing the sagittal suture from the right oblique or transverse diameter, respectively, into the anteroposterior diameter of the mother's pelvis with the occiput directly anterior and the brow in the hollow of the sacrum of the mother's pelvis. This is evidenced externally because the delivered body also rotates, thereby bringing the bisacromial diameter of the shoulders into the horizontal plane of the mother and the sacrum into a direct anterior position (i.e., the back of the baby is upward and the baby is facing down).	9. Facilitate rotation of the head to an occiput anterior: a. Grasp the baby by placing your hands on the baby's hips as you did for Step 6. b. Monitor the rotation of the head as it is externally evidenced. c. Do not allow the unusual happening of rotation of the head to an occiput posterior as evidenced by rotation of the back posteriorly. If this rarity should begin to occur: d. Counteract by rotating the baby so its back is anterior. Rotation of the head posteriorly so that the occiput is posterior and the chin is facing the symphysis pubis makes delivery of the head extremely difficult and dangerous. Fortunately this posterior rotation is quite rare.

10. Birth of the head by flexion.	10. The vital assistance needed at this time is to keep the head flexed. This is done by continuing suprapubic pressure and by using the Mauriceau-Smellie-Veit maneuver. This maneuver is performed as follows (see Fig. 15-7):
	a. One hand is introduced into the vagina palmar side up beneath the baby's face.
	  (1) The index finger of this hand is put in the baby's mouth and the back of the finger pressed against the maxilla (upper jaw bone), i.e., against the roof of the mouth.
	  (2) This finger is used to help keep the head in flexion and should *never* be used for traction.
	  (3) Care must be taken that the finger does not slip so that pressure and/or traction is applied against the mandible (lower jaw bone) and the base of the tongue since this could cause serious injury.
	  (4) The remainder of the hand is used to support the body of the baby as the baby is positioned astride your arm.
	b. Your other hand is placed on the upper back of the baby with your index finger hooked over one shoulder on one side of the neck and your middle finger hooked over the other shoulder on the other side of the baby's neck.
	  (1) This hand will be used for exerting traction.
	  (2) Place your hooking fingers away from the neck insofar as possible to avoid pressure on the cervical or brachial nerve plexuses.
	  (3) Grasp the shoulders with your thumb and remaining fingers.
	c. Apply downward and outward traction with your hand on the baby's shoulders until the suboccipital region (hair line) can be visualized under the symphysis pubis.
	d. Now apply upward traction while elevating the body of the baby so that the curve of Carus is followed for the sequential birth of the chin, mouth, nose, eyes, brow, anterior fontanel, posterior fontanel, and occiput as the head remains flexed for birth.
	e. Birth of the head is controlled by the pressure of your hands. If it is too fast and the head pops out, intracranial damage may result; and if it is too slow, hypoxia becomes a concern.

TABLE 15-1.   (Continued)

Mechanism of labor	Hand maneuvers

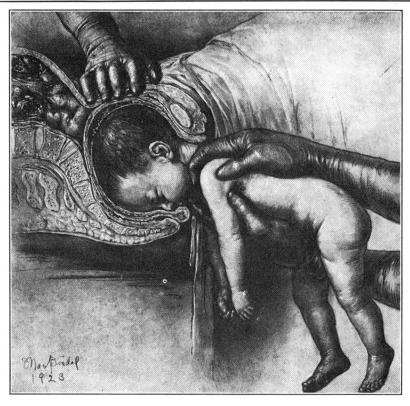

FIGURE 15-7.   Mauriceau-Smellie-Veit maneuver and suprapubic pressure for delivery of the head in a breech presentation. (Reproduced by permission from J. A. Pritchard and P. C. MacDonald. *Williams Obstetrics, 15th.* New York: Appleton-Century-Crofts, 1976.)

for birth of the buttocks, birth of the shoulders, and birth of the head.

Before the actual delivery begins, the following should have taken place:

1. Complete cervical dilatation.
2. Elimination of any question about the adequacy of the pelvis.
3. Emptying of the bladder.
4. Cutting of an episiotomy if you determine the need for one. The need for an episiotomy depends on the estimated fetal weight and the relaxation of the perineum. If an episiotomy is to be performed, choose the type of incision which will give you the most room for manipulative maneuvers (this is usually a mediolateral incision). You can cut an episiotomy at any time during the delivery, even after the buttocks are delivered, if you determine the need for additional room to complete the birth.
5. Effective maternal pushing effort.
6. Readiness for a full-scale newborn resuscitation effort.

7. Positioning so there is plenty of room for lateral flexion and downward traction, that is, lithotomy position either in stirrups or at the edge of a bed.

8. Notification and presence or immediate availability of your consulting physician. If this is an emergency situation in which the nurse-midwife is delivering a woman she or he has not seen before and has not previously had time to examine, the first action of the nurse-midwife is to inform the attending nursing staff of the situation and request that a *stat.* call be placed for the physician. Calls should also be placed for an anesthesiologist or nurse anesthetist and a pediatrician; both must be standing by if needed.

DELIVERY OF A WOMAN WITH MULTIPLE GESTATION

Nurse-midwifery management of the labor and delivery of a woman with multiple gestation is done only in collaboration with the physician and with assurance of the physician's presence for help with the potential problems of neonatal resuscitation, prematurity (higher incidence in multiple gestation), immediate postpartal hemorrhage (resulting from an overdistended uterus), malpresentation of the second twin (higher incidence of malpresentations in multiple gestation), delay in resumption of labor for delivery of the second twin, or need arising for cesarean section such as with locked twins. The nurse-midwife may at some point during her or his career be confronted with the delivery of multiple-gestation infants on an emergency basis. This situation should not arise because of a lack of diagnosis by a nurse-midwife caring for the woman during the antepartal period.

In the event of an emergency the nurse-midwife must know what to do to effect safe delivery of all viable fetuses. For sake of presentation this discussion will be limited to the delivery of twins. The process is repeated for however many fetuses there are. Following are the cardinal points for the labor and delivery of a woman with multiple gestation:

1. Medication during labor should be limited to ataractics (e.g. Vistaril) because of the gestation and size of the fetuses. They are often preterm or small-for-gestational-age — either condition makes medication (analgesics and sedatives) hazardous for them.

2. The woman should have a patent IV.

3. The woman's bladder should be empty at the start of the actual delivery.

4. The physician should be notified and present at the start of the actual delivery.

5. Anesthesia personnel should be notified and on standby.

6. The pediatrician should be notified and present.

7. The woman should be well-positioned in lithotomy position with plenty of room for manipulations.

8. Nursing personnel should be alerted as far in advance as possible because they must prepare multiples of equipment, supplies, forms, and so forth.

9. Preparation for full-scale resuscitation should be completed at the start of the actual delivery.

10. Nursing personnel should be alerted to the probability of an immediate postpartum hemorrhage.

11. The need for an episiotomy depends on the estimated fetal weights, the anticipated need for manipulation if there are fetal malpresentations, and the relaxation of the perineum. If an episiotomy is to be performed, choose the type of incision which will give you the most room for manipulative maneuvers and, in the event of small size or prematurity, will reduce the possibility of intracranial damage. This is usually a mediolateral incision. You can cut an episiotomy at any time during the delivery, for example, after the

first twin is born and during the delivery of the second twin, if you determine such a need.

12. The presentation and position of the babies should be known prior to the start of the actual delivery.

13. Delivery of the first twin is conducted in accord with its presentation and position.

14. Have an assistant direct the second twin into position abdominally as you deliver the first twin.

15. The cord is quickly and securely clamped and cut. There must be no delay in this action because whether or not these are monozygotic twins most likely will not have been diagnosed prior to delivery. The second twin may exsanguinate by bleeding through this cord if they are. Monozygotic (single-ovum) twins usually have one placenta, one chorion, and two amnions (Fig. 15-8).

16. The presentation and position of the second twin are carefully ascertained and the size of the baby is evaluated. If the nurse-midwife has never seen the delivering woman before nor had opportunity to examine her prior to scrubbing for delivery, it may be at this point that the nurse-midwife, in routinely palpating the uterus after the delivery of a baby, discovers the presence of another baby. The immediate action of the nurse-midwife in this situation is to inform the attending nursing staff of the situation and request a *stat.* call be placed for the physician. If the physician will not be able to arrive for some period of time, the nurse-midwife proceeds in this emergency situation as follows, after determination of the presentation, position, and size of the second twin.

17. The fetal heart is closely monitored and the vagina constantly scrutinized for any sign of bleeding while waiting for labor to resume. As long as there is no bleeding or evidence of fetal distress, haste is not indicated. However, a time lag of more than 5 to 10 minutes should not be allowed. This is because the optimum time of birth for the second twin is between 3 to 15 minutes after delivery of the first twin. The reason for this is that advantage must be taken of the just fully dilated cervix before it starts to close again. Also, you wish to deliver the second twin before the placenta starts to separate, a condition

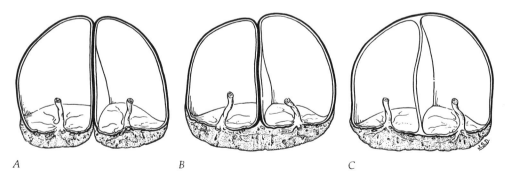

A *B* *C*

FIGURE 15-8. Placenta and membranes in twin pregnancies. A. two placentas, two amnions, two chorions from either dizygotic twins or monozygotic twins (zygotic division occurred within the first 3 days after fertilization); B. same as A., except two placentas fused into single placenta; C. one placenta, two amnions, one chorion from monozygotic twins (zygotic division occurred between the fourth and eighth days after fertilization. (Reproduced by permission from J. A. Pritchard and P. C. MacDonald, *Williams Obstetrics, 15th.* New York: Appleton-Century-Crofts, 1976.)

which demands quick action in order to obtain a viable second baby.

18. With or without labor resumption within the time limit, the presenting part is guided into the true pelvis by a combination of abdominal pressure and vaginal manipulations. Care is first taken to rule out a presenting umbilical cord.

19. Once the presenting part is fixed into the pelvis, rupture the membranes. If the presenting part is a breech or an unengaged head, leave your hand in the vagina to ascertain whether or not the cord has prolapsed. There is less chance of a prolapsed cord if the membranes are ruptured with no pressure (contractions or fundal) behind them and if they are leaked rather than torn. If there has not been resumption of labor up to this time, rupturing the membranes may stimulate contractions to resume.

20. The mother should be encouraged to push.

21. If contractions have still not resumed and the maternal pushing effort is insufficient, an intravenous solution of 1000 milliliters D_5W or D_5RL with 10 IU of Pitocin should be hung and started at a slow drip (12 to 15 drops per minute).

22. Delivery is conducted as usual.

23. Third stage hemorrhage or immediate postpartum hemorrhage is likely (see Chapters 17 and 19 for management of these emergencies).

REFERENCE

1. Morris, W. I. C. Report of societies. *J. Obstet. Gynaecol. Brit. Empire* 62:302, 1955.

BIBLIOGRAPHY

Barnum, C. G. Dystocia due to the shoulders. *Am. J. Obstet. Gynecol.* 50:439, 1945.

Cetrulo, C. L., Freeman, R. K., and Knuppel, R. A. Minimizing the risks of twin delivery. *Contemporary OB/GYN* 9:47, 1977.

Greenhill, J. P., and Friedman, E. A. *Biological Principles and Modern Practice of Obstetrics.* Philadelphia: Saunders, 1974.

Intrapartum Module. Nurse-Midwifery Education Program, University of Mississippi Medical Center, Jackson, Mississippi (Baton Rouge draft), 1976.

Little, W. A., and Friedman, E. A. The twin delivery — factors influencing second twin mortality. *Obstet. Gynecol. Surv.* 13:611, 1958.

Morris, W. I. C. Reports of societies, *J. Obstet. Gynecol. Brit. Empire* 62:302, 1955.

Myles, M. F. *Textbook for Midwives, 8th.* London: Livingstone, 1975.

Oxorn, H., *Oxorn-Foote Human Labor and Birth, 5th.* Norwalk, Conn.: Appleton-Century-Crofts, 1986.

Pritchard, J. A. MacDonald, P. C. and Gant, N. F. *Williams Obstetrics 17th.* Norwalk, Conn.: Appleton-Century-Crofts, 1985.

Reid, D. E., Ryan, K. J., and Benirschke, K. *Principles and Management of Human Reproduction.* Philadelphia: Saunders, 1972.

Rovinsky, J. J., Miller, J. A., and Kaplan, S. Management of breech presentation at term. *Am. J. Obstet. Gynecol.* 115:497, 1973.

Swartz, D. P. Shoulder girdle dystocia in vertex delivery: Clinical study and review. *Obstet. Gynecol.* 15:194, 1960.

Taylor, E. S. *Beck's Obstetrical Practice, 9th.* Baltimore: Williams & Wilkins, 1971.

Taylor, E. S. *Beck's Obstetrical Practice and Fetal Medicine, 10th.* Baltimore: Williams & Wilkins, 1977.

Woods, C. E. A principle of physics as applicable to shoulder delivery. *Am. J. Obstet. Gynecol.* 45:796, 1943.

16

The Normal Third
Stage of Labor

The third stage of labor starts upon completion of the birth of the baby and ends with the birth of the placenta. It is known as the placental stage of labor. The third stage of labor averages between 5 and 10 minutes. However, it is within the realm of normal for the third stage to be of longer duration.

DATA BASE OF THE THIRD STAGE OF LABOR

The components of the data base for determining the well-being of the patient during the third stage of labor are as follows:

1. Continuing evaluation of any previous significant findings.
2. Evaluation of the progress of labor.
3. Continuing evaluation of the mother.
4. Screening for signs and symptoms of third stage hemorrhage. (This content may be found in Chapter 17.)

The processes of the third stage of labor and parameters of normal for this period must be known in order to evaluate the data base.

Although initial evaluation and management of the baby also occurs during the third stage of labor, for the sake of clarity it is not covered in this chapter. Content regarding the baby may be found in the chapters pertaining to the neonate.

Evaluation of the Progress of Labor

The third stage of labor consists of two phases. The first phase is that of placental separation and the second phase is that of placental expulsion. Both separation and expulsion are brought about by contractions which begin again after a brief pause at birth. The contractions had been approximately every 2 to 2½ minutes apart during the second stage of labor. After the birth of the baby, the next contraction may not occur for 3 to 5 minutes. Contractions then follow every 4 to 5 minutes until there has been separation and expulsion of the placenta. After that, the emptied uterus contracts down on itself and remains contracted if the muscle tone is good. Otherwise, recurrent uterine contraction and relaxation constitute afterbirth pains if the muscle tone is not as good.

Placental separation is the result of the abrupt decrease in size of the uterine cavity during and following the delivery of the baby as the uterus contracts down upon the reduced uterine contents. This decrease in uterine size necessarily means a concomitant decrease in the area of placental attachment. The placenta, however, remains the same size. The placenta first tries to accommodate itself to this decrease in uterine size by becoming thicker, but at the site of attachment it is unable to withstand the stress and buckles. The result is a separation of the placenta from the uterine wall, which takes place in the spongiosa layer of the decidua. As the placenta separates, a hematoma forms between the separating placenta and the remaining decidua as a result of bleeding into the intervillous space. This is known as the retroplacental hematoma and may vary considerably in size. While it is the result rather than the cause of placental separation, it does facilitate the completion of placental separation.

After the placenta has separated it descends into the lower uterine segment or into the upper vaginal vault, causing the clinical signs of placental separation to become evident. These are as follows:

1. Sudden trickle or small gush of blood
2. Lengthening of the amount of umbilical cord visible at the vaginal introitus
3. Change in the shape of the uterus from discoid to globular as the uterus now contracts upon itself
4. Change in the position of the uterus as it rises in the abdomen because the bulk of the placenta in the lower uterine segment or upper vaginal vault displaces the uterus upwards

Placental expulsion begins with the descent of the placenta into the lower uterine segment. It then passes through the cervix into the upper vaginal vault, from whence it is expelled. Expulsion of the placenta is by one of two mechanisms. The Schultz mechanism is by far the more common of the two although both are considered normal.

The *Schultz mechanism* of placental expulsion is delivery of the placenta with the fetal side presenting. This is thought to occur when separation begins centrally with corresponding formation of a central retroplacental clot which weights the placenta so the central portion descends first. This, in effect, inverts the placenta and amniotic sac, and causes the membranes to peel off the remainder of the decidua and trail behind the placenta. The majority of bleeding occurring with this mechanism of labor is not visualized until the placenta and membranes are delivered, since the inverted membranes catch and hold the blood.

The *Duncan mechanism* of placental expulsion is delivery of the placenta with the maternal side presenting. This is thought to occur when separation first takes place at the margin or periphery of the placenta. Blood escapes between the membranes and uterine wall and is visualized externally. The placenta descends sideways and the amniotic sac, therefore, is not inverted but trails behind the placenta for delivery.

The memory aid for correctly identifying the mechanisms of placental expulsion is based on the appearance of the two different sides of the placenta. The fetal side is shiny and glistening because its covering is the fetal membranes, while the maternal side is rough and red-looking. Hence the sayings "shiny Schultz" and "dirty Duncan."

Continuing Evaluation of the Mother

Many of the normal physiologic changes occurring during the first and second stages of labor return to prelabor levels during the third stage. These are as follows:

Blood pressure — both systolic and diastolic pressures start to return to prelabor levels.
Pulse — the pulse rate gradually returns to prelabor level.

Temperature — continues to be slightly elevated.

Respirations — return to normal.

Gastrointestinal activity — if not affected by drugs, gastric motility and absorption begin to return to normal activity. It is unusual for there to be any nausea and vomiting during the third stage.

During the third stage of labor the mother's interest in the baby is apparent if the baby is on her abdomen. In the event the baby is not with the mother, she will express her interest and concern with questions: ''Is it all right?'' ''What is it?'' ''How much does she/he weigh?'' She wants to see for herself that her baby is all right and usually is eager to touch and hold her baby (Fig. 16-1). She is elated, proud of herself, relieved, and very tired. She also has concerns for herself and usually asks if she needs stitches. Prepared mothers are also usually interested in the placenta.

Mothers or couples may desire the Leboyer approach to childbirth and transition of the baby from intrauterine to extrauterine life.

The methodology for this is detailed later in this chapter.

MANAGEMENT PLAN FOR THE THIRD STAGE OF LABOR

This part of the chapter deals strictly with the obstetric management of the mother during the third stage of labor. During the third stage of labor the nurse-midwife is also responsible for initial management of the baby (i.e., drying the baby, providing for warmth, assuring a clear airway) and for initial mother-baby-family bonding and relationships. This material is presented elsewhere.

Management of the placental stage of labor can make considerable difference in the amount of blood the mother loses. Mismanagement of third stage is the largest single cause of third stage hemorrhage. Mismanagement of third stage can also be the cause of uterine inversion and its attendant life-threatening shock. Such disastrous complications can be readily avoided

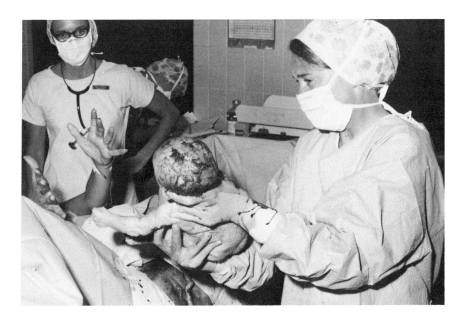

FIGURE 16-1. Nurse-midwife handing baby to mother immediately after birth.

by strict adherence to the following rules:

1. Guard the uterus to keep yourself and anyone else from massaging it prior to placental separation.
2. Do not massage the uterus before placental separation except when partial separation has occurred by natural processes and excessive bleeding is evident. (See Chapter 17.)
3. Do not pull on the umbilical cord before the placenta separates or ever with an uncontracted uterus.
4. Do not try to deliver the placenta prior to its complete separation unless in the emergency situation of third stage hemorrhage. (See Chapter 17.)
5. Become expert in diagnosing placental separation.
6. Discipline yourself in the art of patient waiting and in not feeling pressured into unwise interference with natural processes.

Placental Separation

During initial care of the baby the nurse-midwife must keep one eye on the mother's perineum in order to watch for signs of placental separation and for excessive bleeding. (By the same token, when the nurse-midwife has returned to the mother's perineum to manage third stage she or he must keep one eye on the baby to continually evaluate the baby's well-being.) Upon return to the mother's perineum to manage third stage the first action is to evaluate the progress of labor and the mother's condition. One hand is placed on the mother's abdomen to feel, without massaging, the shape and position of the uterus and whether or not it is contracted.

If cord blood is to be collected, now is the time to obtain the specimens. The easiest non-messy way to obtain cord blood is to guide the cut end of the umbilical cord into the open end of the sterile blood tube and to hold it in position with the fingers of the same hand that is holding the blood tube. The other hand releases the clamp on the cord and is ready to reclamp the cord when the tube is filled. This sequence is repeated for however many blood tubes are being collected. If the end of the umbilical cord is not held in its position in the upper end of the blood tube, it most likely will flip out of the tube when the clamp is released due to the sudden pressure of blood flowing through the depleted cord; this will result in a spray of blood over everyone and everything within about a 3-foot radius.

Some clinicians fairly routinely "drain the placenta" by simply taking the clamp off the umbilical cord and catching the blood either in the foot basin or placental pan. The rationale used for this action is that draining the placenta decreases its volume, thereby facilitating its separation from the uterine wall. This rationale is of questionable validity but there are no known dangers to draining the placenta. It is worth trying if separation is slow and time is extending to the point of concern. The only problem is that blood from the placenta can badly distort upwards the estimation of the total blood loss unless it is collected separately.

The cord is wound around the clamp until the clamp is at the vaginal introitus so that traction can be effectively exerted on the cord when needed. This clamp is held with one hand while the other hand continues to guard the uterus.

"Guarding the uterus" means exactly what the words imply. While your hand is in a position to continually ascertain the shape, position, and consistency of the uterus it is also in a position to keep anyone from massaging the uterus, thereby guarding it and the mother from the complications that can result from such an action. Normal placental separation from the uterine wall is accomplished by the effect of uterine contractions as detailed earlier in this chapter. If the uterus is massaged before the placenta's separation from the uterine wall the chances are high for this action causing a partial separation of the placenta and resulting hemorrhage. The danger of a partial separation is that the uterus, because there is a portion of the placenta still attached to it, is unable to contract sufficiently to ligate and collapse the bleeding vessels interwoven through the muscle fibers in the area where separation has occurred; hemorrhage results. Management of this complication is discussed in Chapter 17.

If you are unsure whether or not the placenta has separated, you can check by using a modification of the Brandt-Andrews maneuver. In this you hold the cord taut at the vaginal introitus with one hand, using the clamp for leverage. With your abdominal hand you bring the tips of your fingers, with your fingers close against each other, straight down into the lower abdomen just above the symphysis pubis and watch what happens to the umbilical cord (Fig. 16-2). If the cord recedes into the vagina

then the placenta is not separated. If the cord has a feeling of give and remains the same or lengthens beyond its position at the vaginal introitus, then the placenta has separated and you may proceed with facilitating placental expulsion.

If you are still unsure whether the placenta is separated there is another method you can use to determine the location of the placenta. In this you again hold the cord tautly with one hand at the vaginal introitus, and with your other hand follow the cord into the vagina with your examining fingers until either you feel where it inserts into the placenta or the cord extends through the cervix and into the uterus beyond your reach. In the latter instance you can assume that the placenta has not separated. In the former instance you will probably find the placenta in or at the cervical

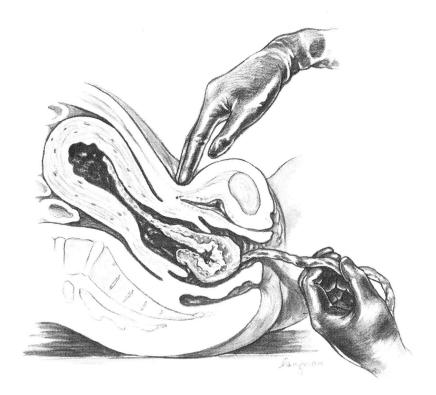

FIGURE 16-2. Checking for placental separation. (Reproduced by permission from J.P. Greenhill and E.A. Friedman. *Biological Principles and Modern Practice of Obstetrics*. Philadelphia: Saunders, 1974.)

os or in the upper vaginal vault and obviously separated. This technique should not be used routinely but reserved for when there is true doubt or concern, because of both the increased risk of introducing infection every time you put your fingers inside the vagina and the possible additional discomfort to the woman. Generally speaking you do not need to use this technique but it is handy to know. It is better, however, to sharpen your diagnostic ability by scrupulous attention to the signs of placental separation.

Placental Expulsion

Once you are sure the placenta has separated you may facilitate the mother's efforts to expel it. This is done by using a combination of the Brandt-Andrews maneuver and controlled cord traction. The abdominal hand assures that the uterus is contracted and braces the body of the uterus. This is done by placing the palmar surface of the hand just above the symphysis pubis and pressing straight down against the uterus with a slight direction toward the umbilicus. At the same time the other hand exerts traction on the cord, using the clamp around which the excess cord is wrapped for leverage. Also, at the same time, you ask the woman to push. It is important to remember that the placenta follows the curve of Carus just as the fetus did. Therefore, the direction of the traction exerted on the cord is first downward and then upward as it comes into view for the actual delivery.

Cord traction is never exerted at any time unless the uterus is contracted. If the uterus is not contracted and the placenta or membranes are adherent to the uterine wall, inversion of the uterus is a potential danger. In such circumstances cord traction may bring not only the placenta but also the attached uterine wall. This is an obstetric disaster and is discussed in the next chapter. Such a disaster is prevented by checking to make sure the uterus is contracted before exerting any degree of cord traction and

by not attempting to deliver the placenta by pulling on the cord before being absolutely sure placental separation has occurred.

Likewise, the cord should never just be pulled. If the placenta has not yet separated it is possible to (1) disrupt the placenta, causing a partial separation and possible hemorrhage; (2) cause an inversion of the uterus as described in the preceding paragraph; or (3) cause the cord to detach from the placenta, thereby requiring manual removal of the placenta and exposing the woman to unnecessary trauma and an increased risk of intrauterine infection.

Bracing of the uterus in the expulsion of the placenta and strict abstinence from using the uterus as a piston to propel the placenta through the vaginal canal has important gynecologic implications. Using the uterus as a piston stretches the cardinal ligaments and may potentiate uterine prolapse in later life, especially if done vigorously or repeated with each childbearing experience. Avoidance of using the uterus as a piston then becomes a preventive measure to uterine prolapse.

It should be noted that placental expulsion is not a problem requiring facilitative efforts by the attendant when natural positions of the mother, such as squatting, are utilized. The positioning of the woman in a flat or slightly elevated recumbent position negates both the down and outward direction of the vagina and the direction of gravity, which are the natural facilitative forces when the woman is in an upright position.

A basin is pressed against the woman's buttocks to catch blood and to hold the placenta when it is born. If the woman is in a lithotomy position the pan is braced between the woman's buttocks and the nurse-midwife's body because the nurse-midwife needs both hands free to manage the third stage of labor. Use of the placenta basin to catch the blood makes it possible to measure the majority of the blood loss and also minimizes mess.

As the placenta is born it is either allowed to slide gently down the side of the placenta basin, which is positioned more on its side at

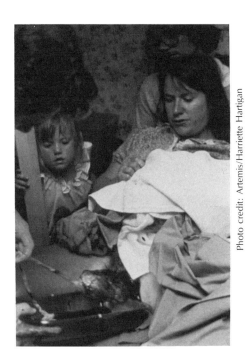

Photo credit: Artemis/Harriette Hartigan

FIGURE 16-3.   Delivery of the placenta.

the vaginal introitus for this purpose, or is delivered into the nurse-midwife's hands at the vaginal introitus. Either way the principle involved is not to let the placenta drop any distance from the level of the vaginal introitus since this might cause the after-coming membranes, which may still be peeling off the uterine wall as the placenta is delivered, to tear and break off and be retained. See Figure 16-3.

The third stage has ended if the membranes immediately follow the placenta and are delivered with the placenta. However, sometimes the membranes trail behind and threaten to break off if tension is applied to them. In such an instance, they may be teased out in one of two ways.

One way is to take a clamp (large Kelly clamp preferably; large ring forceps will do) and place it on the membranes at the vaginal introitus. One hand continues to support the placenta, or the basin with the placenta in it,

in order to prevent tension on the membranes. The other hand manipulates the clamped membranes by gently rocking them up and down and side to side while exerting the slightest bit of traction on them. You are able to judge the appropriate amount of traction inasmuch as you can feel when the steady "give" of the membranes being teased out becomes a "tearing give" instead. As the membranes are gradually teased out, the clamp moves away from the vaginal introitus. Therefore it needs to be periodically reclamped on the membranes at the introitus whenever it gets an inch or two away, because you have better control of manipulating the membranes the closer the clamp is to the vaginal introitus. The process is continued until the membranes are delivered.

The other way to tease out the membranes is to hold the placenta in your hands and turn it over and over. This causes the membranes to twist, thereby having the effect of gradually teasing them out until they are delivered. This method may be more difficult for inexperienced hands because the placenta is slippery and it is not as easy to control the amount of tension on the membranes as it is in the first method.

If the membranes do break off while you are trying to tease them out, third stage is considered ended. Sometimes the torn end of the membranes may be visualized during the cervical inspection and more teased out. The generally accepted management if a portion of the membranes is retained is that this does not warrant uterine exploration to remove them. Uterine exploration is traumatic to the woman and increases the risk of intrauterine infection. Retention of a portion of the membranes is not a cause of hemorrhage as is true for retained placental fragments. While the retained portion of the membranes will eventually be expelled with the lochia, they need to be expelled as soon as possible as their retention does increase the risk of endometritis. To achieve this more rapid expulsion a full methylergonovine (Methergine) or ergonovine (Ergotrate) series should be ordered for the woman: Methergine 0.2 milligrams or Ergotrate 0.2 milligrams every

4 hours for 6 doses. Some clinicians follow this initial series with 0.2 milligrams Methergine or Ergotrate t.i.d. for 3 days. If the estimated portion of membranes retained was a large amount, some clinicians also give an immediate dose of Methergine 0.2 milligrams or Ergotrate 0.2 milligrams intramuscularly unless the woman is hypertensive, in which case it would be contraindicated.

Evaluation of the Mother

The blood pressure and pulse of the mother should be taken at least once during the third stage and more often if the third stage is longer than average or the blood pressure and pulse are either bordering upon or in abnormal ranges. This monitoring not only follows through on evaluation of any previous elevations but is necessary as a means of screening for shock in the event of hemorrhage.

LEBOYER METHODOLOGY

The Leboyer approach to childbirth and to transition of the baby from intrauterine to extrauterine life is geared toward making this transition as atraumatic, painless, and non-frightening as possible for the baby. This requires a reeducation process for parents and professionals alike. A full discussion of the methodology and its effect may be found in Dr. Frederick Leboyer's book, *Birth without Violence* [1]. The following is a listing of specific actions, in sequence, suggested in his book:

1. Extinguish or dim lights to the minimum needed for birth; dim still further after birth. For example, overhead lights or spotlights are not really necessary at this time.
2. Silence. Any essential communication should be done in very low, muted voices toward the end of labor, reducing to a whisper at the time of birth and thereafter.
3. Patience throughout.
4. Support the baby's body without touching the baby's sensitive head during the delivery and place the baby on the mother's abdomen. Normally the baby emits one to three good, clear cries, no more, and settles into breathing. If the cries are not good, clear, and vigorous and the baby is limp, then resuscitation efforts are indicated.
5. Place the baby initially on the mother's abdomen with the limbs underneath the body. After the baby has stretched and the limbs are moving, turn the baby onto one side because this position facilitates relaxation of the limbs. Then, briefly, place the baby on his or her back.
6. Cut the umbilical cord when it has stopped pulsating. The cord is cut immediately if necessary during birth if it is tight around the baby's neck.
7. While the baby is on its abdomen, on the mother's abdomen, the baby's body is massaged, preferably by the mother. Massage is initiated by letting the hands lie motionless yet attentive, responsive, loving. Then a slow, continuous, wave-like massage is done down the baby's back, over and over in measured fluidity.
8. The baby is then placed in a basin for a water bath. The temperature of the water should be 98° to 99°F (36.6° to 37.2°C). The baby is placed in the water extremely slowly and remains in the bath until completely relaxed. This is a good role for the significant other, thereby further involving and bonding this person with the baby. The baby most likely will open his or her eyes during the bath and may also smile and indulge in exploratory play (Fig. 16-4).
9. Remove the baby slowly from the water bath, reimmerse, and then remove from the water again. This facilitates adjustment to gravity.
10. Place the baby on a warmed diaper and

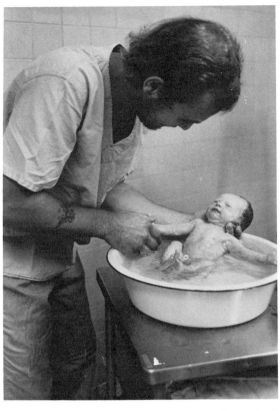

FIGURE 16-4.   Father giving his baby a Leboyer bath.

wrap in warm blankets without restraining the baby's hands.
11. Place the baby on one side with back support provided.
12. The baby is then left alone in stillness.

This does not mean that the baby is no longer under continuing observation. This entire process takes approximately 10 minutes, depending on the length of time in the water bath.

The Leboyer method dovetails nicely with attachment processes, maternal-infant bonding, and the initiation of the parenting continuum. Further contact with the mother, including breast-feeding and eye-to-eye contact, may be smoothly initiated after completion of the Leboyer method.

REFERENCE

1. Leboyer, F. *Birth without Violence.* New York: Knopf, 1976.

Bibliography is at the end of Chapter 19.

17

Third Stage Complications and Management

Third stage complications relate to the placenta and its attachment to the uterus. All are life threatening. The nurse-midwife must know what to do within the limits of her or his capabilities to maintain the woman or resolve the problem while awaiting the physician. Third stage complications discussed in this chapter are third stage hemorrhage, placenta accreta, and uterine inversion.

THIRD STAGE HEMORRHAGE

Third stage hemorrhage is due to partial separation of the placenta. The most common reason for partial separation is mismanagement of the third stage, usually involving uterine massage prior to placental separation. Partial separation may occur naturally during the physiologic separation of the placenta but this stage usually is quickly transient. Partial separation due to massage of the uterus before

the placenta's separation from the uterine wall is not physiologic and carries with it the almost guaranteed result of third stage hemorrhage.

Normally there is some blood loss during the third stage insofar as a sudden trickle or small gush of blood is a sign of placental separation. However, when there is a steady flow of blood and you have located the placenta within the uterus and determined that it has not fully separated (see p. 367), measures for managing third stage hemorrhage need to be instituted immediately. These measures are as follows:

1. Have the nursing staff give the physician a *stat.* call.

2. Thoroughly massage the uterus. Although this should never be done prior to placental separation in a normal situation, it is the first action to take when faced with a partially separated placenta and third stage hemorrhage. This is because a thorough massage

at this time may complete placental separation. This action, with a well-contracted uterus, is combined with controlled cord traction so that as separation is completed delivery of the placenta occurs immediately.

3. While doing step 2, have the nursing staff:
   a. make sure that the IV is patent or start one with a 16-gauge needle if the woman does not have an IV.
   b. draw a type and crossmatch if one has not already been drawn.
   c. watch for signs and symptoms of shock and start monitoring the blood pressure and pulse; lower the head of the bed if indicated.
   d. have Ringer's lactate solution ready to hang if needed for IV infusion.

4. If the placenta has not yet delivered, perform manual removal of the placenta (see Chapter 57). Catheterize the woman first unless you are sure that her bladder is empty.

5. If the nurse-midwife does not know how to perform manual removal of the placenta, the placenta has not yet delivered, bleeding is steadily continuing, and the physician has not yet arrived, then the addition of oxytocin to the IV infusion is order. The purpose for using oxytocin is to contract the uterus in an effort to cause completion of placental separation. Usually this action is delayed unless absolutely necessary. Oxytocin causes the cervix to close, thereby making manual removal of the placenta difficult as well as increasing the incidence of placental retention after its separation. However, an oxytocin preparation which causes intermittent contractions (Pitocin, Syntocinon), is preferred over a preparation which causes a sustained contraction (Ergotrate, Methergine). The former is less likely to cause the cervix to clamp down.

6. If the patient is developing shock and the physician has not yet arrived, order the lactated Ringer's substituted for the D₅W as the solution for the intravenous infusion.

The incidence of third stage hemorrhage is rare *if* third stage is *not* mismanaged. Nevertheless, it can happen, even with the best third stage management. An infectious process with a high temperature during pregnancy increases placental adherence, as does any intrauterine infection, disease processes of the fetal membranes, or previous cesarean section. History of a previous third stage hemorrhage should make you anticipatory, alert, and wary. Third stage hemorrhage will occur when there is a partial placenta accreta.

PLACENTA ACCRETA

Placenta accreta is an abnormal partial or total adherence of the placenta to the uterine wall. In placenta accreta the placenta is directly adherent to the myometrium with either defective decidua or no decidua in between. When the chorionic villi extend further than contact with the myometrium and actually penetrate the uterine wall, the condition is called *placenta increta*. *Placenta percreta* occurs when the chorionic villi invade through the entire uterine wall to the serosa layer. These conditions are rare complications, although placenta accreta does have an increased incidence when the patient has placenta previa.

A partial placenta accreta is first seen as an acute third stage hemorrhage resulting from a partially separated placenta. Clinical diagnosis is made when the placenta's adherence is discovered during attempted manual removal. Definitive diagnosis of placenta accreta is made by microscopic examination. A complete placenta accreta has no signs and symptoms since there is no partial separation and, therefore, no hemorrhage. It is discovered during attempted manual removal of the retained placenta.

Placenta accreta is an obstetric disaster. Any suspicion that a retained placenta is due to placenta accreta requires that the nurse-midwife immediately place an urgent call for the physician. While waiting, the nurse-midwife does all she can to maintain the woman and prepare her for immediate surgery. Under no circumstances should any further attempt be made to remove the placenta as this will only yield greater hemorrhage and possible rupture or inversion of the uterus. The physician probably will manage the care of the woman by performing an emergency hysterectomy.

UTERINE INVERSION

Uterine inversion is the situation in which the uterus literally turns inside out so that the inside of the fundus either (1) protrudes through the cervical os (incomplete), (2) descends to immediately within the vaginal introitus (complete), or (3) extrudes beyond the vulva (prolapsed). In the first two positions, the fundus is felt, upon vaginal examination, as a soft tumor filling the cervical or vaginal orifice. Abdominally, a funnel-like depression may be felt instead of the fundus.

Basically there are three conditions that combine to create a situation favorable to uterine inversion. These are (1) uterine atony, or uncontracted uterus, (2) a patulous, dilated cervix, and (3) fundal pressure or traction caused by pulling on the umbilical cord or placenta.

While it is possible for a uterine inversion to occur spontaneously, it is more likely to be the result of mismanagement of the third stage of labor. In considering the three conditions just mentioned it becomes obvious that it is the third condition over which the most control can be exerted. Uterine inversion can take place as a result of fundal pressure caused by a sudden increase in intraabdominal pressure, such as with coughing. However, it is more apt to occur from any or a combination of the following events, each of which is an act of mismanagement:

1. Applying fundal pressure with a hand on an uncontracted uterus such as might be erroneously done in facilitating expulsion of the placenta if the uterus were wrongly being used as a piston.

2. Having the mother push to help expel the placenta without first checking to see that the uterus was contracted.
3. Exerting cord traction prior to placental separation.
4. Pulling on the placenta during manual removal prior to total placental separation.

In approximately three-quarters of the cases of uterine inversion the placenta is completely or partially attached to the uterine fundus. Spontaneous uterine inversion fortunately is an extremely rare obstetric accident.

The major result of uterine inversion is shock. Excessive bleeding and severe uterine pain may or may not be present. Diagnosis is made by observation of the uterine lining outside the vulva or by findings upon vaginal and abdominal examination. Uterine inversion should be suspected and a diagnostic vaginal examination performed if the woman goes into shock after delivery without obvious reason.

In the event of uterine inversion the physician is notified immediately and the woman is maintained and treated for shock until the physician arrives. The physician probably will manage the care of the woman by treating for shock and by repositioning the uterus. Repositioning of the uterus can be done manually if inversion is diagnosed and the manipulation is performed immediately after the inversion occurs. However, if there has been a time interval between inversion and diagnosis, which can happen in insidious cases during the postpartal period, then operative procedures will be required in order to reposition the uterus.

Manual repositioning of the uterus is accomplished by placing one entire hand in the vagina with the fingertips circumferentially at the junction where the uterus has turned on itself and the inverted fundus in the palm of the hand. Pressure is then applied with the palm of the hand on the fundus and the fingertips on the uterine walls. The fingertips walk up the uterine walls as the fundus is repositioned. Care must be taken not to puncture or rupture the soft uterine wall. At the same time the entire uterus is lifted high out of the pelvis, above the level of the umbilicus, and held there for several minutes. This puts tension on the uterine ligaments which keeps the uterus reinverted. This procedure is usually quite painful, and deep anesthesia is desirable. However, the nurse-midwife should know this technique and use it, without anesthesia, in the event that arrival of a physician is going to be delayed. Most nurse-midwives will never see this complication.

_____

Bibliography is at the end of Chapter 19.

18

The Normal Fourth Stage of Labor

The fourth stage of labor begins with the birth of the placenta and ends one hour later. It is, in fact, the first hour of the postpartum period. While labor and the intrapartal period have technically ended, the first postpartal hour is often referred to as the fourth stage of labor. This is because it is a critical time of initial recovery from the stresses of labor, requiring close observation of the patient, and because a portion of this hour will be spent in activities directly related to the intrapartal period. These activities may include the following:

1. Evaluation of the uterus
2. Cervical, vaginal, and perineal inspection and evaluation
3. Inspection and evaluation of the placenta, membranes, and umbilical cord
4. Repair of episiotomy and lacerations, if any

In addition, vital signs and other physiologic manifestations are evaluated as indicators of recovery from the stresses of labor.

Throughout this period another activity of paramount importance is ongoing. This is the beginning of family relationships (Fig. 18-1). It is during this hour that the baby is in the taking-in phase. Facilitation of this phase and ensuring the mother's participation in it are vital to the bonding process. Such facilitation and participation presupposes a mother and baby neither of whom is in jeopardy. Continuing evaluation of the baby's vital signs and physiologic manifestations are imperative and also ongoing during the fourth stage of labor. Continuing evaluation of the baby is discussed in the chapters on the neonate.

DATA BASE OF THE FOURTH STAGE OF LABOR

Information needed for the evaluation and management of the care of the mother during the first hour postpartum, and knowledge of the taking-in phase of the newborn and the maternal-child bonding process are the components of the data base for the fourth stage of labor.

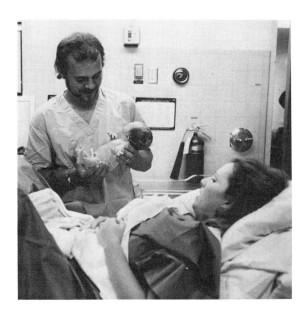

FIGURE 18-1.   Father-baby early bonding.

The Uterus

After delivery of the placenta, the uterus is normally found in the midline of the abdomen approximately two-thirds to three-fourths of the way up between the symphysis pubis and the umbilicus. (See Fig. 24-1, p. 477). A uterus found above the umbilicus is indicative of blood clots in the uterus which need to be expressed and expelled. A uterus found above the umbilicus and to one side, usually the right side, indicates a full bladder. In such an instance the bladder must be emptied. A full bladder displaces the uterus from its position and prevents its contracting as it should, thereby allowing a greater amount of bleeding.

The uterus should be firm (hard) to the touch. A soft, boggy uterus is a hypotonic uterus that is not contracting as it should and, therefore, more bleeding is occurring than should be. Uterine atony is the major cause of immediate postpartum hemorrhage. A firm uterus is indicative of effective uterine hemostasis. Uterine hemostasis is effected by con-traction of the uterus. When contracted the entwining muscle fibers in the myometrium serve as ligatures to the open blood vessels at the placental site and bleeding is controlled naturally. Normally thrombi do not form in the blood vessels in the myometrium but rather form in the distal blood vessels in the decidua. This arrangement of ligation occurring in the myometrium and thrombosis occurring in the decidua is important because it prevents the release of thrombi into the systemic circulation from the myometrial veins.

The Cervix, Vagina, and Perineum

The cervix, vagina, and perineum are inspected primarily for lacerations and secondarily for bruising. Since inspection of the cervix is an uncomfortable procedure for the mother it is done only when indicated, as discussed later in this chapter.

Immediately after delivery of the placenta the cervix is patulous, thick, and floppy. If there was a pronounced anterior lip during labor it is obvious during cervical inspection because it is more edematous than the rest of the cervix.

The Placenta, Membranes, and Umbilical Cord

Necessary data for inspection and evaluation of these structures includes identification of the different types of placentas and cord in-sertions. This content is covered along with the description of how to do placental in-spection in Chapter 55.

Repair of Episiotomy and Lacerations

Repair of episiotomies and lacerations entail a knowledge of perineal muscle structure, types of stitches, hemostasis, and wound healing. All of this content is included in Chapter 60.

Physiologic Status

Many of the physiologic changes that occur during the intrapartal period return to prelabor levels and stabilize during the first hour postpartum. Other physiologic manifestations of the fourth stage of labor result from, and are an aftermath of, the stresses of labor. In order to evaluate the status of the mother one must know what is normal.

Vital Signs

The blood pressure, pulse, and respirations should stabilize at prelabor levels during the first hour postpartum. Monitoring of the blood pressure and the pulse is important during the fourth stage of labor as one means of detecting shock resulting from untoward blood loss. The temperature continues to be slightly elevated with normal being less than a 2° (Fahrenheit) increase, or below 100.4°F (38°C).

Chill

It is not uncommon for a shaking chill to occur during the fourth stage of labor. It is considered within the realm of normal in the absence of infection. Most likely it is an aftermath of, and due to, the release from the nervous tension and the energy put out during labor and delivery.

Gastrointestinal System

Any previous nausea and vomiting should have ended. Primarily the mother is thirsty during the fourth stage of labor, and she may be, or shortly will be, hungry also.

Renal System

A hypotonic bladder with urinary retention and bladder enlargement is not uncommon. This is due to trauma caused by pressure and compression placed on the bladder and urethra during labor and delivery. This trauma is lessened if the bladder was kept empty during labor. It is important for the bladder to be emptied because a full bladder displaces the uterus and decreases its ability to contract properly. A poorly contracted uterus increases the amount of bleeding and increases the severity of afterpains.

MANAGEMENT PLAN FOR THE FOURTH STAGE OF LABOR

Evaluation and Management of the Uterus

The first action of the nurse-midwife after the placenta has been delivered is to evaluate the consistency of the uterus and to massage it if it is anything less than firm. The nurse-midwife also ascertains the need for an oxytocic drug and orders it given if indicated.

Use of Oxytocic Drugs

An oxytocic drug is one that stimulates uterine contractions. A number of factors should be considered in using oxytocic drugs during the immediate postpartum period. They include the following.

Determination of Need. Determination of whether or not there is a need for an oxytocic drug is based on the following:

1. Uterine consistency. The uterus should be well contracted, feeling firm and hard to touch.
2. Potential for the uterus to relax even if it is presently firm. A uterus is more apt to relax if:
   a. the uterus has been overdistended, as when there has been multiple gestation, polyhydramnios, or a large baby.
   b. the patient had a Pitocin induction or augmentation.
   c. labor and delivery have been rapid and precipitous.
   d. the patient is a grand multipara.
   e. there is a history of uterine atony during previous childbearing experience.
   f. the first and second stage of labor were prolonged.

3. Availability of someone, other than yourself, to monitor uterine consistency and amount of lochia flow and to massage the uterus.
4. Whether or not the membranes were completely delivered.
5. Whether or not the mother initiates breast-feeding immediately (see Fig. 18-2).

Mother's Preference. The woman may have made a prior statement of preference for having or not having an oxytocic drug.

Action and Effect. The action and effect of the different oxytocic drugs must be considered. The synthetic forms of the posterior pituitary hormone oxytocin (Pitocin, Syntocinon) stimulate intermittent contractions. They have little to no effect on the blood pressure *if* given intramuscularly or added to IV fluids. These are the drugs of choice in most situations.

The natural and synthetic ergot preparations — ergonovine (Ergotrate) and methylergonovine (Methergine), respectively — stimulate a sustained, tetanic contraction. Both of these drugs potentiate a hypertensive condition and may cause blood pressure increases in normotensive women because of their peripheral vasoconstrictive effect. However, of the two drugs, Methergine is less likely to cause a blood pressure elevation than Ergotrate, and if it does, the elevation will not be as high.

Therefore, if the woman is bleeding excessively as a result of uterine atony (which indicates a need for a drug that will stimulate a sustained contraction) but there is concern for a possible hypertensive effect, Methergine would be the drug of choice for the nurse-midwife to select if the intermittent contractions Syntocinon will produce are not felt to be sufficient for control of the degree of uterine atony present. The management of the care of the woman, and therefore the selection of the oxytocic drug, in the presence of a severe

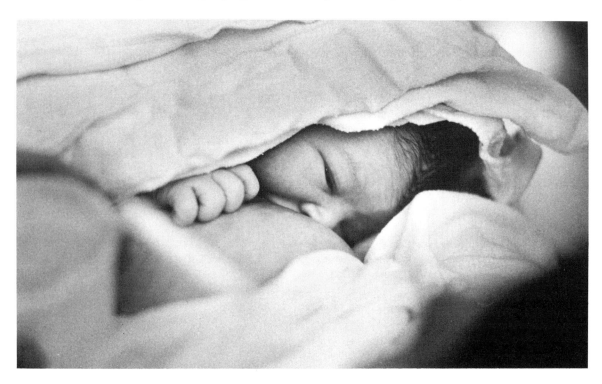

FIGURE 18-2. Breast-feeding within the first hour of life.

hypertensive condition, would be a decision of the physician.

Drugs with the action of stimulating intermittent contractions may be used to supplement those effecting a sustained contraction by adding them to an IV infusion which will last over time or may be used by themselves when bleeding is not excessive but the uterus is tending to relax.

Dosage and Route. The standard single dose for each oxytoxic drug is as follows:

Ergotrate — injection: 0.2 milligram (1 cc.)
             tablets: 0.2 milligram per tablet
Methergine — injection: 0.2 milligram (1 cc.)
             tablets: 0.2 milligram per tablet
Pitocin — injection: 10 U.S.P. units (1 cc.)
Syntocinon — injection: 10 U.S.P. units (1 cc.)

Ergotrate and Methergine injection are intended for intramuscular use. Ergotrate can be given intravenously but this is *not* recommended. Methergine can also be given intravenously but such use is *warned against* as this may cause sudden hypertension and a cerebrovascular accident. *At no time should either of these drugs be given prior to the birth of the baby* because a sustained contraction at that time could have the effect of killing the baby (by sustained uteroplacental insufficiency) and rupturing the uterus, thereby endangering the life of the mother. A single 0.2 milligram intramuscular dose of either Ergotrate or Methergine is the effective amount. This may be repeated in 2 to 4 hours if needed. More than this does not increase the effectiveness of either of these drugs in the event of hemorrhage but would unnecessarily increase the risk of undesirable side effects.

Pitocin and Syntocinon injection may be given intramuscularly or added to intravenous fluids for a prolonged effect by intravenous infusion. *At no time should either drug be given "IV push."* This practice is fraught with cardiovascular danger and is actually counterproductive to the lifesaving results desired in controlling immediate postpartal hemorrhage, the circumstance for which it is most often ordered.

The administration of Pitocin or Syntocinon, 10 units intramuscularly or 20 units diluted in 1000 milliliters of intravenous fluid, has no demonstrable cardiovascular effect. However, intravenous injection (IV push) of even as small an amount as 0.5 unit elicits a pattern of hypotension and tachycardia. The extent of the hypotension and tachycardia and length of time before recovery to preinjection level are directly proportional to the dosage given. The larger the amount of Pitocin or Syntocinon given, the greater the blood pressure reduction for a longer period of time. There can be nearly a 40 to 50 percent reduction in blood pressure when the dosage is 10 units. This is sufficient to put a patient into shock, if not already there, or to endanger the life of the mother if she is already in shock. Such an action is counterproductive to the desired results.

The idea of giving a combination of Ergotrate or Methergine and Pitocin or Syntocinon intravenously, thinking that their opposite actions would counteract each other, is erroneous. Instead, the patient sequentially responds to the synthetic oxytocin with hypotension and then to the ergot preparation with hypertension.

The use of oxytocic drugs in invaluable in controlling postpartal uterine bleeding. The desired action, however, can be obtained rapidly by way of the intramuscular route for the ergot preparations or by way of the intramuscular or diluted intravenous infusion routes for the synthetic oxytocin drugs, and without the cardiovascular dangers involved in direct intravenous administration of any of these drugs.

Inspection, Evaluation, and Repair of the Cervix, Vagina, and Perineum

Once the nurse-midwife is assured that the uterus is well contracted she or he inspects the perineum, lower vagina, and periurethral area for bruising, hematomas, lacerations, and bleeders and evaluates the condition of the episiotomy if one was cut.

Inspection of the Cervix and Upper Vaginal Vault

The nurse-midwife then decides whether or not to inspect the cervix and upper vaginal vault. This decision is based on whether or not there are any indications for making such an inspection. Indications include the following:

1. The uterus is well contracted but there continues to be a steady trickle or flow of blood from the vagina.
2. The mother was pushing prior to complete dilatation of the cervix.
3. The labor and delivery were rapid and precipitous.
4. There was manipulation of the cervix during labor, such as manually pushing back an edematous anterior cervical lip.
5. Traumatic procedures were necessary, such as a forceps delivery.
6. Second stage or delivery was, or was potentially, traumatic (e.g., prolonged shoulder dystocia, a large baby).

Usually in normal, spontaneous, vaginal deliveries none of these indications are present and it is not necessary to do a cervical and upper vaginal vault inspection. However, if any of the indications are present the nurse-midwife should not hesitate to perform this inspection and ascertain the need for any repair of these structures. Some clinicians advocate routine inspection of the cervix using the rationale that this then rules out the possibility of a cervical laceration as the cause if the woman bleeds excessively 2 hours after the delivery. Development of skill in doing this inspection thoroughly but rapidly is important since it can be uncomfortable or painful for the woman. The technique is discussed in Chapter 56.

Repairs

The repair of any lacerations or of an episiotomy is done after examination of the placenta. This is so a repair is not stressed if uterine exploration for retained placental fragments is necessary. The uterus is checked again for consistency and repair is begun. Basic stitches used in the repair of lacerations, manipulation of the needle holder and suture, and the step-by-step repair of a midline episiotomy, mediolateral episiotomy, and lacerations are detailed in Chapter 60.

Inspection and Evaluation of the Placenta, Membranes, and Umbilical Cord

Even though the nurse-midwife may have done a quick, cursory inspection of the placenta, membranes, and umbilical cord as they were delivered, it is essential to do a thorough inspection and examination of them at this time before repairing any lacerations or an episiotomy. This is because, if during your examination of the placenta you determine that the uterus needs to be manually explored because of a retained placental fragment, it needs to be done as soon as possible since it has the potential for causing a hemorrhage. Also, it is undesirable to place stress on any repair work, which would necessarily happen, if any were done prior to the uterine exploration. How to examine the placenta, membranes, and umbilical cord is detailed in Chapter 55.

Finishing in the Perineal Area

When all inspections, and repairs, if necessary, are completed there are three last actions to take before the woman puts her legs together. The first action is to recheck the uterus for consistency, watch the effect of uterine massage on the amount of vaginal blood flow, and express any blood clots. The second action is to do one last vaginal examination to assure removal of any forgotten 4 × 4s, massage the lower uterine segment, check for uterine inversion, and check any repair work. The third and final action is to wash off the mother's entire perineal area including the perineum, vulva, inner thighs, buttocks, and rectal area following the same principles as observed when initially washing off the perineum before delivery. The reason for this final washing is the woman's comfort. Probably there is dried blood on these areas. This can be sticky and irritating and simply washing all blood and other fluids off will make her feel less messy and more comfortable.

A perineal pad is then placed against the perineum and the mother puts her legs together. In some settings a perineal pad is not used and a large absorbent bed pad (Chux) placed under the mother is used exclusively to catch the vaginal drainage. This is done in the belief that a perineal pad may irritate stitches and that the back-and-forth movement of the pad with the mother's movements increases the risk of introducing contamination from the rectal area to the vaginal area. No known studies that support this latter idea have been done. Most women will feel more comfortable and less messy if they have a perineal pad to catch the vaginal drainage. A perineal pad is also necessary if the woman is ambulatory.

If the woman was in lithotomy position it is important to remove both legs from the stirrups at the same time in order to avoid undue back strain and discomfort which may occur if one leg is down and the other is still up in a stirrup. It is also helpful to have her put her legs together while they still are in the air with you supporting them and bicycle them down, with your help, to a resting position. This stimulates circulation to the legs and makes the transition of position less abrupt and more comfortable.

Continuation of Monitoring and Evaluation

Throughout the remainder of the fourth stage of labor the mother's vital signs, uterus, bladder, lochia, and perineum are monitored and evaluated. This monitoring is maintained until all are stabilized within normal range.

Vital Signs

Monitoring of the mother's vital signs — her blood pressure, pulse, and respirations — during the fourth stage of labor began when they were recorded immediately following delivery of the placenta. They are subsequently evaluated every 15 minutes until stable at prelabor levels or more frequently if indicated.

The temperature is taken at least once during the fourth stage of labor and hydration is evaluated. The mother most likely will be thirsty and if all is progressing normally she should be encouraged to take fluids such as water, juices, and tea or coffee with sugar. After her condition has stabilized within the limits of normal, which will usually be by the end of this first hour postpartum, she may also eat solid foods. However, what she eats may be limited by what is available in the setting.

If she has a shaking chill and no signs of infection (remember that a temperature elevation within 2° F of normal is normal) it will quickly pass if the following measures are implemented:

Warmth — blankets, preferably warmed blankets if available. This feels good even on the hottest of days in the hottest of settings.

Reassurance — usually consisting of an explanation of why she is shaking uncontrollably combined with a massive dose of praise for her performance during labor and delivery.

Relaxation techniques — controlled breathing and progressive relaxation technique, if known.

Uterine Contractility and Lochia

Monitoring of uterine contractility and the amount of lochial flow should be simultaneous inasmuch as they are directly related. The amount of vaginal bleeding should be minimal if the uterus is well contracted. If the uterus tends to be boggy the amount of lochia will be moderate to large. If the uterus is boggy the woman may be bleeding excessively or hemorrhaging. Watch the perineum for any increase in bleeding or expulsion of clots while you manipulate the uterus. This enables you to evaluate the relationship between the two.

In order not to stretch the cardinal ligaments it is necessary to support the uterus when giving it a thorough massage. This is done by grasping the lower portion of the uterus through the abdominal wall just above the symphysis pubis and holding it in place with one hand while massaging it with the other hand. Effective massage involves massaging more than just the anterior slope of the fundus. The entire fundus — top, anterior slope, lateral slopes, and posterior slope — should be massaged when the uterus needs massaging. This should be done quickly with a gentle but firm touch after forewarning the woman that you may hurt her and why it is necessary. The need for such thorough massage can be circumvented if the uterus is never allowed to soften or get boggy. Softness can be prevented if someone keeps a hand on the uterus during the first postpartal hour, maintaining its firmness with a light massage whenever it begins to soften. While this is not generally practical and within the limits of realities for nursing personnel in the usual situation, there is someone who can do it. Teaching the mother how to keep her own uterus firm with constant contact and light massage has large returns in terms of her own feeling of participation and knowledge in caring for her body, lessened bleeding, and reduced need for periodic thorough massage (which also means less discomfort for her).

Bladder

The bladder must be evaluated and emptied if it is full and displacing the uterus. Bladder hypotonicity may cause the woman not to feel a desire to void. Catheterization, which carries with it a significant risk of infection, is to be avoided except when all inducements to void

fail and it is essential to empty the bladder in order for the uterus to better contract and reduce bleeding. Putting the woman on a bedpan, running water over her perineum, having her dabble her fingers in water, having her listen to the sound of running water, applying light suprapubic pressure, and having her practice perineal relaxation may work in getting her to void; but the most effective and comfortable method is simply to assist her to the bathroom. There is no contraindication to walking with assistance at this time if she is not heavily medicated, did not have spinal anesthesia (neither of which will be the case in the normal management of childbirth by a nurse-midwife), or has not had an excessive blood loss.

Perineum

The perineum is evaluated for edema and hematomas. An ice pack to the perineum has the double effect of reducing both discomfort and edema in the presence of an episiotomy or lacerations. This is especially useful if there has been extensive repair, such as third- or fourth-degree perineal repair, or repair in an exceptionally sensitive area, such as the clitoris. For small perineal lacerations a woman may decide she feels more comfortable without the ice pack. If chemical perineal "ice" packs are not available, adequate ice packs can be created by putting crushed ice in a rubber glove or a sandwich bag. All ice packs should be covered with some form of clean cloth or peri-chux before being placed on the perineum.

Mother-Infant-Family Relationships

It must be emphasized again that the fourth stage of labor, the first hour postpartum, is a crucial time for maternal-infant-family relationships and for the start of parent-infant bonding and attachment (Fig. 18-3). During this time a number of interactions take place between the infant and the mother as detailed by Klaus and

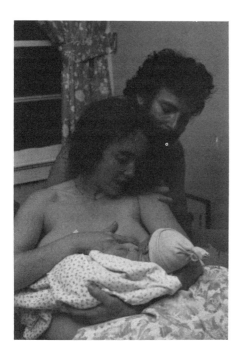

FIGURE 18-3.   Initial breast-feeding during the fourth stage.

Kennell [1]. As discussed for the third stage of labor, in Chapter 16, the Leboyer method of delivery facilitates this bonding for both mother and father with their infant.

The first hour includes a unique period called the maternal sensitive period, during which bonding occurs. The most crucial aspect to the occurrence of bonding is that the mother and baby be together. Behaviors can then be noted that signify beginning attachment — the mother moves from fingertip touching to full palmar contact with stroking and massaging of the baby, the percentage of time spent in the *en face* position increases, the mother uses a high-pitched voice, and so forth.

Family-infant attachment can be facilitated, even in the routines of a hospital that is not geared to family-centered maternity care, by performing the initial physical examination of the baby in the presence of and involving the

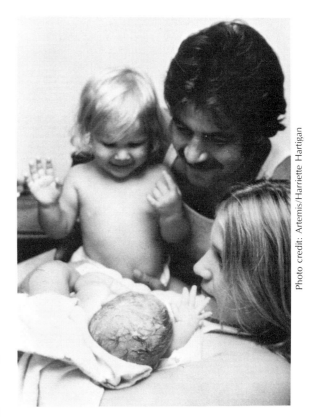

FIGURE 18-4.   Family bonding.

mother and family — showing them unique aspects of their baby, having them touch their baby's head to feel the molding, having them count the baby's fingers and toes, and so forth (Fig. 18-4). Baby holding and breast-feeding can be managed as readily and successfully on a delivery room table as elsewhere.

REFERENCE

1. Klaus, M., and Kennell, J. H. *Maternal-Infant Bonding*. St. Louis: Mosby, 1976.

Bibliography is at the end of Chapter 19.

Photo credit: Artemis/Harriette Hartigan

19

Management of Immediate Postpartum Hemorrhage

Hemorrhage, by definition, is an abnormal loss of blood. In obstetrics this is considered to be a loss of 500 milliliters or more. One does not, however, wait until there has been a loss of 500 milliliters of blood before deciding that the woman may be hemorrhaging and taking action. In fact early action in the presence of excessive bleeding may prevent actual hemorrhage and certainly the life-threatening sequelae of hemorrhage that are first manifested by the signs and symptoms of shock.

Immediate postpartum hemorrhage is that which takes place immediately after completion of the delivery of the placenta, which marks the end of the third stage of labor. In 80 to 90 percent of cases of immediate postpartum hemorrhage the cause is uterine atony. The remaining causes of immediate postpartum hemorrhage which a nurse-midwife might encounter are as follows:

1. Uterine atony resulting from incomplete delivery of the placenta, that is, retained placental fragments or cotyledons. This is also a cause of delayed postpartum hemorrhage.
2. Cervical lacerations.
3. Extensive lacerations of the vagina and perineum.
4. Very rarely, laceration of the lower uterine segment or uterine rupture.

There are a number of other situations in which immediate postpartum hemorrhage may be encountered. However, these are, or relate to, abnormal situations and such women would already be under the management of a physician (e.g., placenta previa, abruptio placentae, cesarean section, deep and prolonged inhalation anesthesia, operative procedures such as version and extraction, prolonged retention of a dead fetus following intrauterine death).

Uterine atony and the possibility of immediate postpartum hemorrhage in essentially normal women usually can be anticipated prior to delivery. The following conditions should alert the clinician to the potential of immediate postpartum hemorrhage due to uterine atony:

1. Overdistended uterus (multiple gestation, polyhydramnios, a large baby)
2. Oxytocin induction or augmentation
3. Rapid or precipitous labor and delivery
4. Prolonged first and second stage of labor
5. Grand multiparity
6. History of uterine atony with previous childbearing

Anticipation of immediate postpartum hemorrhage as a result of uterine atony allows preparatory measures to be taken for avoiding hemorrhage. These preparatory measures include the following:

1. Alert the physician to the possibility so he or she is prepared for a *stat.* call if needed.
2. Alert the nursing staff to the possibility and request that they draw up and have ready to give your order for oxytocic drugs for use immediately after delivery of the placenta.
3. Make sure that an intravenous infusion is started with a 16-gauge needle and that this venous route is patent at the time of delivery. Use 5% dextrose in lactated Ringer's solution.
4. Draw a type and crossmatch preparatory for obtaining blood if needed.
5. Make sure the woman's bladder is empty at the time of delivery.

Bleeding should be minimal due to a well-contracted uterus after delivery of the placenta. If, instead, there is a steady flow (as opposed to a trickle) or gush of blood from the vagina the following steps should be taken to manage this emergency of immediate postpartum hemorrhage:

1. Check the consistency of the uterus. This step is first since 80 to 90 percent of immediate postpartum hemorrhage is due to uterine atony.
2. If the uterus is atonic, massage it in order to stimulate contraction so that the bleeding vessels at the placental site will be ligated.
3. If the uterus fails to contract well immediately with massage:
   a. Do bimanual compression (see Chapter 58). In addition to stimulating contraction of the uterus for reasons stated in Step 2, bimanual compression places continuous pressure on the uterine veins and on the lower uterine segment, which may be, in part, the site of bleeding.
   b. Simultaneously order the administration of oxytocic drugs if they have not already been given, or additional oxytocic drugs to those already given. (See Chapter 18 for discussion regarding the use of oxytocic drugs.)
4. If bleeding obviously is not under control by now:
   a. Have the nursing staff give your physician backup a *stat.* call.
   b. Continue bimanual compression.
   c. Make sure the IV is patent, or have the nurse start one with a 16-gauge needle and 5% dextrose in lactated Ringer's solution to which you have the nurse add 10 units of Pitocin per 500 milliliters of solution. If the woman does have a patent IV, have the nurse add Pitocin to the existing IV solution in the same proportion as just stated.
   d. Have a type and crossmatch drawn, if not already drawn, and sent to the blood bank.
   e. Have the nursing staff monitor the woman's blood pressure and pulse for signs of shock.
5. Examine, or have examined, the placenta to ascertain if any placental fragments or cotyledons were retained and to determine

if a uterine exploration needs to be done.

6. Do a uterine exploration (see Chapter 57). The uterus needs to be completely empty in order to effectively contract.

7. If the uterus is empty and well-contracted but bleeding continues, examine the woman for cervical, vaginal, and perineal lacerations since these may be the cause of the hemorrhage (see Chapter 55). Tie off the bleeders that are the source of hemorrhage and repair any lacerations.

8. If the woman is developing shock (i.e., lowered blood pressure; elevated pulse rate; rapid, shallow respirations; cold, clammy skin), place her in shock position, cover her with warm blankets, administer oxygen, and order the blood to the floor.

9. In extreme and very rare cases when hemorrhage is rampant, the woman's life is imminently in danger, and the physician has not yet arrived, aortic compression can be carried out in relatively thin women. This involves abdominally compressing the aorta against the spine.

In the vast majority of situations in which a nurse-midwife is managing the care of the woman and an immediate postpartum hemorrhage occurs, it is readily controlled with a combination of bimanual compression and oxytocic drugs. Frequently, this is done so rapidly, due to anticipatory alertness and early detection, that excessive blood loss is avoided. Occasionally the nurse-midwife will need to do an intrauterine exploration (Chapter 57). It will be the extremely rare situation not ever seen by most nurse-midwives in which the first seven steps listed here will not be suf-ficient. In such an event the nurse-midwife maintains the woman as outlined in the last two steps until the physician arrives, and then functions under the direction of the physician who assumes management of the situation.

BIBLIOGRAPHY FOR CHAPTERS 16, 17, 18, AND 19

Bonica, J. J. *Principles and Practice of Obstetric Analgesia & Anesthesia*, Vol. 1. Philadelphia: Davis, 1967.

Gimbel, J., and Nocon, J. J. The physiological basis for the Leboyer approach to childbirth. *J. Obstet. Gynecol. Neonat. Nurs.* 6:11, 1977.

Greenhill, J. P., and Friedman, E. A. *Biological Principles and Modern Practice of Obstetrics*. Philadelpia: Saunders, 1974.

Hellman, L. M., and Pritchard, J. A. *Williams Obstetrics, 14th*. New York: Appleton-Century-Crofts, 1971.

Hendricks, C. H., and Brenner, W. E. Cardiovascular effects of oxytocic drugs used postpartum. *Am. J. Obstet. Gynecol.* 108:751, 1970.

Klaus, M., and Kennell, J. H. *Maternal-Infant Bonding*. St. Louis: Mosby, 1976.

Leboyer, F. *Birth without Violence*. New York: Knopf, 1976.

Oliver, C. M., and Oliver, G. M. Gentle birth: Its safety and its effect on neonatal behavior. *J. Obstet. Gynecol. Neonat. Nurs.* 7:35, 1978.

Phillips, C. R. The essence of birth without violence. *Am. J. Maternal Child Nurs.* 1:162, 1976.

Pritchard, J. A., MacDonald, P. C., and Gant, N. F. *Williams Obstetrics, 17th*. Norwalk, Conn.: Appleton-Century-Crofts, 1985.

Rotton, W. N., and Friedman, E. A. Placenta accreta. *Obstet. Gynecol.* 9:580, 1957.

Scupholme, A. Puerperal inversion of the uterus: A case report. *J. Nurse-Midwifery* 27(5):37−40 (September/October) 1982.

20

Out-of-Hospital Birth

It has been only within the twentieth century that the term *out-of-hospital birth* has come into existence. Before 1900 giving birth in-hospital was the rare exception. Fewer than 5 percent of all women were delivered in the hospital and then only because they were desperately sick. Birth happened at home, controlled by women and attended by female midwives.

All this changed in a brief span of time. By 1940 nearly half of all births took place in hospitals and by 1970 the changeover was complete with over 99 percent of births occurring within hospitals. Birth now happened in the hospital, controlled by men and largely attended by male physicians.

Some of the same factors influencing the status of midwives during the late 1800s and early 1900s (see Chapter 2) were also responsible for the move of birth from home to hospital. These factors include the evolution of the male midwife (physician) in the late 1700s and 1800s; the inclusion of obstetrics in medical practice with the concurrent development of lying-in wards for the urban poor for teaching purposes during the late 1800s and early 1900s; the conquest of puerperal fever by Semmelweis with handwashing, which made hospitals more safe; the concerted effort to abolish midwifery in the early 1900s; the evolution and refinement of early obstetric technology such as forceps (1700s), anesthesia (ether, 1847; chloroform, 1853; spinal anesthesia, 1885–1946); analgesia (1902); and infant incubators (late 1800s).

The move into the hospitals brought with it the days of female dependency behaviors and demand for analgesia and anesthesia; of twilight sleep, fear of pain, and ignorance; of centralized nurseries; and of separation of baby from mother and mother from the family. Only the rural poor, still attended by uneducated "granny" midwives and too poor either to afford medical insurance or to pay cash, were denied access to the "comfortable, pain-free" childbirth promulgated by the hospitals during this period of transition of birth into the hospital [1, p. 44].

The early nurse-midwifery services were home birth services (Frontier Nursing Service,

1925; Lobenstine Midwifery Clinic, 1931; Tuskeegee School of Nurse-Midwifery, 1941; Catholic Maternity Institute, 1944). Nurse-midwives did not move into the hospitals until the mid-1950s. This was a deliberate and successful effort to gain access to the public hospitals because these hospitals were where the majority of women cared for by nurse-midwives were now giving birth [2, p. 349]. It was also part of moving into educational institutions for the placement of nurse-midwifery educational programs (Columbia University, 1955; Johns Hopkins University, 1956; Yale University, 1956; the move of the Maternity Center Association School of Nurse-Midwifery into Downstate Medical Center, State University of New York, 1958).

The early expression of consumer dissatisfaction with hospital childbearing practices and routines began in the 1940s. The mid-1940s saw the development of rooming-in in an effort to reverse the separation of mother and baby from each other and from the family (see Chapter 24). Grantly Dick-Read wrote *Childbirth without Fear* in 1944. Herbert Thoms wrote *Understanding Natural Childbirth* in 1950. Maternity Center Association developed preparation for parenthood and childbirth classes and teaching materials such as *The Birth Atlas* during the 1940s and 1950s. Marjorie Karmel wrote *Thank You, Dr. Lamaze* in 1959 and the birth of psychoprophylaxis and a variety of childbirth theories and methods was underway. The late 1950s and the 1960s and early 1970s also saw consumers and professionals joining together to form national organizations supportive of their beliefs in natural, prepared childbirth. Examples include the International Childbirth Education Association (ICEA), the American Society for Psychoprophylaxis in Obstetrics (ASPO), La Leche League International, the National Association of Parents and Professionals for Safe Alternatives in Childbirth (NAPSAC), and many smaller organizations.

The natural evolution of consumer discontent with hospitals was to remember that childbirth had not always been in hospitals. The organizational alliances of consumers and professionals began to focus not only on promoting change within hospitals but also on the acceptance of out-of-hospital birth and the utilization of midwives.

CHARACTERISTICS AND PRINCIPLES

There are still segments of the population who deliver out of hospital because of inability to gain access to all the resources and facilities of the health care system (e.g., migrant workers, rural poor). For the vocal individual consumer, consumer groups, and the aforementioned national organizations, however, out-of-hospital birth is a matter of choice and educated, participatory decision making. These are knowledgeable consumers who are disenchanted with what the health care system has to offer in maternity care and services. The result has been conflict which has raised issues of power, control, responsibility, economics, and safety for both in-hospital and out-of-hospital birth settings and for consumers and health care professionals and providers alike.

Out-of-hospital birth has two locales: home and birth center. If one were to look at the control and responsibility assumed by the consumer on a continuum, the continuum would stretch from the hospital delivery room at one end to home birth at the other. There are two important breaks in this continuum where transference of power to the consumer takes place. The first break is when birth moves out of hospital. The second break is when it moves from a freestanding out-of-hospital childbirth center to home birth. In each instance the consumer moves further away from external regulations and policies which are imposed upon her childbirth experience. It should be recognized, however, that there are women who do not wish to assume the control and responsibility that comes with out-of-hospital birth or who for other reasons choose to deliver in the hospital even when out-of-hospital options are available to them. It should be recognized also that there are women in out-of-hospital settings who abdicate responsibility to the attending professional; and there are women in the hospital setting who assert their rights for control and responsibility even though it is harder to do so in an institution.

Safety has been the issue most used to obfuscate the other issues in out-of-hospital birth. This does not negate the fact that safety is a valid concern. It is a concern, however, that has valid answers. There are five criteria that must be met in order to ensure safety in out-of-hospital birth settings and to draw comparisons with in-hospital birth settings. These are as follows:

1. Attendance by a qualified heath care professional
2. Strict adherence to stringent screening and transfer criteria
3. Provision of care appropriate to the setting
4. Immediately available transport system
5. Immediately accessible consulting physician and hospital arrangements

The details in criteria 2 and 3 are critical in determining safety in practice in an out-of-hospital setting. For example, criterion 2 would exclude women with a breech presentation, multiple gestation, or a previous cesarean section from delivering in an out-of-hospital setting. Criterion 3 would specify the emergency equipment which would be present in the setting and procedures which would *not* be done in an out-of-hospital setting (e.g. paracervical blocks, oxytocin induction or augmentation).

The American College of Nurse-Midwives (ACNM) has taken the professional leadership in promoting the development of safe out-of-hospital birth settings. In 1979, ACNM published *Guidelines for Establishing a Home Birth Service* and *Guidelines for Establishing an Alternative Birth Center* (out-of-hospital). ACNM based its action on the experience, statistics, and demonstrated safety of nurse-midwives in out-of-hospital birth settings since 1925.

Basic knowledge and skills learned in a nurse-midwifery education program are applicable in all birth settings. As in any setting, certain skills and techniques are more refined in an out-of-hospital setting. These include those which develop from having more flexibility in facilitating different labor and birth positions and having siblings as well as other family members and support people present at birth. Working in nonhospital settings also refines your ability to obtain clinical data from your observations (visual and auditory) and from use of your hands.

OUT-OF-HOSPITAL BIRTH CENTERS

Definitions and Models

There is no commonly accepted definition of an out-of-hospital birth center. There are considerable variations among birth centers, for example, as to whom the attendants are, what procedures may take place within the birth center, what the screening criteria are for women who wish to deliver there, and what equipment may be present. It is important, therefore, to ascertain the woman's or couple's expectations regarding a birth center in order to determine whether the one under consideration can meet their expectations. It is also important that they know precisely what equipment (for monitoring, delivery, emergencies, and transport) is available as this varies from one birth center to another. Some birth centers may be too "high tech" for some consumers as some professionals have simply substituted one institution for another institution.

Out-of-hospital birth centers are either freestanding or under the jurisdiction of a hospital. Freestanding birth centers are those which are both physically and administratively separate from a hospital. A birth center may be physically separate from a hospital but is not freestanding if it is on hospital property, or owned by the hospital, or under the administration of a hospital. Most out-of-hospital childbirth centers are freestanding [2, p. 352].

There are two models of freestanding, out-of-hospital childbirth centers: the *closed* model and the *open* or *community* model. The closed model is a birth center which is owned and used by a single private practice of certified nurse-midwives and/or physicians. Only their patients may be delivered at their birth center. Such a birth center is usually a facility for prenatal, postpartal, interconceptional, and well-woman gynecologic care as well as care during labor and delivery.

An open model is a community facility owned by a separate corporation of individuals. It is available to all women who have health care providers with practice privileges at the birth center. While such a childbirth center may serve as a community resource on childbirth (library resources, center for childbirth education classes, etc. — see Fig. 20-1) it is primarily a facility for care during labor and delivery (Fig. 20-2). Women receive their prenatal, postpartal, and gynecologic care in the offices of their health care providers and deliver at the birth center. There may or may not be an "in house" practice that provides prenatal and postpartal care at the birth center.

The term *alternative birth center*, or *ABC*, is very confusing as it has been used to refer to

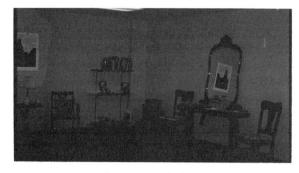

FIGURE 20-1. Classroom of the Family Childbirth Center, New Haven, Connecticut.

both in-hospital and out-of-hospital birth centers. You must, thus, be a discriminating reader of the literature in order not to draw comparisons between two very different types of birth centers in significantly different locales which have been called the same thing.

History

The first established freestanding out-of-hospital childbirth center was La Casita at Catholic Maternity Institute in Sante Fe, New Mexico. It was started in the mid-1940s by graduates of the Maternity Center Association School of Nurse-Midwifery who were medical mission sisters. It closed in the mid-1960s. During the 1940s and 1950s there were also a number of so-called maternity hospitals or homes which were often associated with residential care for

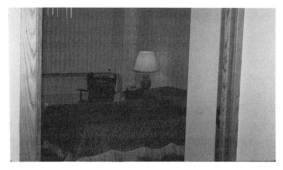

A

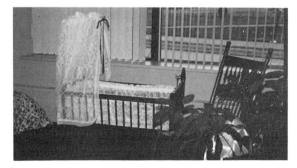

B

FIGURE 20-2. The Family Childbirth Center, New Haven, Connecticut. A. birth room; B. birth room.

unwed mothers at that time. Most of these closed during the late 1950s to mid-1960s.

In 1972, Su Clinica Familiar, a migrant health clinic in southern Texas, expanded its services to include delivery in their clinic setting and became the first out-of-hospital childbirth center in current history. Maternity Center Association, in New York City, opened its precedent-setting Childbearing Center in 1975 (see Fig. 20-3).

In 1980, the Office of Migrant Health in the Bureau of Community Health Services of the United States Public Health Service contracted with the American College of Nurse-Midwives for the provision of guidelines and consultant help in establishing childbirth centers associated with their clinics.

In 1981, the Cooperative Birth Center Network, a program of Maternity Center Association of New York which was funded by the John A. Hartford Foundation, began collecting data on birth centers and establishing a network for the collection and dissemination of information regarding birth centers. Recognizing the need for standards in the face of a proliferating number of childbirth centers, the Cooperative Birth Center Network underwent a metamorphosis in 1983 to become a nonprofit membership organization called the National As-

sociation of Childbearing Centers (NACC). One function of this organization is the development of standards and criteria for care and safety in childbirth centers. By 1984 the NACC reported that over 126 out-of-hospital childbirth centers had opened in 35 states and were the site of delivery for approximately 15,000 babies. Over 300 more childbirth centers were then in the planning stages.

Characteristics

Although childbirth centers in most states have to meet a large numer of bureaucratic regulations, they have a different ambience from an in-hospital birth center. This difference in tone and mood is present whether the birth center is in an existing health clinic, an office building, or a renovated old Victorian house. Although in many senses a childbirth center is a facility, which imposes certain institutional characteristics, the ambience is of a noninstitutional setting with a homey environment and comfortable surroundings in what becomes a familiar place prior to birth (Fig. 20-4). Policies are designed for flexibility and are geared towards helping women and couples to have the kind of childbirth experience they want within the

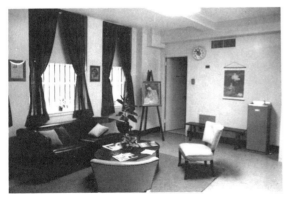

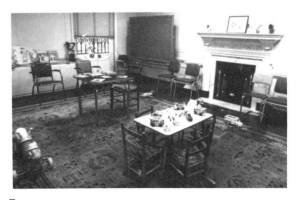

A

B

FIGURE 20-3.   The Childbearing Center of the Maternity Center Association. A. the family room; B. a multi-purpose room used for group discussion and as a playroom for children accompanying their parents. (Courtesy of the Maternity Center Association, New York, New York. Photographs by Paco North.)

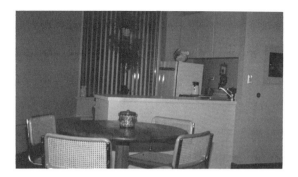

FIGURE 20-4.   Kitchen in the Family Childbirth Center, New Haven, Connecticut.

boundaries of stringent safety screening and transfer criteria. Emergency and transport equipment are on site and immediately accessible although well hidden from view.

Freestanding out-of-hospital childbirth centers promote the concept of safe, satisfying, and cost-effective childbirth. The cost-effectiveness of the closed model freestanding childbirth center run by certified nurse-midwives has been well documented. Maternity Center Association collaborated with New York Blue Cross/Blue Shield in studying the cost of MCA's Childbearing Center (CBC) compared to aggregated data on hospital maternity care costs. This study showed that "CBC costs have been repeatedly found to be about 40 percent less than the cost of conventional care for normal childbirth" [3, p. 1055]. Reasons for such cost-effectiveness include the following:

1. The philosophy of the nurse-midwife to facilitate natural, normal processes results in the use of expensive diagnostic and treatment technology and interventions only when indicated.
2. The fact that only healthy women with uncomplicated pregnancies deliver in a childbirth center means that there is no need for costly equipment in the childbirth centers other than emergency equipment.
3. The fact that an out-of-hospital childbirth center does not bear overhead costs for anything except its own services.

Cost-effectiveness studies on open model childbirth centers or on closed model childbirth centers run by health care professionals other than certified nurse-midwives have not yet been done.

For some nurse-midwives who have never worked in an out-of-hospital setting the move from the hospital, especially a tertiary medical center, to a freestanding out-of-hospital birth center may be a frightening thought, although not as disconcerting as moving into home birth since a birth center is still the professional's territory. For them there is a great deal of security in the hospital where there are other professionals to call upon for help and unlimited resources and equipment. Out-of-hospital birth centers require reliance upon your own clinical judgment without the built-in security of "discussion-in-passing" of a situation with several others. This self-reliance sharpens the concept of consultation with your consulting physician. It also makes you feel more acutely the responsibility and accountability inherent in the role of a nurse-midwife. From this comes (1) a surety of knowing who you are as a nurse-midwife managing the care of healthy women with uncomplicated pregnancies and (2) confidence in your abilities in such a setting.

HOME BIRTH

A primary difference between the two out-of-hospital birth settings is that a childbirth center is still the professional's territory, to which a woman comes. A home birth takes place in the woman's territory, to which the nurse-midwife goes. This is a fundamental difference which involves different *responsibilities* for the woman or couple and different planning, approaches, and methods of providing care by the nurse-midwife. These will be detailed in this section.

Developing A Partnership

The relationship of a home birth couple and a

nurse-midwife is essentially that of a partnership. As stated earlier in this chapter, the home is the birth setting in which the woman or couple can have the greatest amount of control over their childbirth experience. It is also the setting for which they must assume the greatest amount of responsibility for their own childbirth experience and for the care the mother and baby receive. The principles of self-care are most fully applicable to home birth couples. The outcome is an immense awareness of their own capability. The strength of women who have accepted full responsibility for their childbearing is palpable and powerful.

In developing a partnership a woman or couple must first make the decision to deliver at home. This is a decision in which influence may be exerted by family members, especially mothers and mothers-in-law. The greatest amount of influence, however, is exerted by the partner or husband. This is important because it is to him that the woman will turn for support and strength when she feels vulnerable or weak. He must, therefore, be as firmly committed as she is (but not more committed) and a full participant in the process. A difficult and poor situation can develop if he is more committed to a home birth than she is. There needs to be an equal commitment by both partners by the time the woman is at term.

Factors which couples consider in making the decision to deliver at home include the following:

1. Normalcy of the pregnancy
2. Previous hospital experience
3. Availability of alternatives both in and out of hospital
4. Availability of their preferred health care provider in different birth settings
5. Safety for the woman in and out of hospital
6. Safety for the baby in and out of hospital
7. Availability of what they want in another setting (hospital or out-of-hospital birth center), such as:
   a. presence of significant others
   b. no restriction as to the number of others they want present
   c. presence of siblings (no age restrictions) for birth as well as during labor and postpartum
   d. no strangers without prior introduction and permission to be in room
   e. ability to assume responsibility for their baby's birth
   f. no shave
   g. no enema
   h. no intravenous infusion
   i. no restriction of activity
   j. no electronic fetal monitoring
   k. availability of a bathtub
   l. no artificial rupture of membranes
   m. no analgesia or anesthesia
   n. no transfer to a delivery room
   o. no restriction on birth position
   p. no episiotomy
   q. gentle birth (low lights, quiet or soft music, Leboyer bath for baby)
   r. delay of eye prophylaxis
   s. no separation of mother and baby
   t. early initiation of unlimited breast-feeding
8. Amount of control of the situation they perceive they will have
9. Degree of participatory decision making they perceive they will have
10. Amount of responsibility they perceive they will have
11. Smells, noise, and cleanliness of a setting
12. Their desire to be at home in familiar surroundings
13. The trust they both have in her body

Women and couples thus choose home birth for a variety of reasons. It is essential that the nurse-midwife ascertain exactly what their expectations are of the nurse-midwife, of their responsibilities, and of the home birth experience in order to determine if these expectations are realistic and if they fit with the nurse-midwife's clinical standards and expectations of the relationship within the partnership being forged between them. Examples of standards and expectations the woman or couple may have of the nurse-midwife include the following:

1. Acknowledgement of their acceptance of responsibility
2. Acknowledgement of their control and decision making
3. Provision of knowledge for their utilization
4. Recognition of being a guest, albeit a welcome, invited guest, in the home
5. Establishment of clinical standards and expectations
6. Provision of prenatal, delivery, and postnatal care
7. Provision of a positive mental attitude
8. Appreciation of the strengths of the woman and of her partner if he is present

The nurse-midwife in the partnership facilitates the efforts of the woman or couple in their childbirth experience and sets the clinical standards and expectations of the relationship. The setting of clinical standards and expectations clarifies the partnership and the responsibilities of each partner within the relationship. Standards and expectations may vary from practitioner to practitioner. Examples of standards and expectations the nurse-midwife may have of the woman and couple include the following:

1. Must meet screening criteria for normalcy and for home birth
2. No smoking
3. No "recreational" drugs
4. No analgesics
5. Assumption of responsibility for:
   a. keeping prenatal care appointments
   b. keeping the nurse-midwife informed of any life changes
   c. complying with the agreed-upon plan of care
   d. obtaining pediatric care
   e. doing specified reading
   f. attending childbirth education classes
   g. confronting and resolving their fears
   h. preparing siblings for their participation
   i. preparing invited participants for their responsibilities
   j. attending La Leche League meetings antepartally
   k. making an accurate, detailed map to the home
   l. making emergency plans and posting them by each telephone
   m. knowing where the hospital is and the fastest route for getting there
   n. having a full gas tank
   o. purchasing the specified supplies
   p. purchasing and installing an infant car seat
   q. paying fees for care
   r. having a clean house
   s. controlling pets at the time of labor and delivery
6. Anticipatory agreement to transfer to the hospital if the nurse-midwife believes this is indicated or the condition of the woman or baby meets transfer criteria
7. Acknowledgement of the expertise and decision making of the nurse-midwife and the physician consultant

These standards and expectations should be written and may be referred to in a general informed-consent form. Because of national controversy and adverse publicity about home birth, and often local physician opposition, many home birth practitioners have their clients sign an informed consent. This informed consent is signed by the woman or couple and details the controversies; lists the possible complications associated with childbirth; lists the emergency equipment the nurse-midwife brings to the home; grants permission for examination, treatment, and transfer as indicated in the professional judgment of the nurse-midwife and consulting physician; and states their acceptance of responsibility for the consequences of childbearing and the decision to deliver at home attended by a Certified Nurse-Midwife.

Such a consent form is in keeping with the philosophy that a home birth couple should be fully knowledgeable about all possibilities — positive and negative — relating to childbirth at home, and should have confronted and addressed their fears, planned for all eventualities, and accepted responsibility for their actions. The nurse-midwife serves as facilitator, guide, educator, and provider of care. Thus, the partnership is forged.

The Woman's/Couple's Preparations for the Birth

Preparation for birth involves considerable time, thought, energy, planning, and activity. All the activities listed under item 5 in the immediately preceding list of standards and expectations the nurse-midwife may have of the woman/couple are part of their preparation for birth. These will be elaborated on in this section.

Keeping prenatal care appointments, complying with the agreed-upon plan of care, keeping the nurse-midwife informed of any life changes, and obtaining pediatric care are basic to the provision of maternal and newborn care. Professional monitoring of health and well-being is essential to health promotion and illness prevention and continual assurance that screening and transfer criteria are being met.

Education and knowledge are essential for a home birth couple. They need to know as much as they can about the anatomic, physiologic, and psychologic processes taking place and what they can do to help themselves. The provision of a list of books with a recommended number to read is useful. This list should include books on pregnancy, birth, breastfeeding, sibling presence at birth, and early parenting. In addition, some nurse-midwives want all their clients to read a particular book on home birth.

Childbirth education classes take on a different meaning for most home birth couples. Most women having a home birth find the usual childbirth education classes superficial, not useful, and at times misleading. These women express the need for knowledge, as knowledge dispels fear and answers the "what ifs." They express the need to know that labor is going to hurt. They feel that the set pattern of various psychoprophylactic methods are not functional for them as it turns them away from an internal focus of feeling, experiencing, and coping, to an external forcus with too much to remember and do. They prefer a more eclectic approach which emphasizes their inner strengths and helps them slow down and relax.

Listening to home birth women talk is like hearing a return to the work of Grantly Dick-Read. In his 1944 book, *Natural Childbirth*, Read articulated that fear causes tension which in turn causes pain which in turn causes more fear and thus a vicious cycle is established. He projected that the fear-tension-pain cycle could be broken by knowledge which would reduce or eliminate fear and thus tension and pain. His method was expanded by a physiotherapist, Helen Herdman, who added relaxation techniques to also aid in the reduction of tension and thus of pain.

Childbirth education for home birth couples includes an open discussion, confrontation, and subsequent dispelling of their fears about having a home birth. These fears need to be clearly separated from fears about childbirth. Complications, emergencies, the "what ifs," and dealing with other people's negative reactions are all explored and thoroughly discussed. Explanations of exactly what problems can occur and what can and cannot be done about each possible situation in the home setting are given. Recognition that the hypothetical complications envisioned in their "what ifs" are *not* normal and that their own history *is* one of normalcy gives them reassurance and strength; at the same time they grow in their recognition of the responsibility they have assumed and in their acceptance of it.

Childbirth education classes also include an exploration of the class members' motivations for having a home birth; other psychological issues as they pertain to home birth (i.e., anxiety, intuition, fears, guilt, pain, responsibility, sexuality); very specific details about what goes into a birth plan (e.g., who will be there, doing what, how notified; photography; music); preparations and supplies for birth; the emergency plan; and what to expect after the birth of the baby. The class members also serve the function of being a support group. Attending a series of La Leche League meetings and a night of birth films completes the educational activities. The La Leche League meetings provide the woman with the opportunity to observe how to breast-feed, how different babies nurse, and how different mothers and babies relate to each other.

Making an accurate, detailed map to the home is an obvious necessity. Another essential document is the emergency plan posted by each telephone. A very useful emergency backup plan worksheet and form for emergency numbers is in *Special Delivery* [4]. The woman or couple should make "practice runs" to their backup hospital to learn the fastest route, where to park, where to enter the building, and so on in case this should become necessary. A cardinal rule of responsibility is making sure that the gas tank in the car that will be used for emergency transportation is always at least half full (or contains more than enough fuel for the distance).

Purchase of the specified supplies should be completed by the thirty-sixth week of gestation. Appendix I at the end of this chapter is a sample list of supplies to be purchased by the woman/couple. It is very important that these items be singly purchased rather than a check made out to a supply house for a kit. The rationale for the single purchases is to focus on each purchase — what it is for and how it may be used. This again reinforces the responsibility the woman or couple have assumed and their knowledgeable participation. All parents should purchase an infant car seat.

A clean house and pet control are obvious responsibilities. Pet control requires some thought, depending on what the pet is and its usual care and limitations.

Preparation is also required for those who will be present for the birth. If there are children, then not only do they need preparation but also an adult needs to be designated as primarily responsible for them. This adult needs preparation as well for the labor and birth and for his or her role. Sibling preparation classes should be attended together by the parents, the children, and their adult helper. Other participants should also be prepared. This preparation includes assumption of their responsibility:

1. Not to smoke
2. Not to bring any animals
3. To wear clean clothes
4. To be informed, preferably to have attended a night of birth films with the woman or couple
5. To know and respect the expectations the woman or couple have
6. To have a positive mental attitude (a feeling that supports the birthing mother, respects her integrity in what she is doing, and trusts the normal physiologic processes and the body's capability for giving birth)

The selection of participants should be made with great care and thought. Aside from all the reasons a woman or couple may have for inviting someone to participate in this experience, the attitude of these individuals toward out-of-hospital birth must be determined. Fear of an out-of-hospital birth has no place at a home birth. No one must be allowed at a home birth who might convey fear to the birthing mother.

The Nurse-Midwife's Preparations for the Birth

Preparation for the birth by the nurse-midwife includes:

1. Continual screening to be certain that the woman meets criteria for normalcy
2. Plans for transfer to the hospital if this should become necessary, including contact with the backup hospital and preparation of the nursing staff
3. A home visit during the thirty-sixth week of gestation (details are given later in this chapter)
4. Checking for adequacy and functioning of the supplies and equipment the nurse-midwife takes with her to the home

In addition to stringent criteria for normalcy there are other criteria that a nurse-midwife may require for a home birth. These vary from practitioner to practitioner but may include the following:

1. Compliance with the plan of care, including attendance at childbirth education classes and La Leche League meetings
2. Compliance with assumption of responsibilities — purchase of supplies, making of an emergency plan, and so on
3. Positive attitude toward the capabilities of the woman's body
4. Appropriate psychological motivation for a home birth
5. Compliance with practice standards regarding smoking, drug use, nutrition, and so forth

The nurse-midwife remains observant for any other clues that the woman or couple are (or are not) psychologically attuned to a home birth.

Plans for transfer to the hospital include the procedure to be used if transfer should become necessary. The physician consultant is contacted and arrangements made for meeting him or her at the designated backup hospital. Transfer takes place in the woman's or couple's car that has the sufficiently full gas tank. The importance of the attitudes of the nursing staff at the hospital cannot be overemphasized. It is

well worth the nurse-midwife's time and effort to have cultivated a relationship with the nurses at the backup hospital and provided education and information about her practice and home birth. A prepared and involved nursing staff can greatly facilitate the goals of the home birth woman or couple to be accepted, to keep the family unit together, and to leave the hospital as soon as possible.

The home visit during the thirty-sixth week serves a number of purposes and enables the nurse-midwife to:

1. Use the map and directions to the home and assure that she or he can find it.
2. Become familiar with the layout of the house and its facilities for birth (bedroom, bathroom, kitchen, telephone).
3. Check that all supplies are purchased and ready for use.
4. Check that the emergency plan and telephone numbers are posted by each telephone in the house.
5. Assess the arrangements for pet control and where the animals will be during birth.
6. Discuss the completed arrangements for any siblings.
7. Assess the preparations for having a baby in the family. Unless there are ethnic or cultural beliefs to the contrary, by the thirty-sixth week names for the baby should be selected, baby clothes and care supplies purchased, and plans made for the baby's place in the home. Look for signs of life and nurturing in the house, such as plants, music, fish, and animals, as a reflection of the attitude of the woman or couple towards bringing new life into their home.

The home visit is also part of the continual screening for normalcy and appropriate preparations for a home birth. If these are found lacking then the nurse-midwife needs to be clear that this is *not* an appropriate woman or couple for a home birth.

Appendix II at the end of this chapter contains a list of supplies and equipment that the nurse-midwife takes with her to the home. Critical in this listing are the emergency supplies and equipment; these are marked with a dagger.

The Birth

To understand *home* birth, you need to go into different families' *homes.* One of the facts I want you to know and really understand is how different each family's environment is. Their values, priorities, and even the ways in which family members relate to each other are all reflected in the home. You get so much more information about people when you see them in their own environments. I also want you to get the idea — I think this is crucial — that when we take all these very different people and put them all into the identical environment of a hospital, we have enormously changed the quality and the character of the birth experience. [5]

The advantages of being at home become obvious during the labor and delivery of a home birth. From the beginning, courtesy prevails. It is the woman's or couple's home and you are a guest in their house. They act like it and you act like it. Having their own unconfined space and control in their own surroundings facilitates relaxation and promotes confidence, pride, and capability. The intimacy and the ability to cope with labor her own way in her own setting foster the woman's reliance upon herself and her partner. Being able to have the persons they want with them is both their decision and a means of sharing and enhancing family bonds.

When active labor begins the woman or couple prepares for birth by doing the following:

1. Contacting the nurse-midwife
2. Making the bed with two sets of sheets with the plastic shower curtain liner (Appendix I) between
3. Getting out three pans for boiling water for instruments, eye drops (depending on type of prophylaxis used), and tea
4. Calling the invited participants

As the nurse-midwife you bring into the home birth situation not only clinical knowledge, skills, and judgment but also a positive attitude of confidence and belief in the birth process and the capability of woman's body, mind, and spirit. With the woman's and participants' help, you set up your supplies and equipment (Appendix II) along with what they have purchased (Appendix I). Water is boiled in the pans in the kitchen and the instruments, bulb syringe, and shoelaces are sterilized. If you have an autoclave in your practice then only the bulb syringe the woman or couple has purchased and the shoelaces will need sterilization. All is in readiness and the birth transpires.

The home setting is also a natural setting for sibling participation in and learning about the normal birth process. The little girl in Figure 20-5 was not sure at first that she wanted to get her fingers into the blood and fluid, so she put on a glove "like the midwife." She shortly changed her mind and discarded the glove when more of the baby's head appeared.

Early Parenting, Postpartum, and Follow-up

In keeping with the responsibility the woman or couple has assumed, it is important that they be the ones to first clean and dress their baby. Instruction may be needed but you should check your impulses to do this yourself. This deliberate action is also in keeping with the philosophy that if the mother or parents are well cared for they will be capable of caring for their baby. *Caretaking of the baby is the responsibility of the parents.*

A home visit is made by the nurse-midwife within 24 hours after birth. Physical assessment of both the mother and baby is done.

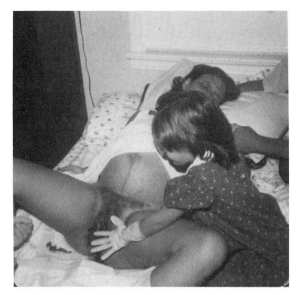
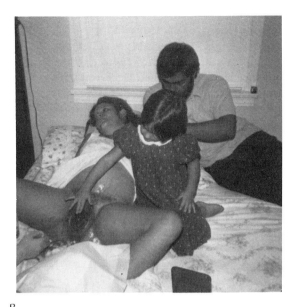

A

B

FIGURE 20-5. Sibling participation in home birth. A. learning about birth; B. touching the baby's head.

Assessment is also made of the developing family relationships, adequacy of help in the home, infant caretaking abilities, and timing of the appointment with the pediatrician. The family is seen again at 2 weeks and 6 weeks postpartum in the nurse-midwife's office.

Follow-up thereafter is in accord with the woman's needs for interconceptional care. Most nurse-midwife home birth practitioners also have some form of monthly group get-together which mothers attend as long as they want. Topics of interest and sharing are the basis for the content of these meetings. Those interested may attend parenting or family support groups.

The Nurse-Midwife in Home Birth

Throughout this section on home birth, the responsibilities of the nurse-midwife have been enumerated. This segment is for the purpose of discussing the differences you will experience when moving out of the hospital, especially from a tertiary medical center, to a home birth setting.

Responsibility becomes the key word. The hospital setting tends to diffuse responsibility among a number of people. As the woman or couple assume responsibility you both relinquish and acquire it. It is in the home birth setting that you may feel most keenly the professional responsibility and accountability you have undertaken. Even though you and the woman or couple share responsibility for whatever happens during a home birth, if an unfortunate event or tragedy occurs you will be held solely and visibly responsible, professionally and legally, by the community. The development of the partnership between the woman or couple and the nurse-midwife, thus, is critical. Also critical is the need to really get to know this woman, couple, or family as a unit in the larger context of their life and how they work together. While this is also true for in-hospital birth, it becomes a screening criterion for home birth. How a woman lives her life will be reflected in how she gives birth. Her trust and belief in herself and her capabilities will affect the course of labor [6].

You will experience a different professional growth from that which you gain in the hospital. Your point of view may be altered with a resulting mixture of conflict and clarity regarding clinical issues and parameters of normal to be resolved. The effects of the uniqueness of each individual woman's life upon her childbearing experience and the course and progress of labor are more visible because the psychological processes are allowed to unfold without environmental hindrance or physical interventions. Growth for the nurse-midwife in home birth also "has to do with being intimately involved with people as part of the intimate process that birth *is*, rather than putting it into an artificial structure" [7].

You must be very exact and certain of your clinical skills, abilities, and findings as this is all you have with which to work. Then you must trust your own knowledge and judgment as you apply them to the individual woman's own labor process. For some nurse-midwives this is an exciting challenge. For others it is frightening. For at least one nurse-midwife it was freeing:

I was in a setting where no one could impose external parameters and policies; where I could use my clinical judgment and conclude that all was normal. There was no one around to tell me otherwise, to try to fill me with negativism and doubt, or to tell me I was wrong. [8]

REFERENCES

1. Burst, H. V. The influence of consumers on the birthing movement. In J. Strawn (Issue Ed.). *Topics in Clinical Nursing: Rehumanizing the Acute Care Setting* 5(3):42–54 (October) 1983.
2. Burst, H. V. Alternative birth settings and providers. In J. McCloskey and H. Grace (Eds.). *Current Issues in Nursing, 2nd.* Boston: Blackwell Scientific Publications, 1985.
3. Lubic, R. W. Childbearing centers: Delivering more for less. *Am. J. Nurs.* 83(7):1053–1056, 1983.
4. Baldwin, R. *Special Delivery: The Complete Guide to Informed Birth.* Berkeley, Calif.: Celestial Arts, 1979.
5. Kier, J. Personal communication, August 23, 1983.
6. Kier, J. Personal communication, October 6, 1983.
7. Melnikow, S. Personal communication, October 7, 1984.
8. The author. Personal notes, October 8, 1983.

BIBLIOGRAPHY

Adamson, G. D., and Gare, D. J. Home or hospital births? *JAMA* 243(17):1732–1736, May 2, 1980.

Allgair, A. Alternative birth centers offer family centered care. *Hospitals* 52:97–105, 1978.

American College of Nurse-Midwives. *Guidelines for Establishing a Home Birth Service.* Washington, D. C.: ACNM, 1979.

American College of Nurse-Midwives. *Guidelines for Establishing an Alternative Birth Center* (out-of-hospital). Washington, D. C.: ACNM, 1979.

Anderson, S., and Simkin, P. *Birth through Children's Eyes.* Seattle, Wash.: Pennypress, 1981.

Annas, G. J. Homebirth: Autonomy vs. safety. *The Hastings Center Report* (August) 1978, pp. 19–20.

Aylsworth, S. Birthing environments: Historical background. In Summer, P. E., and Phillips, C. R. (Eds.). *Birthing Rooms: Concept and Reality.* St. Louis: Mosby, 1981, pp. 1–11.

Baldwin, R. *Special Delivery: The Complete Guide to Informed Birth.* Berkeley, Calif.: Celestial Arts, 1979.

Bauwens, E., and Anderson, S. Home births: A reaction to hospital environmental stressors. In Bauwens, E. (Ed.). *The Anthropology of Health.* St. Louis: Mosby, 1978, chapter 6.

Bennetts, A., and Lubic, R. W. The free-standing birth centre. *Lancet*, February 13, 1982, pp. 378–380.

Burnett, C. A., III et al. Home delivery and neonatal mortality in North Carolina. *JAMA* 244(24):2741–2745, December 19, 1980.

Burst, H. V. Alternative birth settings and providers. In McClosky, J. and Grace, H. (Eds.). *Current Issues in Nursing, 2nd.* Boston: Blackwell Scientific Publications, 1985.

Burst, H. V. Harmonious unity. *J. Nurse-Midwifery* 22(3):10–11 (Fall) 1977.

Burst, H. V. Our three-ring circus. *J. Nurse-Midwifery* 23:11−14 (Fall) 1978.

Burst, H. V. The influence of consumers on the birthing movement. In Strawn, J. (Issue Ed.), *Topics in Clinical Nursing: Rehumanizing the Acute Care Setting* 5(3):42−54 (October) 1983.

Cameron, J. et al. Home birth in Salt Lake City, Utah. *Am. J. Public Health* 69(7):716−717 (July) 1979.

Carroll, M. H. Starting a childbearing center in your community. In Stewart, D., and Stewart, L. (Eds.). *Compulsory Hospitalization or Freedom of Choice in Childbirth?* Marble Hill, Mo.: NAPSAC Reproductions, 1979.

Conklin, M., and Simmons, R. *Planned Home Childbirths: Parental Perspectives.* Health Monograph Series, No. 2. Lansing, Mich.: Michigan Department of Public Health, 1979.

Devitt, N. The transition from home to hospital birth in the United States, 1930−1960. *Birth Family J.* 4:47−58, 1977.

DeVries, R. G. Image and reality: An evaluation of hospital alternative birth centers. *J. Nurse-Midwifery* 28(3):3−9 (May/June) 1983.

Epstein, J. et al. A safe homebirth program that works. In Stewart, D., and Stewart, L. (Eds.). *Safe Alternatives in Childbirth.* Chapel Hill, N. C.: NAPSAC Publications, 1976.

Ernst, E. K. M. et al. The continuum concept: Home, hospital and birth center care within a single (Ob-Gyn/nurse-midwifery) service. In Stewart, D., and Stewart, L. (Eds.). *Compulsory Hospitalization or Freedom of Choice in Childbirth?* Marble Hill, Mo.: NAPSAC Reproductions, 1979.

Ernst, E. M., and Gordon, K. A. Fifty-three years of home birth experience at the Frontier Nursing Service, Kentucky: 1925−1978. In Stewart, D., and Stewart, L. (Eds.). *Compulsory Hospitalization or Freedom of Choice in Childbirth?* Vol. 2. Marble Hill, Mo.: NAPSAC Reproductions, 1979.

Estes, M. N. A home obstetrical service with expert consultation and back-up. *Birth Family J.* 5(3):151−157, (Fall) 1978.

Faison, J. et al. The childbearing center: An alternative birth setting. *Obstet. Gynecol.* 54(4):527−532, 1979.

Fullerton, J. The choice of in-hospital or alternative birth environment as related to the concept of control. *J. Nurse-Midwifery* 27(2):17−22 (March/April) 1982.

Gabel, H. D. Alternative birth centers: Fact or fan-tasy. *Va. Med. J.* 104(11):771−772, 1977.

Gordon, I. T. The birth controllers: Limitations on out-of-hospital births. *J. Nurse-Midwifery* 27(1):34−39 (January/February) 1982.

Hazell, L. A. *Birth Goes Home.* Seattle, Wash.: Catalyst Press, 1974.

Hazell, L. A. Study of 300 elective home births. *Birth Family J.* 2(1):11−18, 1974−1975.

Hosford, E. Implementing a medically sound childbearing center: Problems and solutions. In Stewart, L., and Stewart, D. (Eds.) *21st Century Obstetrics Now!* Chapel Hill, N. C.: NAPSAC, 1977.

ICEA Position Paper on Planning Comprehensive Maternal and Newborn Services for the Childbearing Years. Minneapolis, Minn.: International Childbirth Education Association, 1983.

Karmel, M. *Thank You, Dr. Lamaze.* Philadelphia: Lippincott, 1959.

Kier, J. *Decision Making for the Place of Birth: Home or Hospital.* Unpublished master's thesis. New Haven, Conn.: Yale University School of Nursing, 1982.

Kier, J. *Woman's Guide to a Stress-Free Pregnancy and Creative Childbirth.* Houston, Texas: Butterfly Books, 1985.

Kitzinger, S. *The Complete Book of Pregnancy and Childbirth.* New York: Knopf, 1980.

Krutsky, C. *Home Births: A Review of the Pertinent Issues.* Unpublished independent study paper. New Haven, Conn.: Yale University School of Nursing, 1982.

Lubic, R. W. Alternative patterns of nurse-midwifery care. 1. The childbearing center. *J. Nurse-Midwifery* 21(3):24−25 (Fall) 1976.

Lubic, R. W. Childbearing centers: Delivering more for less. *Am. J. Nurs.* 83(7):1053−1056, 1983.

Lubic, R. W. Evaluation of an out-of-hospital maternity center for low-risk patients. In Aiken, L. H. (Ed.). *Health Policy and Nursing Practice.* New York: McGraw-Hill, 1980, chapter 6.

Lubic, R. W. The impact of technology on health care — The childbearing center: A case for technology's appropriate use. *J. Nurse-Midwifery* 24(1):6−10, 1979.

Lubic, R. W. The Maternity Center Association's childbearing center. *J. Reprod. Med.* 19(5):293−294, 1977.

Lubic, R. W. Comprehensive maternity care as an ambulatory service — Maternity Center Association's birth alternative. *J. N. Y. State Nurses Assoc.* 8(4):19−24, 1977.

Lubic, R. W. The childbearing center: A demonstration project in out-of-hospital care. *J. Nurse-Midwifery* 21(3):24–25, 1976.

Lubic, R. W. & E. K. M. Ernst. The childbearing center: An alternative to conventional care. *Nurs. Outlook* 26(12):754–760, 1978.

Maternity Center Association. *Mothers' Classes and Preparation for Natural Childbirth.* New York: MCA, 1949.

Mehl, L. E. Home delivery research today — A review. *Women and Health* 3–11, 1976.

Mehl, L. E. Research on alternatives in childbirth: What can it tell us about hospital practice? In Stewart, L., and Stewart, D. (Eds.). *21st Century Obstetrics Now! Vol. 1.* Marble Hill, Mo.: NAPSAC, 1977.

Mehl, L. E. Statistical outcomes of homebirths in the U. S.: Current status. In Stewart, L., and Stewart, D. (Eds.). *Safe Alternatives in Childbirth.* Chapel Hill, N. C.: NAPSAC, 1976.

Mehl, L. et al. Outcomes of elective home births: A series of 1146 cases. *J. Reprod. Med.* 19(5):281–290 (November) 1977.

Murdaugh, A. Experiences of a new migrant health clinic. *BCHS* 1977.

Nielsen, I. Nurse-midwifery in an alternative birth center. *Birth Family J.* 4(1):24–27, 1977.

Parma, S. A family-centered event? Preparing the child for sharing in the experience of childbirth. *J. Nurse-Midwifery,* 24(3):5–10 (May/June) 1979.

Read, G. D. *Childbirth without Fear.* New York: Harper & Brothers, 1944.

Reinke, C. Outcomes of the first 527 births at The Birthplace in Seattle. *Birth* 9(4):231–238 (Winter) 1982.

Report of the Birth Center Task Force. Massachusetts Health Systems Agency, Area IV, March, 1980.

Rice, A., and Carty, E. Alternative birth centers. *Can. Nurse* 73:31–34, 1977.

Ritchie, D., and Swanson, L. A. Childbirth outside the hospital — The resurgence of home and clinic deliveries. *Am. J. Mat. Child. Nurs.* (November/December) 1976, pp. 372–377.

Rothman, B. K. Anatomy of a compromise: Nurse-midwifery and the rise of the birth center. *J. Nurse-Midwifery* 28(4):3–7 (July/August) 1983.

Sagov, S. E., Feinbloom, R. I., Spindel, P., and Brodsky, A. *Home Birth: A Practitioner's Guide to Birth Outside the Hospital.* Rockville, Md.: Aspen, 1984.

Searles, C. The impetus toward home birth. *J. Nurse-Midwifery* 26(3):51–56 (May/June) 1981.

Stewart, D. Home: The traditional safe place for birth. In Stewart, D. (Ed.). *The Five Standards for Safe Childbearing.* Marble Hill, Mo.: NAPSAC, 1981.

Stewart, D., and Stewart, L. (Eds.). *Compulsory Hospitalization or Freedom of Choice in Childbirth? Vol. I, II, and III.* Marble Hill, Mo.: NAPSAC, 1979.

Thoms, H., Roth, L. G., and Linton, D. *Understanding Natural Childbirth.* New York: McGraw-Hill, 1950.

White, G. A comparison of home and hospital delivery based on 25 years' experience with both. *J. Reprod. Med.* 19(5):291–292 (November) 1977.

Zabrek, E., Simon, P., and Benrubi, G. The alternative birth center in Jacksonville, Florida: The first two years. *J. Nurse-Midwifery* 28(4):31–36 (July/August) 1983.

APPENDIX I

SAMPLE LIST OF SUPPLIES TO BE PURCHASED BY THE WOMAN OR COUPLE PREPARING FOR HOME BIRTH*

Large maternity sanitary pads

Sanitary belt

Clean bed linen — 2 sets

Tongs — 1 pair (optional)

Sterile gloves (specify size and number)

Sterile gauze squares (4 × 4) individually packaged — 2 boxes (25/box)

Mirror (8 × 10 inches)

Large trash bags — 2

Small white baby-shoe shoelaces — 1 pair — or umbilical cord tape

Bulb (ear) syringe (3-ounce size)

Antiseptic solution — 1 small bottle

Topical anesthetic spray or squirt bottle — 1

Large disposable underpads (Chux or Sears) — 40 to 50

Hydrous or anhydrous lanolin — 1 small bottle

Ice bag (optional)

Heating pad (optional)

---

* Other items are brought by the nurse-midwife to the home (see Appendix II).

Flexible straws (optional)
Shower curtain liner (for bed protection)
Flashlight *with batteries* and extra batteries
Hooded towels for baby at time of
    delivery — 2
Baby diapers and clothes
Thermometer
Camera, if desired
Tape recorder and tape, if desired
Videocassette recorder (VCR), if desired
Eye drop prophylaxis (according to state
    law) — get prescription filled

APPENDIX II

SAMPLE LIST OF SUPPLIES AND
EQUIPMENT THE NURSE-MIDWIFE TAKES
TO A HOME BIRTH*

Map of city and surrounding area
Map to house
Blood pressure cuff
Stethoscope
Fetoscope
Doptone
Flashlight or lantern and batteries
Penlight
Fish scales and sling
Urine dipsticks (for glucose, protein, ketones)
Nitrazine paper
Urinary catheter
Fleets enema
Sterile gloves
Scissors — 2
Clamps — 2
Hemostats — 2
Sponge forceps
Ring forceps — 2

Needle holder
Package of sterile towels
Alcohol swabs or wipes
†Tourniquet
†Blood tubes — red-top and purple-top
†IV tubing
†Intravenous fluid — 5% dextrose in lactated
    Ringer's solution
†Adhesive tape
Amnihooks
†Intravenous catheters (16-gauge)
Lidocaine HCl (Xylocaine), 1% solution — 50
    milliliter multiple dose vial
Suture — 2-0, 3-0, and 4-0 chromic gut
Needles — various gauges and lengths
Syringes — various sizes but at least 3-, 5-,
    and 10-milliliter
†Ambu bag with infant mask
†Small oxygen tank
†Oxygen tubing
†Oxygen masks — infant and adult
DeLee suction catheter with mucus trap
†Laryngoscope with infant blade
†Infant endotracheal tubes and stylet
†Oral airways — infant and adult
Eye prophylaxis (according to state law)
Vitamin K or analogue
Methergine in 0.2 milligram vials and tablets
Pitocin in 10 IU vials
Birth certificates
Labor, delivery, and postpartal record forms
Statistics record form
Smelling salts — spirits of ammonia or amyl
    nitrate

---

* Other items are purchased by the woman or couple
(see Appendix I).
† Denotes emergency supplies and equipment.

IV

Management of the Newborn

Second Edition Revision by

Mary Kathleen McHugh, C.N.M., M.S.N.
Lecturer, Nurse-Midwifery Program
University of Pennsylvania
Staff Nurse-Midwife
The Birth Center, Bryn Mawr, PA.

Original text by
Joy M. Brands, R.N., C.N.M., M.P.H. and Mary I. Banigan, R. N., Ph.D.

21

The Normal Neonate

The perinatal period is a time of risk for the fetus and newborn. While perinatal statistics refer specifically to the time between 28 weeks gestation and 28 days after birth (the neonatal period), the perinatal period has come to take on broader boundaries to include the time from conception through pregnancy and the neonatal period. It is a period during which all mothers, whether normal or high-risk, are concerned for the well-being of their child.

THE PERINATAL JOURNEY

The needs of the fetus for an optimal intrauterine existence and extrauterine adaptation are summarized in the following instructions to the fetus:

Choose parents that are sound and healthy. If possible, find two that are of good socioeconomic status. It is preferable that they are neither too short nor too tall, and not overweight. Your mother should be Rh positive and have a regular menstrual cycle. Your mother-to-be should not smoke, take drugs, nor seek medication. Your parents' family background must be genetically impeccable. They should seek good antenatal care and look for a safe place to be delivered. If you could order your own environment, request not to be born early or late. Keep your membranes intact until you are sure you are on the way into the world. Position yourself so that you will enter the world headfirst. Once you have arrived, breathe quickly before they cut your cord. Ask to be dried, kept warm, and given time to adjust to the new environment. Ask to meet your parents so you can start getting acquainted with them. With these goals in mind, you will have the best chance to survive all of the risks of your perinatal lifetime.

The purposes of a perinatal health care program are to make available to each family the best possible advice and care before conception and during the antepartum, intrapartum, and immediate postnatal periods and to prevent or treat causes of maternal, fetal, and neonatal morbidity and mortality. Every conceptus should have the opportunity to progress to its genetic potential and to accomplish this in a manner acceptable to the parents and optimal for the fetus (Fig. 21-1).

The improvement and maintenance of peri-

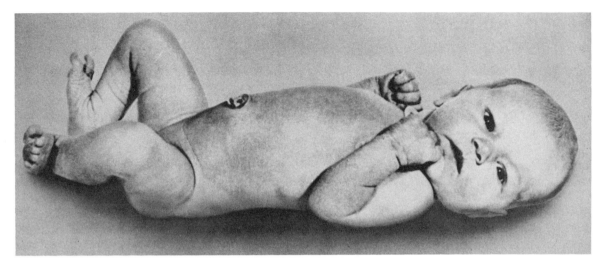

FIGURE 21-1. The normal newborn. (Reproduced by permission from *The Birth Atlas*. New York: Maternity Center Association.)

natal health care service is the responsibility of all those involved in maternal-child health. The combined efforts of nurse-midwives, nurses, physicians, and others from the ancillary services should bring about a more conscious effort toward the provision of quality services for perinatal health care. For instance, if a universally adequate diet could be assured, the incidence of prematurity would be drastically reduced. Then there would be fewer fragile babies born; there would be fewer deaths from such acute conditions as respiratory distress syndrome; and there would be fewer survivors left with permanent neurological deficits.

The management of the potentially or acutely ill mother and newborn usually is not recognized as an integral part of nurse-midwifery practice. However, an understanding of the pathology in the mother, fetus, and newborn will prepare the nurse-midwife to make appropriate decisions for consultation or referral and to manage emergency situations until more qualified help arrives. The knowledge of factors that contribute to high-risk conditions in the fetus will enable the nurse-midwife to anticipate the level of care that should be provided for the mother and her infant. Therefore, a chapter on high-risk conditions in mother or fetus and newborn is included in this part on the neonate (Chapter 23).

EXTRAUTERINE ADAPTATION

The neonate must change its entire life-style upon delivery. He or she must go from complete dependence to an independent state. All the systems in the nondistressed full-term neonate are adequate to adapt to extrauterine life immediately after delivery. This complex process of change and instability is known as the transitional period. It is the nurse-midwife's responsibility to know, understand, be aware of, and assess the changes that take place as the neonate goes through its transitional period. Assessment of findings along with the action taken must be charted. Appropriate medical consultation or referral is required when deviations are noted. The physiologic and psychosocial changes and factors involved in extrauterine adaptation are discussed here.

Respiratory Changes

The respiratory system is the system most challenged in the change from intrauterine to extrauterine environment. Upon arrival into an atmospheric environment there is an immediate demand on the neonate for respiration. The organ responsible for fetal respiration prior to delivery is the placenta. Upon delivery the lungs change from a liquid-filled state to a system well prepared for and capable of respiration.

The phenomenon that occurs to stimulate the neonate to take the first breath is still unknown. It is believed to be a combination of biochemical changes and a number of physical stimuli to which the neonate is subjected, such as cold, gravity, pain, light, and noise, which cause excitation of the respiratory center.

The first active breaths of air, once taken and sustained, set in motion a nearly inexorable chain of events that:
1. Converts the fetal to the adult circulation
2. Empties the lung of liquid
3. Establishes the neonatal lung volume and the characteristics of pulmonary function in the newly born infant. [1, p. 78]

The primary concern at the time of delivery is the establishment of respiration. The prompt onset of breathing is essential to subsequent mental and physical development.

When the head is delivered, mucus drains from the nares and mouth. Many neonates gasp and even cry at this time. Therefore, suctioning the mouth and nares with a bulb syringe to prevent aspiration of mucus or amniotic fluid may be necessary as soon as the head is accessible (Fig. 21-2). More mucus will be noted as the body is compressed during delivery. This release of fluid allows air to be taken into the lungs.

Gentle rubbing of the neonate's back, flicking the sole of the foot, or vigorous drying of the infant to reduce heat loss are sufficient aids in stimulation of respiration. If stimulation is too vigorous, such as slapping or exposure to extreme cold, it becomes distressful and tends to inhibit respirations.

There is variation in the respiratory pattern with onset of respiration. Respirations fluctuate and are not stable for a period of time. There are, however, certain normal and abnormal responses for which to look in the newborn. A respiratory rate consistently greater than 60 per minute, with or without flaring, grunting, or retractions is clearly abnormal at 2 hours of life. Other normal and abnormal responses are indicated in Table 21-1.

Circulatory Changes

The blood flow from the placenta is stopped by the clamping of the umbilical cord. This eliminates the placental supply of oxygen and forces the neonate to obtain oxygen from the lungs. This alters the path of blood flow and causes changes in blood volume, pressure, and chemical composition. The onset of respiration increases the arterial oxygen pressure

TABLE 21-1. Normal and Abnormal Respiratory Responses

Normal	Abnormal
Average rate: 40/min.	—
Range: 30–60/min.	—
Diaphragmatic and abdominal breathing	Intercostal retractions, retractions of the xyphoid
Obligate nose breather	Flared nostrils
—	Grunting on expiration

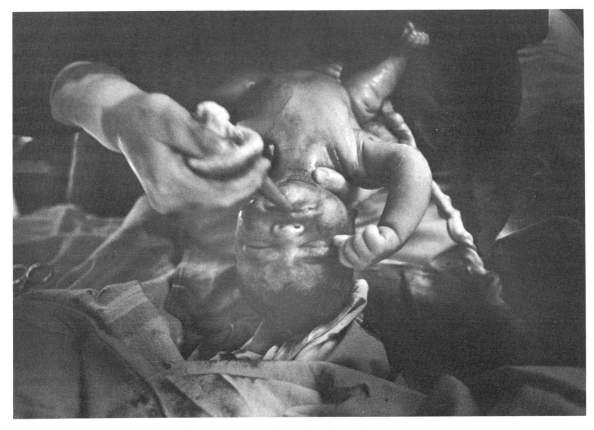

FIGURE 21-2. Newborn at mother's introitus with cord still attached.

(pO_2). This increase in oxygen causes a vaso-dilatation of pulmonary arterioles and an abrupt decrease in pulmonary resistance. The following anatomic changes then follow (see Fig. 21-3):

A much larger amount of blood is pumped into the pulmonary arteries by the right ventricle and a smaller amount passes through the ductus arteriosus. The ductus arteriosus begins to atrophy and eventually is known as the ligamentum arteriosum.

As the pulmonary circulation increases, more blood is returned from the lungs to the left atrium. Increase in pressure in the left atrium causes the foramen ovale to close. Placental circulation ceases to function when the umbilical cord is tied. The ends of the hypogastric arteries atrophy, and are known as the hypogastric ligaments.

The ductus venosus becomes occluded and is known as the ligamentum venosum. The umbilical vein becomes obliterated and is known as the ligamentum teres. [2, pp. 5–6]

Thermal Regulation *(Thermogenesis)*

One of the first things people knew about the neonate was that he or she had to be kept warm. But how warm is warm? Because of a large body surface area and poor thermal regulation, the neonate loses heat instantly at

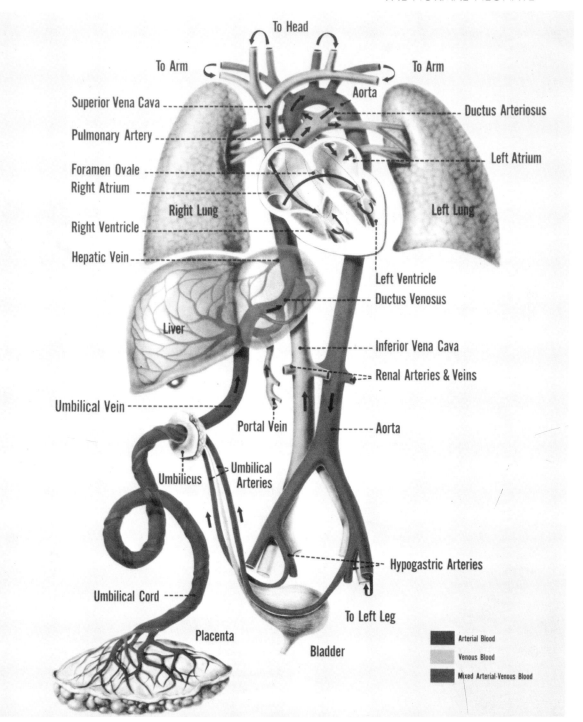

FIGURE 21-3.   Fetal-newborn circulation. (Reproduced by permission from *Fetal Circulation*, Nursing Education Series #1. Columbus, Ohio: Ross Laboratories, 1957.)

birth. Specific ways in which the neonate loses heat are:

1. Evaporation — whenever the skin becomes wet in a relatively dry room or incubator
2. Radiation — when heat is transferred from the body surface to cooler surfaces not in actual contact with the body
3. Convection — with the movement of air currents over the infant's skin
4. Conduction — when heat is lost from the surface of the body to other objects in direct contact with the skin

The newborn will attempt to conserve heat by peripheral vasoconstriction and adoption of a flexed posture. However, the neonate is also capable of producing heat through both general and brown fat metabolism. Brown fat is located in the upper thorax, in the axillae, and beneath the skin in the upper part of the back. This fat is different from white fat in that, if the neonate is cold, the autonomic nervous system triggers the brown fat deposits to release and metabolize the stored fat. The white fat, or ordinary adipose tissue, acts as a reservoir for potential energy and cannot be utilized as readily as brown fat. Brown fat is a limited resource which is rapidly depleted during periods of cold stress.

The neonate uses up energy at the time of delivery. If the delivery room is 15°F cooler than the intrauterine temperature, the neonate will lose 200 kilocalories per minute through evaporation, convection, and radiation. Washing or placing the baby in an unwarmed crib causes further heat loss. Heat loss can be minimized by having the room where the baby is born warm, drying the neonate as soon as possible after delivery, wrapping the baby in a warm blanket and placing him or her in a warm crib or next to the mother. Particular care must be taken to prevent heat loss from the head, which can represent 25 percent of a neonate's surface area.

According to *Hospital Care of Newborn Infants*,

Each infant must have his own thermometer. Deep or core temperatures can be determined in either the rectum or the axilla. The site should be recorded and consistently used in making serial measurements. Moreover, because of inconsistencies in the accuracy of clinical thermometers, the same thermometer (whether glass or electronic) should be used in serial measurements made in an individual infant. Consistency in the technique of measurement will improve the ability to interpret recorded fluctuations in temperature. [3, p. 108]

There is no magic temperature that is adequate for all neonates. Therefore a balance must be maintained between the amount of heat produced and the amount of heat lost. Normal body temperature for an infant is 97.7 to 99.5°F, or 36.5 to 37.5°C.

Acid-Base Balance

Before delivery the fetal acid-base balance is controlled via the placenta through the maternal lungs and kidneys. This is ended with birth. The neonate is born with an oxygen debit and elevated carbon dioxide pressure (pCO_2) levels. Usually the neonate compensates for this with increased respiratory efforts within the first hour of life, thus bringing the pCO_2 to within normal limits. Healthy term babies achieve normal limits whereas a stressed baby, regardless of the cause of stress, is less able to do this. Table 21-2 indicates some of the changes that take place.

Blood Volume Changes

Although a considerable portion of the total blood volume is in the placenta and umbilical vessels during fetal life, neither the amount nor the percentage of the total volume has been measured during human fetal life.

According to indirect measurements, the term placental circuit contains approximately 125 to 150 ml. of blood at the moment of birth, which can be

TABLE 21-2.   Normal Blood Gases For Age

Age	pO₂	pCO₂	pH	Base excess	Hct.
Fetus before labor	25	40	7.37	−2	55
Fetus at end of labor	20	55	7.25	−5	55
Newborn at term — 10 min.	50	48	7.20	−10	55
Newborn at term — 1 hour	70	35	7.35	−5	60
Newborn at term — 1 week	75	35	7.40	−2	55
Newborn premature — 1 week	60	38	7.37	−3	47

compared with a total blood volume of approximately 300 ml. in the term baby a few hours after birth. The average blood volume of the newborn is estimated to be 85 ml. per kg. body weight consisting of 41 ml. of plasma and 44 ml. of red blood cell mass. [4, p. 228]

There is a notable difference in the blood volume of an infant whose cord is clamped immediately after delivery (78.0 milliliters per kilogram of body weight) and one for whom the cutting of the cord is delayed (98.6 milliliters per kilogram).

Glucose Balance

The fetus receives a constant supply of glucose from the mother through the placenta. This glucose is the major source of energy for the fetus, and the brain is dependent on it. Without glucose, central nervous system damage occurs. Since the fetus is dependent on a constant source of glucose in utero, this basic need is present at the time of delivery. The glycogen store in the neonate is an adequate source of energy, but for a few hours only.

The normal newborn glucose levels are 50 to 60 milligrams per 100 milliliters. A check on blood levels is as follows:

50–60 mg./100 ml. — normal
    40 mg./100 ml. — regard with suspicion
    30 mg./100 ml. — needs greater concern
    20 mg./100 ml. — indication for therapeutic intervention

The blood glucose level falls in the normal neonate after birth. It usually reaches its lowest level in 1 to 2 hours but is considered normal if it is above 40 milligrams per 100 milliliters. The blood glucose remains low until feedings have begun, then begins to rise. In some institutions blood glucose is measured routinely on all newborns. In other institutions blood glucose is checked only if there is evidence of maternal problems or the fetus or neonate has been assessed as high risk.

Clinical manifestations of hypoglycemia in order of severity are as follows:
Mild: apathy, abnormal cry, hypothermia, irregular respirations, refusal to feed
Moderate: apnea, cyanosis, marked tremors, limpness, three or more mild signs
Severe: convulsions (three or more moderate) [5, p. 7]

A blood glucose measurement should be done if any of these clinical signs are present.

The lack of glucose in sufficient quantity to be utilized by tissue, especially that of the central nervous system, constitutes hypoglycemia. Clinical signs may occur even in the presence of blood glucose levels normally considered to be adequate [6, p. 423]. When this occurs, the possibility of another problem such as central nervous system damage, hypocalcemia, or drug withdrawal should be explored.

There are various test-strip methods for bedside determination of blood glucose. Meticulous attention must be paid to proper technique to insure accurate results. The following is the procedure for Dextrostix determinations.

1. Indications
   a. small-for-gestational-age infants
   b. infants of diabetic mothers
   c. infants with erythroblastosis fetalis
   d. prematures
   e. asphyxiated infants
   f. cold-stressed infants
   g. infants with central nervous system hemorrhages and malformations
   h. infants with rare developmental and genetic disorders (galactosemia) who are subject to develop hypoglycemia during and after transfusions (exchange, reduction, etc.)
2. Equipment
   a. alcohol wipe
   b. microlancet
   c. cotton ball
   d. Dextrostix strip and color chart
3. Procedure
   a. rub infant's heel with alcohol wipe and let it dry.
   b. puncture lateral edge of foot (inside or outside) with microlancet, deep enough to obtain free flow of blood (Fig. 21-4).
   c. freely apply a large drop of blood to Dextrostix strip; use enough blood to sufficiently cover entire reagent area on printed side of slip.
   d. wait exactly 60 seconds.
   e. wash blood off strip for 1 to 2 seconds (gentle stream of water).
   f. hold strip close to color chart and read results within 1 to 2 seconds after washing.
   g. place cotton ball over infant's heel to stop bleeding.
   h. record Dextrostix results.
   i. notify physician if result is less than 45 or greater than 130.
   j. confirm a low Dextrostix reading with blood glucose test from the laboratory (treatment should not be withheld during the wait for values to return from the lab).

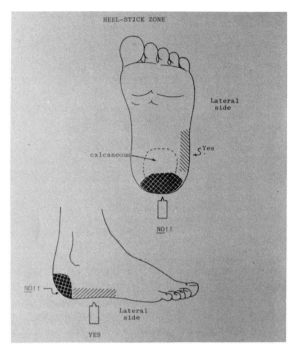

FIGURE 21-4.   Diagram showing heel-stick zone on newborn.

4. Cautions
   a. strips that have brownish discoloration or do not match the "O" color block on the chart are not to be used.
   b. Dextrostix strips are good 4 months after initial opening.

Gastrointestinal Tract Function

The gastrointestinal tract is relatively inactive during fetal life. Variable amounts of amniotic fluid are swallowed and absorbed, and the production of meconium begins.

At the time of delivery, the neonate is capable of both secretory and absorptive activities. Stern illustrates the regional specialization and functions of the gastrointestinal tract [6, p. 840].

Mouth — chewing, moistening, preliminary starch digestion

Stomach — mixing, liquefaction, formation of acid curd, beginning adjustment of tonicity, preliminary protein digestion, absorption of alcohol

Duodenum — chyme rendered isotonic with blood, emulsification of fats, pH raised to neutral, preliminary digestion and absorption of carbohydrate, fat, and protein

Jejunum — final brush border digestion; main absorptive site for carbohydrate, fat, and protein; water absorbed passively with nutrients and sodium chloride, absorption of many vitamins and minerals

Ileum — sodium reabsorbed against gradient; water reabsorbed with sodium chloride; reserve nutrient absorption; absorption of bile salts and Vitamin B_{12}; chloride-bicarbonate exchange

Colon — final salt and water absorption, chloridebicarbonate exchange, storage prior to evacuation.

Renal Function

The urinary system is immature at the time of delivery and the volume of urine is low. Most newborns urinate at the time of delivery or sometime within the first 12 hours. If the newborn does not urinate by the end of 24 hours, a physician should be notified for investigation of the problem.

The first urine is characteristically hypotonic and may contain acetone and protein. This reflects the prenatal status of the kidneys which are required to excrete rather large volumes of water, while the placenta serves the function of metabolic excretion. At birth the glomerular filtration rate is relatively low and the kidney is incapable of adjusting to sudden changes in water and electrolyte balance. [7, p. 310]

Hepatic Function

The maternal liver provides the majority of hepatic functions for the fetus in utero. Many functions of the neonate's liver are not fully mature at birth. For example, the ability to conjugate bilirubin is suboptimal and this contributes to neonatal physiological jaundice.

The liver is the only organ that breaks down glycogen for release into the general circulation. It also can utilize noncarbohydrate sources for glucose production (gluconeogenesis) when necessary. The release of this glucose enables the neonate to survive until external food sources are provided.

Blood-clotting factors II, VII, IX, and X are synthesized in the liver and drop to low levels by the third day of life. Synthesis of these factors is dependent on healthy liver function and adequate provision of vitamin K, which can be absorbed from the gut and utilized by the liver.

Immune System Changes

The neonate has an impaired ability to react to invading organisms. On a cellular level there is a decreased ability of leukocytes to concentrate where necessary. These leukocytes are less bactericidal and phagocytic. At the humoral level the newborn has low or nonexistent levels of the immunoglobulin antibodies IgM, IgE, and IgA. The neonate is born, however, with IgG antibodies acquired from the mother, which confer protection from some specific diseases. These is a slow rise of immunoglobulin levels after 3 months of age to levels of older children.

Laboratory Tests and Values

Local laboratories should be contacted for normal values as well as types of tests used. It has been noted that specific values change from laboratory to laboratory because of their individual methods of testing. Tests which should be inquired about include hemoglobin, hematocrit, blood type (ABO and Rh), bilirubin, glucose, calcium, direct Coomb's test, and phenylketonuria (PKU) and thyroid screening tests.

Psychosocial Factors

The newborn infant enters the world with an ability to respond to and even control the environment into which he or she is placed. Since infants are born with the capacity to shut out stimuli after repeated trials, they can be selective about the stimuli to which they will respond. The stimuli should be meaningful for the infant. Selection of specific stimuli should be chosen to promote specific types of responses from the infant.

In the awake and alert state, the infant has the ability to follow visually an inanimate object that is placed within the field of vision. When the infant responds to an animate object (the parent's face) the parent will respond to the infant in a reciprocal fashion. When the voice is presented at the same time that the face is within the visual field, the infant will follow and be able to turn toward the sound of the voice when the parent's face is out of the field of vision. When parents talk to their infants, the response is significant. The infant learns to discriminate between the voices of parents and those of strangers. As the infant's hearing develops, he or she will soon be able to distinguish the day-to-day sounds of the environment.

THE TRANSITIONAL PERIOD

The transitional period is the time the individual infant requires to stabilize to extrauterine independence. This stabilization is facilitated by the infant's capacity for adaptation and environmental assistance. The period of transition is divided into three stages: the first is the period immediately after birth and lasts approximately 30 minutes, the second is the interval lasting from 30 minutes until about 2 hours after birth, and the third continues from 2 hours after birth until the baby is around 6 hours old. During this time assessments are made of heart rate, respiratory rate, temperature, mucus, neurologic function (which includes activity, reactivity, tone, and posture), and bowel function (which includes peristalsis and passage of meconium). These assessments are summarized in Table 21-3.

The infant is stressed through the process of birth and should be allowed to stabilize

TABLE 21-3. The Transitional Period: Recovery and Activity Periods in the Neonate

Observe*	First Activity Period (First Period of Reactivity): Birth−30 min.	Rest Period (Second Period of Reactivity): 30 min.−2 hr.	Second Activity Period (Third Period of Reactivity): 2−6 hr.
Color	Brief cyanosis	Flushing with crying	Swift color changes
Respirations	Rapid, grunting retractions	Decreased	Irregular with rest periods
Heat sounds	Rapid	Decreased	Increased
Activity	Active Eyes open Muscle tone increased Alert	Sleeping	Variable alertness
Mucus	Drooling Vomiting	Absent	Oral
Bowel	Sounds present	Absent	Sounds appear Meconium passed

* These observations by the nurse-midwife can be done in the nursery or at the mother's bedside so the mother can be involved in the evaluation of her infant.

before extensive examinations or procedures are performed. In the normal neonate procedures to be deferred include bathing, circumcision, or a fatiguing complete physical and neurologic examination. All infants need time to adjust to the physiologic and psychologic changes required during the early hours following birth. The time frame of the transitional period is altered if the infant was significantly distressed or if there was an excessive use of drugs.

The First Period of Reactivity

The first period of reactivity lasts from birth to 30 minutes. During this time the heart rate is rapid and cord pulsation is present. The newborn's color can be described as transient cyanosis or acrocyanosis. Respirations are rapid at the upper end of the range of normal, and rales and rhonchi are present. The rales should disappear by 20 minutes of age. There can be flaring of the alae nasi with grunting respirations and retractions. The presence of mucus usually is due to expulsion of retained lung fluid. This mucus is thin, clear, and may have small bubbles.

The newborn's temperature falls to the lower end of the range of normal. After it was demonstrated that a neonate's temperature could be affected by the environment of the delivery room, the need for the newborn to be in a neutral thermal environment was recognized.

During the first period of reactivity following birth the newborn's eyes are open and the baby manifests alert behavior. Since the mother is also alert at this time the initial contact between mother and infant should be facilitated. The practice of enabling the mother to hold the infant at this time aids in the acquaintance process. The infant focuses visually on the mother when she is in the appropriate field of vision (Fig. 21-5). There is increased muscle tone with the upper extremities flexed and the lower extremities extended, allowing the infant to mold itself into the mother's body while being held.

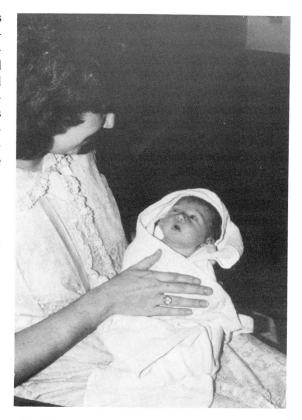

FIGURE 21-5. Mother-baby interaction.

The infant frequently has a stool immediately after birth, and bowel sounds are present at about 30 minutes of age. Bowel sounds indicate the digestive system is capable of functioning. The presence of stool alone, however, does not indicate that peristalsis is present.

The Second Period of Reactivity

The second reactivity period lasts approximately from 30 minutes to 2 hours of age. The newborn's cardiac rate is decreased to less than 140 beats per minute. A murmur can be heard; this is merely an indication that the ductus arteriosus has not closed and is not considered an abnormal finding. The skin is flushed during drying.

The infant's respiratory rate becomes more

regular with clear lung sounds. The temperature, which has been falling, reaches the lower end of the range of normal. The infant is in its first sleep and is relatively unresponsive. At this time the mother may be in a recovery room, and the infant continues the stabilization process in the recovery nursery. In ideal situations the mother and infant recover in the same room. The infant appears relaxed and sleeping. Bowel sounds usually are diminished.

In the past it was common practice to bathe the infant immediately after birth. The wiser and safer procedure is to allow the body temperature to stabilize. A reasonably healthy infant can be compromised by exposure to unnecessary cold stress.

The Third Period of Reactivity

During the third period of reactivity, from 2 to 6 hours of age, the heart rate is labile and there are swift changes in color, which are related to environmental stimuli. The respiratory rate is variable and related to activity. Mucus which may be present at this time may interfere with adequate feeding, particularly if the mucus is excessive. The presence of large amounts of mucus may be an indication of a problem. Bile-stained mucus is always a sign of illness in the newborn infant and feeding should be delayed until the cause has been investigated thoroughly.

Peristalsis is variable and the infant may pass meconium; however, some infants do not have stools during the first 12 hours. The absence of peristalsis in the infant that has bile-stained mucus is a sign of bowel obstruction or ileus and requires prompt attention.

REFERENCES

1. Nelson, N. The onset of respiration. In Avery, G. (Ed.), *Neonatology.* Philadelphia: Lippincott, 1975.
2. *Fetal Circulation.* Nursing Education Series #1. Columbus, Ohio: Ross Laboratories, 1957.
3. Committee on Fetus and Newborn. *Standards and Recommendations for Hospital Care of Newborn Infants, 6th.* Evanston, Ill.: American Academy of Pediatrics, 1977.
4. Clark, A. L., and Affonso, D. D. *Childbearing: A Nursing Perspective.* Philadelphia: Davis, 1976.
5. Pildes, R., Cornblath, M., Warren, I., et al. A prospective controlled study of neonatal hypoglycemia. *Pediatrics* 54:5, 1974.
6. Stern, L. Disturbances in glucose, calcium, and magnesium homeostasis. In Avery, G. B. (Ed.). *Neonatology: Pathophysiology and Management of the Newborn.* Philadelphia: Lippincott, 1975.
7. Thomas, J. B. *Introduction to Human Embryology.* Philadelphia: Lea & Febiger, 1968.

Bibliography is at the end of Chapter 23.

22

Evaluation and Management of the Neonate

IMMEDIATE ASSESSMENT AND RESUSCITATION

Apgar Scoring

The best single immediate assessment of the physical well-being of the neonate is the Apgar scoring system (Table 22-1). It provides an adequate evaluation and predicts the outcome of the neonate. This assessment is performed at 1 and 5 minutes following birth, preferably by someone other than the person responsible for the delivery.

Apgar scoring is based on five signs ranked in order of importance and a scoring of 0 through 10. With absence of cardiac activity, a heart rate below 100, or the absence of respiratory effort, *the Apgar scoring must be stopped immediately, resuscitation initiated, and help sought.*

The five signs and methods of evaluation for these are as follows:

1. Heart rate — check apical pulse, using a stethoscope and counting for 30 seconds.

2. Respiratory effort — when checking the heart rate, note the respiration; if it is shallow, listen with stethoscope to chest.
3. Muscle tone — this is checked by flexion and response of extremities: note flexion; straighten extremity and note response to return flexion.
4. Reflex irritability — this is done by tickling the nostril or flicking the sole of the foot and looking for facial or foot changes.
5. Color — check for the presence or absence of cyanosis; good places to check are the fingernails, palms of hands, soles of feet, tongue, lips, and mucous membranes (acrocyanosis, if not prolonged, is not uncommon).

The Apgar scoring system should be used as an anticipatory guide for the management of the neonate. The 1-minute Apgar indicates what degree of resuscitation is needed.

There is an air of excitement and concern at the time of delivery. It is imperative to have adequate operational equipment ready before

TABLE 22-1. Apgar Scoring Chart

Sign	0	1	2
Heart rate	*Absent	*Slow (below 100)	Over 100
Respiratory effort	*Absent	Weak cry Hypoventilation	Good strong cry
Muscle tone	Limp	Some flexion of extremities	Well flexed
Reflex response:			
1. Response to catheter in nostril (tested after oropharynx is clear)	No response	Grimace	Cough or sneeze
2. Response to foot slap	No response	Grimace	Cry and withdrawal of foot
Color	Blue, pale	Body pink, extremities blue	Completely pink

* Indicates immediate management required.

the delivery. The equipment is worthless if personnel are unable to use it. In case of an emergency, the nurse-midwife must be prepared to give emergency treament until the appropriate medical help arrives. The parents should be told what is happening if resuscitation is necessary — what is being done and why. This alleviates some of their anxieties, if the problem is minimal. If the problem is severe, they will know that all possible is being done.

The 5-minute Apgar has a direct relationship to neonatal morbidity and mortality. The risk of neonatal death is increased with a low Apgar. Death within the first 48 hours of life can be expected if the Apgar is 0 to 1 at 5 minutes of life. Low birth weight adds to this risk. With both low birth weight and a low Apgar score there is a noticed incidence of neurologic abnormalities when checked at 1 year of age [1, pp. 71–72].

The 5-minute Apgar should be used also in making a decision about whether the neonate may stay with the mother following delivery or should be sent to the nursery for additional care.

Rationale for Resuscitation

The three major goals of resuscitation are to encourage and maintain the neonate's airway, breathing, and circulation. These goals are best achieved in a thermoneutral environment. Prompt correction of hypoxia and poor circulation and the provision of warmth will minimize glucose usage and reduce the risk of hypoglycemia.

Careful intrapartum assessment of the fetal heart rate patterns can alert the nurse-midwife to the probable need for resuscitation. The fetus undergoing prolonged periods of asphyxia may make gasping attempts followed by apnea in utero. At birth weaker gasps may be followed by a last gasp and secondary period of apnea (Fig. 22-1). The heart rate falls dramatically and, without intervention, the infant dies. The infant born in secondary apnea cannot be revived with suctioning and tactile stimulation; ventilation and perhaps also cardiac massage are required.

The asphyxiated infant has low blood oxygen levels, elevated carbon dioxide, and lower blood pH (acidosis). This condition contributes

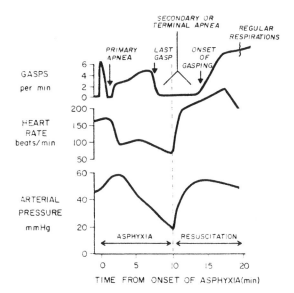

FIGURE 22-1. Changes in physiologic parameters during asphyxiation and resuscitation of the rhesus monkey fetus at birth. (Reproduced by permission from G. S. Dawes. *Foetal and neonatal physiology.* Chicago: YearBook, 1968, p. 149.)

to vasospasm of pulmonary arterioles and increased resistance to blood flow in the lungs after birth. The weak gasps of the asphyxiated newborn cannot overcome this resistance and establish adequate respirations. As the hypoxia continues, the heart rate slows and the myocardium contracts ineffectively. Blood pressure drops and systemic circulation slows, leading to organ damage.

Degrees of Resuscitation

Resuscitative requirements vary with the infant's condition at 1 minute of age.

1. The baby with an Apgar score of 7 to 10 has a blood pH of 7.20 to 7.40. This baby has minimal depression, and a normal transition period can be expected.

   a. suction the oropharynx and then the nose to clear the airway and provide tactile stimulation (see Table 22-2).

   b. dry the infant and provide warmth: apply warmed blankets to the baby on the mother's abdomen, or use radiant warmer.

   c. continue to observe transition closely.

2. The baby with an Apgar score of 4 to 6 has a blood pH of 7.09 to 7.19 (moderate acidosis). This baby has moderate depression probably reflecting a period of primary apnea.

   a. dry the infant.

   b. place infant under radiant heat source.

   c. suction the oropharynx and then the nose to clear the airway and provide tactile stimulation; give free-flow oxygen by face mask.

   d. if the infant is still apneic or has a heart rate below 100, begin positive pressure ventilation by face mask attached to an anesthesia bag or self-inflating bag with an oxygen reservoir; both give nearly 100% oxygen (see Table 22-3).

   e. continue free-flow oxygen after infant has established good respiratory effort.

3. The infant with an Apgar score of 0 to 3 has a blood pH of 7.00 or below (severe acidosis). This baby has severe depression reflecting secondary apnea.

   a. suction the infant to clear the airway.

   b. dry the infant.

   c. place infant in work area under radiant heat source.

   d. begin positive pressure ventilation.

   e. if adequate ventilation does not ensue with bag and mask, perform endotracheal intubation (see Table 22-4).

   f. if heart rate is less than 60 after 30 seconds of adequate ventilation, begin cardiac massage (see Table 22-5 and Fig. 22-2); continue massage until infant can sustain heart rate over 80 with ventilation alone.

TABLE 22-2.   Suctioning

Equipment:	1.	Bulb syringe or DeLee mucus trap #8 or #10.
Method:	1.	Suction oropharynx, then nose, since stimulation of nasal mucosa may cause reflex inhalation of pharyngeal mucus.
	2.	DeLee trap may be used for gastric and tracheal suctioning.
Precautions:	1.	Prolonged suctioning may traumatize mucosa, and cause laryngospasm and vagal stimulation that leads to profound bradycardia.
	2.	An old, soft bulb won't provide adequate suction.

TABLE 22-3.   Positive Pressure Ventilation

Equipment:	1.	Anesthesia bag with pressure gauge (manometer) *or* self-inflating bag with oxygen reservoir attachment.
	2.	Infant- and premature-size face masks.
	3.	Stethoscope.
	4.	Feeding tube.
	5.	Source of humidified oxygen with flow meter.
Method:	1.	Suction nares and oropharynx to clear secretions.
	2.	Place infant's head in a neutral position (when hyperextended, air enters esophagus).
	3.	Place mask over nose and mouth, making sure seal is tight.
	4.	Pressure for first breath should be 40−50 cm. H_2O.
	5.	Subsequent breaths need about 25 cm. H_2O or whatever the lowest pressure is that will allow you to see the chest wall expanding.
	6.	Ventilate 40−50 times per minute for 2−3 minutes.
	7.	Have assistant auscultate anterior upper lobes of the lungs for aeration.
	8.	Continue to provide free-flow O_2 by face mask after infant has established respirations.
Precautions:	1.	Inadequate ventilation may be caused by poor seal around mask, flexed or hyperextended neck, or inadequate pressure of ventilation.
	2.	Face mask pressure near the infant's eyes can cause tissue damage.
	3.	Positive pressure ventilation will cause air retention in the stomach. After bagging for a brief period of time, vent the stomach by passing a feeding tube. Any gastric contents should also be emptied. If bagging is going to continue over time (e.g., while awaiting a transport team), stop momentarily to slip a tube into the stomach to vent the stomach and prevent or reduce distention. Secure tube in place while continuing to ventilate.

Resuscitation Equipment

Resuscitation equipment should be available in the delivery room and nursery area in close proximity to oxygen and suction outlets. The equipment and medications should include those that will provide for adequate ventilation or resuscitation, thermoregulation, hypoglyce-mia, fluids and electrolytes, plasma expanders or blood volume replacement, and cardiac stimulation.

A list of essential equipment includes the following:

1.   Well-lighted area of sufficient height for easy infant intubation

TABLE 22-4. Endotracheal Intubation

Equipment:	1.	DeLee suction catheters.
	2.	Endotracheal tubes, various sizes with adapters.
	3.	Laryngoscope with blades.
	4.	Positive pressure bag.
	5.	Towel.
	6.	Tape.
Method:	1.	Place infant with head in slightly extended position; may place towel under infant's shoulders.
	2.	Introduce laryngoscope at the right corner of the mouth.
	3.	Advance 2 to 3 cm. while rotating it to midline and moving tongue to left.
	4.	When tip of blade is between the base of the tongue and the epiglottis a slight elevation will expose the glottis (sometimes a gentle compression of the external larynx by an assistant will more easily expose the glottis).
	5.	Insert the endotracheal tube at the right side of the mouth and through the vocal cords, being sure the insertion is easily visualized (the tube must be small enough to allow an air leak, i.e., room around it; this space insures easy expiration and reduces the risk of tissue damage).
	6.	Suction secretions if needed.
	7.	When the endotracheal tube is inserted, hold it firmly but gently in place and withdraw the laryngoscope slowly.
	8.	Attach the endotracheal tube to the adapter on the bag.
	9.	Ventilate with oxygen by bag; assistant should check for adequate ventilation of both lungs with stethoscope.
Precautions:	1.	If you have difficulty with the procedure, remove laryngoscope and ventilate with mask; try again in 2 minutes.
	2.	If tube is passed too far into the airway, it enters into the mainstem bronchus and breathing sounds on the left decrease. If this occurs, withdraw slowly until breath sounds on the left increase.
	3.	If tube is left in place, suction as necessary when excess secretions are detected (possibly every 30−60 minutes) with a sterile suction catheter.

2. Radiant heat source for prevention of cold stress
3. Battery-powered heart rate monitor
4. Stethoscope
5. Laryngoscope with infant blades — size 0 and 1
6. Magill forceps
7. Endotracheal tubes — several sizes
8. DeLee suction catheter
9. Suction catheter
10. Positive pressure bag or equivalent with several sizes of infant masks
11. Adapters
12. Umbilical catheter tray
13. Medications:
    a. sodium bicarbonate
    b. epinephrine
    c. 50% dextrose
    d. glucagon
    e. heparin
    f. nalorphine hydrochloride (Nalline)
    g. naloxone hydrochloride (Narcan)
14. Syringes and needles
15. Microcrit
16. Dextrostix
17. Skin preparation solutions:
    a. povidone-iodine (Betadine)
    b. saline
    c. alcohol
    d. benzoin

TABLE 22-5. Cardiac Massage

Method:	1.	Place infant on a firm surface.
	2.	Use either the two-finger technique or the thumb technique, illustrated in Figure 22-2. Place fingers on the middle third of the sternum. Do not raise fingers off chest between compressions or you will lose your place.
	3.	Depress sternum to a depth of ½–¾ inch at a rate of 100–120 per minute.
	4.	Coordinate heart compression with ventilation. Count aloud: "One and two and three and ventilate." Repeat.
	5.	Assess effectiveness by having third person check femoral or carotid pulse
	6.	Discontinue when infant can maintain heart rate above 80 by ventilation alone.
Precautions:	1.	Make sure to coordinate respirations with compressions. If both are done simultaneously, the infant may suffer a pneumothorax.
	2.	In order for resuscitation to be effective, adequate ventilation must be maintained throughout cardiac massage.

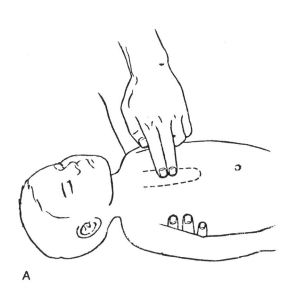
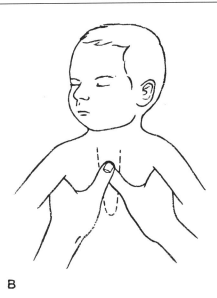

A

B

FIGURE 22-2. A. two-finger technique for cardiac massage; B. thumb technique for cardiac massage. (Reproduced by permission from R. S. Bloom, C. Cropley, and G. Peckham. Principles of neonatal resuscitation. In R. Polin and F. Burg [Eds.]. *Workbook in Practical Neonatology*. Philadelphia: Saunders, 1983, p.16.)

18. Tape
19. Oxygen and tubing
20. Extra batteries and bulbs

One of the best means of keeping equipment conveniently located is to design a resuscitation board for the wall of delivery rooms and nurseries. The board is mounted close to suction and oxygen outlets. Equipment and medications are placed in plastic bags and hung from hooks in appropriate labeled spaces.

EVALUATION OF THE NEONATE

The following evaluation of the full-term neonate is a compilation of the most useful aspects of several newborn appraisals [2–6]. A form for charting findings is given in Figure 22-3.

Physical Examination

Infants must be examined nude in a warm, comfortable environment. Any deviations from the normal findings here require medical consultation or referral.

General Appearance
The neonate changes rapidly, differing from hour to hour, day to day, and week to week. The following should be found in the normal baby (Fig. 22-4):

1. Body symmetrical and cylindrical in contour
2. Head large in proportion to rest of body
3. Small hips
4. Narrow chest
5. Protruding abdomen

Measurements
Variations in measurements may occur but relationships are consistent. The following shows average measurements:

1. Head circumference — 13½ inches (34.3 centimeters)
2. Chest measurement — 12½ inches (31.7 centimeters)
3. Crown-rump length — 13½ inches (34.3 centimeters)
4. Crown-heel length — 20.0 inches (50.8 centimeters)

Weight
As a general rule, males weigh more than females, whites are heavier than nonwhites, and second babies are heavier than first babies. Other normal observations include the following:

1. Loss of 5 to 10 percent of birth weight in the first 3 days.
2. Recovery of birth weight by 7 to 10 days.
3. Gain of 4 to 8 ounces per week.
4. Doubling of birth weight by 6 months.
5. Size depends on heredity, maturity, amount of subcutaneous fat, and maternal nutrition.

Activity
General body movements are symmetric and include sneezing, yawning, sucking, rooting, swallowing, grasping, responding to sound, blinking, and crying.

Crying
Listen to the infant's cry. Variations indicate the following:

1. Persistent, weak cry — the infant is sick and must be referred to the physician.
2. Persistent, high-pitched cry — possible intracranial injuries; medical consultation is required.
3. Persistent, inconsolable cry — refer to the physician.
4. Cry stops when baby is picked up — normal.

Color
Melanin pigmentation is present in varying degrees at birth. The color of the epidermis darkens with exposure to light in infants of dark-pigmented parents. If the infant is pink with bluish nailbeds, palms, and soles and the extremity color improves with activity, the infant is normal. However, if this coloring becomes worse with activity, watch for cyanosis around the mouth and fingernail beds. It may be due to intracranial hemorrhage, cardiac problems, or central nervous system involvement. If the infant becomes jaundiced at any time throughout hospitalization, a bilirubin test is required and the cause must be investigated.

Skin
The skin has a velvet softness and elastic texture

Examination of the Neonate

Name   Birthdate   EGA

Parents   EDD

Prenatal problems:
    Medications:

Labor and delivery:
    Medications:

General appearance:

Measurements:
    Head   Weight
    Chest   Apgar 1 min.
    Length   5 min.

Activity and cry:

Color and Skin:

Head: Genitals and anus:
    Symmetry
    Fontanels, sutures   Back:
    Eyes
    Nose   Reflexes:
    Ears   Moro
    Mouth   Tonic neck
                                                Palmar grasp
Neck: Walking/stepping
                                                Eyes
Extremities: Blink
                                                  Corneal
Chest: Mouth
    Heart   Rooting
    Lungs   Sucking
    Breasts   Plantar
                                                Babinski
Abdomen:

Formula or breastfeeding and eating patterns:

Awake-sleep patterns:

Urine and stools:

Added comments:

FIGURE 22-3. Form for use in the examination of the neonate. The sample form shown here is useful in charting the findings during the physical and neurological examinations of the neonate.

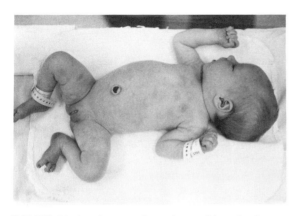

FIGURE 22-4.   A normal newborn. Note body proportions.

as a result of subcutaneous fat; however, dryness and peeling are normal. Observe the infant for the following conditions:

1. Edema — backs of hands and feet, legs below knees, pubic area, face around eyes, lateral aspects of thighs. Will last one week or more; the cause is unknown and the edema will disappear spontaneously.
2. Milia papules on nose, chin, and cheeks. Pinhead sized, they appear about the second day and disappear spontaneously early in the second week. These are sebaceous cysts and no treatment is necessary. See Figure 22-5.
3. Flea-bite dermatitis — closely resembles flea bites. There is a blanched, wheellike appearance, and tiny vesicles may develop at the site of the papules. Minute amounts of clear fluid may be exuded which may lead to the erroneous diagnosis of impetigo. The rash appears on the diaper area, abdomen, thorax, and back. No treatment is necessary and the rash will disappear.
4. Vascular nevi
   a. stork bites — dilatation of capillary vessels and minute arteries; found at the nape of the neck and extending over the lower occipital area, between the eyebrows, on upper eyelids, and around

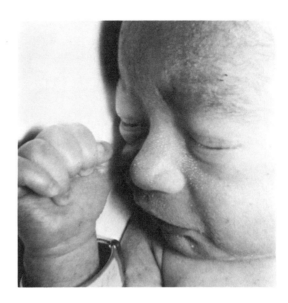

FIGURE 22-5.   Milia on nose and chin of a newborn.

   the nose. They fade and are usually indistinguishable by the second year.
   b. Strawberry mark — bright red spot, may be present at birth or appear within the first 6 weeks. May increase in size for a few months but not after 12 months of age. Most will spontaneously regress and disappear by 10 years of age. No treatment is necessary. It may appear anywhere on the baby's body.
   c. Port wine mark — smooth, flat, superficial angioma, varies in size from a few millimeters to an area that covers most of the face and neck. Those less intensely colored often disappear spontaneously in infancy or early childhood. Treatment is usually very difficult and undertaken only on the more extensive lesions.
5. Pigmented nevi — moles, from light brown to black; present at birth or appear during the first 5 years of life. No treatment is necessary.
6. Mongolian spots — bluish or slate-colored pigmentation over sacrogluteal area; can

extend over entire dorsal area of body; common in Black infants, those of Mongolian ancestry, Indians, and Eskimos; rare in Caucasians. This coloring fades in time and is not associated with Down's syndrome.

7. Marbling — irregular mosaic areas outlined by pinkish or faintly purplish capillary network; appear when body surface is exposed to cold and disappear when body is warmed.

8. Harlequin color — seen only in neonates, but rarely. A deep red color develops in the dependent half of the body when the baby is lying on one side; lasts from 1 to 20 minutes; has no pathological significance.

9. Trauma — firm areas of induration in subcutaneous tissue. The skin may be reddened or purplish. Discoloration disappears spontaneously within 6 to 8 weeks. Mainly caused by forceps injuries and found on cheeks, neck, back, and thorax.

10. Deep blue face with pink body. Noticed following tight nuchal cord. Disappears spontaneously in 24 to 48 hours.

Head

Examine the head for the following:

1. Temporary asymmetry as a result of molding. Overlapping of cranial bones should be noted. Should not overlap after first few hours following delivery since the head readjusts to normal position rapidly.

2. Fontanels:
   a. anterior — diamond-shaped; closes at 12 to 18 months. May be overlapping after delivery.
   b. posterior — triangle-shaped; closes in 6 to 8 weeks; may feel closed after delivery because of overlapping sagittal suture.
   c. sagittal suture — may be overlapping after delivery due to molding.

d. bulging fontanels indicate intracranial pressure.
e. depressed fontanels indicate dehydration.
f. if the anterior fontanel is closed and the sagittal suture appears stenosed, there is possible craniostenosis.

3. Caput succedaneum — swelling on the scalp resulting from pressure of the cervix; disappears in 24 to 48 hours; crosses suture lines, and the position depends upon intrauterine position during labor and delivery.

4. Cephalhematoma — subperiosteal bleeding, does *not* cross suture lines; has hard edges around the soft center; does not disappear for several weeks; is caused by pressure during delivery. Check carefully for enlargement. See Figure 22-6.

Eyes

Eyes should not be forced open for the examination. The following observations should be made:

1. Puffy — aggravated by silver nitrate; common after forceps delivery.

2. Pupils react to light. Unequal size may be due to brachial plexus paralysis; ptosis may also be present.

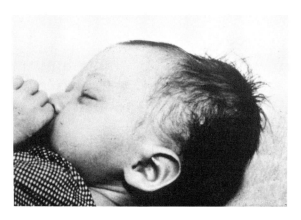

FIGURE 22-6.   Cephalhematoma in a newborn.

3. Movement of eyes not coordinated, and transient strabismus and nystagmus observed. These conditions should be investigated if still present at 6 months.
4. Opaqueness — suggests cataract formation or possibly a tumor.
5. Almond-shaped eyes — if present concomitantly with other signs, Down's syndrome should be suspected.
6. Subjunctival hemorrhage — small patch or patches of red within the sclera. Usually absorbs in 2 to 3 weeks.
7. Red reflex — the eye is examined directly with flashlight or ophthalmoscope, which causes the pupil to glow with a reddish light as the red of the retina is reflected through the lens. The color should be orange-red and uniform; dark spots indicate increased intracranial pressure and opaque spots indicate cataracts.
8. Ptosis of the eyes or lids — may indicate nerve damage.
9. Purulent discharge from eyes — should be cultured.

Nose
Nasal breathing is natural and instinctive in the newborn period. Undue restlessness, crying, and choking indicate nasal obstruction; the infant should be observed when feeding for signs of respiratory distress.

Ears.
Check the ears for the following:

1. Presence of canal should be verified.
2. Infant reacts to loud noises.
3. Size and shape are hereditary factors.
4. In Down's syndrome, the ear lobes are deformed, with the upper margin of the pinna rolled down and thickened.
5. Ears low and subnormally shaped — congenital malformation of the kidneys or Potter's syndrome. See Figure 22-7.
6. In the presence of autosomal chromosome

abnormalities (trisomy 15 and 18), ears are low set.

Mouth
The following should be noted when examining the mouth:

1. Cleft lip or palate.
2. Epstein's pearls — normal finding. Disappear in about 4 weeks spontaneously; found on the palate at the junction of the hard and soft palate. These are inclusion cysts and they rupture spontaneously.
3. Facial nerve paralysis — characterized by asymmetry of the mouth when open, especially when crying (Fig. 22-8).
4. Since any teeth present usually are loose, they should be removed because of the possibility of aspiration.
5. Large amounts of saliva or pooling of saliva — first symptom of tracheoesophageal fistula. *Note:* First feeding of any newborn must be observed very closely for signs of tracheoesophageal (TE) fistula.

Neck
Check the neck for the following:

1. Head is freely movable.
2. Neck webbed on shoulders may indicate Down's syndrome or Turner's syndrome.
3. Tightness of muscles on one side or lump on the side may indicate a torticollis.
4. Fat pad on back of neck may be normal, a lipoma, or associated with Down's syndrome.
5. Brachial palsy or fractured clavicle — reflexes absent on side of fracture, arm remains extended when lying on back; immobilization of affected side for 1 week usually is adequate.

Extremities.
Check arms, hands, legs, and feet as follows:

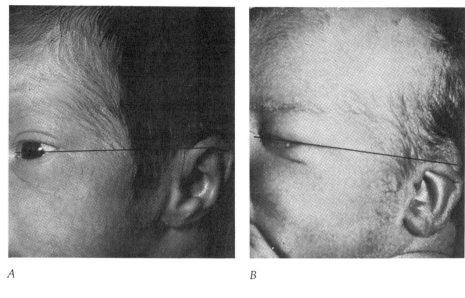

A   B

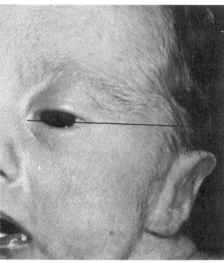

C

FIGURE 22-7.   Judging ear position. A. normal position; B. twisted or pseudo low-set ears; C. true low-set ears. (Reproduced by permission from Variations and *Minor Departures in Infants*. Evansville, Ind.: Mead Johnson, 1978.)

1. Arms
    a. should be of equal length when extended.
    b. infant should move both arms equally well and resist having arms extended.
2. Hands
    a. a single deep, sharp, transverse palmar crease (simian line) along with a flat

and stubby thumb and a short little finger which is concave on the medial side — found in mongolism (Down's syndrome). A single palmar crease alone does not always denote Down's syndrome. See Figure 22-9.

b. fingers — may show webbing, poly-

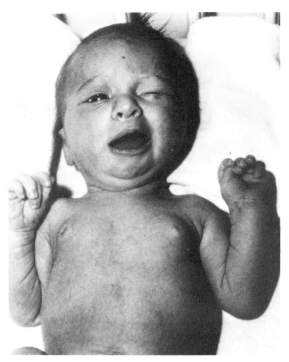

FIGURE 22-8. Facial nerve paralysis in a newborn.

dactylism (extra digits — more frequent in Blacks) and syndactylism (too few digits — more common in toes than fingers).

c. nails — fingernails well developed in most instances, extending beyond finger tips.

3. Legs
   a. should be of equal length when extended.
   b. with knees flexed, legs should abduct to table in froglike position. Dislocated hip is suspected if abduction is asymmetrical, and inguinal folds and thigh creases are not symmetrically placed, and hip click is present.
   c. if legs are persistently limp, it is indicative of spinal cord lesion.

4. Feet
   a. freely movable; if not, may be positional or indicative of clubbed feet.
   b. toes — may show webbing, polydactylism, or syndactylism. The first and second toes are widely separated in Down's syndrome.

Chest

The following observations should be made of the chest:

1. Respiration (evaluation of respiratory status; see Silverman-Anderson index, Table 22-6).

   The scoring used in the Silverman-Anderson Index is just the opposite of that used in Apgar scoring. The index of respiratory distress is determined by grading the criteria so that a total of 0 indicates no respiratory distress, and a total of 10 indicates severe distress. The score is reached by adding the score given in each of the five categories that best describes the infant at the time of observation.

2. Breasts
   a. engorgement — commonly seen in both sexes, due to maternal hormones; usually occurs at 3 days of age (Fig. 22-10). By the end of the first week, the nipples may secrete a milklike substance resembling colostrum or milk. No attempt should be made to express this fluid since doing so may cause mastitis.
   b. supernumerary nipples — relatively common, but glandular tissue usually does not accompany the extra nipples.

3. Heart
   a. rates — normal heart rates are 120 to 160 beats per minute; the first 30 minutes of life, the heart beat is rapid; from 30 minutes to 2 hours, the rate decreases; and after 2 hours it is more rapid again. They should all be within normal range.
   b. murmurs — heard for short period of time; if longer than 48 hours, investigate.
   c. rhythm — arrhythmias noted after 72 hours may be indicative of abnormality. Areas to be auscultated are sternoclavicular junction, second right intercostal space, pulmonic area, anterior pericardial area, apical area, epigastric area, and ectopic areas [2].

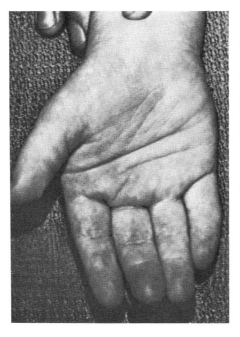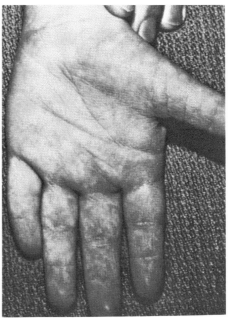

FIGURE 22-9. Hands in mongolism (Down's syndrome). (Reproduced by permission from *Variations and Minor Departures in Infants.* Evansville, Indiana: Mead Johnson, 1978.)

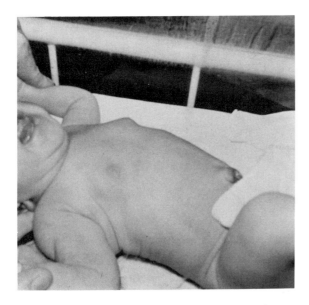

FIGURE 22-10. Breast engorgement in a newborn.

Abdomen

The following should be observed about the abdomen:

1. Should look round and protruding.
2. Cord — dry and odorless; separates in 7 to 10 days; should have one vein and two arteries. Any questionable deviation requires laboratory examination. If any odor is present, or if any reddened areas around the umbilicus are noted, a culture should be done.
3. Hernias
   a. umbilical — defect in muscle, usually closes over by 2 to 3 years.
   b. inguinal — 90 percent are found in males, usually must be repaired surgically.
   c. diaphragmatic — may be fatal.
4. The liver is palpable up to 2 centimeters below the costal margin.

TABLE 22-6.   Silverman-Anderson Index: Observation of Respirations

Grade (score)	Upper chest	Lower chest	Xyphoid retractions	Nares dilatation	Expiratory grunt
0 (0 points)	Synchronized	No retractions	None	None	None
I (1 point each)	Lag on inspiration	Just visible	Just visible	Minimal	Stethoscope only
II (2 points each)	Seesaw	Marked	Marked	Marked	Naked ear

Modified from W. A. Silverman and D. H. Anderson. A controlled clinical trial of effects of water mist on obstructive respiratory signs, death rate and necropsy findings among premature infants. *Pediatrics* 17:1, 1956.

5. The spleen is sometimes palpable, as is the bladder.
6. Infants are born with diastasis recti abdominis.

Genitalia
Female and male genitalia should be examined for the following:

1. Female
   a. large, edematous labia (Fig. 22-11).
   b. grayish-white mucus discharge from vagina, lasting about 2 weeks.
   c. blood-streaked discharge is normal; frank bleeding is not.
   d. hymenal tag apparent; shrinks and disappears by end of neonatal period.
2. Male
   a. edema of scrotum frequently present at birth; disappears within 1 to 2 weeks (Fig. 22-12).
   b. foreskin of penis is slightly retractable.
   c. testicles may or may not be present in scrotum.
   d. urethral meatus should be at end of glans; deviations indicate hypospadias or epispadias.
   e. hyperpigmented external genitalia and nipples present with what appears to be undescended testicles and marked hypospadias, may actually be a hypertrophied clitoris in a female with adrenogenital syndrome.

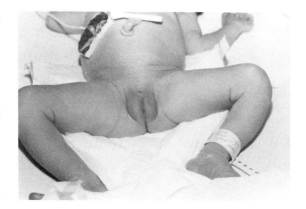

FIGURE 22-11.   Edematous labia in a newborn.

Back
Observe the back for the following:

1. Spinal defects must be noted. A dimple in the coccygeal-sacrococcygeal area may denote a pilonidal cyst, sinus opening, or spina bifida.
2. Neonate should be able to turn head to either side when in a prone position.

Anus
Presence of a perforate anus must be verified. A soft red rubber catheter is gently inserted in the rectum if no stools have been passed. *Do not* use your finger.

Character of stools
The character of the stools changes during the

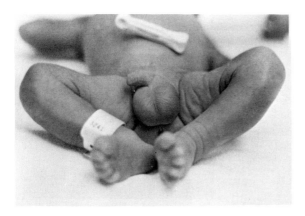

FIGURE 22-12. Edematous scrotum in a newborn.

first few days and then differs according to type of feeding. These changes and differences are:

1. First stool — meconium — dark greenish-brown, almost black, sticky semisolid substance; usually continues for 1 to 3 days.
2. Transitional stools — 3 to 5 days, contain last trace of meconium and early feedings; yellowish-brown.
3. After fifth day, character and color of stool depend on infant feedings.
   a. breast feeding — stools bright golden yellow, small soft mushy curd, fairly homogenous with little form but not watery; nonoffensive odor; baby has stool two to five times a day during first few weeks.
   b. bottle feeding — stools pale yellow, hard, homogenous with pasty formed cheesy curds, somewhat offensive odor; baby has stool one to four times a day during first few weeks.
4. Constipation stools are small, dry, very hard, and difficult to pass. The infant may not have a stool for 2 to 3 days.
5. Diarrhea stools are liquid, green, and foul smelling. A "water ring" will be left on the diaper after a stool. The infant may have five, six, or more stools a day.

Urine
First voidings may be dilute. Unusual colors or odors may be clues to inborn errors of metabolism, and a medical consultation is needed. All infants should void within 24 hours.

Collecting Culture Specimens

Sometimes cultures are required because of your observations. They should be done immediately and sent to the laboratory.

Purpose: To obtain uncontaminated specimens for culture in order to identify an organism causing an existing infection.

Indications: Suspicion of infection from any area suspected of harboring an undesirable organism.

Equipment:
1. Culture tubes with media: for culturing umbilical artery catheter or endotracheal tubes and tips
2. Culturettes: for swab of nose, umbilicus, skin, wound drainage, throat, eyes, ears, and so forth
3. Culture tube or sterile container (dry): for stool
4. Tongue blade or popsicle stick (for stool culture)
5. Bacteriology information slip that includes the following:
   a. date, time, and source of specimen
   b. patient's diagnosis and any antibiotics currently being given
   c. type of study requested (e.g., routine culture and sensitivity)

Procedure:
1. Nasal, umbilical, and skin cultures: remove applicator from culturette tube, using plastic top to hold applicator end; gently swab area to be cultured with applicator; for eye culture, swab the corner of the eye; for suspected amnionitis, swab the inner ear. Replace inside culturette tube and break

fluid vial as directed on package. Attach lab slip and send to laboratory.

2. Stool cultures: scrape stool specimen into sterile container or dry culture tube using tongue blade or popsicle stick; attach lab slip and send to laboratory.

3. Infant cultures are taken as indicated of any area suspected of being infected.

4. Initial results are obtainable within 24 hours after the sample is sent to the laboratory.

Neurologic Examination

Head circumference should be included in the neurologic examination, particularly if the infant is preterm. Evidence of increasing head size or separation of the sutures should be noted. The fontanel is considered to be under pressure if it is bulging while the infant is in an upright position and not crying. Suture lines are generally separated in the preterm infant but usually adjacent in term infants.

The assessment of the infant for the purpose of determining neurologic and behavioral competency is an important part of the total assessment of the infant. The focus is on those positive things within the makeup of the infant that contribute to future adjustment to extra-uterine life. The neurologic evaluation is equally as important as the respiratory and circulatory assessments. Frequently the infant transmits neurological messages to the effect that one of the other systems may be in crisis. It is important that the professional providing care for the neonate be aware of the subtle and more obvious signals that a problem is developing. Continuous and frequent observations of the infant's behavior are essential to an accurate assessment. It is in this way that change can be demonstrated and documented. The total neurologic assessment proceeds in an orderly fashion.

Level of Alertness

An infant born earlier than 28 weeks gestation is in a state of persistent stupor, but after 28 weeks the infant can be awakened with minimal stimuli, remains in an alert state for several minutes, and demonstrates spontaneous movement. At 32 weeks gestation, stimulation is no longer necessary. Frequently the infant lies with eyes open and keeps them open while making spontaneous roving eye movements. Spontaneous head turning can be observed and the infant's movements are more pronounced. At 37 weeks gestation the level of alertness increases as well as the frequency of the periods of alertness. At this time the infant demonstrates vigorous crying during periods of wakefulness. Movements at this time are smoother and more coordinated in the lower extremities than before.

When born at term, the infant responds to distinct visual and auditory stimuli. The infant focuses on an object within the visual field and demonstrates both vertical and horizontal visual following. Infants respond readily to the human face as well as to brightly-colored or shiny objects. The alerting response in the infant tends to diminish with repeated trials due to the ability to shut out stimuli.

Examination of behavior should be performed when the infant is in his or her most alert state and can respond to the limit of capabilities. The infant's state of alertness depends on physiologic variables such as hunger, nutrition, degree of hydration, and the time within the wake-sleep cycle of the infant. Brazelton [7, p. 571] categorizes these states as follows:

Sleep states:

1. *Deep sleep* is characterized by regular breathing, closed eyes, and no spontaneous activity except startles or jerky movements at quite regular intervals. External stimuli produce startles with some delay.

2. *Light sleep* is characterized by closed eyes

with observable rapid eye movements under closed lids. There is low activity level, with random movements and startles. Movements are likely to be smoother and more monitored than in the deep-sleep state. The infant responds to internal and external stimuli with startle equivalents, often accompanied by a change of state. The infant's respirations are irregular with sucking movements observed periodically.

Awake States

3. *Drowsy or semi-dozing state* is characterized by open or closed eyes, the eyelids fluttering. The activity level is variable with mild startles from time to time. The infant reacts to sensory stimuli, but the response is often delayed. There will often be a change in state after stimulation. The infant's movements usually are smooth.

4. *Alert state* is demonstrated by a bright look. The infant seems to focus attention on the source of stimulation, such as an auditory or visual stimulus. The infant's motor activity is at a minimum.

5. *Eyes open* is accompanied by considerable motor activity. The infant will have thrusting movements of the extremities. The infant reacts to external stimulation with an increase in startles or motor activity.

6. *Crying* is characterized by intense crying which is difficult to break through with stimulation.

The optimal states for observing behavior are the awake states, when the infant's eyes are open. Crying does not interfere with the observations. The time immediately after a feeding should not be used because the infant is too sleepy. Immediately before a feeding the infant is too distracted to demonstrate optimal functioning.

Cranial Nerves

The evaluation of cranial nerve function includes vision, pupillary response, extraocular movement, hearing, sucking, and swallowing.

At 28 weeks gestation, the infant consistently blinks to light. By 32 weeks, eye closure to bright light persists as long as the light is present. At 37 weeks, the infant demonstrates visual following consistently and turns toward a soft light.

Although the infant's pupils react to light as early as 29 weeks gestation, consistency is not accomplished until approximately 32 weeks. The premature infant's eyes are often disconjugate with one or the other eye deviating 1 or 2 millimeters. At 32 weeks gestation, the infant is capable of spontaneous roving eye movement, but tracking movements occur later in gestation. At first, eye movements are rather jerky and gliding until the infant is approximately 3 months of age. Extraocular responses can be elicited by spinning the baby in a vertical position. The eye deviates in a direction opposite to the spin. The infant may not keep his or her eyes open during the early hours of life due to edema, but the eye movements can be observed behind the closed lids.

Spontaneous facial motility is of great importance in the identification of cerebral lesions or nerve injuries. The contours of the infant's mouth should be observed during crying for bilateral symmetry of the facial muscles. The observer should notice the position of the face at the onset of movement as well as at its final amplitude.

By 28 weeks gestation, infants have been observed to startle in response to auditory stimulation. The older infant manifests hearing ability by cessation of motor activity, change in respiratory pattern, and opening of the mouth and eyes. Some babies do not respond initially but will respond after resting or under more favorable conditions. The well-organized infant responds to auditory stimuli by turning the head toward the sound and making searching excursions with the eyes.

Sucking requires the function of the fifth, seventh, and twelfth cranial nerves and swallowing requires the ninth and tenth. By 32 to 34 weeks gestation, the normal infant is able to maintain a concerted action for productive oral feeding. However, since the preterm infant may not perform consistently in this way, consideration should be given to the length of time of the feeding and the amount taken in relation to caloric requirements.

Reflexes

Moro Reflex. The most commonly used evaluation of the neurological status of the newborn is the Moro reflex, or embracing reflex. In normal infants the response is symmetrical and disappears by 2 to 4 months. The Moro reflex consists predominantly of abduction and extension of the arms with hands open and the thumb and index finger semiflexed to form a C. Leg movements may occur, but they are not as uniform as the arm movements. With return of the arms toward the body the infant either relaxes or cries.

Care must be taken to elicit a Moro reflex and avoid "startles". Acceptable ways to elicit a Moro reflex include the following:

1. The examining table is struck near the head of the baby.
2. A semisitting infant is allowed to fall backward (onto the examiner's open hand) from an angle of 30°.
3. The table is jarred suddenly.
4. A loud noise or handclap is utilized.

If the following deviations are found with the Moro reflex test, medical consultation is required.

1. Absence of the reflex indicates possible intracranial lesions.
2. Asymmetrical response may indicate birth injury involving the brachial plexus, clavicle, or humerus.
3. Abnormal persistence of embrace gesture indicates hypertonicity.
4. Persistence of entire Moro reflex after 4 months indicates delay in neurological maturation.

Tonic Neck Reflex. A positional reflex is not always noted. The infant is placed on his or her back and the head is turned to the side. The arm and leg on the same side extend and the opposite arm and leg flex; thus the infant assumes the fencing position. The head is turned to the opposite side and the same reaction should occur. The response may be present or absent in the newborn and, if present, lasts about 2 or 3 months. If it persists longer than this time and is constant, it usually is pathological and often indicates neurological dysfunction.

Palmar Grasp Reflex. With the baby supine and the head in midline, the fingers of the examiner are placed in both the infant's hands and the surface of the palms pressed. There should be flexion of all the infant's fingers around the examiner's. Asymmetric intensity or symmetrical weakness in the grasp is significant. If there is no response, the midline position of the head should be checked. Infants who hold so tightly that they can be picked up and held by their grasp alone may present a hyperkinetic reaction. This reflex diminishes, weakens, and disappears after 3 months. Complete absence of the reflex may be found in brain damage.

Walking/Stepping Reflex. The baby is held so that the sole of the foot touches a flat surface. This should stimulate a stepping or dancing movement with both legs (Fig. 22-13). This reflex is present at birth and gradually disappears after 3 or 4 weeks.

Reflexes of the Eyes. Reaction to light is elicited easily by shading one eye with the examiner's hand for a moment or two, followed by withdrawal. Asymmetry in the pupil or poor response to light suggests neurologic dysfunction.

1. Blink reflex. A bright light is shone suddenly at the infant's eyes. Normally a quick closure of the eyes and a slight dorsal flexion of the head are elicited. With im-

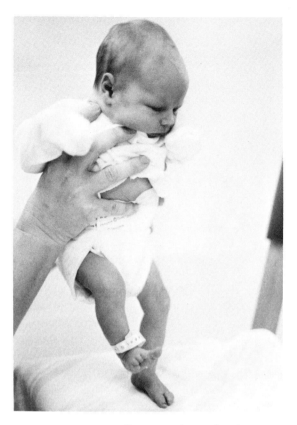

FIGURE 22-13. Walking/stepping reflex in a newborn.

paired light perception this response is absent.

2. Corneal reflex. When the eyes are open, the cornea is touched lightly with a piece of cotton, with care to avoid touching eyelids or lashes. Normally the eyes close. The absence of this response denotes lesions of the fifth cranial nerve.

Reflexes of the Mouth

1. Rooting response. The corner of the infant's mouth, the upper lip, and the lower lip are touched in turn with the finger. Upon stimulation the head turns toward the stimulated side, the mouth opens, the tongue moves to the point of stimulation, and the infant tries to suck on the stimulating object. A baby whose hunger has been satisfied will turn away from the stimulation. There is also a positive correlation between the levels of alertness and the rooting response.

2. Sucking response. When the examiner's index finger is placed in the infant's mouth, rhythmical sucking movements will be felt. The following should be noted:
   a. stripping action of the tongue forcing the finger upward and back
   b. rate
   c. suction
   d. grouping of sucks

Sucking is often less intense and less regular during the first 3 to 4 days. Poor sucking may be noted in apathetic or hyperactive babies and is the first indication of other problems such as sepsis.

Plantar Reflex. The examiner's thumbs are pressed against the balls of the infant's feet. There should be a flexion of all toes (Fig. 22-14). The absence of this response is correlated with defects of the lower spinal cord. Asymmetries should be noted. This reflex disappears in 2 to 3 year.

Babinski Reflex. The lateral aspect of the sole of the infant's foot is scratched, going from heel to toes. This must be more than pressure; if not, a plantar reflex instead of a Babinski reflex will be elicited. The Babinski reflex shows a dorsal flexion of the big toe with spreading of the smaller toes (Fig. 22-15). It is present in the newborn and disappears between the ninth and eighteenth months. A poor response may be due to nervous system immaturity; absence of the response may be from defects of the lower spinal cord.

NUTRITION AND FEEDING

The nutritional needs of the newborn are simple

but very important. These needs include water and nutrients consisting of carbohydrates, proteins, fats, vitamins, and minerals. Ready-to-use commercially prepared formula leaves no room for error relative to the appropriate proportion of nutrients and fluid requirements of the newborn. When instructions are carefully followed, the fluid content in powdered formula preparations will be appropriate. Formulas prepared at home, such as condensed canned milk mixed with corn syrup and water, do require knowledge of newborn requirements since there are no instructions provided. Generally the normal 6- to 7-pound newborn requires approximately 120 calories per kilogram per day. This is provided for in 20 calories per ounce of formula or 380 milliliters of fluid. Condensed evaporated whole milk may be deficient in sugar for some infants. The resulting constipation may be prevented or cured with the addition of sugar, preferably corn syrup. Dried powdered milk usually is fat free and thus will not provide newborns with the fat they need for metabolism. Although it is easier to use, the commercially-prepared formula may be more expensive. The money-conscious mother may prefer to prepare her own formula. She will need guidance as to when to increase calories and what volume of fluid will be appropriate as the infant matures. There is no absolute resolution to the problem of mothers who are unable to prepare formula appropriately, who have insufficient means to purchase ready-to-use formula, and who, for one reason or another, are not breast-feeding. These problems have to be dealt with on an individual basis.

Many mothers are provided instructions on the use of vitamin supplements upon discharge from the hospital. It is necessary to know which vitamins, and the amounts of each, are contained in the formula preparation being used. It is possible for the infant to receive dangerously high dosages of vitamins A and D. Should the mother choose to change formulas, the addition of or deletion of vitamins may be

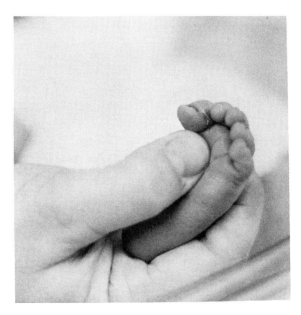

FIGURE 22-14.   Plantar reflex in a newborn.

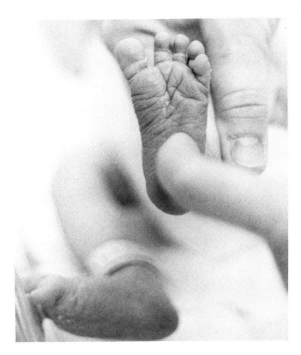

FIGURE 22-15.   Babinski reflex in a newborn.

necessary. All mothers should be cautioned to read the labels of formula and vitamin preparations. The ingestion of iron may create problems in some newborns and result in constipation or diarrhea. Under such circumstances the need for iron before 6 months of age should be evaluated carefully.

Mothers often ask if warming bottles prior to feeding is necessary. Some infants tolerate well and even appear to enjoy a refrigerator-cold bottle. Others will prefer a warm bottle or experience increased problems with gas when given a cold bottle.

There is no need to sterilize bottles for full-term infants. Thorough cleaning with detergents, hot water, and brushes should be emphasized. Leftover formula may be refrigerated and used for the next feeding provided that it has not been out of the refrigerator for too long. Excess milk can be used in family food preparation.

Nursery policies may regulate the time and content of the first infant feeding. It may be appropriate to give the infant water before offering the first formula feeding, to rule out tracheoesophageal fistula. Water is given because if it is aspirated it will be absorbed. A sterile spoon or dropper may be substituted for a nipple when a breast-feeding infant is given this water.

The demand feeding schedule seems totally appropriate to meet the individual newborn's needs. The demand for less than 2 or more than 5-hour intervals between feedings should be explored. Small infants may need more frequent feedings, whereas the larger infants may take more per feeding and not feed as often. The lethargic infant who does not want to feed within the 5-hour period should be watched. This infant may have neurologic or other physical problems.

Newborns should be held in a position comfortable for both the infant and mother. Some mothers prefer a semisitting position with the baby resting in the curve of the arm, very much as if breast-feeding. Stroking the

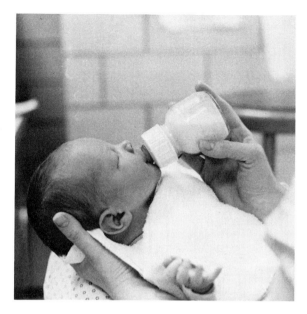

FIGURE 22-16. Proper position of bottle with milk filling nipple and neck of bottle.

baby's lip with the nipple allows the baby to root for the nipple and grasp it. The baby will be much more relaxed than if the nipple is forced into the mouth. The bottle is held so that the milk is in the nipple and neck of the bottle (Fig. 22-16). This keeps the infant from swallowing any more air than necessary.

An infant who has cried for a period of time before the feeding may have swallowed enough air to need burping prior to feeding or after taking a swallow or two of formula. Many infants will suck on their fingers or anything else that comes in contact with their lips or mouth, swallowing air and requiring burping accordingly. As the baby increases in age, a toleration for more formula before burping is acquired. Burping or bubbling can be done several ways and the mother should use the method most comfortable to her and the baby. She can place the baby over her shoulder, set the baby upright in her lap while supporting the chest and jaws with one hand, or lay the baby over her legs while patting or rubbing the back to bring up the bubble of air (Fig. 22-17).

The mother should be told that it is normal for a small amount of formula to be regurgitated. This is common in the first few days after birth due to irritation of the gastric mucosa by foreign material ingested at birth. Later it is due to overflow that relieves a distended stomach after feeding. It can also indicate the infant has taken too much formula or taken it too rapidly. This knowledge will help alleviate some of the anxiety the mother may have if the baby spits up a small amount of formula. She may also want to keep an extra diaper or cloth handy. The spitting up or regurgitation of milk after feedings should not be confused with vomiting. Vomiting is a forceful emission of a large quantity of milk. This may occur at any time and usually is followed by other symptoms. Anatomic defects should be considered and medical consultation is needed in cases of persistent vomiting.

Hiccups also are common and are more annoying to the mother than to the infant. They are due to spasmodic contractions of the diaphragm caused by irritation from regurgitation of gastric contents. Usually a few swallows of water to wash down the irritating material help. These contractions stop soon. Some babies are more prone to hiccups than others.

Many babies sleep intermittently after feeding. Some babies apparently require less sleep and the postfeeding period becomes one of activity. This can prove to be a good get-acquainted period for both the mother and her infant.

Fluid imbalance in the infant quickly leads to electrolyte imbalance. Therefore, anorexia, excessive vomiting, and diarrhea lead to dehydration and electrolyte imbalance.

References to specialized feeding techniques in the newborn and premature infants such as gavage, nasojejunal feedings, and hyperalimentation are included in the bibliography.

It is important in infant feeding that food not be withheld too long. The quantity of feeding should not be increased too rapidly. Infants with respiratory rates above 60 per minute and those with hypothermia should not be nipple-fed. Infants receiving assisted

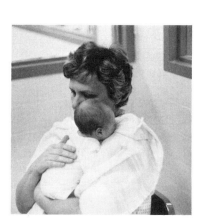
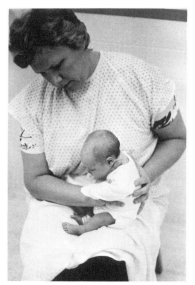
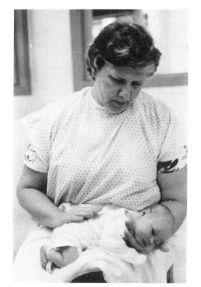

FIGURE 22-17. Different methods of burping a baby.

ventilation with mask and bag or those who are apneic should not be bottle-fed. Infants who have been delivered of mothers with hydramnios or infants with excessive mucus should not be fed until a tube has been passed into the stomach to assure patency. Extrauterine adaptation should be normal before the first feeding. The gastric capacity of the small infant is limited, so small babies need small amounts of formula at frequent intervals. When spitting or regurgitation occurs, there is an increased risk of aspiration. If spitting up is noted, the volume of formula per feeding and time intervals between feedings should be reduced. The mother must be encouraged during feedings and given support and help in understanding the infant with feeding problems.

When there are no problems with feedings, this usually indicates that mother and infant are doing well. Successful feedings provide the basis for a warm and trusting relationship that develops between the mother and her infant. If a mother and infant are having a problem, the possibility of pathology should be investigated.

Difficulties in feeding can result from a firm nipple with small holes or a mother who is unfamiliar with feeding infants. A very hungry infant cries more and may create anxiety in the mother. An approach the nurse-midwife can use to help this mother with anxiety is to model a feeding for her, sit beside her and talk with her while feeding, showing her how to relax and feed, reinforce her role as a mother, and help her to be aware of clues from her infant that he or she is comfortable. This kind of assistance may be needed once or during several feedings.

REFERENCES

1. Korones, S. B. *High-Risk Newborn Infants, The Basis for Intensive Nursing Care, 3rd.* St. Louis: Mosby, 1981.
2. Alexander, M. M., and Brown, M. S. *Pediatric Physical Diagnosis for Nurses.* New York: McGraw-Hill, 1974, p. 137–138.
3. Arnold, H. W. et al. Transition to extrauterine life. *Am. J. Nurs.* 65:77, 1975.
4. Desmond, M. M. et al. The clinical behavior of the newly born. *J. Pediatr.* 62:307, 1963.
5. Desmond, M. M. et al. The transitional care nursery: A mechanism for preventive medicine in the newborn. *Pediatr. Clin. North Am.* 13:651, 1966.
6. Moore, M. L. *The Newborn and the Nurse.* Philadelphia: Saunders, 1972, p. 117.
7. Brazelton, T. B. Behavioral assessment of the neonate. In Clark, A. L., and Affonso, D. D. *Childbearing: A Nursing Perspective.* Philadelphia: Davis, 1976.

Bibliography is at the end of Chapter 23.

23

Perinatal Problems

RISK ASSESSMENT DURING PREGNANCY

It is commonly believed that, by identification of the high-risk pregnant patient, the incidence of poor neonatal outcome can be reduced significantly. A high-risk pregnancy is considered to be one in which some factor in the maternal environment or past medical history represents a risk to fetal well-being. Strides have been made to reduce the perinatal complications of mothers with diabetes and Rh isoimmunization, but there are a number of other less apparent factors that contribute to poor fetal outcome.

Several methods have been introduced to apply scoring systems to the various problems that can occur during the prepregnancy, antenatal, intrapartum, and neonatal period that place the infant at risk for a healthy survival. Many women considered high-risk during pregnancy or prepregnancy bear healthy infants. Others considered low-risk during pregnancy become high-risk during the intrapartum period. Goodwin and colleagues' descriptions of low risk and high risk are as follows:

The pregnancy of a 23-year-old Para 2, 5'6" tall woman weighing 120 pounds. She and her husband live near a hospital. There were no complications in the previous pregnancy which terminated more than two years prior to the present pregnancy. She has had several antenatal examinations. Her hemoglobin is presently 12 gm. There has been no bleeding during the present pregnancy, nor is there history of renal disease, bacteriuria or hypertension. The glucose tolerance shows a normal curve.

A high-risk pregnancy is described as that of a 39-year-old woman, Para 8, who is 5'0" tall. Her blood pressure is 160/110 and her weight is 170 pounds. Her last hemoglobin was 9 gm. She and her family live in an isolated community. She has had a history of having had two premature infants and one stillbirth. She lost a baby at 11 months of age. There was some bleeding earlier in the present pregnancy. She has chronic pyelonephritis with decreased renal function, and has an abnormal glucose-tolerance curve. [1, p. 458]

The scoring technique is intended to be a rough, practical assessment in any given pregnancy of the potential for increased risk to the unborn fetus. The following conclusions can be drawn from this method: if a woman manifests none of the adverse conditions or risk factors embodied in the description, the probability of perinatal death is remote; perinatal deaths are usually associated with a number of adverse conditions which combine to produce an unfavorable environment. Congenital anomalies seem to account for a considerable number of fetal deaths associated with poor prenatal scores.

It is felt that risk assessment must be tied to action and much of the action involves regionalization. A major contribution to such a program is the development of a centralized community (or regional) hospital-based newborn intensive care unit. Concentration of the high-risk infant care programs in hospitals specially staffed and equipped to provide optimal care is a proven life saving mechanism for infants at risk [2]. Researchers have demonstrated that critically ill newborns treated with the best available techniques survive with significantly less damage than was the case in previous decades [3].

Factors in High-Risk Pregnancy

Maternal Risk Factors
Maternal risk factors that contribute to the prediction of high-risk infants are grouped in the following categories:

1. Any *previous pregnancy* that resulted in fetal morbidity or mortality, such as spontaneous abortion, premature or postmature birth, stillbirth or neonatal death, anomalies or mental retardation, including cerebral palsy and learning disabilities, epilepsy, fetal or neonatal exchange transfusion
2. *Maternal medical complications,* such as cardiovascular disease, renal disease, chronic hypertension, metabolic disorders including diabetes (or family history of diabetes) and thyroid disease, pulmonary disease, and sickle cell disease
3. *Maternal infections* which can cross the placental barrier or be contracted via direct exposure as the infant traverses the birth canal, such as toxoplasmosis, histoplasmosis, rubella, influenza, genital herpes,

malaria, encephalitis, tuberculosis, hepatitis, gonorrhea, cytomegalic inclusion disease, coxsackievirus B, chlamydia, and syphilis.
4. *Drugs,* including alcohol and smoking
5. *Maternal age* over 35 or under 15
6. *Pregnancy-induced hypertension*
7. *Severe anemia* (hemoglobin 9 grams per 100 milliliters, hematocrit 30 percent)
8. *Grand multiparity*
9. *Deviations in reproductive anatomy and physiology,* such as abnormal pelvic shape or size, abnormal uterine configuration, stenosed or incompetent cervix, precipitous or prolonged labor, premature rupture of the membranes, previous caesarean section.
10. *Placenta and umbilical cord problems,* such as placenta previa, abruptio placentae, bleeding from a marginal sinus, unusually long or short cord

Fetal Risk Factors
Fetal risk factors include fetal problems such as a fetus that is too large or too small, malposition or malpresentation, shoulder dystocia, multiple pregnancy, fetal bradycardia or tachycardia, and any anomalies.

Environmental Factors
Environmental factors include those factors in the delivery room environment that will assist the infant during the transition to extrauterine life. Since there are a limited number of potential neonatal problems that are diagnosed prior to delivery, every maternity service must have proper equipment and experienced personnel available to care for the neonate until vital signs are established.

Once a mother has been diagnosed as being at risk for potential neonatal complications, proper referrals should be made to have care provided whenever possible at an institution where appropriate physical facilities, services, and personnel are continuously available to manage complications. Several maternal conditions will be discussed in reference to problems in the neonate. Since detailed discussions are beyond the scope of this chapter, only the cardinal signs will be addressed to emphasize the need for the nurse-midwife to be able to make appropriate judgments in regard to proper referrals.

Infants who can be identified prenatally as needing to be delivered in a perinatal center or transferred immediately after birth are infants of mothers who are insulin-dependent diabetics, Rh sensitized, infected, moderate to severe toxemics, placental bleeders in the third trimester of pregnancy or candidates for babies with recognizable malnutrition syndromes or postterm or preterm delivery (less than 36 weeks gestation).

INFANTS BORN TO HIGH-RISK MOTHERS

Infants of Mothers with Multiple Pregnancy

Multiple pregnancy is associated with increased risk for both the mother and her fetuses. Premature labor resulting from spontaneous rupture of membranes, abruptio placentae, and intrapartum hemorrhage occurs more often in multiple pregnancy than with a single pregnancy. Frequently one or more of the infants has been compromised during fetal life and may be at risk for intrauterine growth retardation, twin-to-twin transfusion, and other complications related to intrauterine growth retardation.

Infants of Rh-Sensitized Mothers

It is important that women who are Rh sensitized be delivered in centers that are equipped to supply specialized care for the mother and infant at the time of delivery. These infants need prompt oxygenation and provision of adequate red cell volume to allow for oxygen transport to the tissues. Endotracheal intubation and ventilation may be necessary to provide adequate lung expansion.

The infant should be evaluated continuously for other problems that may occur, such as congestive heart failure, acidosis, hypoglycemia, and a rapidly rising serum bilirubin. The infant may be in critical condition.

Infants of Mothers with Polyhydramnios

Polyhydramnios is the accumulation of amniotic fluid in excess of 2 liters. It occurs with increased frequency in diabetic pregnancies. There is a significant association of polyhydramnios with fetal anomalies, especially those of the upper gastrointestinal tract and central nervous system. Other complications include maternal respiratory embarrassment, premature rupture of the fetal membranes, prolapse of the cord, premature labor, and infants that are small for gestational age.

Infants of Mothers with Moderate to Severe Pregnancy-Induced Hypertension

Neonatal problems that should be anticipated in the infant born of the mother with pregnancy-induced hypertension are prematurity and intrauterine growth retardation resulting from decreased uterine blood flow. There is also an increased incidence of abruptio placentae associated with the hypertensive state of the mother. Hypotonia arising from hypermagnesemia secondary to therapy may present a major problem in the immediate neonatal period.

Preexisting decreased uterine blood flow can be intensified during labor and result in fetal asphyxia in the intrapartum period. Preparations should be made for immediate resuscitation of the infant. Other causes of asphyxia are prematurity and convulsions or oversedation of the mother. Intensive care is imperative for the infant so it can be observed closely for signs of respiratory distress, hypoglycemia, or central nervous system complications.

Infants of Mothers with Placental Bleeding in the Third Trimester

Because of the high neonatal mortality associated with placental bleeding, labor and delivery should be carried out in a center where the problems of both the mother and infant can be anticipated and promptly managed. Premature delivery often follows significant placental site hemorrhage. As a result there is disruption of the fetoplacental blood supply, and hypovolemia followed by shock and asphyxia can result. This requires immediate resuscitation and provision for restoration of blood volume. Sustained respiratory support is necessary, as is provision for monitoring blood gases and recognition of central nervous system damage.

Infants of Diabetic Mothers

The excessive weight gain in the fetus of the diabetic mother is the result of increased body fat and glycogen deposition in the viscera (see Fig. 23-1). The large infant may be traumatized during delivery, resulting in intracranial bleeding or asphyxia, or both.

Hypoglycemia may result when the glucose value falls precipitously to levels that are lower than in normal infants. Hypoglycemia usually occurs during the first 6 hours of postnatal life; however, later onset may also be seen, especially in infants who are unable to tolerate oral feedings. When the placental glucose supply is suddenly interrupted by cutting the umbilical cord, hyperinsulinism results and hypoglycemia occurs. Feedings should be started early and, if the infant is unable to tolerate them, intravenous feeding should be chosen.

The diabetic mother's infant who is large

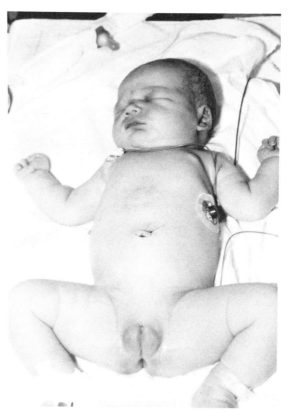

FIGURE 23-1. Large-for-gestational-age infant of a diabetic mother.

for gestational age may also be preterm and at greater risk for respiratory distress syndrome. Respiratory distress syndrome has been found with greater frequency in infants of diabetic mothers than in other infants of comparable gestational age, suggesting that prematurity may not be the single underlying factor of respiratory distress syndrome [4, p. 304].

Infants of diabetic mothers are also at higher risk for many congenital anomalies and hyperbilirubinemia. Frequently they are polycythemic with hematocrits of 65 percent or greater. If the infant exhibits clinical symptoms of polycythemia a partial exchange transfusion may be necessary.

INFANTS AT RISK BECAUSE OF SIZE AND AGE

Estimation of gestational age

An accurate determination of gestational age is essential in determining an infant's risk status. Until recently birth weight was the sole criterion used to assign a low- or high-risk label. Adequate methods have now been found to ascertain gestational age after birth. A properly done gestational age examination allows the nurse-midwife to classify the newborn according to age, size, and size in relation to age. Since infants in different categories often have different potential problems it is crucial that the nurse-midwife understand the technique of gestational age assessment.

The Ballard scale for assessment of gestational age [5] is an abbreviated version of the original examination formulated by Dr. Lilly Dubowitz and colleagues. This scale incorporates estimates of neurologic and physical maturity in a format designed to minimize handling of the infant. The gestational age examination must be done precisely according to directions. Practice is essential. Chapter 61 contains the explanation and procedure for doing this gestational age assessment.

Once gestational age has been assessed the infant's weight, length, and head circumference are plotted on charts denoting the 90th, 50th, and 10th percentiles by gestational age for each of these measurements (see Chapter 61). A determination can then be made that the infant is appropriate, small, or large for gestational age (AGA, SGA, LGA).

The final classification of risk status merges both these assessments. The infant will be referred to as preterm, term, or postterm *and* AGA, SGA, or LGA (see Chapter 61).

Preterm infants

Infants born prior to 38 weeks of gestation have an increased risk of mortality and morbidity. The less mature the infant the higher the risk. Transfer in utero is safer and less expensive and involves less separation from the mother than transfer after delivery. Transfer prior to birth also ensures intensive care from the moment of delivery and a lower mortality rate.

Preterm infants are predisposed to respiratory problems like hyaline membrane disease and recurrent apnea. Often a patent ductus arteriosus persists. Their decreased subcutaneous fat renders them susceptible to hypothermia. Metabolic problems like hypoglycemia, hypomagnesemia, and hyperbilirubinemia are common. Preterm babies are susceptible to infections and conditions resulting from hypoxia, such as necrotizing enterocolitis and intracranial hemorrhage. The infant who is in an intensive care nursery will have the benefit of early diagnosis and treatment.

Postterm Infants

Postterm infants are at risk for asphyxia, meconium aspiration, central nervous system damage, early development of hypoglycemia, and pulmonary hemorrhage. If placental dysfunction produces severe asphyxia, death can occur in utero.

Large-for-Gestational-Age Infants (LGA)

The LGA infant will fall above the ninetieth percentile in measurements of the head, height, and weight [6, p. 403]. Infants born to parents who are large tend to be large. Infants who are LGA have a greater incidence of transposition of the aorta. The mean weight of these infants has been found to be 3450 grams as compared to 3140 grams for infants with all other congenital heart disease. The chief and immediate problem in the infant who is LGA is birth trauma such as fractured bones, cephalhematoma, cervical or brachial plexus palsy, and subdural hematoma. These babies may be prone to hypoglycemia.

Small-for-Gestational-Age Infants (SGA)

The infant is considered small for gestational age when its weight, height, and occipitofrontal head circumference fall beneath the tenth percentile. An adverse intrauterine environment can result in slowed fetal growth. The causes include congenital anomalies, nutritional deficiency in the mother, and maternal infection. The most serious causes are those related to fetoplacental insufficiency as found in diabetics with vascular impairment and mothers with hypertension. Women with pregnancy-induced hypertension frequently have such severe involvement that the fetus is deprived of essential nutrients and fails to grow. Smoking has accounted for a number of infants with birth weights lower than the mean by 100 to 200 grams.

The infant that is small for gestational age appears thin and wasted. There is little subcutaneous tissue. While weight is low, length quite often is not affected and head size may be normal. The infant usually is alert and very hungry. The SGA infant performs in a more mature manner than the preterm infant of comparable size.

SGA infants are prone to neonatal asphyxia, particularly those infants that are markedly undernourished. Frequently the infant has been severely deprived in utero and asphyxia occurs before delivery. The stress of labor uses up most of the available stores of glycogen, leaving the infant depleted and therefore subject to hypoxia in utero and at the time of delivery. Meconium aspiration occurs by the infant's breathing in utero, as a result of the asphyxiated state.

Polycythemia has been described by several authors. Although it is of unknown origin, chronic intrauterine hypoxemia has been suggested. Not all infants are symptomatic. Those who may need treatment have tachypnea, grunting, and tachycardia.

Because of differing body composition and basal metabolic rate, the usual tables for neutral thermal environments, which are based on weight, do not apply for SGA infants. The isolette settings should be determined by closely monitoring the infant's temperature and the ambient temperature of the environment. The infant's skin temperature should be maintained between 36°C and 36.5°C (96.8° and 97.8°F) [7].

Hypoglycemia, with blood glucose concentrations of less than 20 milligrams per 100 milliliters, is seen frequently during the first 12 hours of life. Blood sugar should be monitored carefully and an early feeding regimen commenced. Intravenous infusion of 10% glucose may be necessary. The SGA infant requires more calories than a preterm infant. Frequently it will be necessary to give this infant as much as 150 to 180 calories per kilogram of body weight per day.

Congenital anomalies occur more frequently in SGA infants than in any other category. The more severe the growth retardation the greater the chance of an anomaly. The SGA baby with a normal-sized placenta should be regarded as at particular risk for having a congenital anomaly. To facilitate early detection, close attention must be paid to all aspects of the physical examination [8, p. 84].

INFECTIONS OF THE NEONATE

As discussed in Chapter 21, the immune system of the newborn is immature at the time of birth. All infants are at risk for infection but particular risk is carried by preterm infants, infants with low Apgar scores who require invasive resuscitation, and infants born with congenital anomalies. Infants may acquire an infection prior to birth, during labor (by organism ascent through the vagina), during the passage through the birth canal, and after birth (from care givers and nursery factors [9, p. 271]).

Infections such as congenital rubella, cytomegalic inclusion disease, toxoplasmosis, congenital varicella, coxsackievirus, syphilis, and hepatitis are usually transmitted to the fetus through the placenta. Symptoms vary with the disease but babies with congenital viral infections are frequently small for gestational age and may exhibit early-onset jaundice, anemia, and hepatosplenomegaly. In the cord blood there may be elevated levels of the immunoglobulin IgM. An abnormally high cord IgM level suggests intrauterine infection but its absence does not rule out infection.

When the maternal tissues have been infected or colonized with organisms, the infant may become infected with the organism at the time of delivery. Maternal tissues may be infected with organisms that are nonpathogenic to the mother, such as staphylococci and group B beta-hemolytic streptococci, but pathologic to the fetus. Other organisms such as *Chlamydia*, *Candida*, and *Neisseria gonorrhoeae* cause maternal and neonatal damage.

The amount of risk incurred when the amniotic membranes have been ruptured for longer than 24 hours is unclear. It is known that bacteria rarely penetrate intact membranes. However, in situations where there is prolonged rupture of membranes there are often other simultaneous factors that increase the likelihood of infection such as long labor, multiple vaginal examinations, and use of internal monitors. A maternal amnionitis with uterine tenderness, discharge, and fever predisposes the neonate to infection.

The infant with sepsis can present widely varying symptoms. Symptoms involving the respiratory, gastrointestinal, and central nervous systems may be present. The neonate may have trouble maintaining body temperature. Vomiting may be accompanied by abdominal distention. Central nervous system symptoms include lethargy, irritability, jitteriness and tremors. Seizure activity is manifested by apnea, abnormal eye movements, or sucking movements with increased salivation. Respiratory symptoms include cyanosis, irregular respirations, and tachypnea. Any infant with a single episode of cyanosis requiring oxygen is suspected of having an infection.

The infant with possible sepsis should have a complete physical examination and cultures of the urine, blood, and spinal fluid. Surface cultures of the skin are useless because they reflect surface colonization and contamination only. A complete blood count and chest x-ray are useful.

The astute nurse-midwife will notice the subtle indications of sepsis and refer the infant to physician management.

RESPIRATORY PROBLEMS

Evaluation and Immediate Treatment

The infant's respiratory status is initially evaluated at birth. Respiratory effort and color are part of the Apgar scoring system used in evaluating the immediate resuscitation needs of the newborn, as was discussed in Chapter 22. Subsequent evaluation of the infant's respiratory status is best done through observation of the resting or sleeping infant. The infant's color and respiratory quality can be observed more accurately in the quiet infant.

There are five cardinal signs and symptoms of a respiratory problem:

1. Tachypnea (respiratory rate persistently above 60 per minute) — the most common sign of a respiratory problem in the newborn
2. Retractions of the sternum and intercostal spaces
3. Expiratory grunting
4. Cyanosis in room air
5. Apnea

The Silverman-Anderson Index scoring method, discussed in Chapter 22, evaluates retractions and expiratory grunting.

Retraction of the accessory muscles of respiration indicates that the infant is having a problem in stabilizing the thorax to improve lung inflation. When the primary muscles of respiration are stressed, the infant facilitates breathing and ventilation by calling on the accessory muscles of respiration, such as the intercostals and the sternocleidomastoids. In severe retractions, the sternum is forced inward during inspiration. The infant may be compromised from hyaline membrane disease (respiratory distress syndrome), obstruction of the upper airway, or choanal atresia.

The sound the infant makes when exhaling against a closed glottis is called expiratory grunting. It is the infant's attempt to prolong alveolar expansion and maintain oxygenation. Grunting occurs at the onset of expiration. The infant with hyaline membrane disease customarily adopts a grunting type of breathing.

The infant may have rapid respirations and not be cyanotic or may be cyanotic and not have rapid respirations. Peripheral cyanosis generally includes only the extremities and circumoral areas. Central cyanosis involves the entire body and mucous membranes.

Cyanosis may be of pulmonary, cardiac, central nervous system, or metabolic origin. Cyanosis that is pulmonary in origin involves problems with ventilation of the respiratory system (e.g., hyaline membrane disease) and will improve when the infant cries or when oxygen is administered. Cyanosis that is cardiac in origin involves problems within the circulatory system and will worsen when the infant cries; administration of 100% oxygen will not induce changes in the blood pO_2 or the infant's color. This is indicative of a significant right-to-left shunt from congenital heart disease. Cyanosis that is of central nervous system origin or due to certain metabolic problems (e.g., hypoglycemia) may be manifested by a combination of cyanosis and apnea.

Apnea is a frequent problem in the newborn infant, particularly the preterm infant. Apneic spells in small babies are related to the irregular respiratory pattern known as periodic breathing. This occurs in 25 to 50 percent of premature babies, and irregularities of respiration occur at one time or another in nearly all small babies. Periodic breathing is more frequent in the more immature baby and becomes less frequent after 36 weeks of gestational age [10].

Periods of not breathing that last more than 20 seconds and those accompanied by bradycardia and cyanosis are defined as apneic spells. Bradycardia and cyanosis, followed by hypotonia and unresponsiveness, usually occur after 45 seconds. The heart rate and respiratory rate should be monitored in all preterm infants. Monitors are customarily set to sound when the heart rate drops below 100 and the respiratory rate below 20. At these levels, stimulation can be provided before the rates drop to more critical levels.

Monitoring, however, does not replace observation. Careful documentation of the episode and those events immediately preceding the episode should be done. Respiratory causes of apnea are those related to feeding, such as aspiration. Vagal response at the time the nasogastric tube is inserted can result in apnea in the premature. Apnea resulting from metabolic derangements are due to hypoglycemia, hypocalcemia, acidosis, and marked hyperbilirubinemia. A full-term infant who has a single episode of apnea should have a thorough physical and diagnostic workup immediately because of the association with group B beta-hemolytic streptococcal sepsis.

Apneic spells in the neonatal period have been considered as possible forerunners of brain injury. Deuel [11] observed marked suppression of the EEG pattern during apneic spells, which suggests cerebral hemispheric and perhaps diencephalic dysfunction.

There are myriad causes of respiratory problems. A decision regarding the cause of observed respiratory distress must be made as soon as possible in order to avoid ensuing asphyxia and collapse of the infant. The nurse-midwife, therefore, must consult with a physician when respiratory distress is first observed. Depending on the cause, this may occur any time during the first week of life.

Pulmonary causes of respiratory problems include:

1. Transient tachypnea of the newborn (TTN)
2. Respiratory distress syndrome (RDS), otherwise known as hyaline membrane disease (HMD)
3. Meconium aspiration
4. Pneumothorax
5. Pneumonia
6. Pulmonary hemorrhage
7. Upper airway obstruction (e.g., choanal atresia)
8. Space-occupying lesion (e.g., diaphragmatic hernia)

The first four of these are more common than the others and are discussed in this chapter.

Other causes of respiratory problems include:

1. Cardiac — congenital heart disease
2. Metabolic — metabolic acidosis, hypoglycemia, hypothermia, hypocalcemia
3. Central nervous system — hemorrhage, edema, drugs
4. Circulatory — acute blood loss, hyperviscosity, marked hyperbilirubinemia
5. Infectious — sepsis caused by group B beta-hemolytic streptococci and other bacteria

While awaiting physician management the nurse-midwife should begin immediate treatment of the signs and symptoms of respiratory distress. Resuscitation was discussed in Chapter 22. The cardinal components of a clear airway, adequate oxygenation, maintenance of bodily warmth, and continuing evaluation of the infant are essential at any time.

Oxygen should be administered and blood gases obtained. A normal pO_2 (50 to 70 millimeters of mercury) should be maintained.

While waiting for blood gas determinations, follow the rule of thumb for adequate oxygenation that the baby be pink (except when the problem is cardiac in origin) regardless of the percentage of oxygen it takes to do this. The infant who is having respiratory problems is at risk for hypothermia and requires a neutral thermal environment.

The nurse-midwife should also start obtaining a data base which will facilitate a diagnosis of the problem as quickly as possible. In addition to ordering blood gases, the nurse-midwife should also determine blood glucose and calcium levels, start serial hematocrits or hemoglobins, carefully review the maternal prenatal and intrapartal history, check the infant's vital signs, and continue evaluation of the infant's respiratory status.

Physician management includes diagnosis and treatment of the cause of the respiratory distress. During this time conservation of energy can be promoted by offering feedings by gavage or even stopping feedings and maintaining the infant with intravenous feedings until the infant's condition is stabilized. An accurate assessment of the respiratory status should be performed at frequent intervals.

Transient Tachypnea of the Newborn

Sometimes transient tachypnea occurs in mature infants with no specific problems. It is felt that the pathogenesis is delayed absorption of fetal lung fluid trapped in the interstitial space. Usually the outcome is good. The infant usually has an elevated respiratory rate. This may be as rapid as 120 per minute without other signs of respiratory distress such as grunting or retractions. Occasionally the infant will be cyanotic in room air but responds readily when given small amounts of oxygen. The infant improves rapidly. It is wise not to feed these infants but to maintain them with intravenous fluids until the respiratory rate is below 60 and the infant no longer needs oxygen for support. The first feedings should be by gavage to conserve the infant's energy.

Respiratory Distress Syndrome (Hyaline Membrane Disease)

Premature infants are highly susceptible to the development of respiratory distress syndrome (RDS). It is extremely rare for an infant past 38 weeks gestation to have hyaline membrane disease (HMD). Mothers at risk for having infants that develop respiratory distress syndrome are those with diabetes, pregnancy-induced hypertension, and histories of other premature births or respiratory distress. The use of amniocentesis to predict lung maturity is widely used to determine the lecithin-sphingomyelin ratio. As the infant matures, the amount of lecithin increases in relation to the sphingomyelin. A mature lung is associated with a lecithin-sphingomyelin ratio of 2:1 or greater. Severe RDS can be expected when the ratio is between 1:1 and 2:1.

The symptoms begin at or shortly after birth. Respiratory distress after 4 hours of life is not due to hyaline membrane disease. The infant is tachypneic with a respiratory rate above 60. Intercostal and sternal retractions may be mild to severe. The infant has flaring of the alae nasi and grunting expirations. On auscultation of the chest, air exchange is noted to be poor and breath sounds are diminished or inaudible. Optimal ventilation should be maintained by proper positioning, mechanical ventilation, thinning of the secretions, and prompt removal of secretions from the infant's respiratory tract.

Meconium Aspiration

Fetal aspiration of meconium-contaminated amniotic fluid is thought to be due to hypoxia in utero, which is accompanied by increased respiratory activity. Usually this relates to an interruption in maternal-fetal oxygen transport either from placental insufficiency or a sudden traumatic event in utero such as cord prolapse or placental separation.

The presence of foreign material in the trachea or lungs of the newborn results in severe asphyxia. The lungs fail to expand at delivery due to meconium blockage of large and small airways. This results in impaired air exchange, hypoxia, and acidosis. A chemical pneumonia can result. The pulmonary blood vessels become rigid and persistent fetal circulation results.

As soon as the head is delivered the mother should be instructed not to push while thorough suctioning of the mouth, throat, and nares is performed with a DeLee suction catheter. After the delivery of the body the vocal cords should be visualized by laryngoscope. If the cords are stained, the infant should be intubated, lavaged with normal saline, and then suctioned to remove the meconium from the respiratory passages. Normal saline serves as a wetting agent in liquifying the thick meconium.

Positive pressure ventilation should be avoided until the infant is suctioned, since this will only push the foreign material further into the lungs and further compromise the infant. After being stabilized in the delivery room, the infant should be taken to an intensive care nursery where 24-hour nursing surveillance can be provided (see Fig. 23-2). The infant should be observed frequently for respiratory status.

Pneumothorax

Pneumothorax can be caused by overdistention and rupture of the alveoli resulting from mechanical stresses associated with initiation of breathing at birth. More commonly it is due to overinflation of the lungs during resuscitation. First, there is overdistention of the distal air sacs, followed by rupture of the sacs and escape of air into the interstitial spaces. Subsequently there will be rupture of air into the pleural space.

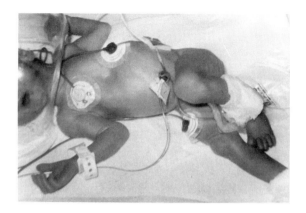

FIGURE 23-2. Infant being monitored.

The infant looks, and is, acutely ill. The respiratory rate increases with accompanying cyanosis. There is an increased anteroposterior diameter of the chest. On auscultation there is a shift of apical cardiac impulse. The chest is hyperresonant to percussion. Chest roentgenography should be done immediately and the infant placed in an oxygen environment. The pneumothorax should be aspirated. For severe involvement a chest tube is inserted and attached to suction. The infant should be cared for in an intensive care nursery, but transport is inappropriate until the infant is stabilized and in condition to be moved.

NEONATAL SEIZURES

The nervous system of the newborn infant functions primarily at the spinal cord and brainstem levels. A seizure is a symptom of a central nervous system disturbance which may result from either local or systemic causes. Seizures in the full-term newborn and preterm infant frequently are associated with other disease processes and are of concern since they may cause irreversible brain damage.

Since seizures in the preterm neonate are demonstrated differently from those of the full-term newborn or adult, they frequently go unnoticed. Neonatal seizures are manifested in varied, subtle forms. Therefore, recognition of seizures depends upon an astute nursery staff. Seizures manifest themselves by brief tonic extensions of the body, episodes of limpness, clonic movement of one extremity, eye rolling, or episodes of apnea or tremors. An infant with seizures of any form should have a thorough neurological workup.

Seizures in the newborn are due to perinatal complications such as trauma, hypoxia, fetal distress, or cerebral contusion. Hemorrhage frequently occurs in preterm infants following severe respiratory distress and acidosis. A large percentage of seizure disorders result from central nervous system infection or generalized sepsis.

Metabolic disorders that result in seizures include hypoglycemia, hypocalcemia, and hypomagnesemia. The infant may have seizure-like activity when the blood glucose level falls below 15 milligrams per 100 milliliters. The infant will show similar activity when the blood calcium level reaches 7 milligrams per 100 milliliters or less. Differentiation between hypocalcemia and hypoglycemia should be made early by Dextrostix determination of blood sugar. If the Dextrostix reading is less then 25, a blood glucose should be drawn. The infant should be given glucose and water if the Dextrostix reading is below 45.

Other causes of seizures are inborn errors of metabolism such as galactosemia, phenylketonuria, or pyridoxine deficiency. Narcotic withdrawal after maternal addiction is a frequent cause of seizures in the newborn period. When the mother's history of addiction is well known, withdrawal in the newborn can be quickly identified. Kernicterus is one of the conditions that has the most grave outcome for the infant; however, since the advent of RhoGAM, the incidence has decreased sharply. Infections caused by rubella, toxoplasmosis, or cytomegalovirus, and bacterial meningitis can cause early seizures.

The infant with seizures, regardless of the cause, requires attention to thermoregulation, adequate ventilation, oxygen if cyanosis develops, and close observation. It is necessary to make accurate documentation of the events preceding the seizure and description of the length of time the activity lasted and the parts of the body and extremities that were involved.

The most widely used drug for the control of seizures is phenobarbital. A dosage of 20 milligrams per kilogram of body weight, administered slowly intravenously, should be used initially. The infant should be placed on a maintenance dosage of 5 milligrams per kilogram of body weight daily [12, p. 146]. Many clinicians agree that any infant who has had a seizure episode outside the neonatal period should remain on the anticonvulsive therapy for 1 to 2 years [13].

Neonatal seizures may take many forms, with tonic-clonic movements being the least common type. The treatable causes of seizures should be evaluated before standard anticonvulsants are used. Although the mortality rate is high, survivors have a significant chance of being normal [14, p. 293].

JAUNDICE IN THE NEWBORN

Jaundice is the most common newborn problem the nurse-midwife will encounter. Some 30 percent of healthy newborns will develop what is termed physiologic jaundice and in others, jaundice will represent a disease state [15].

Physiologic jaundice represents both an overproduction of bilirubin and inefficient excretion during the first week of life. Bilirubin is formed mainly from the heme proteins that result from the catabolism of aged hemoglobin. The red blood cells of neonates have shorter life spans, so at any time there are more of them being broken down. In order for this excess bilirubin to be excreted it must be bound to albumin and transported through the plasma to the liver. Excess bilirubin traveling in the plasma and not bound to albumin can be deposited in fatty tissues like the brain. In rare cases this results in the encephalopathy known as kernicterus. Bilirubin is released from the albumin at individual liver cells (hepatocytes) and diffuses across the cell membrane with the help of a carrier protein.

In the liver bilirubin becomes water soluble. It is conjugated or joined to a glucuronic acid with the help of the enzyme uridine diphosphate (UDP) — glucuronyl transferase. It is then actively transported out of the liver through the biliary system and into the duodenum. In the bowel another enzyme, beta-glucuronidase, breaks apart the bilirubin diglucuronide. The bilirubin is now converted by intestinal bacteria to easily excreted types of bilirubin. However, this unconjugated bilirubin in the bowel can be easily reabsorbed into the systemic circulation while awaiting excretion. This reabsorption is termed the enterohepatic shunt.

There are some aspects of physiologic jaundice which cannot be changed by the care giver. The relative immaturity of the liver can cause a deficiency of carrier proteins, enzyme glucuronyl transferase, and glucuronic acid. The excess production of bilirubin secondary to the breakdown of red blood cells is also unchangeable. The care giver can, however, make a case for introducing feedings early in life. Early feedings encourage bacterial colonization of the bowel and peristalsis. The unconjugated bilirubin is more quickly excreted and not reabsorbed.

There are many disorders that can cause nonphysiologic, or pathologic, jaundice. Infections, liver disease, metabolic disease, and hemolytic disease all involve jaundice. Polycythemia and extravascular blood collection (hematomas and cerebral hemorrhage) also are causes of jaundice. Of these, the hemolytic disorders due to fetal and maternal blood group incompatibility, especially of the ABO type, are most common.

In physiologic jaundice the peak bilirubin levels are reached on the third to fourth day of life and 95 percent of infants will be below 15 milligrams per 100 milliliters [16, p. 77]. The following guidelines will assist the nurse-midwife in identifying infants at risk for pathologic jaundice:

1. Cord bilirubin greater than 2 milligrams per 100 milliliters
2. Jaundice visible in the first day of life
3. Jaundice associated with anemia
4. Increase in serum bilirubin of greater than 5 milligrams per 100 milliliters per day

Infants at risk will be followed by a pediatrician with serial bilirubin levels, complete blood counts, direct and indirect Coombs' tests, and careful history and physical examinations.

The need for treatment of physiologic jaundice in term, well babies has become controversial in recent years. Phototherapy utilizes blue fluorescent light at a specific wavelength. It breaks down bilirubin in the skin and produces an isomer of bilirubin which can be excreted via the liver. Phototherapy also increases bowel peristalsis. Some unanswered concerns have arisen regarding its effect on cell growth and DNA [17, p. 258]. Some side effects of phototherapy include insensible water loss, lactose intolerance with diarrhea, and retinal damage in unprotected eyes. Physiologic jaundice is almost always self-limited; however, there may be an occasional infant in whom the body response is so sluggish that treatment is necessary. It is unclear at what bilirubin level healthy term babies sustain central nervous system damage, although the risk rises at greater than 20 milligrams per 100 milliliters.

INFANTS WITH ANOMALIES

Congenital Heart Disease

During the third to eighth weeks of fetal life, as the heart develops from a tube to a four-chambered organ, it is particularly vulnerable. There are some maternal factors such as diabetes and rubella that predispose to anomalies, as does a close family history of congenital

heart disease. Many of the chromosomal abnormalities involve heart defects; as many as 30 percent of Down's syndrome babies are affected. Approximately 90 percent of congenital heart disease is felt to be of multifactorial origin, involving both genetic predisposition and exposure to an environmental factor such as a virus or drug [18].

There are many kinds of heart defects. They are usually classified into two major categories: cyanotic and acyanotic. The first indications of acyanotic heart disease frequently are the symptoms of volume overload characteristic of congestive heart failure. Some heart disease combines cyanosis with congestive heart failure. Congenital heart disease does not always present itself in the immediate newborn period and in some cases not until late infancy.

Most acyanotic heart disease involves lesions that produce symptoms of congestive heart failure (CHF). CHF results when the left ventricle does not adequately empty itself after each ejection of blood; the cardiac output decreases and eventually pulmonary symptoms arise secondary to venous congestion. This situation can occur when the outflow of blood from the ventricle is diminished, as in coarctation of the aorta or mitral and aortic valve atresia. An irregular heart rhythm can also lead to poor cardiac output. Another common cause of acyanotic heart disease is patent ductus arteriosus. In this condition the ductus remains patent after birth, causing a shunting of blood from the aorta back into the lungs. This may overburden the left side of the heart and lead to congestive heart failure.

Cyanosis is the most common symptom of heart disease in the newborn and reflects the circulation of blood whose hemoglobin is not saturated with oxygen. Cyanosis usually results from the shunting of blood from the right to the left side of the heart before the blood is oxygenated in the lungs. Tetralogy of Fallot is a common cyanotic heart condition involving the shunting of blood through a large ventricular septal defect. In the condition called persistent fetal circulation, blood is shunted through a patent foramen ovale. In transposition of the great arteries the aorta arises in the right ventricle and circulates unoxygentated blood returning to the heart back into the systemic circulation, while the pulmonary artery arises in the left ventricle.

Symptoms of congenital heart disease vary with type. The nurse-midwife should be suspicious of full-term babies exhibiting decreased activity and difficulty maintaining adequate nursing. Cyanosis must be observed in a good light and, in heart disease, usually gets worse with crying. A cold infant will give a false impression of cyanosis. A newborn in transition may have a normal peripheral cyanosis of hands and feet. More accurate is assessment of the tongue, lips, and trunk skin color.

Infants may demonstrate tachypnea of greater than 50 breaths per minute at rest or hyperpnea of consistent very deep but unlabored respirations. Respiratory symptoms such as nasal flaring, grunting, and retractions are common, as is sweating.

On palpation absent femoral pulses, a grossly enlarged liver, or a prominent precordial thrill is suggestive of congenital heart defect. Various murmurs may be present although serious heart disease can exist without murmurs. The nurse-midwife must bear in mind the variations in time of onset of symptoms and the variable nature of the symptoms themselves [19].

Nurse-midwifery management consists of immediate consultation with a pediatrician and supportive care. The infant in congestive heart failure may need to be positioned in a semi-Fowler's position and the cyanotic infant often seems better in the knee-chest position. Oxygen may help some infants. Feedings often must be withheld and an intravenous infusion initiated.

Esophageal Anomalies

Normally the fetus swallows amniotic fluid while in utero. The infant with esophageal stenosis is not able to assimilate fluids swallowed and tends to regurgitate the fluid, which increases the amount of amniotic fluid. The infant born with tracheoesophageal fistula may be small for gestational age. Five types of esophageal malformations have been described. Type A (Fig. 23-3A) is an esophageal atresia with a tracheoesophageal fistula connecting to the lower pouch. Type A occurs more frequently than the other types. The infant has excessive oral mucus, which is an overflow from the blind upper segment of the esophagus. Respiratory distress occurs gradually as the mucus spills over into the trachea from the esophagus.

In type B (Fig. 23-3B) there is an isolated esophageal atresia with no tracheal communication. The infant has excessive mucus and respiratory distress as in Type A. There is an absence of gas in the bowel. A catheter cannot be passed into the stomach. When a soft catheter is used for the examination, it frequently curls up in the end of the pouch, thus giving the examiner a false diagnosis. A lateral x-ray of the neck may demonstrate air in just the upper esophageal pouch.

Type C (Fig. 23-3C) is an isolated esophageal fistula referred to as the H-type. This is more difficult to diagnose. The infant has coughing or cyanosis with feeding and frequent episodes of aspiration pneumonia. New techniques for roentgenography of infants have been used for easier diagnosis of the H-type fistula.

Type D (Fig. 23-3D) is a double fistula. Both upper and lower pouches of the esophagus communicate with the trachea. The infant with the Type D anomaly presents at birth with coughing, choking, and pneumonia. There will be gas present in the bowel on roentgenography. Saliva drains directly into the lungs, increasing pulmonary complications.

Type E (Fig. 23-3E) has an upper pouch fistula: the upper portion of the esophagus communicates with the trachea. The lower pouch remains blind. Infants with type E anomalies have increased mucus and gradually increasing respiratory distress from the mucus flowing directly into the trachea. The infant

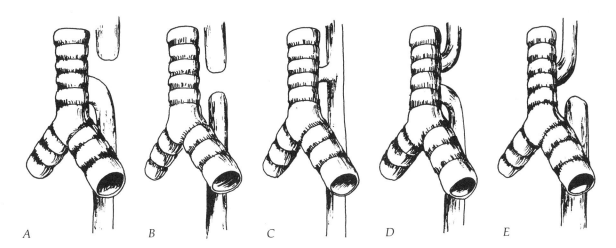

FIGURE 23-3.   A. esophageal atresia with a tracheoesophageal fistula; B. isolated esophageal atresia with no tracheal communication; C. isolated esophageal fistula (H-type); D. double fistula; E. upper pouch fistula.

chokes continually. The abdomen will have a scaphoid contour with no gas in the bowel.

Once the diagnosis of esophageal stenosis or fistula is suspected, the infant should be given nothing by mouth and should be placed in an isolette and measures taken to conserve energy and prevent hypothermia. The infant should be in a 30° head-up position with oxygen provided. Once stabilized, the baby needs to be moved to an intensive care nursery, where 24-hour nursing management can be provided.

Diaphragmatic Hernia

Between the eighth and tenth weeks of fetal life the diaphragm is formed and the coelomic cavity divides into the abdominal and thoracic components. During the same stage of morphogenesis the gastrointestinal tract undergoes its major development, elongating into the umbilical pouch and rotating as it descends into the abdominal cavity. Any alteration in these two interrelated processes leads to a diaphragmatic hernia. The extent of the herniation will determine the severity and timing of

the symptoms. The herniation will compress the lung.

The infant has severe respiratory distress with poor chest movement and cyanosis from the moment of birth. Usually the abdomen is small and scaphoid because the bowel is displaced from the abdomen into the chest. Occasionally, peristaltic sounds can be heard in the chest. Breath sounds in the affected hemithorax are absent, with displacement of the point of maximal impulse. The lung on the affected side is compressed and often hypoplastic. Dependence on diaphragmatic respiration, and the right-to-left shunt through a lung incapable of exchanging gases, precipitate hypoxia and acidosis.

The nurse-midwife who delivers an infant with severe respiratory distress should be aware of the possibility of diaphragmatic hernia and should initiate emergency measures until medical help can arrive. Assisted ventilation and oxygen therapy should be started. Assisted ventilation should be initiated by endotracheal tube *only*: when a mask is used the air will be displaced into the stomach and enlarge it, leading to further compromise of the lungs. Gastric drainage should be maintained for deflation of the gastrointestinal portion residing in the lung cavity. The infant should be maintained in a 30° upright position. Careful attention should be given to fluid requirements.

Intestinal Obstruction

An obstruction may occur at any site along the intestinal tract and may be partial or complete. Infants who have more than 20 milliliters of gastric fluid on aspiration at birth must be suspected of having a high gastrointestinal obstruction. If the passage of meconium is delayed longer than 24 hours, a lower gastrointestinal obstruction is suspected. As the infant's condition becomes obvious, abdominal distention develops with absent or decreased bowel sounds and vomiting of bile-stained material. The infant soon develops respiratory distress from pressure of the distended abdomen on the diaphragm.

The infant should be transferred to an intensive care nursery. Management while waiting for transfer should include careful attention to temperature regulation and decompression of the stomach. Oxygen should be provided. The use of oxygen is encouraged for any infant with abdominal distention; this serves to increase the oxygenation of the intestinal tract. Since the infant is given nothing by mouth and is losing fluid through vomiting, fluid and electrolytes should be started to maintain the normal requirements and to replace the amount lost through vomiting.

Imperforate Anus

Imperforate anus results from a failure of differentiation of the urogenital sinus and cloaca. It is seen in about 10 percent of babies that have esophageal atresia and tracheoesophageal fistula. Imperforate anus is considered to be high or low, depending on the level to which the rectal pouch has descended. The abnormal anatomy may consist of stenosis of the anal opening, an unformed anus, or the combination

of unformed anus and atresia of the rectum. A mild form of imperforate anus is caused by membrane covering the anal opening. Fistulas may exist between the terminal rectum and the perineum, vagina, or urinary tract. A high imperforate anus is suspected when no fistula is present on the perineum. Instead, the fistula usually communicates with the posterior urethra. Meconium is expelled through the penis of the male infant. In some instances the fistula communicates with the outside of the scrotum.

Once the diagnosis of imperforate anus is made, management is directed at preventing severe abdominal distention. The infant is not fed. If the abdomen is distended the stomach should be compressed by nasogastric suction. Fluids and electrolytes are provided for maintenance and replacement of fluids lost by suction. Careful attention should be given to adequate oxygenation and thermoregulation while awaiting surgical consultation and diagnostic studies.

Hirschsprung's Disease

Hirschsprung's disease is frequently referred to as aganglionic megacolon. There is a congenital absence of parasympathetic ganglion cells in one segment of the colon or, sometimes, the entire colon. The denervated segment is narrowed and the proximal, uninvolved colon is dilated.

The common early symptom in the neonate is failure to pass meconium in the first 24 hours of extrauterine life. This is rapidly followed by abdominal distention, vomiting, and respiratory distress. In some neonates, symptoms do not become severe until after the immediate newborn period and start with constipation.

Diagnosis is made by x-ray and biopsy of the affected portion of the colon. The immediate treatment is colostomy. Resection of the denervated portion of the colon is usually delayed until the infant is 6 months of age.

Meconium Ileus

A condition that shows symptoms early in the neonatal period and requires the knowledge and skill of the nurse-midwife is meconium ileus. Meconium ileus may or may not be a genetic disorder but is felt to be the earliest manifestation of cystic fibrosis which is a genetic disorder. Meconium ileus results from the inability of the infant to pass abnormally thick, tenacious meconium in the terminal ileum. The infant has the same types of symptoms as infants with other types of small bowel obstruction. Treatment for this condition should be done in an intensive care nursery.

In the past, surgical intervention was required for relief of the obstruction. More recently it has been shown that rectal installation of meglumine diatrizoate (Gastrografin) often eliminates the obstructing bolus of meconium [20]. Gastrografin is a radiopaque contrast material that contains a wetting agent (Tween 80) in which the thick meconium is soluble. If Gastrografin can be successfully advanced through the microcolon and into the obstructed distal ileum there is reasonable expectation that meconium will be passed spontaneously, relieving the obstruction [21]. Because of the hyperosmolarity of Gastrografin, dehydration secondary to fluid shifts into the lumen of the intestine must be prevented [22]. The infant's hydration is maintained throughout the procedure with intravenous fluids. Frequently Gastrografin installation needs to be repeated. If Gastrografin installation fails, the meconium will need to be removed surgically.

Genetic Disorders

The likelihood that a neonate will have a genetic disorder increases if the mother is 35 years of age or older. Genetic disorders may be expected if there are predisposing epidemiological or medical factors associated with genetic disorders or a family history of a genetic disorder. Mothers in this age group may or may not avail themselves of opportunities for antenatal diagnosis, so it is important for the nurse-midwife to give special attention to the previous pregnancy history of the patient.

Maternal age is a primary factor in several disorders resulting from polygenic or multifactoral etiologies, while paternal age has greater influence in certain autosomal dominant disorders. In disorders that are genetically transmitted the likelihood of occurrence in other family members is increased.

The genetic disorders affecting the newborn infant are too extensive to cover in this text. References to medical genetic textbooks for complete coverage of genetic disorders are found in the bibliography.

Down's Syndrome

The most common of the chromosomal abnormalities is trisomy 21, or Down's syndrome. Affected infants present a clinical picture in which all or varying numbers of these findings are noted: narrow face; eyes slant up and outward; epicanthal folds are present; iris is speckled; nose is broad-bridged; tongue is thick, fissured, and protruding; palate is high and arched; ears are small and square; neck is webbed; hands are stubby; there is a clearcut simian line; fifth middle phalanx is short or missing. (See Figs. 23-4 and 22-9.)

These infants may present feeding problems because of their tongues and high palates, along with incoordinate sucking and swallowing. Often there is a considerable amount of mucus. Other problems should be considered since many of these infants have other anomalies also. Congenital heart disease and gastrointestinal anomalies occur most frequently. Mental retardation is present in varying degrees in most of these infants and they are subject to numerous illnesses. They usually require a lifetime of care.

DRUGS AND THE NEONATE

The effect of drugs on the fetus has been under

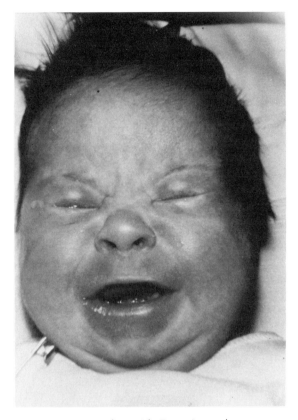

FIGURE 23-4.   Infant with Down's syndrome.

intense study over the past several years. When it was determined that certain drugs taken during pregnancy have deleterious effects on the fetus it was recommended that no drugs be taken during this time. The period of greatest fetal danger from teratogenic drugs is the first trimester, when systems are developing. Following the first trimester, risks are reduced for developmental damage but may be increased for functional disorders.

It is best that no drugs be used during pregnancy unless absolutely necessary. If used, the smallest amount over the shortest period of time is recommended. The drugs of choice include those that have the least deleterious effect on the fetus while producing maximum effect on maternal disease control or cure. Illness which may be life threatening to the mother or the fetus requires appropriate treatment to prevent damage from the disease process.

The intensity and duration of drug use depend upon the absorption, distribution, metabolism, and excretion of the drug, and the interaction between the drug and specific tissue receptors. Drugs administered to the pregnant woman cross the placenta in response to physiochemical characteristics of the drug, physiological properties of the placental tissue, and the maternal and fetal blood flow through the placenta. There is an increase in uterine blood flow as pregnancy approaches term, but there is a decrease in proportion to the weight of the fetus as it increases in size. The decreased blood flow during contractions may impede the passage to the fetus of significant amounts of drugs such as anesthetics and analgesics. Although this can be considered a protection for the fetus, it may also be reponsible for retention over longer periods of time of drugs that are already present in the fetal circulation.

Understanding drug disposition and action on the fetus is essential for the nurse-midwife who is managing the patient throughout pregnancy and delivery. Education of the consumer about the effects of over-the-counter drugs is an important topic of discussion in prenatal classes. There is need for more definitive research on the teratogenic effects of drugs. It may be extremely difficult to evaluate the teratogenic effects of many drugs, since fetal anomalies may be highly associated with a disease process for which the drug is being administered. Diabetes and seizure disorders are good examples.

Self-Administered or Over-the-Counter Drugs

There is increasing concern about the teratogenic effects of drugs on the fetus. The relationship of congenital anomalies and Thalidomide is well known. Unfortunately there is minimal information about the possible or actual teratogenic effects of over-the-counter drugs available to the consumer. Although the consumer is much more conscious than in the past of drug problems in relation to pregnancy, many are unaware of those which might be associated with self-medication, including vitamin and mineral supplements.

An excessive amount of vitamin A is associated with urinary tract anomalies, eye pathology, cleft palate, and syndactylism; excess vitamin D is associated with fetal hypercalcemia, mental retardation, and cardiac anomalies. Harsh laxatives may cause uterine contractions. The fetus absorbs iodine throughout pregnancy after the twelfth or fourteenth week. Excess iodine may result in the arrest of brain development. Some cough syrups and asthma preparations contain iodine. Although there is some information on possible teratogenic effects of over-the-counter drugs, the dose necessary to produce defects by many drugs is not indicated and is not known at present.

Among the mild analgesics, aspirin is used liberally throughout pregnancy, and no obvious toxic effects have been reported. Controversy continues regarding the relationship between salicylates and malformations [23]. Studies have demonstrated evidence of platelet dysfunction and decrease in the activity of Factor XII in the cord blood of newborn infants whose mothers took more than 5 grains of acetylsalicylic acid in the week before birth. Three of the 14 aspirinexposed infants manifested a platelet dysfunction [24]. Another case reported related severe gastrointestinal bleeding in an infant in whom the defect of platelet function was determined [25]. An accurate pharmacokinetic study of salicylate elimination by an infant who received the drug throughout gestation has been published [26]. The normal newborn had a significant concentration of the drug in plasma (25 milligrams per 100 milliliters), which was excreted over 5 days' time at a slower rate than in adults but faster than that of the infant of a mother who takes an occasional aspirin before delivery.

Some pregnant women unknowingly seek immunizations from their local health department. They should be advised that live virus vaccine may affect the fetal neurological system. Therefore flu, polio, measles, smallpox, and yellow fever vaccines are not recommended during pregnancy. There are no known risks to killed virus vaccines.

Smoking

There are approximately 4000 different compounds in cigarette smoke. Carbon monoxide and nicotine are currently thought to be the two most detrimental compounds in smoke. Nicotine in significant concentrations has been measured in the amniotic fluid of smoking mothers [27]. Smoking as few as two cigarettes per day reduces fetal breathing movements in otherwise normal pregnancies [28]. Multiple studies have linked low birth weight, prematurity, and perinatal mortality to maternal cigarette usage during pregnancy [29]. Nicotine may produce vasoconstriction of uterine circulation with consequent reduction in placental exchange [30].

Drug Addiction

Narcotic addiction has remained the most serious problem to the fetus. Maternal use of 6 to 12 milligrams of heroin daily usually results in the development of the withdrawal syndrome in the newborn. It has been reported that stillbirths occur more frequently in these pregnancies; the amniotic fluid frequently shows the presence of meconium, which increase the likelihood of meconium aspiration. The stillbirths and meconium staining of the fluid may be due to variable periods of intrauterine hypoxia during periods of stress in the pregnancy when the heroin-addicted mother and fetus, lacking the drug, experience withdrawal symptoms [31]. Methadone has also been associated with addiction of the fetus. Observations are contradictory, but some researchers state that withdrawal symptoms from methadone are more frequent and prolonged than in newborns of heroin addicts [32].

Frequently the drug-addicted mother has not had prenatal care and may go through an entire hospitalization without the staff's being aware of the addiction or her lack of prenatal care. Addiction and low birth weight are the most common complications of infants of addicted women. Most addicted infants will show signs of withdrawal within the first 48 hours of life, but symptoms have been delayed as long as 5 days in some infants. This delay is more serious because the infant may have symptoms at home for a period of time before treatment can be initiated. General symptoms in the neonate include irritability, high-pitched cry, restlessness, increased appetite, vomiting, diarrhea, and nasal congestion.

Alcohol

Jones and Smith [33] reported altered growth patterns in infants born of chronic alcoholic women (fetal alcohol syndrome). Alcohol must be considered teratogenic when used to excess. Maternal ingestion of alcohol close to delivery produces toxic symptoms in the infant. Ethanol is a central nervous system depressant and causes interference with the cardiorespiratory adaptation of the newborn.

Anomalies found in infants of chronic alcoholic women are microcephaly, with head circumference below the third percentile for gestational age, short palpebral fissure, small cheekbones, prenatal and postnatal growth deficiency, congenital heart defects, congenital hip dislocation and other joint anomalies, and altered palmar crease patterns.

Other Drugs

There are thousands of prescription drugs available to pregnant women in the United States. The individual nurse-midwife must avail herself of current pharmacology textbooks, newsletters, and the *Physicians' Desk Reference* in order to have accurate, current knowledge with which to advise women needing medication. For some medications such as warfarin (Coumadin), diphenylhydantoin (Dilantin), and tetracycline, clear-cut evidence has shown fetal risk. For most medications, risks are not known or the quality of research is so poor that inferences of safe or not safe cannot be made.

Antibiotics

Dicloxacillin is tightly bound to serum albumin (at therapeutic levels). Low cord-blood levels and insignificant amniotic fluid levels are found due to the small free diffusible fraction that crosses the placenta.

About 40 per cent of methicillin is bound to albumin and crosses the placental barrier easily. A significant concentration of the drug is found in the fetal and amniotic fluid concentration.

Ampicillin and penicillin reach the amniotic fluid after some delay. They reach the amniotic fluid through fetal urine, which allows recirculation of the drug in the fetus.

Tetracycline, which accumulates in the fetal skeleton when given early in pregnancy, will result in a decrease in skeletal growth. Discoloration of teeth occurs when the drug is administered during the second trimester. This dental effect is thought to be associated with hypoplasia of the enamel.

Streptomycin reaches the fetus rapidly and minor degrees of acoustic nerve damage may be common.

Anticonvulsant Drugs

Diphenylhydantoin (Dilantin) has been found to produce coagulation defects, and some cases of cleft lip and palate have been reported [34].

Infants of mothers who have received phenobarbital have experienced withdrawal symptoms similar to those seen in neonates of opiate-addicted mothers. The onset of symptoms occurs later than those caused by opium derivatives, thus the infant may not have symptoms until 2 weeks after birth. Defects have been reported in the offspring of mothers taking phenobarbital.

Antihypertensive Drugs

Reserpine has resulted in respiratory depression in the newborn at birth, followed by stuffy nose and lethargy.

Magnesium sulfate has been used extensively in the treatment of patients with preeclampsia. High levels of magnesium in the fetus have been reported. Hypermagnesemia produces neonatal respiratory depression. A decrease in serum calcium has been observed in newborns with high serum magnesium levels [35].

Analgesics and Anesthesia

Barbiturates and Narcotic Analgesics

Most barbiturates cross the placenta rapidly, and the equilibration of drug level in the maternal circulation and that of the fetus occurs within minutes. There is a possibility of neonatal depression when thiopental is used as an anesthetic for cesarean section. Depression does not occur when thiopental is used in a vaginal delivery since the amount of drug transferred is not as great as in cesarean section. Protein binding influences the amount of drug available for transfer across the placenta. The narcotic analgesics such as meperidine transfer rapidly across the placenta into the fetal bloodstream and reach a peak concentration of 80 to 130 percent of maternal levels after an intramuscular injection. At that time a greater proportion of metabolites of meperidine is present in maternal serum, which may cause toxicity to the fetus.

Regional Anesthesia

The drugs used for regional anesthesia are water-soluble salts of lipid-soluble alkaloids and may be divided according to their chemical structure into two groups, esters and amides. The ester group, an example of which is procaine, has a slow onset of action, short duration of pharmacologic effect, and penetrates poorly into tissues. The amides, such as bupivacaine, lignocaine, mepivacaine, and prilocaine are most commonly used in conduction anesthesia because of rapid onset of action and prolonged duration of pharmacological effect. Both esters and amides cross the placenta. The amides are poorly metabolized by the fetus and eventually are excreted relatively unchanged as mepivacaine in the urine.

Questions arise as to the fetal complications associated with paracervical block anesthesia. When sustained maternal hypotension occurs, fetal bradycardia and varying degrees of depression result. These usually are transitory problems. A more serious problem arises when the infant receives an excessive amount of the drug via maternal circulation or direct injection; this can result in severe depression and possible death. The risk of serious difficulties indicates that the total amount of "-caine" drugs should be evaluated prior to reinjection. Time lapse between injections should be included in this evaluation.

Spinal anesthesia has no direct effect on the fetus because the amount of the drug used is too small to achieve toxic levels. When neonatal depression occurs following spinal anesthesia, it is thought to be due to maternal hypotension. Lidocaine and mepivacaine may cause fetal bradycardia and subsequent acidosis in the infant. Rapid absorption of the anesthetic into the blood vessels perfusing the placenta results in immediate transfer into the fetal circulation [36].

General Anesthesia

General anesthetics such as the gaseous anesthetics are rapidly transferred to the fetus.

For example, within 90 seconds of maternal administration, cyclopropane has been found in cord blood [37]. Methoxy-fluorane, which dissociates poorly and is highly lipid, is also transferred early. Within 2 minutes of maternal administration, umbilical vein levels of methoxyfluorane have been found to be 60 percent of the concentration present in maternal blood [38]. Studies of placental transmission of nitrous oxide have shown that the average concentration in cord blood approaches 50 percent of the maternal drug concentration. Cyclopropane in concentrations of 3 to 5 percent does not produce ill effects in the fetus.

REFERENCES

1. Goodwin, J. W., Duane, J. T., and Thomas, B. W. Antepartum identification of the fetus at risk. *Can. Med. Assoc. J.* 101:458, 1969.
2. *Toward Improving the Outcome of Pregnancy.* Committee on Perinatal Health, National Foundation-March of Dimes, 1976.
3. Mandelkorn, T., and Alden, R. R. Morbidity and mortality of infants weighing less than 1000 grams in an intensive care nursery. *Pediatrics* 50:40, 1972.
4. Pildes, R. S. Management of acute metabolic problems in the neonate. In Aladjem, S. (Ed.). *Perinatal Intensive Care.* St. Louis: Mosby, 1977.
5. Ballard, J. et al. A simplified assessment of gestational age. *Pediatr. Res.* 11:374, 1977.
6. Lubchenco, L. O. et al. Intrauterine growth in length and head circumference as estimated from live births at gestational age from 26–42 weeks. *Pediatrics* 37:403, 1966.
7. Babson, S. G. Feeding the low-birth-weight infant. *J. Pediatr.* 76:694, 1971.
8. Sweet, A. Classification of the low-birth-weight infant. In Klaus, M., and Fanaroff, A. (Eds.). *Care of the High-risk Neonate.* Philadelphia: Saunders, 1979.
9. Speck, W. et al. Neonatal infections. In Klaus, M., and Fanaroff, A. (Eds.). *Care of the High-risk Neonate.* Philadelphia: Saunders, 1979.
10. Parmalee, A. H., and Stern, L. Maturation of respiration in prematures and young infants. *Neuropediatrics* 3:294, 1972.
11. Deuel, R. K. Polygraphic monitoring of apneic spells. *Arch. Neurol.* 28:71, 1973.
12. Clancy, R. Neonatal seizures. In Polin, R., and Burg, F. (Eds.). *Workbook in Practical Neonatology.* Philadelphia: Saunders, 1983.
13. Freeman, J. M. Neonatal seizures — diagnosis and management. *J. Pediatr.* 77:701, 1970.
14. Prichard, J. S. The character and significance of epileptic seizures in infancy. In Kelloway, P., and Peterson, I. (Eds.). *Neurologic and Encephalographic Correlative Studies in Infancy.* New York: Grune & Stratton, 1964.
15. Cashore, W., and Stern, L. The management of hyperbilirubinemia. *Clin. in Perinatol.* 11:2, 1984.
16. Cashore, W. Neonatal hyperbilirubinemia. In Polin, R., and Burg, F. (Eds.). *Workbook in Practical Neonatology.* Philadelphia: Saunders, 1983.
17. Poland, R., and Ostra, E. Neonatal hyperbilirubinemia. In Klaus, M., and Fanaroff, A. *Care of the High-risk Neonate.* Philadelphia: Saunders, 1979, p. 258.
18. Morgan, B. Incidence, etiology and classification of congenital heart disease. *Pediat. Clin. North Am.* 25:4, 1978.
19. Shor, V. Congenital cardiac defects: Assessment and case-finding. *Am. J. Nurs.* (February) 1978.
20. Noblett, H. R. Treatment of uncomplicated meconium ileus by Gastrografin enema, a preliminary report. *J. Pediatr. Surg.* 4:190, 1969.
21. Randolph, J. G., and Altman, P. Surgery in the neonate. In Avery, G. B. (Ed.). *Neonatology: Pathophysiology and Management of the Newborn.* Philadelphia: Lippincott, 1975.
22. Rowe, M. I., Seabram, G., and Weinberger, M. Gastrografin-induced hypertonicity: The pathogenesis of a neonatal hazard. *Am. J. Surg.* 125:185, 1973.
23. Nelson, M. M., and Forfar, J. O. Associations between drugs administered during pregnancy and congenital abnormalities of the fetus. *Br. Med. J.* 1:523, 1971.
24. Bleyer, W. A. et al. Studies on the detection of adverse drug reactions in the newborn. 1. Fetal exposure to maternal medication. *JAMA* 213: 2046, 1970.
25. Haslam, R. R. et al. Hemorrhage in a neonate possibly due to maternal ingestion of salicylate. *J. Pediatr.* 84:556, 1974.
26. Garrettson, L. K. et al. Fetal acquisition and

neonatal elimination of a large amount of salicylate. *Clin. Pharmacol. Ther.* 17:98, 1975.

27. Van Vunakis, H., Langone, J. J., and Milunski, A. Nicotine and cotinine in the amniotic fluid of smokers in the second trimester of pregnancy. *Am. J. Obstet. Gynecol.* 120:64, 1974.

28. Manning, F., Wyn Pugh, E., and Boddy, K. Effect of cigarette smoking on fetal breathing movements in normal pregnancies. *Br. Med. J.* 1:552, 1975.

29. Meyer, M. B., Jones, B. S., and Tonascia, J. A. Perinatal events associated with maternal smoking during pregnancy. *Am. J. Epidem.* 103:464, 1976.

30. Yaffe, S. J., and Juchau, M. R. Perinatal pharmacology. *Ann. Rev. Pharmacology* 14:219, 1974.

31. Blinick, G., Wallach, R. C., and Jerez, E. Pregnancy in narcotic addicts treated by medical withdrawal. *Am. J. Obstet. Gynecol.* 105:997, 1969.

32. Rajegouda, B. K. et al. Methadone withdrawal in newborn infants. *J. Pediatr.* 81:532, 1972.

33. Jones, K. L., and Smith, D. W. Recognition of the fetal alcohol syndrome in early infancy. *Lancet* 1:1267, 1973.

34. Mirkin, B. L. Dyphenylhydantoin placental transport, fetal localization, neonatal metabolism and possible teratogenic effects. *J. Pediatr.* 78:329, 1971.

35. Savory, J., and Monif, G. R. G. Serum calcium levels in cord sera of the progeny of mothers treated with magnesium sulfate for toxemia of pregnancy. *Am. J. Obstet. Gynecol.* 110:556, 1971.

36. Shinder, S. M., and Way, E. L. Plasma levels of lidocaine in mother and newborn following obstetrical conduction anesthesia. *Clin. Application Anesth.* 29:951, 1968.

37. Moya, F., and Smith, B. E. Uptake, distribution, and placental transport of drugs and anesthetics. *Anesthesiology* 26:465, 1965.

38. Siker, E. S. et al. Placental transfer of methoxyfluorane. *Br. J. Anesth.* 40:588, 1968.

BIBLIOGRAPHY FOR CHAPTERS 21, 22, AND 23

Aladjem, S., and Brown, A. *Clinical Perinatology.* St. Louis: Mosby, 1974.

Aladjem, S., and Brown, A. *Risks in the Practice of Modern Obstetrics.* St. Louis: Mosby, 1975.

Aladjem, S. and Brown, A. (Eds.). *Perinatal Intensive Care.* St. Louis: Mosby, 1977.

Alexander, M. M., and Brown, M. S. *Pediatric History Taking and Physical Diagnosis for Nurses, 2nd.* New York: McGraw-Hill, 1979.

Alford, C. A. Immunoglobin determinations in the diagnosis of fetal infection. *Pediatr. Clin. North Am.* 18:199, 1971.

Apgar, V. et al. Evaluation of the newborn infant: Second repeat. *JAMA* 168:1985, 1958.

Arnold, P. et al. Transition to extra-uterine life. *Am. J. Nurs.* 65:77, 1965.

Avery, G. B. (Ed.). *Neonatology: Pathophysiology and Management of the Newborn, 2nd.* Philadelphia: Lippincott, 1981.

Babson, S. G. Feeding the low birth-weight infant. *J. Pediatr.* 79:694, 1971.

Babson, S. G., Benson, R. C., Pernoll, M. L., and Benda, G. I. *Management of High-Risk Pregnancy and Intensive Care of the Neonate.* St. Louis: Mosby, 1975.

Ballard, J. et al. A simplified assessment of gestational age. *Pediatr. Res.* 11:374, 1977.

Barnard, C. N., and Louw, J. H. The genesis of intestinal atresia. *Minn. Med.* 39:745, 1956.

Barnett, C. et al. Neonatal separation: The maternal side of interactional deprivation. *Pediatrics* 45:197, 1970.

Battaglia, F. G., and Lubchenco, L. O. A practical classification of newborn infants by weight and gestational age. *J. Pediatr.* 71:159, 1967.

Behrmann, R. E. (Ed.). Neonatal-Perinatal Medicine: *Diseases of the Fetus and Infant.* St. Louis: Mosby, 1982.

Bergsma, D. Contemporary genetic counseling. *Birth Defects* 9:1, 1973.

Besch, N. et al. The transport baby bag. *N. Engl. J. Med.* 284:121, 1971.

Bleyer, W. A. et al. Studies on the detection of adverse drug reactions in the newborn. 1. Fetal exposure to maternal medication. *JAMA* 213:2046, 1970.

Blinick, G., Wallach, R. C., and Jerez, E. Pregnancy in narcotic addicts treated by medical withdrawal. *Am. J. Obstet. Gynecol.* 105:997, 1969.

Bloomfield, D. K. Fetal deaths and malformation associated with the use of Coumarin derivations in pregnancy. *Am. J. Obstet. Gynecol.* 107:883, 1970.

Boyer, D. B. Routine circumcision of the newborn: Reasonable precaution or unnecessary risk? *J.*

Nurse-Midwifery 25(6):27–31 (November/December) 1980.

Brazelton, T. B. Behavioral assessment of the neonate, In Clark, A. L., and Affonso, D. D. *Childbearing: A Nursing Perspective.* Philadelphia: Davis, 1976.

Brazelton, T. B. *Neonatal Behavioral Assessment Scale.* Philadelphia: Lippincott, 1973.

Broussard, E. R. Maternal perception of the neonate as related to development. *Child Psychiatr. Hum. Dev.* 1:16, 1970.

Burstein, I., Kirch, R. A. H., and Stern, L. Anxiety, pregnancy, labor and the neonate. *Am. J. Obstet. Gynecol.* 118:195, 1974.

Cashore, W., and Stern, L. The management of hyperbilirubinemia. *Clin. in Perinatol.* 11:2, 1984.

Cashore, W. Neonatal hyperbilirubinemia. In Polin, R., and Burg, F. *Workbook in Practical Neonatology.* Philadelphia: Saunders, 1983.

Chase, D., Brady, J., and Chir, B. Ventricular tachycardia in a neonate with mepivacaine toxicity. *J. Pediatr.* 90:127, 1977.

Clancy, R. Neonatal seizures. In Polin, R., and Burg, F. *Workbook in Practical Neonatology.* Philadelphia: Saunders, 1983.

Clark, A. L. and Affonso, D. D. *Childbearing: A Nursing Perspective, 2nd.* Philadelphia: Davis, 1979.

Clausen, J. P. et al. *Maternity Nursing Today.* New York: McGraw-Hill, 1973.

Collins, E., and Turner, G. ASA during pregnancy. *Lancet* 2:797, 1976.

Committee on Fetus and Newborn. *Standards and Recommendations for Hospital Care of Newborn Infants, 6th.* Evanston, Ill.: American Academy of Pediatrics, 1977.

Committee on Perinatal Health (American Academy of Family Physicians, American Academy of Pediatrics, American College of Obstetricians and Gynecologists, American Medical Association). *Toward Improving the Outcome of Pregnancy.* National Foundation-March of Dimes, 1976.

Cornblath, M., and Schwartz, R. *Disorders of Carbohydrate Metabolism in Infancy.* Philadelphia: Saunders, 1976.

Desmond, M. M. et al. The clinical behavior of the newly born. *J. Pediatr.* 62:307, 1963.

Desmond, M. M. et al. The transitional care nursery: A mechanism for preventive medicine in the newborn. *Pediatr. Clin. North Am.* 13:651, 1966.

Deuel, R. K., Polygraphic monitoring of apneic spells. *Arch. Neurol.* 28:71, 1973.

Drage, J. S., Kennedy, C., and Schwarz, B. K. The Apgar score as an index of neonatal mortality. *J. Obstet. Gynecol.* 2:22, 1964.

Dubowitz, L. M. S., Dubowitz, V., and Goldberg, C. Clinical assessment of gestational age in the newborn infant. *J. Pediatr.* 77:1, 1970.

Ettinger, B. B. et al. Intrapartal evaluation of the fetus, effects of drugs on the fetal heart rate during labor. *J. Obstet. Gynecol. Nurs.* 5:41, 1976. (Supplement).

Fardig, J. A. A comparison of skin-to-skin contact and radiant heaters in promoting neonatal thermoregulation. *J. Nurse-Midwifery* 25(1):19–28 (January/February) 1980.

Fetal Circulation. Columbus, Ohio: Ross Laboratories, 1957.

Freeman, J. M. Neonatal seizures: Diagnosis and management. *J. Pediatr.* 77:701, 1970.

Garrettson, L. K. et al. Fetal acquisition and neonatal elimination of a large amount of salicylate. *Clin. Pharmacol. Ther.* 17:98, 1975.

Galloway, K. Early detection of congenital anomalies. *J. Obstet. Gynecol. Nurs.* 2:37, 1973.

Gennser, G., and Marshal, K. Maternal smoking and fetal breathing movements. *Am. J. Obstet. Gynecol.* 120:861, 1975.

Giacoia, G. P., and Yaffee, S. J. Drugs and the perinatal patient. In Avery, G. B. (Ed.). *Neonatology: Pathophysiology and Management of the Newborn.* Philadelphia: Lippincott, 1975.

Goodwin, J. W., Dunne, J. T., and Thomas, B. W. Antepartum identification of the fetus at risk. *Can. Med. Assoc. J.* 101:458, 1969.

Gravecki, F. M., and Ponate, R. S. Drugs used in pregnancy. *Nebraska Med. J.* 60:348, 1975.

Griess, F. C. Obstetric anesthesia. *Am. J. Nurs.* 71:67, 1971.

Guidelines for Perinatal Care. American Academy of Pedratrics and American College of Obstetricians and Gynecologists, 1983.

Haslam, R. R. et al. Hemorrhage in a neonate possibly due to maternal ingestion of salicylates. *J. Pediatr.* 84:556, 1974.

Hervada, A. R. Nursery evaluation of the newborn. *Am. J. Nurs.* 67:1669, 1967.

Hey, E. M., and Katz, G. The optimal thermal environment for naked babies. *Arch. Dis. Child.* 45:335, 1970.

Hill, R. M. et al. Infants exposed in utero to antiepileptic drugs, a prospective study. *Am. J. Dis. Child.* 127:645, 1974.

Hill, R. M. Will this drug harm the unborn infant? *Southern Med. J.* 76:1476, 1974.

Hobel, C. J., Hyvarinen, M. A., Okada, D. M., and Oh, W. Prenatal and intrapartum high risk screening *Am. J. Obstet. Gynecol.* 117:1, 1973.

Hypoglycemia in the Newborn. The National Foundation-March of Dimes, 1976.

Jaaskelainen, M. K., and Saxon, L. Maternal influenza, drug consumption and congenital defects of the C.N.S. *Am. J. Obstet. Gynecol.* 118:815, 1974.

Jones, K. L., and Smith, D. W. Recognition of the fetal alcohol syndrome in early infancy. *Lancet* 1:1267, 1973.

Kanto, W. P., Jr. Dealing with respiratory distress. *Emerg. Med.* October, 1977, p. 67.

Karlsson, K., and Kjellmer, I. The outcome of diabetic pregnancies in relation to the mother's blood sugar level. *Am. J. Obstet. Gynecol.* 112:213, 1972.

Kilderberg, P., and Winters, R. Infant feeding and blood acid-base status. *Pediatrics* 49:801, 1972.

Klaus, M., and Fanaroff, A. *Care of the High-Risk Neonate, 2nd.* Philadelphia: Saunders, 1979.

Korones, S. B. *High Risk Newborn Infants: The Basis for Intensive Nursing Care, 3rd.* St. Louis: Mosby, 1981.

Levy, E., Cohen, A., and Fraser, F. C. Hormone treatment during pregnancy and congenital heart defects. *Lancet* 2:323, 1970.

Lewis, O. The culture of poverty. *Sci. Am.* 215:21, 1966.

LoPresti, J. M., and Altman, R. P. Meconium ileus: Operative therapy and pulmonary complications in the newborn. *Clin. Proc. Child Hosp.* 28:221, 1972.

Lubchenco, L. O. et al. Infections in the newborn. In Kempe, C. H., et al. (Eds.). *Current Pediatric Diagnosis and Treatment, 3rd.* Los Altos, Calif.: Lange Medical Publications, 1974.

Lubchenco, L. O. et al. Intra-uterine growth in length of head circumference as estimated from live births at gestational ages from 26–42 weeks. *Pediatrics* 37:403, 1966.

McLean, F. H. Assessing gestational age. *Can. Nurse* 68:23, 1972.

Mandelkorn, T., and Alden, E. R. Morbidity and mortality of infants weighing less than 1000 grams in an intensive care nursery. *Pediatrics* 50:40, 1972.

Mann, L. I. Effects of alcohol on fetal cerebral function and metabolism. *Am. J. Obstet. Gynecol.* 120: 845, 1976.

Manning, F., Wyn Pugh, E., and Boddy, K. Effect of cigarette smoking on fetal breathing movements in normal pregnancies. *Br. Med. J.* 1:552, 1975.

Manning, F. A., and Feyerabend, C. Cigarette smoking and fetal breathing movements. *Br. J. Obstet. Gynecol.* 83:262, 1976.

Meyer, M. S., Jonas, B. S., and Tonascia, J. A. Perinatal events associated with maternal smoking during pregnancy. *Am. J. Epidem.* 103:464, 1976.

Mirkin, B. L. Dyphenylhydantoin placental transport, fetal localization, neonatal metabolism and possible teratogenic effects. *J. Pediatr.* 78:329, 1971.

Mirkin, B. L. Drug therapy and the developing human ... Who cares? *Hosp. Form.* 10:530, 1975.

Moore, M. L. *The Newborn and the Nurse.* Philadelphia: Saunders, 1972.

Morgan, B. Incidence, etiology and classification of congenital heart disease. *Pediat. Clin. North Am.* 25:4, 1978.

Moya, F., and Smith, B. E. Uptake, distribution, and placental transport of drugs and anesthetics. *Anesthesiology* 26:465, 1965.

Naeye, R. Relation of poverty and race to antenatal infection. *N. Engl. J. Med.* 283:555, 1970.

Nelson, M., and Forfar, J. Association between drugs administered during pregnancy and congenital abnormalities in the fetus. *Br. Med. J.* 1:523, 1971.

Neonatal Thermoregulation. The National Foundation-March of Dimes, 1976.

Nitowsky, H. Prenatal diagnosis of genetic abnormality. *Am. J. Nurs.* 71:1551, 1971.

Noblett, H. R. Treatment of uncomplicated meconium ileus by Gastrografin enema, a preliminary report. *J. Pediatr. Surg.* 4:190, 1969.

Obstetrics, Gynecologic and Neonatal Functions and Standards. The Nurses Association of the American College of Obstetricians and Gynecologists, 1974.

Osward, D. F., Phibbes, R., and Fox, J. S. Diagnostic use of infant cry. *Biol. Neonate* 13:68, 1968.

Parmalee, A. H., Wenner, W. H., and Schulz, H. R. Infant sleep patterns: From birth to 16 weeks of age. *J. Pediatr.* 65:577, 1964.

Parmalee, A. H. Sleep cycles in infants. *Devel. Med. Child Neurol.* 2:794, 1969.

The Pediatric Clinics of North America, 17:1, 1970.

Pierog, S., and Ferrara, A. *Medical Care of the Sick Newborn, 2nd.* St. Louis: Mosby, 1976.

Pildes, R. S. Management of acute metabolic problems in the neonate. In Aladjem, S. (Ed.). *Perinatal Intensive Care.* St. Louis: Mosby, 1977.

Pildes, R. et al. A prospective controlled study of neonatal hypoglycemia. *Pediatrics* 54(1):5–14 (July), 1974.

Pipes, P. *Nutrition in Infancy and Childhood.* St. Louis: Mosby, 1977.

Poland, R., and Ostra, E. Neonatal hyperbilirubinemia. In Klaus, M., and Fanaroff, A. *Care of the High-risk Neonate.* Philadelphia. Saunders, 1979.

Prichard, J. S. The character and significance of epileptic seizures in infancy. *Neurologic and Encephalographic Correlative Studies in Infancy.* New York: Grune & Stratton, 1964.

Rajegouda, B. K. et al. Methadone withdrawal in newborn infants. *J. Pediatr.* 81:532, 1972.

Randolph, J. G., and Altman, P. Surgery in the neonate. In Avery, G. B. (Ed.) *Neonatology: Pathophysiology and Management of the Newborn.* Philadelphia: Lippincott, 1975.

Reed, B., Sutorius, J., and Coen, R. Management of the infant during labor, delivery, and the immediate neonatal period. *Nurs. Clin. North Am.,* 6:3, 1971.

Rowe, M., Seagram, I., and Weinberger, M. Gastrografin-induced hypertonicity: The pathogenesis of a neonatal hazard. *Am. J. Surg.* 125:185, 1973.

Rudolph, A. M. *Pediatrics, 17th.* Norwalk, Conn.: Appleton-Century-Crofts, 1982.

Sahin, S. The multifaceted role of the nurse as genetic counselor. *Am. J. Mat. Child Nurs.* (July/August) 1976, p. 211.

Savory, J., and Monif, G. R. G. Serum calcium levels in cord sera of the progeny of mothers treated with magnesium sulfate for toxemia of pregnancy. *Am. J. Obstet. Gynecol.* 110:556, 1971.

Shinder, S. M., and Way, E. L. Plasma levels of lidocaine in mother and newborn following obstetrical conduction anesthesia. *Clin. Applic. Anesth.* 29:951, 1968.

Shor, V. Congenital cardiac defects: Assessment and case-finding. *Am. J. Nurs.* (February) 1978.

Siker, E. S., Wolfson, B., Stewart, W. D., et al. Placental transfer of methoxyfluorane. *Br. J. Anesth.* 40:588, 1968.

Silver, H., Kempe, C. H., and Bruyn, H. B. *Handbook of Pediatrics, 10th.* Los Altos, Calif.: Lange, 1973.

Silverman, W., and Parke, P. C. Keep him warm. *Am. J. Nurs.* 65(10):81, 1965.

Simpson, J. L., and Gerbie, A, B. The impact of genetics on perinatal intensive care. In Aladjem, S., and Brown, A. *Perinatal Intensive Care.* St. Louis: Mosby, 1977.

Sinclair, J. Heat production and thermoregulation in the small-for-date infant. *Pediatr. Clin. North Am.,* 17:147, 1970.

Smith, S. E. Drugs and pregnancy. *Nurs. Times* 71:1948, 1975.

Speck, W. et al. Neonatal infections. In Klaus, M., and Fanaroff, A. *Care of the High-risk Neonate.* Philadelphia: Saunders, 1979.

Stahlman, M. Acute respiratory disorders in the newborn. In Avery, G. B. (Ed.). *Neonatology: Pathophysiology and Management of the Newborn.* Philadelphia: Lippincott, 1975.

Standards for Obstetric-Gynecologic Services, 6th. American College of Obstetricians and Gynecologists, 1985.

Stanley, K. et al. Local regional anesthesia during childbirth: Effect of newborn behaviors. *Nurs. Digest.* 4:26, 1976.

Sureau, C. The stress of labor. In Aladjem, S., and Brown, A., *Clinical Perinatology.* St. Louis: Mosby, 1974.

Sweet, A. Classification of the low birthweight infant. In Klaus, M., and Fanaroff, A. (Eds.). *Care of the High-risk Neonate.* Philadelphia: Saunders, 1979.

Thomas, J. B. *Introduction to Human Embryology.* Philadelphia: Lea and Febiger, 1968.

Van Vunakis, H., Langone, J. J., and Milunsky, A. Nicotine and cotinine in the amniotic fluid of smokers in the second trimester of pregnancy. *Am. J. Obstet. Gynecol.,* 120:64, 1974.

Vidyasagar, D. Respiratory failure and ventilatory assistance. In Aladjem, S., and Brown, A. (Eds.). *Perinatal Intensive Care.* St. Louis: Mosby, 1977.

Waechter, E. H., and Blake, F. G. *Nursing Care of Children.* Philadelphia: Lippincott, 1976.

Wennberg, H. What to do when the infant is jaundiced. *Med. Times* 99(11):172, 1971.

Yaffe, S. J., and Juchau, M. R. Perinatal pharmacology. *Annual Rev. Pharmacol.* 14:219, 1974.

Yashiro, K. et al. Preliminary studies on the thermal environment of low-birth-weight infants. *J. Pediatr.* 82:991, 1973.

Young, E., Killam, A., and Greene, J. Disseminated herpes virus infection: Association with primary genital herpes in pregnancy. *JAMA* 103:2731, 1976.

V Management of the Postpartal Period

24

The Normal Puerperium

The postpartal period is the time from the delivery of the placenta and membranes (marking the end of the intrapartal period) to the return of the woman's reproductive tract to its nonpregnant condition. Note that this is to the nonpregnant, not prepregnant, condition as is often said erroneously. The prepregnant condition is gone forever — the most strikingly so after the first pregnancy and childbirth experience but also true with each subsequent experience in relation to the prepregnant state of the organs each time.

This period also is called the puerperium, and the woman progressing through the puerperium is called a puerpera. The puerperium lasts approximately 6 weeks.

DATA BASE OF THE PUERPERIUM

The components of the data base for determining the well-being of the postpartal woman are as follows:

1. Continuing evaluation of any significant findings or developments during the ante-partal and intrapartal periods.
2. Evaluation of the physiologic and anatomic changes of the puerperium.
3. Evaluation of the woman's vital signs and other physical signs, symptoms, and changes.
4. Evaluation of the woman's behavioral changes and psychologic responses to childbearing.
5. Continued screening for signs and symptoms of obstetric or medical complications. See Chapters 9 and 14 for the data base necessary to do this screening.

In order to evaluate any of the components of the data base that is collected you must know what the parameters of normal are for the specific pieces of information obtained for each component.

Physiologic and Anatomic Changes of the Puerperium

Although the term involution has been used at times to refer to the retrogressive changes taking place in all of the organs and structures of the reproductive tract, it is more often meant to refer specifically to the retrogressive changes in the uterus that lead to its reduction in size. For the sake of clarity it is best to limit the definition of puerperal involution to the uterus and simply refer to what happens to all other involved bodily organs and structures as "changes."

Uterus

Involution of the uterus involves the reorganization and shedding of the decidua/endometrium and the exfoliation of the placental site as evidenced by the decrease in size and weight and change in location of the uterus and by the color and amount of the lochia. The amount of lochia and the rapidity of involution are not affected by the administration of a series of ergot preparation (Ergotrate, Methergine). Involution is hastened if the mother is breast-feeding.

The decidua remaining inside the uterus after separation and expulsion of the placenta and the membranes consists of the zona basalis layer and a portion of the zona spongiosa layer of the decidua basalis (at the placental site) and the decidua parietalis (lining the remainder of the uterus). This remaining decidua reorganizes into two layers as the result of invasion by leukocytes: a degenerating, necrotic, superficial layer, which will be cast off as part of the lochial discharge, and a healthy, functional, deep layer next to the myometrium. The latter layer consists of the remnants of the basilar endometrial glands in the zona basalis layer, from which will come regeneration of the endometrium by proliferation of the epithelium of these glands. Regeneration of the endometrium is completed by the middle or end of the third postpartal week except at the placental site.

Complete regeneration of the endometrium at the placental site takes approximately 6 weeks. This is accomplished by inward extension of the proliferating epithelium from the sides of the site, from the surrounding uterine lining, and from beneath the placental site from the remnants of the basilar endometrial glands in the decidua basalis. This growth of endometrium, in effect, undermines the thrombosed blood vessels at the site, causing them to slough and be cast off in the lochial discharge. Thus, the uterine lining is renewed without being functionally crippled from scarring.

The uterus, immediately after delivery of the baby, placenta, and membranes, weighs approximately 1100 grams (2 pounds 7 ounces) and is approximately 15 × 12 × 8 to 10 centimeters in length, width, and thickness, respectively. This is roughly about two to three times the size of the nonpregnant, multiparous uterus. Subsequently, the uterus weighs approximately 500 grams by the end of the first postpartal week, 300 to 350 grams by the end of the second postpartal week, 100 grams by the sixth postpartal week, and its usual nonpregnant weight of 70 grams by the eighth week postpartum.

This rapid decrease in size is reflected in the changing location of the uterus as it descends out of the abdomen and again returns to being a pelvic organ. Immediately after delivery the top of the fundus is approximately two-thirds to three-fourths of the way up between the symphysis pubis and the umbilicus. It then rises to the level of the umbilicus within a few hours. It remains at approximately the level of, or one finger-breadth below, the umbilicus for a day or two and then gradually descends into the pelvis, being abdominally nonpalpable above the symphysis pubis after the tenth day. While there is individual variation of the location of the umbilicus in relation to the symphysis pubis and individual variation in the breadth of the fingers from examiner to examiner, thereby creating a range of normal in the descent and daily location of the fundal height, there is enough similarity to allow the generalization of uterine descent as illustrated in Figure 24-1.

Any time the top of the fundus is above the

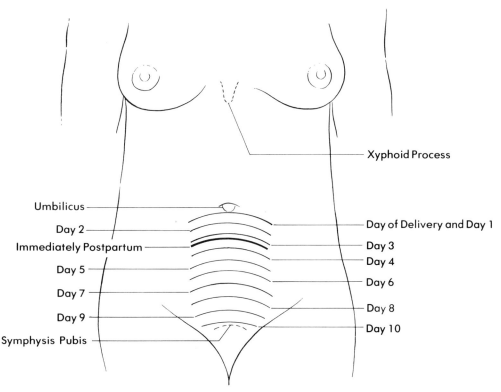

FIGURE 24-1. Fundal height and uterine involution.

umbilicus, the following should be considered: filling of the uterus with blood or blood clots in the early postpartal hours or displacement of the uterus by a distended bladder at any time postpartal (especially if also displaced to the right upper quadrant).

The reduction in the size of the uterus does not decrease the number of muscle cells. Instead, each cell has a dramatic decrease in size as it rids itself of excess cellular material. How this is done is not known.

The large uterine blood vessels of pregnancy are no longer needed because such a rich blood supply for a large area is not applicable for the nonpregnant uterus. These blood vessels degenerate and become obliterated with resorption of the hyaline deposits. They are thought to be replaced by the development of new blood vessels with smaller lumina.

Immediately after delivery the cervix is extremely soft, flabby, and floppy. It may be bruised and edematous, especially anteriorly if there was an anterior lip in labor. It looks congested, reflecting its great vascularity. It assumes a loose form and readily admits two to three fingers. It regains some of its form within the first day and becomes less soft. The cervix continues to admit two fingers for about a week but thereafter admits one finger with difficulty, and even it is stopped now at the internal os. The external os has assumed its nonpregnant form by the fourth postpartal week. This form is determined by parity and the presence of lacerations.

The broad and round ligaments, which accompanied the uterus during its increase in size, are now lax as a result of the extreme stretching. This accounts for the easy displacement of the postpartal uterus by the bladder. By the end of the puerperium the ligaments have regained their nonpregnant length and tension.

Lochia

Lochia is the name given to the uterine discharge that escapes vaginally during the puerperium. As it changes color it changes its descriptive name: rubra, serosa, and alba. Lochia rubra is red because it contains blood. It is the first lochia that starts immediately after delivery and continues for the first 2 to 3 days postpartum. Lochia rubra contains primarily blood and decidual tissue.

Lochia serosa is the next lochia. It starts as a paler version of lochia rubra and is serous and pink. It ends approximately 7 to 8 days later as a pink-yellow-white color as it makes the transition into becoming lochia alba. Lochia serosa contains primarily serous fluid, decidual tissue, leukocytes, and erythrocytes.

Lochia alba is the last lochia; it starts about the tenth postpartum day and dwindles to nothing in another week or so. It is creamy white and consists primarily of leukocytes and decidual cells.

Lochia has a characteristic odor not unlike that of menstruation. This odor is strongest in the lochia serosa. It is made still stronger if mixed with perspiration and must be carefully differentiated from a foul odor indicative of infection.

Lochia begins as a heavy discharge in the early postpartum hours. Subsequently it decreases to a moderate amount as lochia rubra, a small amount as lochia serosa, and a scant amount as lochia alba. It is common for a woman to have a small amount of lochia while lying down and to flood when she gets out of bed. This occurs because the discharge pools in the upper vaginal vault in the recumbent position and then drains out of the vagina with the positional change of standing up. This positional change affects the direction of the vagina in relationship to the pull of gravity. Pooling may cause some clotting, particularly on the day of delivery. The average total amount of lochial discharge is approximately eight to nine ounces (240 to 270 milliliters).

Vagina and Perineum

The immediate postdelivery vagina remains quite stretched, may have some degree of edema and bruising, and gapes open at the introitus. In a day or so it regains enough tone that it does not gape so widely and is no longer edematous. It is now smooth-walled, larger than usual, and generally lax. Its size decreases with return of the vaginal rugae by about the third postpartal week. It will always be a little larger than it was prior to the first childbirth. However, perineal muscle tightening exercises will restore its tone and enable deliberate tightening of the vagina to considerable degree at will. This can be accomplished by the end of the puerperium with daily practice.

The torn hymen heals by scar formation, leaving several tissue tags called myrtiform caruncles (carunculae myrtiformes).

Abrasions and lacerations of the vulva and perineum heal readily, including those needing repair. (See Chapter 60.)

Breasts

Lactation is normally and naturally initiated in all puerperal women unless effectively prohibited by a lactation suppressant. For breastfeeding mothers there are two physiological mechanisms involved: (1) the production of the milk and (2) the secretion, or let-down, of the milk. For those women who do not breastfeed and either do not receive a lactation suppressant or receive one that fails in its action, only the first mechanism of milk production will be initiated. The let-down reflex is activated by the baby's sucking at the breast.

The neurohormonal physiology of milk production is not completely understood. It is thought, however, that the placenta with its high concentration of estrogen and progesterone inhibits the production of prolactin, which is essential for lactation. This would explain why the woman does not produce milk throughout her pregnancy. The effect of the increased levels of estrogen and progesterone during pregnancy does have a preparatory effect because these hormones are responsible for the hypertrophy of the alveoli and lobules (primarily by progesterone) and of the ductal system (by estrogen).

There is a sudden dramatic fall in the estrogen and progesterone levels at the time of delivery of the placenta. This allows the anterior pituitary to produce prolactin. Whether this is a direct action on the pituitary gland or, more likely, an effect on the hypothalamus to inhibit its release of prolactin-inhibiting factor, is not known. It is thought that the hypothalamus constantly releases a prolactin-inhibiting factor that controls the release of prolactin from the pituitary. This action of the hypothalamus, thus, must be suppressed in order for prolactin to be released and lactation initiated by its action on the acini (secretory) cells lining the alveoli. After initiation of lactation, its subsequent continuation is dependent on the suckling stimulus of the baby to the breast. The release of prolactin-inhibiting factor is suppressed by the suckling stimulus. This allows for the increased, or continuing, release of prolactin from the anterior pituitary.

·The secretion, or let-down, of the milk is an exquisite blend of neurologic, hormonal, and psychologic factors in which the latter can totally inhibit and frustrate the others and also frustrate the baby and mother. This has the potential of becoming a vicious cycle — the more frustrated the mother the greater the inhibition of the let-down reflex. Any negative emotions will inhibit this mechanism (e.g., fear, anger, embarrassment, anxiety) as will the presence of pain.

The expulsion of milk from the alveoli through the ducts to the lactiferous sinuses (see Fig. 24-2) is initiated by the baby's sucking, which stimulates the production of oxytocin by the posterior pituitary. Oxytocin enters the circulating blood which in the breasts causes the contraction of the myoepithelial cells surround-

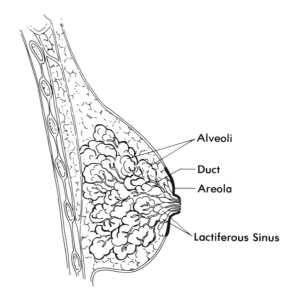

FIGURE 24-2.   Anatomy of the lactating breast.

ing the alveoli and ducts. The contraction of these cells expels the milk out of the alveoli, through the ductiles, to the lactiferous (storage) sinuses where it is now readily accessible to the baby by compression of the sinuses as the baby sucks. The sucking propels the milk the final distance through the lactiferous ducts into the baby's mouth. The movement of milk from the lactiferous sinuses is called the let-down and is felt by the woman as a specific event. Eventually the let-down can be triggered without the actual sucking of the baby, by the mother's simply hearing a baby cry or thinking about the baby. This again points out the influence of the emotions on this mechanism. In such an event the milk may stream from the breasts and leak onto the mother's clothing. As the milk demand and supply stabilizes and lactation is well established, this profuse ejection of milk from the breasts is less apt to happen.

The let-down is essential to successful breast-feeding. Without it the baby can suck and suck but will obtain only a fraction of the milk potentially available in the breast. Should this failure of let-down occur repeatedly, with subsequent failure to empty the breasts, the carefully orchestrated mechanism will be out of balance and cease to function and lactation will end.

The first substance the baby obtains from the mother's breasts after delivery is colostrum. This is immensely valuable to the baby. It contains twice as much protein as the later milk, supplies antibodies to innumerable viral and bacterial diseases, and has a milk laxative effect which facilitates the passage of meconium. Colostrum is slightly thick, sticky, and of a yellowish color because it contains fat globules. The milk "comes in," on the average, by the third to fifth postpartum day. The production of milk is much more rapid if the woman has done the breast preparation exercises of massage, manual expression, and nipple rolling (see Chapter 48); was able to breast-feed the baby within the hour of birth; and was able to have the baby suckle frequently thereafter. In such an event the milk will most likely come in 24 to 48 hours.

Colostrum gradually converts to milk that is somewhat thin, has a sweet taste, and is bluish in color. Milk also contains antibodies and gives immunity to a number of diseases. It is often called the ideal food for babies.

Vital Signs and Other Physical Signs, Symptoms, and Changes

Vital Signs

The *blood pressure* should be stabilized within the realm of normal.

The *temperature* should return to normal from its slight elevation during the intrapartal period and become stabilized within the first 24 hours postpartum. (See "Puerperal Morbidity" and "Differential Diagnosis" under "Puerperal Infection" in Chapter 25 for definition and possible interpretations of any temperature elevations after the first 24 hours and for a discussion of temperature elevation associated with dehydration during the first 24 hours postpartum.)

The *pulse* rate should be within the realm of normal during the puerperium unless affected by a prolonged and difficult labor or by an excessive blood loss. Any pulse rate above 100 during the puerperium is abnormal and may be indicative of infection or delayed postpartal hemorrhage (see Chapter 25). Some women may have what is called a puerperal bradycardia. This occurs immediately after birth and may extend into the early postpartal hours. Such women may have a pulse rate as low as 40 to 50 beats per minute. Any number of reasons have been given as possible causes, but none has been proven. Its only significance is that it is not a harbinger or indication of disease but, rather, a sign of well-being.

Respirations should be within the realm of normal.

Renal System Changes

The renal pelves and ureters, which were stretched and dilated during pregnancy, return to normal by the end of the fourth postpartal week.

Immediately postpartum the bladder is edematous, congested, and hypotonic, which may result in overdistention, incomplete emptying, and excessive urine residual unless care is taken to encourage periodic voiding even when the woman does not feel like it. Rarely is the urethra obstructed but it is insensitive by virtue of trauma during labor. Unless a urinary tract infection develops, the effects of trauma during labor on the bladder and urethra diminish within the first 24 postpartal hours.

Approximately 40 percent of postpartal women have nonpathologic proteinuria from immediately postdelivery to up to the second day postpartum. To be valid the specimen must be obtained as a clean-catch specimen or from catheterization in order not to be contaminated by the protein-laden lochia. A nonpathologic condition of proteinuria can be assumed only in the absence of signs and symptoms of a urinary tract infection or pre-eclampsia.

There is considerable diuresis starting shortly after delivery and lasting up to the fifth day postpartum. The urine output may be more than 3000 milliliters per day. This is thought to be one of the means the body uses in ridding itself of the increased extracellular water (interstitial fluid) that is a normal part of pregnancy. Other routes are used also and this is the explanation for a rather profuse perspiration that may occur during the early postpartum days.

Weight Loss

Women lose an average of approximately 12 pounds at the time of delivery. This loss represents the accumulated weight of the baby, placenta, and amniotic fluid. Another 5 pounds is lost during the first postpartal week as a result of fluid loss, largely through diuresis. Most women have returned to their prepregnant weight by the end of the puerperium.

Gastrointestinal Changes

Women cared for by nurse-midwives frequently are hungry and ready for a regular (or special) meal of their choice an hour or two after delivery.

Constipation may be a problem in the early puerperium due to lack of solid foods during labor and self-restraint in defecation. The woman may practice self-restraint because her perineum is sore or because she lacks knowledge and is afraid she will rip open and tear out her stitches if she has a bowel movement.

Abdominal Wall

The abdominal striae are never eradicated completely but they do change to fine, silvery-white lines.

The abdominal walls are flabby after delivery because of their stretching during pregnancy. All puerperal women have some degree of diastasis recti, which is the separation of the rectus muscles of the abdomen. How severe this diastasis is depends on a number of factors including the woman's general condition and muscle tone, whether the woman exercised faithfully to regain her abdominal muscle tone and close the diastasis after each pregnancy, her parity (regaining complete muscle tone becomes increasingly difficult with increasing parity), the rapidity of her pregnancies (whether or not there was time for her to regain her muscle tone before being into another pregnancy), and pregnancies that have overdistended her abdomen (e.g., multiple gestation). These factors also determine how long it will take her to regain her muscle tone. It takes longer to regain muscle tone from a diastasis that is 5 fingerbreadths wide than it does from a diastasis that is 2 fingerbreadths wide. In the latter instance, it is possible to have closed the diastasis by the end of the puerperium. (See "Diastasis" under "Postpartal Abdominal Examination" in Chapter 41 for how to evaluate, measure, and motivate a woman to exercise in relation to diastasis recti.) If abdominal wall muscle tone is not regained, the space between the rectus muscles fills in with peritoneum, fascia, and fat. Subsequent pregnancies then do not have the necessary muscle support, which accounts for the pendulous abdomen often seen in multiparas. This condition may lead to extreme back pain for the woman and difficulties with fetal engagement at the time of labor and delivery.

Hematologic Changes

The leukocytosis which elevated the white blood cell count to 15,000 during labor remains elevated for the first couple of days postpartum. It may further increase to 25,000 to 30,000 without being pathologic if the woman had a prolonged labor. However, the various types of possible infections should be ruled out in the presence of such a finding.

The hemoglobin, hematocrit, and erythrocyte count vary widely in the early puerperium as a result of vacillating blood volume, plasma volume, and red cell volume levels. This, in essence, renders the hematocrit ineffective as an evaluative measure of blood loss for at least

2 to 4 days postpartum. However, there is a rule of thumb that says if the hematocrit in the first day or two postpartum is lower by two or more percentage points than the hematocrit done upon entry into labor, there has been a sizable blood loss. Roughly two percentage points is the equivalent of a unit (500 milliliters) of blood loss. There is a reduction of approximately 1500 milliliters in total blood volume during delivery and the puerperium. Of this, approximately 200 to 500 milliliters is lost during delivery, another 500 to 800 milliliters during the first postpartal week, and the last 500 milliliters over the remainder of the puerperium.

Normal nonpregnant levels for all the constituents of the blood are reached by the end of the puerperium.

Behavioral Changes and Psychologic Response to Childbearing

Postpartum Blues

Postpartum (after baby) blues are largely a psychologic phenomenon of the woman who is separated from her family and from her baby. This happens most often in hospitals with rigid visiting policies, inflexible nursery policies, and no provision for rooming-in. In such a situation, early discharge decreases the incidence and severity of postpartum blues.

There is also a physiologic basis for postpartum blues. The rapid hormonal changes taking place as the body returns to a nonpregnant state and as the lactation cycle is either established or suppressed have been implicated as a causative factor of the labile emotions characteristic of postpartum blues. The labile emotions are also enhanced by any physical discomforts (e.g., after-birth pains, stitch pain) and lack of sleep.

Postpartum blues usually occur around the third to fifth day postpartum. They range from a mild form of feeling "down," through being easily upset and unexplainably sad, to frequent bouts of crying for reasons the woman is generally unable to articulate. Postpartum blues should not be confused with either maternal rejection or postpartum psychosis.

There is a real sense of physical loss experienced by the woman after birth. This may result in a grief process which would explain some of the depression and its manifestations the woman may have. She has lived intimately with her baby for approximately 9 months, of which she was fully aware of the baby's presence inside her body for approximately 5 months. She has lived with internal movements, turnings, and kicks; fetal quiet periods and active periods; and having to adapt her dietary patterns, clothes, and self-image to the growing baby inside her. Abruptly this living presence inside her is gone and she experiences a real sense of loss, which she may express as feeling "empty." Immediate and continuing contact with her baby, with the physical closeness this involves, is most effective in easing this loss.

The woman may also feel the loss of center-stage status. Throughout her pregnancy she has been the center of attention, with most comments directed to her and numerous questions asked about how she was feeling, what she was thinking, what she was eating, wearing, planning, and so forth. Again abruptly, her baby is now the center of attention. Hospital visitors go to the nursery; ooh, aah, and coo; talk about who the baby looks like and who the baby was named after; and bring presents for the baby. Seldom does a new mother receive a gift that is solely for her, and it is almost unheard of that the new father receives a gift. Yet what a difference such thoughtfulness and recognition can make in the self-concept and image of these new parents at the time they are assuming their role and responsibilities of nurturing and parenting. Again, there is a grief process due to a perceived loss of attention and caring. Childbearing which does not separate the woman from her family and in which family members remain caretakers largely mitigates such a reaction.

The processes involved in postpartum blues leave the woman extremely vulnerable to feelings of insecurity and inadequacy in her new role as a mother. This compounds any lack of self-confidence and makes the woman overly sensitive to any comments or behavior she interprets as critical of her abilities to care for her child. Her self-confidence is enhanced with continuing doses of genuine praise for any and all accomplishments in her handling and caring for her baby. Most importantly, the experienced caretaker (nurse, grandmother, sister, whoever) will achieve more by working through the mother rather than taking direct care of the baby. Nothing deflates an inexperienced, awkward new mother more than watching a skilled, confident nurse doing routine caretaking of her baby (e.g., diapering, bathing, dressing). It is far more helpful to assist the mother in her own efforts in caretaking.

Grief

Grief is the psychologic response an individual has to loss. Grief process consists of the identified stages or phases of this response. Grief work, a term coined by Lindemann [1], refers to the task of moving through the stages of the grief process to a resolution of the grief in the formation of new significant relationships. Grief is normal. Grief work is essential to keeping grief normal. Failure to do grief work, usually because of the individual's desire to avoid the intense pain and distress of grief and its full emotional expression, often leads to a morbid, or pathologic, grief reaction.

Grief varies considerably according to what the loss is and the perception and involvement of the individual with whatever is lost. "Loss" may run the gamut from the loss evolving from the cancellation of a planned-for event (e.g., a picnic, a trip, a party) to the death of a loved one. How severe a loss is depends on the perception of the individual who has suffered the loss. The degree of loss to the individual is reflected in the response to the loss. For example, a death may induce a small or large grief response, depending on the relation and involvement of an individual with the person who has died.

Maternity losses include those which involve losing the baby (abortion, miscarriage, stillbirth, giving the baby up for adoption); having a viable baby but with loss of expectations (prematurity, congenital deformities/abnormalities); or having a normal baby meeting expectations of perfection but with the act of birth precipitating the losses discussed as causative factors of postpartum blues (loss of internal intimacy with the baby, loss of attention). An important loss sometimes overlooked accompanies the change from the exclusive woman-man relationship to that of mother-father-child.

The manifestations and feelings of grief in adults are quite uniform and the process follows a definite pattern. There is, however, considerable movement between the stages of grief, with the intensity of the first and second stages diminishing as grief work is done and movement is made toward resolution.

The first stage of grief is shock, the phase of the individual's initial response to the loss (Fig. 24-3). Behavioral manifestations and feelings include the following: denial, disbelief, despair, anger, fear, anxiety, guilt, emptiness, aloneness, loneliness, sadness, isolation, numbness, crying, introversion, irrationality, hostility, hatred, bitterness, acute awareness, lack of initiative, mechanical actions, alienation, betrayal, abandonment, frustration, rebellion, and lack of concentration. Physical manifestations include waves of somatic distress lasting 20 to 60 minutes, sighing, weight loss, anorexia, fitful sleep, fatigue, restlessness, haggard and drawn appearance, tightness in the throat, choking, shortness of breath, nagging and tormenting chest pain, internal quivering, generalized weakness, and specific weakness in the legs.

The second stage of grief is suffering, the phase of reality (Fig. 24-4). Acceptance of the

For Our Emily

Sweet Emily,
in eager dreams,
in giddy accord
we wished for you.

In delicious tenderness,
in fiery loving
we made you.

In blossoming roundness,
in serene closeness
we grew you.

In joyous preparation,
in gladsome anticipation
we awaited you.

In unbelieving shock,
in agony of grief
we lost you.

And now, in wrenching sorrow,
in aching emptiness
we must part from you and learn to live
without you.

    Lois Lake Church, mother
    April 7, 1984

So much anticipation and so much joy
so much hard work and concentration
so great an effort.
Such breathing energy
such loving unity
such caring teamwork
breathing
inhale
exhale
in and out
then urgent, necessary pushing,
thrusting forth, stretching,
straining till no straw might be added.
A beautiful and magnificent effort
finally ends: through!
Triumphant!
And lovely,
O, so lovely
but absolutely silent
and terrible.

    Allan Southworth Church, father
    April 1984

FIGURE 24-3. Poems written by parents demonstrate initial response to loss. Emily was stillborn. (Used by permission of Lois Lake Church and Allan Southworth Church.)

fact of the loss and adjustment to the realities this imposes occur during this period (e.g., adjustment to the environment without the presence of the loved one, acceptance of the fact of a deformity and necessary adjustments in living and plans because of it). During this time there is preoccupation with and idealization of the lost object. The events leading to and surrounding the loss are relived over and over again. The why, what if, and how questions are repeatedly asked and entail feelings of anger, guilt, and fear, respectively. The pain of loss is felt in its totality, in prolonged reality, and in the memories each day, date, and event evoke. Full expression of emotion is essential to a healthy resolution. Crying is a common form of release. The pain of suffering comes in waves — frequently, less frequently; anticipated, unexpectedly — the intensity of the pain relinquishing with agonizing slowness. During this time life goes on as does the suffering individual's routine involvement in

---

Not Mine

Powdery scent, apricot-soft skin
of someone else's infant;
toddler-round cheeks and sturdy legs,
damp hair clinging in curls
to nape of neck —
child of another woman's body.
Father swooping his girl aloft,
voices bubbling, blending in glee —
not my husband, nor my child.
Babydoll sprawled on car's seat
— not my daughter's,
nor tiny dress of calico,
painstakingly smocked, lovingly pressed.
Not of my family, the long hair
to braid and beribbon,
the child of my gender
to nurture to womanhood.
Mine only, the big-belly memories,
mine the not-to-be-fulfilled dreams.

Lois Lake Church, mother
July 15, 1984

FIGURE 24-4. Poem by mother of recent stillborn demonstrates reality and suffering. (Used by permission of Lois Lake Church.)

it. As the individual continues to do grief work, preoccupation with the loss gradually changes to anxiety about the future.

The third stage of grief is resolution, the phase of establishing new significant relationships. During this period the loss is accepted, adjustment is completed, and the individual is again fully functional. This progress results from the individual's reinvestment of emotions into other significant relationships. Reinvestment of emotions *does not* mean that the loss has been replaced. Rather, it means that the individual is capable of reinvesting in and forming other significant relationships. With resolution the actions of the individual are by free choice whereas during suffering they were forced either by social convention or internal restlessness.

Behavioral manifestations of a morbid, or pathologic grief reaction include avoidance and distortion of normal emotional expression of grief, agitated depression, psychosomatic conditions, acquisition of the symptoms of the last illness of the deceased, activities which are detrimental to the individual's social or economic existence, lasting loss of acceptable patterns of social interaction, morbid attachment to the possessions of the deceased, and persistent loss of self-esteem.

When the maternity loss is death it is essential that the parents experience the reality of the baby's existence in order for them to then

O Emily, we wanted to show you
    the world's wonders,
    but now your sweet blue eyes
    will never see
    the glories of the sunset,
    the miracle of spring's first flowers,
    your papa's loving face.

We wanted to help you know
    the sounds we love,
    but now your tiny ears
    will never hear
    a lacy fugue of Bach,
    the morning song of birds,
    your brothers' laughter.

We wanted you to taste
    all of life's flavors,
    but now your rosebud mouth
    will never know
    the sweet milk I have for you,
    a plump juicy raspberry,
    the tang of ocean waves.

We wanted you to touch and try
    all textures and tasks,
    but now your graceful hands
    will never
    play a note of music,
    stroke a cat's fur,
    slip trustingly into mine.

Our Emily, we wanted to teach you
    how to love,
    but you already know
    the love that created you,
    the joy that nurtured you,
    the strength that birthed you,
    And these will be yours forever.

        In love and sorrow,
        your mama,
        Lois Lake Church
        April 17, 1984

accept the reality of the baby's death. Otherwise, the entire pregnancy-life-death sequence is subject only to fantasy, imagination, and a dream-mirage type of illusion which is difficult to grasp and even more difficult to accept and resolve. Women periodically fantasize about pregnancy, birthing, and parenting (regardless of whether desired or not desired) throughout life, including long before actual conception and childbearing. Conception and recognition of the fact of pregnancy (wanted or unwanted) reawaken, activate, or accentuate these fantasies. Quickening intensifies them as a living presence makes itself known. The fantasies now take on aspects of specific physical and personality characteristics of the child, dreams of parent-child interactions, and projections of the child's growth, maturity and life. Often there is family and environmental reorganization in preparation for the expected baby. Then death — and there is no solace for the grief over the now empty womb. The loss is not only the actual baby but also the loss of all the dreams and fantasies extending far into the future (Fig. 24-5). There is also a real sense of loss of part of one's self, which enhances the feeling of worthlessness to which all who grieve are vulnerable. Actions which help the parents experience the reality of the baby's existence and thus facilitate healthy grieving include seeing and touching the dead baby, naming it, and having some form of funeral and burial service.

When the maternity loss is a loss of expectations of a perfect child due to deformities or abnormalities then it is essential that the parents grieve the loss of their perfect child and all the fantasies and dreams they had in relation to their baby's expected appearance and potential (if this will also be affected). This grieving is essential in order for them to be free to accept and bond themselves to their imperfect child.

FIGURE 24-5.   Untitled poem by mother of stillborn demonstrates the loss of dreams and fantasies. (Used by permission of Lois Lake Church.)

This is a long, painful process that takes place over time. Parents of a child with anomalies also suffer loss of self-esteem during their grief process resulting from their perception that their child's imperfection reflects negatively upon themselves. Resolution includes acceptance of each family member's individual characteristics, development, and potential as separate from one's own.

Actions by health professionals which help the parents to grieve and thus facilitate their attachment to the imperfect child include providing a safe, patient, listening, noncondemning, facilitative environment for ventilation of their negative feelings and hostility toward, and rejection of, their baby as well as anger toward the hospital, health care professionals, God, themselves, and others. It is important also to accept the other behavioral manifestations of grief, such as parents' needs for repeatedly reliving and retelling their experience and feelings, and for full and accurate information. Other actions include the health professional's acceptance of the baby, recognition of the baby's individuality and other characteristics, and genuine caring for the imperfect baby. Professionals should take cues from the parents as to their readiness to care for their infant and then ensure that their initial caretaking experiences are as positive as possible. It is important to encourage and facilitate the sharing of grief, caretaking, and open communication between the parents, and to provide resources of knowledge and help for the most realistic coping with whatever the problem is insofar as the child is concerned, insofar as the parents are concerned, and insofar as any siblings are concerned. Professionals can also help the couple identify and make good use of existing family and cultural sources of support. The parents should be referred for genetic counseling if indicated.

Siblings in the home should be told the truth about the loss so they have an honest explanation of their parent's behavior. Otherwise, they may fantasize that they are the cause of a horrible, unknown problem. Siblings need to be told and assured that whatever has happened is not their fault and that they are still important, loved, and cared for.

The first major responsibility of the nurse-midwife in the event of a loss is to immediately share this information with the parents. Mothers sense instantly when something is not right at birth; there is a stillness in the room, an unnatural quietness and sadness in those attending the woman. In the event of death, there are no baby sounds. She has a right to as much information as we have — then, not later. Suppression of this information results in the cruelty of the woman's knowing something is wrong and being left to the torture of her imagination and uncertainty. Truth and reality are far more gracious.

The nurse-midwife should also encourage and create a safe environment for emotional expression of grief. This means arranging privacy and taking the time to stay with the parents, to share in their grief, to cry with them, and to listen. This is a continuing commitment to the parents and time should be planned for recurring visits to listen as they relive their experience, to provide knowledge of the grief process and of the facts pertaining to their loss, and to assess that their grieving is healthy and without manifestations of a pathological reaction.

MANAGEMENT PLAN FOR THE PUERPERIUM

Management of the puerperium includes management of the early puerperium, guidance for the remainder of the puerperium, and conducting the 4- to 6-weeks postpartum examination. Nurse-midwifery management during the puerperium includes responsibility for the following:

1. Continuing evaluation and management of the well-being of the woman

2. Relief from postpartal discomforts
3. Assistance with breast-feeding
4. Facilitation of parenting
5. Anticipatory guidance and instruction
6. Continuing screening for complications (this content may be found in Chapter 25)

Management of the first hour postpartum was covered as management of the fourth stage of labor in the intrapartal management portion of this book (Chapter 18). Management of the early puerperium refers to management of the woman while she is in the hospital after delivery or for a minimum of 1 or 2 days postpartum in nonhospital settings.

Postpartal care has often been slandered as dull, boring, and routine. Nothing could be further from the truth when you get involved in the very different experience each woman has had and is having and her needs for help, including those for instruction and guidance. When mother and baby are together this care is vitalized by the presence of the baby. This also makes teaching easier and more thorough.

Continuing Evaluation and Management of the Well-Being of the Woman

Evaluation of the Early Puerperium
During the early puerperium the woman is seen at least once daily. The following chart review, history, and physical examination are done at each visit to ascertain the woman's well-being and to screen for complications.

1. Chart review
   a. record of antepartal and intrapartal course (if not known or if this is your first visit with the woman)
   b. number of hours or days postpartum
   c. previous orders and progress notes
   d. record of temperature, pulse, respirations, and blood pressure postpartally
   e. laboratory reports
   f. medication record
   g. nurses' notes

2. History
   a. ambulation — how much? with ease? with or without assistance? any dizziness when ambulating?
   b. voiding — frequency? amount (large, average, small)? hesitancy? pain (dysuria)?

   Pain with urination must be carefully differentiated as to whether the pain or burning is before or as the urine comes out, or after it hits the "outside" (perineum). If it is the latter, it probably is due to irritation of the urine on the episiotomy or laceration repair site(s) or, in their absence, on minute abrasions, and is not a symptom of a urinary tract infection.

   c. bowel movements — number? amount? consistency?

   Because it is a common fear it is useful to also ask women who have stitches if they have any concerns about hurting themselves if they have a bowel movement. A majority of women who have not learned this before do have a fear of tearing out their stitches and ripping open with a bowel movement. Such a fear can cause real inhibition of bowel function and subsequent problems of constipation, impaction, hemorrhoids, and so forth. When asked, these women will often say that they envision their repair as one row of stitches holding everything together. Their fear is readily dispelled with a simple explanation of the layers of stitches involved in a repair (see Chapter 60) and assurance that because of this it is impossible for their fear to come true with normal rectal stretching and bearing down for a bowel movement.

   d. appetite — heartburn? nausea? vomiting?

   A lack of appetite in the hospital often is due to dislike of the food served rather than to the symptoms asked about. This needs to be differentiated.

e. any discomforts or pain? — location? when? type of pain? what relieves or aggravates the pain?

f. any concerns? — about herself? about her baby? about others?

g. any questions about anything?

h. if breast-feeding, how is the breast-feeding going for her and for her baby? reaction to her breast-feeding by significant others?

i. what does she think about her baby?

If at all possible, it is good to time one of your visits to coincide with part of the time the baby is with the mother (if she is not in rooming-in). The value of this is that it enables you to evaluate the mother-baby interaction for normality (screening out maternal rejection) and for the abilities and comfort of the mother in handling her baby, which may indicate areas of learning needs.

j. how does she feel about her labor and delivery experience?

This is probably one of the most crucial questions you can ask the mother in the early puerperium and is a subject which should be initiated and thoroughly discussed at least once during this time. It gives her the opportunity to talk out her feelings (positive and negative). It also gives you the opportunity to identify any misinformation or misconceptions she might have about the experience and to clarify and correct these.This can make all the difference in her viewpoint of her experience and residual long-range psychologic effects.

3. Physical examination

a. blood pressure, temperature, pulse

b. throat, if indicated, for any evidence of irritation or infection

c. breasts and nipples (see "Variations of the Breast Examination for the Postpartal Patient" in Chapter 40)

d. auscultation of lungs, if indicated, for sounds of an upper respiratory infection

e. abdomen — for:
(1) bladder
(2) uterus
(3) diastasis
See "Postpartal Abdominal Examination" in Chapter 41.

f. CVA tenderness — see Chapter 42; note method C

g. lochia — for:
(1) color — rubra, rubra/serosa, serosa, serosa/alba, alba, other
(2) amount.
The flow of lochia should be checked at the time of any uterine manipulation as well as by asking the woman for an accounting of the number of pads she has worn in a specified time period (such as your last visit) and how saturated they were.
(3) odor

h. perineum — for:
(1) healing:
(a) edema
(b) inflammation
(c) hematomas
(d) suppuration (pus)
(e) wound separation or dehiscence (bursting open)
(f) stitches coming out
(g) ecchymosis (bruising)
(2) hemorrhoids

Examination of the perineum requires good visualization, that is, exposure and light. The woman should be positioned with the bottom of her feet together, knees bent, and legs apart. Let her ease into this position. Pain in doing so is informative. A penlight is invaluable in checking the perineum and should be an indispensable item of equipment for making a postpartum visit. Another helpful item of equipment is a large mirror which can be positioned so the woman can see her own perineum if she so desires. This often dispels a number of fears and misconceptions.

For examining the posterior end of a repair (especially if lengthy) and the anal area for external hemorrhoids, visualization may be best, especially if the woman is obese, if the woman turns onto whichever side is more comfortable for her. Gentle separation of the buttocks then reveals and gives good exposure to the area desired.

   i. extremities — for:
      (1) varicosities
      (2) calf tenderness and heat
      (3) edema
      (4) Homan's sign
      (5) reflexes, if indicated; see Chapter 43.
Examination of the legs is easily and smoothly accomplished in the following manner. One leg at a time, the woman places her foot flat on the bed with her knee somewhat bent. Using both of your hands on either side of her leg, feel the calf for tenderness and heat. Inspect the entire leg for varicosities. Inspect and palpate for ankle and pretibial edema.

Then ask her to straighten her leg out on the bed so you can check for Homan's sign. Place one hand on her knee, applying gentle pressure in order to keep the leg straight. With your other hand, firmly dorsiflex her foot. If there is calf pain with this action the sign is positive.

Management of the Early Puerperium

The routine postpartal orders, which are signed in the labor and delivery suite and accompany the woman to the postpartal unit, vary from setting to setting. Usually they consist of some standard management items. To these may be added other orders that pertain to the individual woman and her condition. Variation between routine orders from setting to setting is due largely to variations in the realities in each setting. Each postpartal order constitutes a management decision. This will be discussed with each postpartal order in the presentation that follows. Those marked with an asterisk are most apt to be found on the routine postpartal orders in all settings.

1. Transfer to _____.

    This common order is frequently implicit and thus not found on printed routine orders for normal patients.

*2. Bedrest for _____ hours, then out of bed with assistance × _____, then ambulatory p.r.n.

    This order will vary by virtue of the intrapartal course, the mother's condition, philosophy of the clinician, type of analgesia and anesthesia, and so on. For example, a woman who had a long, difficult labor and is exhausted, who hemorrhaged, or who is still groggy from medication is the type of woman for whom the above order is written. The entire order is modified to "Ambulatory p.r.n. with assistance at first" for a woman who entered labor rested, progressed normally, is alert, and whose clinician, like herself, views childbirth as a natural process. A woman who has had spinal anesthesia will also have her order modified to include 6 to 8 hours flat in bed to prevent a spinal headache.

    Each woman should be assisted and accompanied the first time she gets up and thereafter as indicated until she feels no dizziness, weak knees, light-headedness, or any other indication that she might faint or fall. The present-day practice of early ambulation has greatly decreased the incidence of postpartal thrombophlebitis.

*3. Regular diet.

    For a patient who hemorrhaged, the diet order should be changed to "High protein, high iron diet" to facilitate tissue healing and restore iron levels.

*4. Routine perineal care.

It is vital that you know the perineal care routinely used in your setting so you can add to your orders or individual patient teaching as needed. Routine perineal care varies considerably from setting to setting, with a range from meaning essentially nothing in some settings to meaning an elaborate twice-daily washing of the perineum by a nurse using sterile equipment and technique in other settings. It may or may not include b.i.d. or t.i.d. heat lamp treatment or sitz baths or other relief measures for perineal discomfort and healing.

At its minimum, routine perineal care should include patient instruction on how to cleanse herself after defecation (i.e., wipe once per soapy disposable wipe from front to back across the stitches, rinse, pat dry from front to back), provision of supplies and equipment (e.g., paper wipes or disposable washcloths, peri-pitchers or bottles) with which to cleanse herself, and other basic related instructions such as:

a. washing her hands before and after giving herself perineal care

b. not touching her stitch area with her fingers — if uncomfortable or concerned she should either look in a hand mirror reflecting her perineum or call for help.

c. application of the perineal pad snugly enough so it won't slide back and forth with her movements yet not so snugly as to be uncomfortable

d. application and removal of the perineal pad from front to back

e. never touching the side of the perineal pad that will be worn next to her perineum

In all this instruction it behooves you at first mention of it to check the woman's understanding of what you mean by "front to back."

*5. Catheterize in _____ hours if unable to void.

Some clinicians prefer to modify this order to a request that they be notified if the woman has been unable to void in _____ number of hours. A judgment can then be made as to whether or not catheterization is really needed or can be delayed another hour or so while continued efforts are made for her to void. This judgment is based on the obvious amount of bladder distention, its effect on displacement of the uterus and subsequent amount of uterine bleeding, how much fluid intake the woman has had since her last voiding during the intrapartal period, and whether every technique for getting the woman to void has been used. Techniques include assisting her to the toilet, blowing on her thumb, blowing bubbles through a straw in a glass, running water, pouring water over her perineum, drops of peppermint oil in the toilet or bedpan, and concentrating on the relaxation part of the perineal tightening (Kegel) exercise. Catheterization is to be avoided if at all possible because of the increased risk of bladder infection with catheterization.

*6. Empirin Compound #3 every 3–4 hours p.r.n. for pain.

This is the same as APC (aspirin, phenacetin, caffeine) with codeine. Empirin Compound #3 contains 210 milligrams of aspirin, 150 milligrams of phenacetin, 30 milligrams of caffeine, and 30 milligrams of codeine. All routine postpartal orders have some order for an analgesic. Most often it is this one. If the hospital stay is longer than 2 to 3 days, this order is usually changed to Darvon or Darvon Compound at that time.

*7. Seconal 100 mg. p.o. h.s. p.r.n.

All routine postpartal orders have some order for a "sleeper." Most often it is Seconal or Nembutal, both of which are barbiturates with a maximum effect for sedation and sleep and a secondary action of a moderate effect as a tranquilizer.

*8. Milk of Magnesia 30 ml. p.o. h.s.

An order for some sort of laxative is usually found on routine postpartal orders. In settings where the woman stays 3 or more days there may also be an order for a Dulcolax suppository or an enema on the second or third postpartal day if she has not yet had a bowel movement by that time.

Fear of hurting herself or embarrassment over fecal expression during labor and delivery may now result in difficulties with having a bowel movement. Laxatives will not help if this is the problem. Rather, identification of the problem, discussion of her feelings, and sharing obstetric realities with her and how these are viewed by professionals often dramatically alleviates the problem with rather immediate results.

The other factor that must be considered before subjecting a woman to the discomfort of an enema and increased risk of contamination and infection of any perineal wounds, is the woman's normal pattern and frequency of bowel movements.

The above eight orders pertaining to where the patient is located, her ambulation, diet, perineal care, bladder, bowels, pain, and sleep are the most standard of the routine postpartal orders. Other common routine postpartal orders deal with the woman's breasts, uterus, IV, and supplementary vitamins and minerals as follows:

9. Deladumone OB 2 ml. deep IM
   or
   Tace one 72-mg. capsule p.o. b.i.d. × 2 days (or one 12-mg. capsule p.o. q.i.d. × 7 days; or two 25-mg. capsules p.o. every 6 hours × 6 doses)
   or
   No lactation suppressant, which is expressed by simply striking out the printed order if there is one or by not writing an order for a lactation suppressant if there is not a printed order for one.
   Deladumone OB 2 milliliters contains

360 milligrams of testosterone enanthate and 16 milligrams of estradiol valerate. Tace (chlorotrianisene) is an estrogenic substance of which the total amount received by the woman depends on which capsule is ordered for her for how long. On the above listed options, the total amounts are 288 milligrams, 336 milligrams, and 300 milligrams, respectively.

The management decision is whether or not to order a lactation suppressant for a woman who is not breast-feeding and, if so, which one. Factors to be considered in making these decisions include the following:

a. the clinician's judgment regarding the potential risks involved in giving estrogenic substances to a woman, (e.g., predisposition to thromboembolic disease, cancer). Deladumone OB is generally contraindicated in the same women for whom the oral contraceptive pills are contraindicated. The risk of thromboembolic disease is increased during the puerperium.

b. the woman's belief in the effectiveness of the drug. A woman who had a positive experience from a lactation suppressant with a previous birth may want one again this time.

c. the clinician's belief in the effectiveness of the drug

   Most nurse-midwives who have done postpartal home visiting have little to no faith in the effectiveness of lactation suppressants. Their observation is that instead of preventing breast engorgement as claimed, lactation suppressants more often only delay its occurrence to 1 to 1½ weeks postpartum. Thus it is rarely seen in the hospital, which lures professionals limited to hospital practice into assuming that giving a lactation suppressant has solved and eliminated breast engorgement.

   If a lactation suppressant is to be given, timing is important. Deladumone is thought to be more effective if given at the beginning of the second stage of labor or at the very least prior to the birth of the baby. Tace is given postpartally, either as the clinician's drug of choice or if Deladumone was the drug of choice but wasn't given at the proper time.

If a lactation suppressant is given, the woman should be instructed in what to do in the event of breast engorgement in case the lactation suppressant is not effective (see later in chapter).

10. Methergine (or Ergotrate) 0.2 mg. p.o. every 4 hours × 6 doses.

Some clinicians continue the ergot preparation for another 3 days on a t.i.d. basis.

Some clinicians give an ergot preparation as a routine. Others order it only if one or more of the following factors are present:
   a. some portion of the fetal membranes were retained.
   b. the uterus tends to soften and be boggy rather than firm and hard.
   c. an episode of uterine atony occurred immediately after delivery of the placenta.
   d. the woman is a grand multipara.
   e. the woman had an overdistended uterus.
   f. the woman will not have her uterus and lochia closely monitored after the first postpartal hour.

A series of ergot preparation is also given at any point during the puerperium as treatment for subinvolution.

11. Discontinue present IV when finished.

This is a routine postpartal order in settings in which starting an IV upon admission to the labor and delivery suite is a routine. In the event the IV was started for a specific reason rather than being routine or if medication has been added to the IV, frequently oxytocin, then a judgment needs to be made regarding whether the IV should be discontinued when the present fluid is finished or another amount needs to be hung (and, if so, what and at what rate). This judgment is based on whether the original reason for starting the IV still exists or if there is any further need for intravenous infusion of oxytocin.

12. Supplementary vitamins or iron, or both. Specific orders vary. The following are examples:
   a. one multivitamin capsule b.i.d.
   b. one hexavitamin tablet daily
   c. ferrous gluconate 0.3 gm. t.i.d. p.c.
   d. ferrous sulfate 300 mg. t.i.d.
   e. vitamin C 500 mg. daily

Ordering supplemental vitamins and iron depends on the general health status of the woman, trauma and tissue damage incurred during delivery, her hematologic picture upon admission to labor, and the individual clinician's philosophy regarding supplementary vitamins.

Supplementary iron is indicated if the woman hemorrhaged or entered labor with a borderline anemia (10 to 11 grams hemoglobin per 100 milliliters). Supplementary vitamin C is indicated if the woman hemorrhaged or had extensive trauma and tissue damage. Some nurse-midwives believe that supplementary vitamin C should be a routine postpartum order to facilitate wound healing and the body's repair of tissue damage.

Other postpartum orders are specific to women with special needs or conditions. These include Rh-negative women and those having postpartum discomforts or possibly developing a complication. Categorical examples follow.

13. Relief measures for postpartal discomforts. Examples include sitz baths t.i.d. p.r.n.; perineal heat lamp t.i.d. p.r.n., ice packs to perineum p.r.n.; Dulcolax suppository h.s. p.r.n.; witch hazel compresses p.r.n. (See "Relief from Postpartal Discomforts" later in this chapter.)

14. Breast care measures.

What these are will depend on whether the woman is breast-feeding or not. Some settings have routines which can be ordered as "routine breast care" or "routine breast care — breast-feeding." If not, specific measures may be ordered. Examples include:

a. ice packs to breasts p.r.n.

b. heat to breasts prior to breast-feeding

c. exposure of nipples to air for 20 minutes after each breast-feeding

d. ointment (e.g., Masse' Cream, A and D Ointment or A and D Cream, hydrous lanolin) to nipples after exposure to air

e. continuous breast support

   (See breast engorgement in "Relief from Postpartal Discomforts" and "Assistance with Breast-Feeding," both later in this chapter.)

15. Laboratory screening for complications. This is done when indicated. Examples include lochia specimen for culture and sensitivity, clean-catch urine specimen for culture and sensitivity, hemoglobin and hematocrit on the third postpartum day.

16. RhoGam studies

   RhoGam is an Rh immune globulin specific for the D antigen containing anti-D from fractionated plasma of highly sensitized humans. The fraction used is free of the hepatitis virus.

   The Rh-negative mother receives an infusion of Rh-positive blood from the fetus via the placenta during delivery. The action of RhoGam is to suppress the mother's production of antibodies in response to receipt of the Rh-positive antigen. This treatment is based on the fact that active immunity (antibody formation) is suppressed by passive immunization. The purpose for suppression of antibody production in the woman is that it is the presence of D antibodies in the mother that causes hemolytic disease of the new-born (erythroblastosis fetalis) in subsequent pregnancies.

All postpartal women who meet the following criteria should receive RhoGam:

a. she is Rh negative, specifically D and D^u negative.

b. she is not already sensitized and has D antibodies, that is, she has a negative indirect Coombs' test.

c. her baby is Rh positive, specifically D or D^u positive.

d. her baby has a negative direct Coombs' test for anti-D (this test is done on a specimen of cord blood).

If a woman meets these criteria, a cross-match is done of her red blood cells and a 1:1000 dilution of the RhoGam she is to receive (to ensure compatibility and the Rh D and D^u negative status of the woman). The RhoGam package includes the appropriate dilution vial for the dose of RhoGam in that package.

The administration of RhoGam is ordered if the cross-match shows compatibility.

17. One vial of RhoGam to be given intramuscularly within 72 hours after delivery if the mother is Rh negative and not sensitized, and if the baby is Rh positive and the direct Coombs' test is negative.

The Rh immune globulin is given within 72 hours after delivery because this was the cutoff time arbitrarily set by the original investigators for the clinical trials and the substance has been shown to be effective if given within this period of time. It is thought but not proven that it would still be effective if given even longer after delivery. The point is to administer the Rh immune globulin before antibody production begins and the woman is sensitized. The process cannot be reversed once the mother becomes sensitized. It can be prevented.

RhoGam should never be given to the infant, an Rh D or D^u positive woman, or a sensitized woman; it also should never be administered intravenously.

If a woman was given RhoGam antepartally she should receive it again postpartally to protect against sensitization from any fetomaternal bleeding which might have occurred during delivery. RhoGam should be given to all Rh-negative women who are not sensitized upon termination of their pregnancy whether they have a delivery, ectopic pregnancy, or natural or induced abortion. This process (studies and treatment) is repeated with each subsequent pregnancy. Rh immune globulins other than RhoGam are now on the market. Their use involves the same process.

18. Rubella vaccine is given to those women who had a rubella titer of less than 1:10 during the antepartal period. The question has been raised whether to give the rubella vaccine if the woman is also receiving RhoGam, because the RhoGam may suppress the formation of rubella antibodies and thereby make the vaccine ineffective. Whether or not this actually happens, however, is not known. Since there is no contraindication to giving the rubella at the same time as the RhoGam, most clinicians give the rubella vaccine in this circumstance and recheck the rubella titer at a later date to ascertain immunity. This plan is preferable to giving the rubella vaccine at a later date when there is a chance the woman may be pregnant.

Four- to Six-Weeks Postpartum Examination
Although the puerperium lasts approximately six weeks, marking the length of time it takes for the woman's reproductive tract to return to its nonpregnant condition, most experts feel it is possible to evaluate the normality and conclusion of the puerperium at four weeks postpartum. The reason for this change from the traditional 6-weeks postpartum examination is twofold. The change was made as medical professionals acknowledged the fact that most couples were not waiting six weeks as instructed before resuming sexual intercourse and as evidence grew that a small but sizable per-

centage of puerperal women are vulnerable to pregnancy before the end of the puerperium. The consensus was that initiation of a family planning method at 4 weeks postpartum would decrease to a minimum the occurrence of unplanned pregnancy so close to the termination of the previous pregnancy. Such rapid repeated pregnancies are detrimental to both the mother and the resulting baby. These factors also led professionals to send women home from the hospital with contraceptive foam or cream and condoms for protection during the remainder of their puerperium.

The 4- to 6-weeks postpartum examination consists of a complete history, physical, and pelvic examination as outlined in Chapter 3. Any available records of this pregnancy (antepartal, intrapartal, postpartal) should be reviewed. In addition, there is (1) screening for contraindications to any of the methods of family planning, (2) additional history regarding the period of time since last seen in the early puerperium to the present, and (3) additional specifics in the physical and pelvic evaluation which relate to the return of the reproductive tract and body to its nonpregnant state. This additional history and specifics in the physical and pelvic are outlined as follows.

1. Additional history
   a. number of weeks postpartum
   b. general health and well-being — rest, sleep, appetite
   c. coping ability with caring for baby and family adjustments
   d. baby — any problems, feeding, baby in for first checkup and immunizations, health
   e. family adjustments and interactions, feelings towards baby and each other
   f. resumption of sexual intercourse — number of times, contraception used (which one) or not, dyspareunia, enjoyment and satisfaction by herself and by partner, and problems
   g. family planning method desired; previous family planning methods used —

satisfaction, side effects, length of time used, why discontinued

h. calls to nurse-midwife or physician, visits to hospital emergency room or admission or readmission to hospital — why, when, diagnosis, treatment, duration, and present status of problem

i. fever, chills, cold, flu

j. breasts:
   (1) engorgement — when, how long, treatment
   (2) if breast-fed and stopped — when, why
   (3) if breast-feeding — problems, frequency, management, nipples, enjoyment, breast care

k. bladder — frequency, burning (dysuria), urgency, backache, flank pain, suprapubic pain; stress incontinence, use of Kegel exercises

l. bowel — frequency; use of laxatives, stool softeners, or enemas; problems; diarrhea; constipation; incontinence, especially if the woman had a third or fourth degree perineal laceration

m. lochia — duration of each color in sequence, odor, excessive bleeding, clots

n. resumption of menses — if yes, date, duration, amount

o. abdomen — exercises (frequency, which ones), girdle

p. legs — cramps, varicosities, pain, calf heat or tenderness

2. Additional physical and pelvic examination specifics

   a. evaluation of the breasts and nipples of a breast-feeding mother:
      (1) breasts — lactating, adequate support, symmetry or asymmetry reflecting usage.
      (2) nipples — irritation, blisters, cracks, crusts; galactorrhea elicited by palpation only is normal in all postpartal women.

   b. evaluation of the diastasis recti — measurement of separation, progress toward closure. See "Postpartal Abdominal Examination" in Chapter 41.

   c. while inspecting the external genitalia during the pelvic examination, evaluate any episiotomy and perineal, periurethral, or labial laceration repair for healing, discomfort, and artistry. Press firmly against the posterior aspect of the remnants of the hymenal ring in the incisional line and ask if this causes pain. Also ask if there has been dyspareunia if she has had sexual intercourse.

   d. evaluate her pelvic muscle tone by having her tighten around your examining fingers. Also note her ability to do the tightening and inquire about her practice of the perineal tightening (Kegel) exercise.

   e. take special note of the size of the uterus when palpating it. It may be slightly larger than the nonpregnant uterus and is described as a "4 weeks postpartal-size uterus," "6 weeks postpartal-size uterus," and the like. Larger than expected size for the number of weeks postpartum may be indicative of subinvolution. (See "Subinvolution" in Chapter 25.)

If all is within normal limits the evaluation of the woman is summarized as: "Normal ____ weeks postpartum involution." Management of the woman includes this evaluation; any necessary treatments, physician consultations, or referrals; laboratory work (urinalysis, hematocrit, Pap smear, gonorrhea culture); exercises taught; family planning method and instruction; and when she is to be seen next and for what reason.

Relief from Postpartal Discomforts

There are a number of discomforts of the puerperium. While they are considered normal, there is no reason for a woman to have to suffer with them. Each will be discussed in terms of what it is, its causes, and the measures that will give the woman relief from discomfort. Those specific only to breast-feeding mothers (nipple tenderness and cracked nipples) will be discussed in the segment in this chapter on breast-feeding.

After-Birth Pains

After-birth pains, sometimes called after-pains, can be quite painful. They are the continuing sequential contraction and relaxation of the uterus. They are much more common with increasing parity and in women who breast-feed. In the instance of increasing parity the reason for after-pains is a concomitant decrease in uterine muscle tone which causes the uterus to relax and thereby subjects it to recontraction. This is in contrast to the primipara, whose uterine muscle tone is good and whose uterus simply stays essentially contracted without intermittent relaxation. In the instance of breast-feeding women the suckling of the baby stimulates the production of oxytocin by the posterior pituitary. The release of oxytocin not only triggers the let-down reflex in the breasts but also causes the uterus to contract — even the well-contracted uterus of a primipara will contract even more.

The basis for relief of after-birth pains is a continuously well-contracted uterus. The key to effective relief from after-birth pains is an empty bladder. No matter what else you do, if the woman's bladder is not empty, your treatment will be ineffective. The reason for this is the fact that a full bladder displaces the uterus from its normal and proper position. When the uterus is so displaced it is unable to contract as well as it should and it tends to relax, thus prohibiting relief from after-birth pains. Sometimes after-birth pains are totally relieved just by the act of emptying the bladder, especially in a para 1 or 2.

Once the bladder is empty the woman lies prone or, even better, prone with a pillow under her lower abdomen. The prone position places constant pressure against her uterus (the pillow creates even greater pressure) which keeps it contracted and thus eliminates after-birth pains since there is no uterine relaxation. The woman needs to be forewarned that when she first lies on her stomach she will have severe cramps or pain for about 5 minutes before she experiences complete and total relief.

Analgesia can be effective with after-birth pains but not very effective or for very long if the woman's bladder is not emptied. For non-breast-feeders, analgesia generally is not needed because the prone position usually alleviates the after-birth pains of even a grand multipara. However, breast-feeding mothers cannot feed their babies while in a prone position and may need some analgesia. It is important to remember that the let-down essential to breast-feeding is inhibited by pain. The amount of analgesia that gets into the milk will not hurt the baby.

Excessive Perspiration

Excessive perspiration is due to the body's using this route as well as diuresis to rid itself of the excess interstitial fluid that resulted from the normal increase in extracellular water during pregnancy. Relief is simply to keep clean and dry. The woman may want to change her gown frequently, using a hospital gown rather than her own because the former are more absorbent, readily available, and eliminate laundering problems created by multiple changes of her own gowns. Sheets should be changed as necessary. Care must also be taken to assure that the woman is hydrated. Drinking a glass of water during each hour she is awake will assure this.

Breast Engorgement

It is thought that engorgement of the breasts is due to a combination of milk accumulation and stasis and increased vascularity and congestion. This combination results in further congestion by virtue of lymphatic and venous stasis. It occurs on approximately the third postpartal day in both breast-feeding and non-breast-feeding mothers and lasts approximately 24 to 48 hours.

Signs and symptoms of engorgement include the following, which are experienced to a greater or lesser degree by individual women:

1. Woman experiences a sense of increasing breast heaviness or filling the day preceding engorgement.
2. Breasts enlarge from distention.
3. Skin becomes tight, shiny, and reddened.
4. Breasts are warm to touch.
5. Veins become visible.
6. Breasts are tender, throbbing, painful.
7. Breasts feel firm, full, hard.

Because this is not an inflammatory process there is not a temperature elevation ("breast fever" "milk fever") caused by breast engorgement as was once thought.

Relief measures depend on whether or not the woman is breast-feeding. Relief measures for a woman who is not breast-feeding are geared toward relief of discomfort and cessation of lactation. Relief measures for a woman who is breast-feeding aim for relief of discomfort and continuation of lactation. Treatment of engorgement is of particular importance to the breast-feeding mother as unrelieved breast engorgement suppresses the milk supply.

Relief Measures if Not Breast-feeding. There are four "dos" and two "do nots" in managing breast engorgement in the woman who is *not* breast-feeding. These must be taught to, and clearly understood by, the woman regardless

of whether or not she received a lactation suppressant. With the current short hospital stay many women will be home before breast engorgement occurs and need to know what to do when it happens.

The four dos are:

1. *Do give your breasts good support.* Good support is support that lifts the breasts up and in. A breast binder should be used if the woman's bra is too small for this purpose when her breasts are engorged. A breast binder is used with the understanding that it is not to bind, but to firmly support, the breasts. If a binder is not available it is easy to make one by tearing up a pillow case. All that is needed is one long rectangular piece which will go around the woman and two shorter strips to use as shoulder straps (Fig. 24-6).

   The binder is secured with safety pins to fit the woman. A tuck or dart is taken beneath each breast to give support and the ends overlapped and fitted in front. The straps are then attached in front and back.

   If the woman's breasts are pendulous, a long maternity perineal pad placed beneath and along the outer side of the breasts before application of the binder helps to give upward and inward thrust and support (Fig. 24-6). The woman can hold these pads in place while you fit the binder.

   Done this way a breast binder is extremely comfortable for the woman because it imparts support and prevents painful movement.

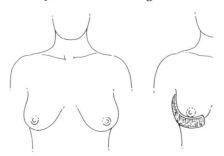
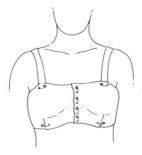

FIGURE 24-6. Breast binder.

2. *Do apply ice bags or packs to the breasts.* Ice relieves discomfort, has a certain numbing effect, and does not encourage milk flow. The idea is for the milk not to flow, as emptying will only stimulate the breast to produce more milk.
3. *Do take analgesics* (e.g., aspirin, Tylenol) to relieve the pain.
4. *Do say to yourself over and over again*: "It will only last 24 to 48 hours. It will only last 24 to 48 hours. It will only last 24 to 48 hours."

The two do nots are:

1. *Do not mash or massage your breasts* in an effort to get the milk out. Such actions will only extend the length of time of breast engorgement and cause residual fullness for months if it becomes a routine practice. Any emptying of the breasts by any means stimulates the breasts to further lactation.
2. *Do not apply heat to your breasts.* Heat dilates the blood vessels and ductile system, causing the milk to flow. This causes some partial emptying but stimulates the breasts to further lactation.

Relief Measures if Breast-feeding. Relief measures for the breast-feeding woman are designed to have the opposite effect on further milk production from those used for the non-breast-feeding woman. In this instance the idea is to get the milk to flow and empty the breasts. This also alleviates the mother's discomfort. The following are relief measures.

1. Carry out prenatal breast preparation — breast massage, manual expression, and nipple rolling. (See Chapter 48.)
2. Begin breast-feeding as soon as possible after delivery.
3. Nurse the baby every 2 to 3 hours without missing any feedings or using any supplements.
4. Use both breasts at each feeding. Start on the breast used last during the previous feeding. This arrangement allows for emptying of each breast. In order to accustom the nipples to the baby's sucking and minimize soreness, the baby should be on each breast 5 to 10 minutes to start with and then build up to complete emptying of one breast (may take 20 minutes) before switching to the other to finish the feeding.

These first four measures are preventive measures. Many breast-feeding mothers who (1) did antepartal breast preparation, (2) began breast-feeding within the hour of delivery, (3) feed frequently thereafter, and (4) use both breasts can avoid having undue breast engorgement. Numbers 3 and 4 also are measures for relief of breast engorgement and continuation of lactation. Other measures include the following:

5. Apply warmth to the breasts, especially prior to each breast-feeding, to promote milk flow. This can be accomplished with warm cloths, warm showers, or a bathtub of warm water full enough so that the breasts will be soaking with the woman in a hands-and-knees position.
6. If there is areolar engorgement, manual expression of the milk to soften the area prior to nursing the baby will help the baby latch on to the nipple properly and easily.
7. Use manual expression of milk to empty the breasts after the baby has nursed if they are still uncomfortably full and engorged after the feeding.
8. Maintain good support to the breasts without any pressure points. This is often supplied by a nursing brassiere which the mother has purchased for use throughout lactation. A breast binder such as described above for the non-breast-feeding mother may be necessary if the nursing bra becomes too tight during engorgement. Pressure points may cause a clogged duct, which will further the problem. It is much more awkward to use a breast binder

since it is not designed for ease in making the breasts accessible for breast-feeding.

9. Put ice bags on the breasts between feedings to reduce swelling and pain.

10. Analgesia, if needed, will not be so much as to affect the baby through what gets into the milk.

Perineal (Stitch) Pain

There are eight perineal comfort measures aimed towards alleviation of discomfort or pain resulting from an episiotomy or laceration and subsequent repair. Before any measures are instituted it is essential to examine the perineum as discussed for the daily physical examination of the postpartal woman. This will tell you if she is experiencing normal pain or if a complication is developing, such as a hematoma or infection. It may also give you an idea of which of the following measures might be most effective; for example, ice packs or witch hazel compresses are best for edema.

An all-important factor to be considered in deciding upon one or a combination of perineal comfort measures is what the woman thinks is going to help her. If her previous experience or a neighbor's or a friend's experience is that one particular measure brings great relief while another one is worthless, then by all means select the one that she believes will work and avoid the one she thinks is worthless. You may be faced at times with simply trying them all, one by one, or in various combinations, before the woman experiences relief. Her comfort is worth the effort. The perineal comfort measures follow.

Ice Pack or Bag p.r.n. If chemical ice packs are not available, an ice bag can be made by filling a rubber glove with crushed ice or ice chips and tying off the glove at the cuff with a rubberband. Glove powder needs to be rinsed off so it does not get into the wound and possibly initiate an infection.

All ice bags or packs should be wrapped in a sterile Peri-Chux, absorbent side out, for the sake of cleanliness to the perineum, protection against an ice burn, and nonmessiness.

Ice bags or packs are applied on a p.r.n. basis. They are most useful for their reducing (reduction of swelling) and numbing effects in the immediate postpartal period as the anesthetic wears off. Ice should always be applied in the event of a third or fourth degree laceration.

Topical Anesthetic p.r.n. Examples of a topical anesthetic are Dermoplast spray, Nupercaine ointment, Americaine spray or ointment, and Surfacaine ointment. If an ointment is to be used the woman should be instructed to wash her hands before applying it. The woman should be instructed not to apply an ointment prior to a perineal heat lamp treatment in order not to be burned. To be safe it is best not to combine these two methods on the same day.

Perineal Heat Lamp 20 to 30 Minutes b.i.d. or t.i.d. The heat increases circulation to the area, which promotes healing. It should not be used in combination with an anesthetic ointment as this may result in a burn. The perineum should be cleaned prior to use of the heat lamp so that lochia does not become dried in the wound closure.

There are various designs of perineal heat lamps. Most have leg supports and may be covered with bedclothes after being properly positioned. The heat is supplied by a light bulb which is usually in a curved, three-sided holder. This directs the heat to the fourth side, which is placed in front of the perineum. Care must be taken that the light bulb is neither too close to the perineum (may burn or be uncomfortably hot) or too far away (ineffective). Approximately 1 foot in distance between the perineum and the light bulb is about right. Check with the woman about what she is feeling in order to make the final adjustment in distance.

Sitz Bath b.i.d. or t.i.d. Many women consider the size bath the most soothing of all the measures. The advent of the disposable, fit-in-the-toilet sitz bath made this a simple, convenient, and comfortable procedure as well, and enables long-term usage because the woman can take it home with her.

A modification of the same idea is to pour warm water over the perineum. This can be a part of routine perineal care after both voiding and defecation. A small pitcher or container facilitates this method.

The warmth of the water for either the sitz bath or for pouring should first be tested on another sensitive but nontraumatized portion of the body, such as the inside of the wrist. The warmth of the water increases circulation and promotes healing. The warmth and motion of the water are also soothing.

Witch Hazel Compresses 20 to 30 Minutes p.r.n.   Witch hazel compresses have the effect of both reducing edema and being analgesic. They are concocted by pouring witch hazel over some 4 × 4 gauze squares in a small cup or basin, squeezing them out to a wet but not drippy state, folding them once, and placing them on the perineum. It is important that the hands of the person doing this be thoroughly washed first.

A variation of this comfort measure is the use of Tucks, which are pads saturated with a mixture of witch hazel, glycerin, and water. These are available commercially.

Analgesia.   (See orders under "Management of the Early Puerperium," earlier in this chapter.)

Rubber Ring.   Use of the rubber ring has been criticized because of its possible interference with circulation. However, properly used, it can bring safe relief when there is considerable positional pressure on the perineal area. The rubber ring should be inflated only enough to relieve this pressure. It should be a large rubber ring and positioned so that there are no pressure points in the pelvic area.

Perineal Tightening.   Doing perineal tighten-

ing, or Kegel exercises, increases circulation to the area and thus promotes healing. It also begins to restore muscle tone to the pelvic musculature. It is one of the most useful perineal discomfort measures and often yields dramatic results in facilitating ease of movement for the woman, and her comfort.

As a perineal discomfort measure, its use is geared towards alleviation of the discomfort and pain a woman has when sitting, especially on a chair, or moving across her bed when getting in and out of bed. In both of these instances her perineal area is subjected to direct pressure and, in the instance of getting in and out of bed, is also subjected to an indirect type of scraping of her stitch area. Perineal tightening draws the affected area up and in, out of reach of direct pressure and indirect scraping, which is now all directed to the gluteal muscles. After being instructed in how to do perineal tightening (see later in this chapter), the woman is told to tighten her perineum, drawing it up and in and maintaining this contracted state, before moving in bed and as she lowers herself onto a chair.

Perineal tightening can have the opposite effect if the woman had a mediolateral episiotomy. Tightening the perineum in this instance pulls on the posterior end of the stitch line since the incision cuts diagonally across the muscles. This can be quite painful.

Constipation

Fears inhibiting bowel function were discussed earlier in this chapter. In addition, constipation may be further aggravated by laxness of the abdominal walls (especially in a multipara who did not do abdominal muscle tightening exercises after each baby) and by the discomfort of a third or fourth degree repair.

Routine postpartal orders to facilitate bowel functioning were discussed earlier in this chapter. In addition, a stool softener, such as Colace, should be ordered for women with a third or fourth degree laceration and repair. If a mild laxative is also needed, Peri-Colace is both a stool softener and a mild laxative.

Hemorrhoids

If the woman has hemorrhoids they may be quite painful for a few days. If they preexisted or developed during pregnancy, they were traumatized and became more edematous during the pushing of the second stage of labor and with pressure of the baby and distention at birth. Relief measures include the following:

1. Ice bags or packs
2. Witch hazel compresses or Tucks

These first two relief measures help reduce the size of the hemorrhoids.

3. Analgesic or anesthetic spray or ointment
4. Heat lamp
5. Warm water compresses

Numbers 4 and 5 are used if the woman does not experience relief with the cold measures. The first four measures were described previously under "Perineal (Stitch) Pain."

6. Stool softener
7. Anusol suppositories
8. Replacement of external hemorrhoids inside the rectum. A lubricated finger cot is used and the hemorrhoids are gently pushed into the rectum. After the hemorrhoids are inserted, the woman tightens her rectal sphincter both to give them support and to contain them within the rectum.

Assistance with Breast-Feeding

A mother who is breast-feeding for the first time is in a vulnerable position and requires support, encouragement, and knowledgeable assistance. She has to make the transition from being insecure, anxious, and full of self-doubt to being self-assured and confident in herself and her capabilities. The purpose of this section is to help you help this new breast-feeding mother and her baby off to a good start, assuming that both the mother and the baby are normal and healthy.

The La Leche League offers the services of experienced women to give help and understanding at all times, day and night, for any breast-feeding mother. They are especially helpful for new breast-feeding mothers and for those in more difficult situations (e.g., mother with cesarean section, multiple gestation, or preterm baby). La Leche League's many helpful publications include its basic book on breast-feeding, entitled *The Womanly Art of Breastfeeding* [2]. The learner is referred to these publications and local meetings of the La Leche League for further self-learning and help for your patients.

Breast-feeding is a learning process for both the mother and baby — learning about themselves, about each other, and about feeding. It is helpful for the mother to view breast-feeding as a learning process; this point of view helps her set more realistic expectations and have a more realistic perspective regarding the initial breast-feeding experience. Even for mothers who have breast-fed before, it is a learning experience. Each baby is different, an individual with his or her own characteristics and personality. The way in which babies suck at the breast varies. However, there is enough similarity in the variations that one set of authors identified types as follows:

1. *Barracudas*: When put to the breast, these babies vigorously and promptly grasp the nipple and suck energetically for from 10 to 20 minutes. There is no dallying. Occasionally this type of baby puts too much vigor into his nursing and hurts the nipple. 2. *Excited Ineffective*: These babies become so excited and active at the breast they alternately grasp and lose the breast. They then start screaming. It is often necessary for the nurse or mother to pick up the baby and quiet him first, and then put him back to the breast. After a few days the mother and baby usually become adjusted. 3. *Procrastinators*: These babies often seem to put off until the fourth or fifth postpartum day what they could just as well have done from the start. They wait till the milk

comes in. They show no particular interest or ability in sucking in the first few days. It is important not to prod or force these babies when they seem disinclined. They do well once they start. 4. *Gourmets or Mouthers*: These babies insist on mouthing the nipple, tasting a little milk and then smacking their lips, before starting to nurse. If the infant is hurried or prodded, he will become furious and start to scream. Otherwise, after a few minutes of mouthing he settles down and nurses very well. 5. *Resters*: These babies prefer to nurse a few minutes and then rest a few minutes. If left alone, they often nurse well, although the entire procedure will take much longer. They cannot be hurried.

There are many babies who fall between these groups and others who fall into groups not described because they are less common. The above grouping serves merely to emphasize the fact that each baby nurses differently, and the course of the nursing will depend on the combination of the baby's nursing characteristics, the mother's personality, and the quality of help from the attending nurse. [3, p. 194]

A baby has a number of reflexes which are pertinent to feeding. These are as follows:

1. Rooting
2. Sucking
3. Swallowing
4. Gag
5. Hunger
6. Satiety
7. Sneezing
8. Hiccupping
9. Regurgitation
10. Burping

While the last nine of these are essential to feeding in general, the first one is particularly useful in breast-feeding. A directed rooting reflex is one in which the baby's head rotates toward the source of cheek stimulation and the mouth opens. In other words if you touch the baby's cheek, he or she will turn the head toward the direction of the side touched. Touching the cheek can be used in getting a baby to turn toward the breast. Aimless rooting is the baby's turning his or her head from side to side seeking, while opening and shutting his or her mouth and making sucking movements. Rooting and sucking movements combined with crying stimulated by the hunger reflex are the indicators, or signs, that a baby is hungry.

The mother should be prepared for each breast-feeding. By this is meant that she be:

1. In a comfortable position, which means any position that is comfortable for her and allows for proper positioning of her baby. This can be accomplished in a side-lying, reclining, or sitting position. Generous use of pillows for support and comfort is most useful.
2. Without discomfort or pain. Her bladder should be empty. Any pain such as afterbirth pains or episiotomy or laceration repair pain should have received comfort measures prior to breast-feeding time.
3. Rested.
4. Assured of available help as she deems necessary.
5. Free of any pressing concerns for the next 20 to 30 minutes.
6. Relaxed. Sometimes a beer or a glass of wine is helpful in promoting relaxation at a time when this is more difficult to achieve.
7. Clean; her hands should be washed and her nipples cleansed. Nipple cleaning is done simply by gently wiping them off with plain water.

The baby's immediate preparation for breast-feeding is to have a clean dry diaper and, if absolutely necessary, to be swaddle wrapped. While freedom of the baby's arms and hands to touch are important to both mother and baby, the active movement of her baby's arms and legs may be too much for a new, inexperienced mother to cope with when she is trying to learn how to hold her baby and hold her breast. A swaddle wrap in such a situation can make the difference between a frustrating, unhappy experience with failure feelings and a successful, happy feeding. Swaddle wrapping, when properly done, may be comforting rather than confining to babies because they feel held close and secure rather than bound. The arms are positioned anatomically in approximation to the body, in other words, flexed at the elbow (see Fig. 24-7). The wrapping is loose enough for freedom of motion of the legs. What has been achieved is control of waving arms. For mothers who need this initially, it will be just a few feedings before they can cope without swaddle wrapping their baby.

Position the baby so that he or she will not be doubled up or have a twisted neck when sucking and so that the head and body are supported. In bringing the baby and the breast together, the following are helpful:

1. Don't thrust the breast in the baby's face since this may be frightening or give the baby a feeling of suffocation. Rather, let the baby find the breast and grasp the nipple.
2. Help the mother learn to hold her breast in such a way as to guide and control the breast and shape it in a way that facilitates the baby's grasping of it. In doing this she must be sure to hold the breast beyond the areolar area so her fingers will not interfere with proper positioning of the baby's mouth and gums on the nipple.
3. Touch the baby's cheek with the nipple so the baby will turn towards the breast (use of the rooting reflex).
4. Express a few drops of colostrum so they are on the surface of the nipple. This provides the baby with instant gratification and reinforces learning.
5. As the baby grasps the nipple, the mother must make sure that the infant has enough of it for proper positioning in the mouth. The baby must grasp more than just the end of the mother's nipple. If not, this will result in a hungry, frustrated, unhappy baby and a frustrated, unhappy mother with sore nipples which may lead to further problems of cracking and an increased risk of mastitis. It is to be remembered that the lactiferous sinuses are located beneath the areolae. The baby must compress these with his or her gums when sucking in

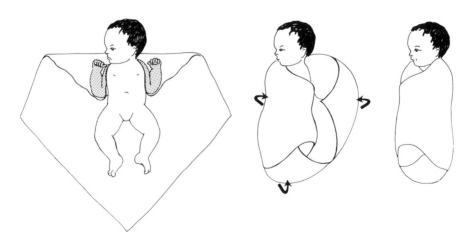

FIGURE 24-7.   Swaddle wrapping.

order to obtain the colostrum or milk. The sequence of movements of compression, sucking, and swallowing is rhythmic and the mother can feel a steady pull which is not felt if the baby is essentially just chewing on the end of the nipple.

6. Once the baby's mouth is properly positioned well onto the areolae the mother releases her grasp of her breast. She now provides breathing space for the baby if needed by pressing with a finger on her breast where the baby's nose is (this is usually necessary only during this learning period and when the breast is engorged). It is to be remembered that the baby is a nose breather.

Breast-feeding should begin as soon as possible after delivery and should be frequent (approximately every 2 hours) thereafter. These early feedings might best consist of approximately 5 to 10 minutes suckling on each breast while the nipples get accustomed to it. This frequent suckling stimulates the production and let-down of lactation and reduces the potential severity of engorgement. Therefore, it is essential that there be no missed feedings, including those at night, in a misguided concern for the mother's rest. She will rest better knowing that her baby is not receiving any bottle feedings, is receiving the benefits of her colostrum, and that her breasts are getting the best possible help by feeding. In a few days the baby should be feeding approximately 20 minutes on one breast (the time it will probably take to empty it) and then finishing the feeding on the other breast. At the next feeding the baby should start on the last breast suckled at the last feeding. A way of remembering is to place a safety pin on the side of the bra covering the breast last suckled. In this way usage of the breasts is continually rotated, thereby assuring both are completely emptied and the balance of demand and supply estab-

lished. By this time the baby will be setting his or her own frequency of feeding.

Babies usually will suck a bit, rest a bit (maintaining their hold on the nipple while they rest), and then suck some more. The mother should be prepared for this so she does not get upset and mistake for disinterest the baby's rest periods. The mother should also be prepared for the strong uterine contraction she will feel when the baby first latches on to her breast.

Suction must be broken before trying to remove the baby from the breast. Pulling the baby off causes injury to the nipple. Suction is broken by slipping a finger into the corner of the baby's mouth and between the baby's gums. Once the suction is broken the baby is easily removed from the breast without injury to the nipple. The baby is then burped and put to the other breast.

Lactation is established and maintained by a combination of the following (Fig. 24-8):

1. Breast-feeding starting as soon as possible after delivery
2. Frequent feedings during the first few days, using both breasts
3. No missed feedings
4. No supplementary feedings
5. Rotation of breasts as the starting and ending breasts to provide for complete emptying of both breasts
6. Tension-free, painless, rested, relaxed mother during feeding times
7. Baby properly positioned on the breast
8. Supportive partner.

After the first few days the baby will settle into his or her individual pattern of feeding frequency. Inherent in this discussion is the absence of rigid scheduling and the assumption of self-demand scheduling (i.e., feeding the baby when he or she is hungry).

The final factor in successful breast-feeding

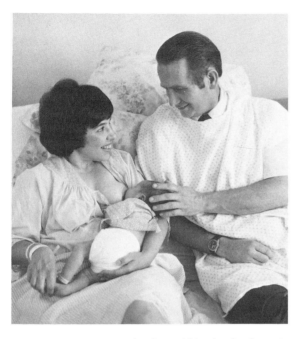

FIGURE 24-8. Breast-feeding within the family unit.

is effective breast care. If the breasts are not properly cared for they can become sore and painful. Nipples will be somewhat tender to start with. They then either become accustomed to the baby's sucking, with concomitant reduction in tenderness, or become truly sore and painful. Soreness is the most common reason why mothers give up breast-feeding during the early stages of breast-feeding.

Breast care and preparation for breast-feeding begin in the antepartal period (see Chapters 7 and 48). Breast care while breast-feeding is as follows:

1. Wash only with water (especially the nipples) — no soap, alcohol, or any other drying agent. Drying agents can lead quickly to cracking of the nipples.
2. Expose the nipples to air for 15 to 30 minutes after a feeding.
3. While exposing the nipples to air, expose them also to sunshine or to a 25-watt light bulb (be careful not to burn the nipples) because this is soothing to tender nipples.
4. Following exposure, rub in a nipple cream, for example, Masse' Cream, A and D Ointment or Cream, hydrous lanolin.
5. Provide good support to the breasts.
6. If the breasts become engorged, care for them as discussed earlier in this chapter under "Relief from Postpartal Discomforts."
7. If the nipples become tender:
   a. enhance the let-down before feeding with warmth as discussed for care of the breasts during engorgement.
   b. nurse on the less sore nipple first until there is let-down, then switch the baby to the sorest nipple to empty that breast, then switch back to the less sore nipple to finish the feeding, empty that breast, and meet the baby's sucking needs.
   c. use a pacifier rather than the end of feedings on the nipples to meet the baby's sucking needs until the nipples are not sore.
   d. breast-feed more frequently for shorter periods of time.
   e. be sure the baby is properly positioned on the breast.
   f. change the baby's position for feeding, which will change the precise pressure points on the nipple; for example, shifting from an arm hold to a football hold varies precisely where the strongest pressure will be exerted on the nipple.
   g. be sure to use a combination of exposure to both air and heat after each breast-feeding, followed by a thorough application of nipple cream.
8. Be sure to break the suction before removing the baby from the breast.

Facilitation of Parenting

Early Attachment and Bonding

It has long been known that animals demonstrate a pattern of behavior in accepting their newborn and that certain intervening variables alter this pattern and end in rejection of their newborn. The description of this behavior as *species-specific* reflects the fact that the pattern of attachment behavior differs from species to species of animals.

How a human mother and father behave toward their newborn is influenced in part by internal factors, which they bring into the situation, and in part by external factors, which occur at the time. The internal factors include how the individuals were cared for by their own parents; their genetic endowments; internalized cultural practices, mores, and values; relationships with each other, families, and significant others; previous pregnancy and bonding experiences; and the identification work done during this pregnancy, including the effect of the course of the pregnancy on this. The external factors include the care received during labor, delivery, and postpartum; the attitudes and behaviors of attendants; the responsiveness of the infant, including the effect of the newborn's condition on this; the practices of the attendants and institutions impinging on the situation; and whether or not there is separation from the baby during the first hours or days of life.

There are basically three sequential time periods during which initial parental attachment and bonding to a specific baby develops and takes place. Each encompasses a series of events. These time periods are (1) the prenatal period, (2) the time of birth and immediately following birth, and (3) the postpartal and early caretaking period. Delineating these three time periods does not negate the influence of the prepregnancy period, both in shaping parental attitudes and role anticipation from birth to present parenthood, and in the thought, plans, and dreams that go into planning a pregnancy; nor the continuing reciprocal responses, strengthening of bonds, and changing roles occurring throughout life after the postpartal period.

The Prenatal Period. It is during the prenatal period that the woman accepts the fact of pregnancy, delineates her mothering identity as separate from that of her own mother's, verifies the pregnancy and identifies the baby as an individual separate from herself, dreams and fantasizes about the baby, and makes preparations for the baby. These psychological processes and events are discussed in Chapter 6. The father experiences a similar sequence of events.

The Time of Birth and Immediately following Birth. This period starts with labor because what happens during labor directly affects the attachment process at birth. The most obvious direct relationship is that of medication. Attachment processes are thwarted if both mother and baby are "sleepy" from medication. The mother's active participation and involvement during labor sets the stage for taking-in and reception of the baby at birth (Fig. 24-9). The bonding which occurs between the mother and the father resulting from the power of the shared labor experience strengthens and facilitates postbirth family bonding.

The actual taking-in and touching of her baby may begin with the mother's touching her baby's head at the introitus shortly before birth. Even when the baby is placed in a skin-to-skin total body contact position on the mother's abdomen immediately after birth or when the mother has reached out for her baby, there is a definite sequence in her touching of the baby. The rapidity of this sequence may vary. The basic direction is from peripheral actions and position inward to central actions and position. This touching sequence starts with the mother's fingertips touching the baby's extremities in an exploratory, questioning manner; progresses to application of her palms to the trunk of the baby and then the encirclement of the baby's trunk with both hands; and ends with the enclosure and encompassing of the entire baby to her own body within her arms.

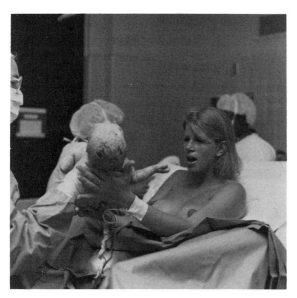

FIGURE 24-9.   Mother receiving her baby at birth.

Other attachment and bonding behaviors in the immediate postbirth period include establishing mutual eye contact and spending time in the *en face* position, talking to the baby in a high-pitched voice, comparing the baby to the baby fantasized and dreamed of during pregnancy (this comparison usually starts with the sex of the baby), and using the baby's name.

These behaviors mesh with the unmedicated newborn's capabilities. This meshing enables a responsiveness that establishes a reciprocal and reinforcing two-way interaction between parent and child. The capabilities of the newborn are facilitated because the baby is in a quiet-alert state during the first hour after birth. This makes the baby receptive to stimuli and constitutes a sensitive time for the baby corresponding to a sensitive time for the mother during the first hour postpartum. The baby has the capability to see at birth and is able to visually follow a moving object at an optimal distance of 10 to 12 inches. This corresponds to the distance the baby is usually held in the *en*

face position and results in reciprocal eye contact and mutual gazing. The high pitched voice of the mother corresponds to the baby's ability to hear especially well in the high-frequency range.

The attachment behaviors of the father also follow an orderly progression. Unlike the mother, who may be in constant intimate contact with her baby, the father is himself peripheral to the central interaction between mother and baby. This is evidenced in the series of behaviors which bring him to the same touching sequence described for the mother and into his own central interaction and bonding with the baby. This series of behaviors starts with a hovering posture over the baby. In this he visually latches on to the baby with an intensity that is only briefly and infrequently diverted during the first few minutes immediately after birth. The father's hands and fingers may be positioned in readiness toward the baby and he gets as close as possible to a face-to-face position with the baby who is in an *en face* position with the mother. He establishes fingertip contact with the baby, leading to palm contact. When he holds the baby he positions himself *en face* for eye contact and mutual gazing (Fig. 24-10).

The Postpartal and Early Caretaking Period. A relationship develops over time and is dependent on the participation of both in the relationship. Reciprocity and reinforcement from circular communication lead to learning what to expect from each other and to the development of trust. Caretaking ability resulting in a healthy, responsive baby inspires fulfillment, confidence, and feelings of competence and success within the caretaker. The satisfied, loved baby learns the feeling of self-worth and gains the confidence to learn and to adapt. Early learning has a direct relationship with early caretaking.

For the inexperienced mother, caretaking may be fraught with anxiety to prove herself a good mother and her concern with skills may

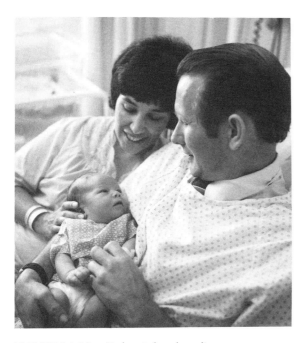

FIGURE 24-10.   Father-infant bonding.

supplant alertness and responsiveness to the baby's cues. Focus on her needs and support, teaching, and anticipatory guidance geared toward building her confidence quickly enables her to comfortably assume caretaking tasks. If the mother's bodily and emotional needs are being met she will be much more able to meet the bodily and emotional needs of her baby.

Questions during the postpartal period (6 weeks) center around caretaking concerns, especially as they relate to feeding, bowels, and trying to ascertain if the baby is sick. A system designed for the caretaker to readily obtain information during the early weeks of caretaking greatly reduces anxiety as well as provides preventive health care for the baby and the family.

Rooming-In

The best possible structure in the hospital for facilitating mother-infant attachment, bonding, parenting, and the family unit is rooming-in.

Rooming-in is not a new concept but one that was lost in the history of maternity care in the United States when childbirth moved inside the hospital and separated the mother and baby from the family and, by and large, from each other. In the mid-1940s a movement began to reverse this separation within the hospital. Opponents' fears of rooming-in because of increased infection have been proven invalid. In fact, the danger is less. The most comprehensive definition of rooming-in was developed at that time at Yale University as follows:

The term rooming-in refers to a hospital arrangement for maternity patients wherein a mother and her new-born are cared for together in the same unit of space. However, its meaning reaches beyond physical facilities and signifies an attitude in maternal and infant care and a general plan of supportive parental education which are based on the recognition and understanding of the needs of each mother, infant, and family. It is a plan to maintain natural mother-infant relationships, to reinforce the potentialities of each mother and infant, and to encourage the family unit. From this broad point of view, then, rooming-in is not to be viewed merely as a specific plan for space arrangement or as a particular kind of equipment or organization, but rather as an integrated, interdepartmental program of professional assistance which is aimed to help parents achieve happy family unity and warm parent-child relationships. [4, p. 484]

There are two administrative versions of rooming in: a rooming-in unit and modified rooming-in. The principles of rooming-in are the same in both (Fig. 24-11). A rooming-in unit is a patient care unit that has been constructed specifically for the purpose of rooming-in. Usually it consists of a two-bed or four-bed room with sufficient space for an equal number of bassinets or cribs and an adjacent nursery. It can be designed so that the adjacent nursery serves more than one room of mothers. It is a self-contained unit and nursing staff assignment is to the unit.

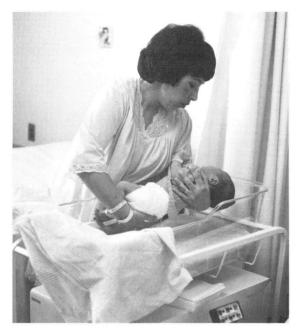

FIGURE 24-11. Rooming-in.

Modified rooming-in utilizes the existing facilities of a centralized nursery separated from the mothers' rooms but changes the policies so that a baby can be transported from the nursery to the mother's room in his or her crib and back to the nursery at will. This requires flexible nursing staff assignment and commitment by all nursings staff to caring for both the mother and the baby either together or separately.

Rooming-in does *not* mean that the baby has to be with the mother every minute of her hospital stay, nor does it mean that the mother assumes sole responsibility for the care of the baby. The latter situation would be unfair, unwise, unsafe, and a sure way to defeat the initiation of rooming-in in a setting. In rooming-in the nursing staff remains responsible for the nursing care of both the mother and the baby. The mother assumes care of her baby as she desires and as she demonstrates the ability

to do so. The setting is ideal for a new, inexperienced mother to learn not only how to care for her baby but also the individuality of her baby and the infant's communication with her in body movement and vocal noises. The experienced mother also benefits from learning the individuality and communication of this baby and rests comfortably having her baby with her, yet knowing that the actual care of her baby can be done by herself or the nurse as she desires so that she can obtain her needed rest and prevent exhaustion.

Rooming-in also is the ideal setting for breast-feeding, because the mother can respond when the baby is hungry and nurse frequently for stimulation of lactation, for involvement of the father, and for beginning parenting (Fig. 24-12). The baby needs the security that comes from prompt attention to its demands and from holding, cuddling, fondling, and nuzzling. These needs must be satisfied if the baby is to be healthy and happy. An inexperienced mother and father may find it difficult both to recognize these needs and to know how to satisfy them. Baby care is a learned skill and art. In rooming-in there is opportunity to get

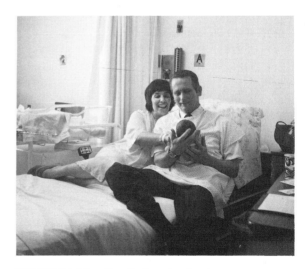

FIGURE 24-12. Family in rooming-in.

to know the baby and the way he or she communicates and to learn how to meet the needs being expressed. The transition from hospital to home in caring for the baby becomes a gradual and natural one instead of a shock. And what a shock it is to a new, inexperienced mother to be home suddenly with a baby she has no idea how to care for and has only seen three or four times a day for approximately 20 minutes, if that often. No wonder such a mother is frightened and anxious, has overwhelming feelings of self-doubt, and is subject to postpartum blues. A rooming-in mother and father go home confident in their ability to care for their baby.

The importance of recognizing the baby's needs and individual behavior lies in the potential for growth when the needs are satisfied and there is collaboration with the individual's growth and development pattern. An impersonal hospital regimen encourages a mother to believe, falsely, in the automatic behavior of her baby to inflexible and mechanical standards, conditions a mother to follow rules instead of being guided by the needs of her baby, and does not allow her to learn that a satisfied baby cries relatively little and will settle into a fairly regular schedule of his or her own in 2 to 3 weeks. Growth and development are fostered when the baby is secure in the warmth and contact that comes from holding and cuddling and when free to eat, sleep, and eliminate according to internal rhythms rather than in accord with a rigid and arbitrary regimen. Parenting begins in respect for and in response to the individual.

Anticipatory Guidance and Instruction

This portion of the chapter is an outline of the topics included in anticipatory guidance and instruction of the postpartal mother during the early puerperium. This does not mean that all women have learning needs for all of this teaching. It does mean that each woman should be apprised of these topics and then instruction given in those in which she feels a need. You cannot assume that because she is a first-time mother she doesn't know anything about these topics. She may have baby care experience through caring for a sibling or other infant relatives. By the same token you cannot assume that because a woman is a multipara she knows all you have to offer. She may need a refresher depending on how many years it has been since her last baby; she may be feeling foggy and insecure in her memory. Also, most professionals who have become mothers don't like to have to rely on themselves; they want to be treated like any other new mother with the right to be taught if they wish without being made to feel like they should already know everything.

The following material is presented in topical outline with only occasional further notations. Most nurse-midwifery students will have done this teaching before either as student nurses or in practice, and there are innumerable pamphlets and books available that detail this instruction. Those who are unfamiliar with this teaching can use the topical outline to identify areas in which they need instruction and use these sources plus observation of classes being given for the information. Some of these sources are listed in the bibliography to this chapter. This outline is divided into three large areas: anticipatory guidance and instruction related to (1) self, (2) baby, and (3) self in relation to others.

Self
1. Perineal care. (This was discussed earlier in this chapter.)
2. Breast care for the breast-feeding mother. (This was discussed earlier in this chapter.)
3. Care of the breasts during breast engorgement. (This was discussed earlier in this chapter.)
4. Abdominal tightening exercises:

a. chin-chest. Start now. (This is discussed under "Diastasis" in Chapter 41.)

b. sit-ups. Start in 2 weeks. Sit-ups should be started with the woman's arms by her sides. When she can do these with ease she should do sit-ups with her hands behind her head; this is more difficult.

c. leg raises. Start in 2 weeks. It is important that she does *not* raise both legs at the same time as this can injure her back. This must be stressed because it is contrary to many exercise booklets.

Remind her that she knows how to check her progress by feeling for closure of her diastasis. She should be encouraged not to rely on a girdle because it does nothing for the problem of lack of muscle tone, as evidenced when she takes the girdle off.

5. Perineal tightening (Kegel) exercise. Start now. The basic aspect of teaching this is in the woman's identification of which muscles she is to tighten. This is best done by having her squeeze and tighten around your fingers during a vaginal examination. However, if you are not doing a vaginal examination when you are teaching her, the most effective way is to have her urinate and "go-stop-go-stop-go-stop-go" during urination. Advise her to take note of which muscle she tightens and uses in order to stop the flow of urine. There is no limit to how often or how many times she does this exercise. The more the better.

6. Rest. Help the woman clarify her priorities. If she has help in the home, encourage her to use this help for household functions, thus leaving her to care for her baby, rather than vice versa.

7. Tub bath or shower as preferred.

8. Wash hair as desired. There are many old wives' tales denying hair washing for several weeks. This places the mother between what she wants to do and what older female relatives tell her she should or should not do. She needs to know that this is her decision to make and that there are no obstetric or medical reasons for not washing her hair.

9. Normality of after-baby blues.

10. Call the nurse-midwife in the event of any of the following:
    a. fever or chills
    b. excessive bleeding
    c. abdominal pain
    d. severely painful lumpy breast
    e. calf pain or heat, with or without leg edema

11. Return for 4- or 6-weeks postpartum checkup.

Baby

1. If being bottle fed:
   a. the preparation and storage of formula
   b. the care and preparation of bottles and nipples
   c. how to hold the baby during feeding
   d. how to hold the bottle during feeding (so the nipple is full, otherwise the baby is getting air)

2. Burping (see Fig. 24-13).

3. Baby bathing, including shampooing.

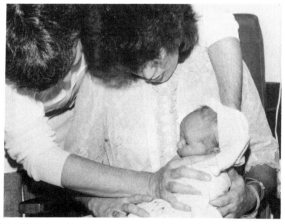

FIGURE 24-13.   Teaching and learning about burping.

4. Dressing:
   a. how to dress (manipulation of clothes and baby)
   b. how much clothing in relation to both environmental and body temperature (the latter as determined by feeling the baby's trunk)
5. Care of circumcision, if applicable.
6. Cleansing and care of penis if not circumcised and if applicable.
7. Care of female perineum, if applicable.
8. Cord care.
9. How to lift, hold, and carry a baby.
10. Diapers — how to change them, what to do with them.
11. Prevention and treatment of diaper rash.
12. Oiling or powdering of baby. Powdering should be limited to what is left on the mother's hands after brushing the powder off of them and should be done at a distance so the baby is not inhaling powder.
13. How to take the baby's temperature and how to read a thermometer.
14. Judicious use of a pacifier.
15. Crying means one or more of the following:
   a. hunger
   b. need for a diaper change
   c. need to be burped
   d. uncomfortable position — needs to be changed
   e. being hurt by something, for example, stuck by a safety pin
   f. need for loving — wants to be held and cuddled
   g. clothes or blanket too tight — needs freedom of motion
   h. sick

The parents should be assured that it is not possible for them to spoil their baby at this time. Quite the contrary, babies whose needs are satisfied will not need to resort to whining and tantrums and to develop the disagreeable personality of the spoiled child.

16. Call the nurse-midwife in the event of any of the following:
   a. fever
   b. diarrhea
   c. respiratory infection
   d. poor feeding
   e. persistent restless crying
   f. yellow color
17. Taking baby for four-week checkup and immunizations.

Self in Relation to Others
1. Sibling rivalry.
2. Husband rivalry.
3. Transitional family relationships.
4. Breast-feeding. (This was discussed earlier in this chapter.)
5. Family planning. See chapters on family planning.
6. Resumption of sexual intercourse:
   a. time of resumption determined by desire and comfort. Women with stitches most likely will not be comfortable enough for sexual intercourse for at least 2 to 3 weeks.
   b. alternate methods of satisfying male and famale sexual needs in the puerperium.
   c. problems of privacy, noninterruption, and the let-down reflex if the woman is breastfeeding.
   d. alternate positions for sexual intercourse which reduce pressure on the repair site.
   e. use of K-Y Jelly for lubrication.
7. Need for time together separate from the baby and away from home.

REFERENCES

1. Lindemann, E. Symptomatology and management of acute grief. *Am. J. Psychiatry* 101:141, 1944.
2. *The Womanly Art of Breastfeeding*. Franklin Park, Ill.: La Leche League International, 1963.
3. Barnes, G. R., Jr. et al. Management of breastfeeding. *JAMA* 151:194, 1953.
4. Jackson, E. B. The development of rooming-in at Yale. *Yale J. Biol. Med.* 25:484, 1952.

BIBLIOGRAPHY

Aaronson, M. Infant nuturance and early learning: Myths and realities. *Child Welfare* 57:165, 1978.

Affonso, D. The newborn's potential for interaction. *J. Obstet. Gynecol. Neonat. Nurs.* 5:9, 1976.

Appelbaum, R. M. The modern management of successful breast feeding. *Pediatr. Clin. North Am.* 17:203, 1970.

Arnold, J. H., and Gemma, P. B. *A Child Dies: A Portrait of Family Grief.* Rockville, Md.: Aspen, 1983.

Barnes, J. et al. Management of breast feeding. *JAMA* 151:192, 1953.

Bishop, B. A guide to assessing parenting capabilities, *Am. J. Nurs.* 76:1784, 1976.

Bonica, J. J. *Principles and Practice of Obstetric Analgesia & Anesthesia.* Philadelphia: Davis, Vol. 1, 1967, and Vol. 2, 1969.

Borg, S., and Lasker, J. *When Pregnancy Fails.* Boston: Beacon Press, 1981.

Cahill, A. S. Dual-purpose tool for assessing maternal needs and nursing care. *J. Obstet. Gynecol. Neonat. Nurs.* 4:28, 1975.

Carr. D., and Knupp, S. F. Grief and perinatal loss: A community hospital approach to support. *J. Obstet. Gynecol. Neonat. Nurs.* March/April, 1985, pp. 130–139.

Catz, C. S., and Giancoia, G. P. Drugs and breast milk. *Pediatr. Clin. North Am.* 19:151, 1972.

Clarke, C. A. The prevention of Rh isoimmunization. *Hosp. Prac.* 8:77, 1973.

Clerk, N. W. (pseud. for C. S. Lewis). *A Grief Observed.* Greenwich, Conn.: Seabury Press, 1963.

Cormon, A. The beginning of the end of sex: The first baby. *Cosmopolitan* October, 1974, p. 188.

Ewy, D., and Ewy, R. *Preparation for Breast Feeding.* Garden City, N. Y.: Dolphin Books/Doubleday, 1975.

Furr, P. A., and Kirgis, C. A. A nurse-midwifery approach to early mother-infant acquaintance. *J. Nurse-Midwifery* 27(5):10–14 (September/October) 1982.

Haire, D. *Instructions for Nursing Your Baby.* Seattle, Wash.: International Childbirth Education Association, 1969.

Haire, D. B. *The Cultural Warping of Childbirth.* Seattle, Wash.: International Childbirth Education Association, 1972.

Harris, A. A public health nurse in rooming-in. *Publ. Health Nurs.* 44:583, 1952.

Hazle, N. R. Postpartum blues: Assessment and intervention. *J. Nurse-Midwifery* 27(6):21–25 (November/December) 1982.

Ilse, S. *Empty Arms.* Long Lake, Minn.: Sherokee Ilse, 1982.

Infant Care. U. S. Department of Health, Education and Welfare. Children's Bureau Publication No. 8, 1963.

Jackson, E. B. The development of rooming-in at Yale. *Yale J. Biol. Med.* 25:484, 1952.

Jelliffe, D. B., and Jelliffe, E. F. P. Breast is best: Modern meanings. *N. Engl. J. Med.* 297:912, 1977.

Jimenez, S. L. M. *The Other Side of Pregnancy: Coping with Miscarriage and Stillbirth.* Englewood Cliffs, N. J.: Prentice-Hall, 1982.

Kayiatos, R., Adams, J., and Gilman, B. The arrival of a rival: Maternal perceptions of toddlers' regressive behaviors after the birth of a sibling. *J. Nurse-Midwifery* 29(3):205–213 (May/June) 1984.

Keith, L., and Berger, G. S. Anti-Rh disease prophylaxis. *Perinatal Care* June, 1978, p. 37.

Keith, L., Halloway, M., and Stepto, R. C. The multiple use of RhoGAM, *J. N. Med. Assoc.* 65:40, 1973.

Kennell, J. H., and Trause, M. A. Helping parents cope with perinatal death. *Contemporary OB/GYN* 12:53, 1978.

Kitzinger, S. *The Complete Book of Pregnancy and Childbirth.* New York: Knopf, 1980.

Klaus, M. H. et al. Human maternal behavior at first contact with her young. *Pediatrics* 46:187, 1970.

Klaus, M. H. et al. Maternal attachment: Importance of the first post-partum days, *N. Engl. J. Med.* 286:460, 1972.

Klaus, M. H., and Kennell, J. H. *Maternal-Infant Bonding.* St. Louis: Mosby, 1976.

Klaus, M. H., Leger, T., and Trause, M. A. (Eds.). *Maternal Attachment and Mothering Disorders: A Round Table.* New Brunswick, N. J.: Johnson & Johnson, 1975.

Kontos, D. A study of the effects of extended mother-infant contact on maternal behavior at one and three months. *Birth Fam. J.* 5:133, 1978.

Kreis, B., and Pattie, A. *Up from Grief.* New York: Seabury Press, 1969.

La Leche League, *The Womanly Art of Breastfeeding.* Franklin Park, Ill.: La Leche League International, 1963.

Lactation: A Programmed Review. Cincinnati, Ohio:

Wm. S. Merrell Company, 1969.

Lepler, M. Having a handicapped child. *Am. J. Mat. Child Nurs.* January/February, 1978, p. 32.

Lin-Fu, J. S. *Prevention of Hemolytic Disease of the Fetus and Newborn Due to Rh Isoimmunization.* Washington, D. C.: U. S. Department of Health, Education and Welfare Publication No. (HSA) 75-5125, 1975.

Lindemann, E. Symptomatology and management of acute grief. *Am. J. Psychiatry* 101:141, 1944.

McDonald, D. L. Paternal behavior at first contact with the newborn in a birth environment without intrusions. *Birth Family J.* 5:123, 1978.

McGowan, M. N. Post partum disturbance ... A review of the literature in terms of stress response. *J. Nurse-Midwifery* 22:27, 1977.

Meara, H. La Leche League in the United States: A key to successful breast-feeding in a non-supportive culture. *J. Nurse-Midwifery* 21:20, 1976.

Murdaugh, A., and Miller, L. E. Helping the breast feeding mother. *Am. J. Nurs.* 72:1423, 1972.

Newton, M., and Newton, N. The normal course and management of lactation. *Clin. Obstet. Gynecol.* 5:44, 1962.

Newton, N. Breast feeding. *Psychology Today* 2(1):34 (June) 1968.

O'Donohue, N. Facilitating the grief process. *J. Nurse-Midwifery* 24(5):16—19 (September/October) 1979.

Panuthos, C., and Romeo, C. *Ended Beginnings: Healing Childbearing Losses.* South Hadley, Mass.: Bergin & Garvey, 1984.

Physiology of Lactation. World Health Organization Technical Report Series, No. 305. Geneva, Switzerland: World Health Organization, 1965.

Pollack, W., Gorman, J. G., and Freda, V. J. Prevention of Rh hemolytic disease. In Brown, E. B., and Moore, C. V. (Eds.). *Progress in Hematology, Vol. 6.* New York: Grune & Stratton, 1969.

Practical Hints for Working and Breastfeeding. Franklin Park, Ill.: La Leche League International, Publication No. 83, 1983.

Pritchard, J. A., and MacDonald, P. C. *Williams Obstetrics, 15th.* New York: Appleton-Century-Crofts, 1976.

Quirk, T. R. Crisis theory, grief theory, and related psychosocial factors: The framework for intervention. *J. Nurse-Midwifery* 24(5):13—16 (September/October) 1979.

Reid, D. E., Ryan, K. J., and Benirschke, K. *Principles and Management of Human Reproduction.* Philadelphia: Saunders, 1972.

Robson, K. S., and Moss, H. A. Patterns and determinants of maternal attachment. *J. Pediatr.* 77:976, 1970.

Rozdilsky, M. L., and Banet, B. *What Now? A Handbook for Couples (Especially Women) Postpartum.* Seattle, Wash.: What Now?, 1972.

Rubin, R. Basic maternal behavior. *Nurs. Outlook* 9:683, 1961.

Rubin, R. *Maternal Identity and the Maternal Experience.* New York: Springer, 1984.

Rubin, R. Maternal touch. *Nurs. Outlook* 11:828, 1963.

Schwiebert, P., and Kirk, P. *When Hello Means Goodbye.* Portland, Ore.: University of Oregon Health Sciences Center, 1981.

Shepherd, S. C., and Yarrow, R. E. Breastfeeding and the working mother. *J. Nurse-Midwifery* 27(6):16—20 (November/December) 1982.

Spock, B. *Baby and Child Care.* New York: Simon & Schuster, 1977.

Sumner, G., and Fritsch, J. Postnatal parental concerns: The first six weeks of life. *J. Obstet. Gynecol. Neonat. Nurs.* 6(3):27 (May/June) 1977.

Varney, H. R. (idem. Burst) Rooming-in. Unpublished paper, 1960.

Waller, H. *Clinical Studies in Lactation.* London: William Heinemann, 1939.

Wiedenbach, E. *Family-Centered Maternity Nursing, 2nd.* New York: G. P. Putnam's Sons, 1967.

Wong, D. L. Bereavement: The empty-mother syndrome. *MCN* 5:385—389 (November/December) 1980.

Ziegel, E., and VanBlarcom, C. C. *Obstetric Nursing, 6th.* New York: Macmillan, 1972.

25

Screening for Puerperal Abnormality and Disposition

The complications of the puerperium presented in this chapter are the more common or well-known complications. Others, rarely seen in practice and requiring earlier involvement of the physician, are not included. Examples of the latter are Sheehan's syndrome, broken coccyx, muscle paralysis in the lower extremities, and separation of pelvic joints. The student interested in these complications is encouraged to pursue these interests in the medical and obstetric textbooks and journals.

The nurse-midwife needs to be thoroughly familiar with the normal physiologic and anatomic changes of the puerperium in order to differentiate the abnormal as early as possible in its development. It is essential that the nurse-midwife be familiar with the signs and symptoms of the more common complications in order to consult, collaborate with, or refer to the physician, depending upon the condition and its severity.

The extended sites of puerperal infection, while fortunately rarely seen today, are included in this chapter. They serve as a reminder of what once was a most feared sequela of the puerperium and can be again if strains of bacteria grow resistant to antibiotics and if professionals become careless about hand washing and aseptic technique. The history of puerperal infection is at the same time tragic and fascinating. Those interested are encouraged to pursue this interest in obstetric literature.

PUERPERAL MORBIDITY

Puerperal morbidity has been defined by the Joint Committee on Maternal Welfare as a "temperature of 100.4°F (38.0°C), the temperature to occur on any two of the first ten days postpartum exclusive of the first 24 hours, and to be taken by mouth by a standard technique at least four times daily." While puerperal morbidity and puerperal infection are sometimes thought of as synonymous, it is incorrect to do so. Puerperal morbidity may be caused by infections and conditions other than puerperal infection. These other causes include dehydration, urinary tract infection, upper respiratory infection, and mastitis.

Differential Diagnosis

Differential diagnosis entails (1) whether evidence of puerperal morbidity is due to puerperal infection or one of the other causes, (2) if a result of puerperal infection, where the inflammatory lesions are, and (3) if a result of another infection, what the offending organism is and what antibiotics it will respond to.

Temperature elevation caused by dehydration usually occurs during the first 24 hours postpartum. This time period is excluded from consideration in determining puerperal morbidity. Dehydration may be present in the first 24 hours as a carryover from decreased fluid intake during labor (especially if labor was prolonged) and compounded by a period of rest and sleep during the early hours of the puerperium. If dehydration continues into the next day postpartum it may confuse the etiologic and symptomatologic picture of temperature elevation. This is prevented by encouraging women to drink at least one glass of water per hour during their waking hours and anytime they awaken briefly from sleep.

Urinary tract infection is difficult to differentiate by signs and symptoms. Its symptoms are similar to those of some types of puerperal infection and moreover may vary widely depending on whether it is a simple cystitis or a fulminating pyelonephritis. Urinary tract infection may cause frequency, low-grade fever with spikes, dysuria, CVA tenderness, flank pain, urgency, and lower abdominal pain. Definitive diagnosis for a urinary tract infection is made by culture of a clean-catch urine specimen demonstrating a significant number of a single type of bacteria (see Chapter 9).

Auscultation of the lungs should be part of the daily postpartum examination of the woman. This examination would disclose the sounds of an upper respiratory infection and point towards this as the cause of temperature elevation, as would the other usual signs and symptoms.

Mastitis produces a rapid elevation in temperature to 103 to 104°F (39.4 to 40°C). The other signs and symptoms of mastitis are detailed later in this chapter.

If a woman has an elevated temperature of more than 100.4°F (38°C) the nurse-midwife does a history and physical examination of the lungs, breasts, urinary tract, and lochia; reviews the chart for evidence of predisposing causes for puerperal infection; obtains urine or lochial specimens, or both, for culture and sensitivity, if indicated; and consults with the physician. If a woman has an elevated temperature of less than 100.4°F, especially within the first 24 hours postpartum, and in the absence of any other indications of illness, the fever most likely is due to dehydration. In such a situation the nurse-midwife should urge the woman to drink one glass of fluid per hour. The woman should also be encouraged to urinate frequently, even if she doesn't feel like it because of hypotonia of the bladder. The frequent urination helps to avoid urine stasis and the increased potential of a urinary tract infection. The woman's temperature must be taken and recorded every 4 hours.

PUERPERAL INFECTION

Puerperal infection is a bacterial infection originating in the reproductive tract during labor or the puerperium. It no longer is responsible for a high incidence of puerperal mortality as it was historically, when it was known as the dreaded childbed fever. However, puerperal infection still is responsible for a high incidence of puerperal morbidity.

Predisposing Causes

The following circumstances predispose the woman to puerperal infection:

1. Prolonged labor, especially with ruptured membranes
2. Prolonged rupture of the membranes
3. Numerous vaginal examinations during labor, especially with ruptured membranes
4. Breaks in aseptic technique
5. Carelessness regarding hand washing
6. Any intrauterine manipulation
7. Extensive tissue trauma, either as an open wound or as tissue devitalization
8. Hematomas
9. Hemorrhage, especially if more than 1000 milliliters
10. Operative delivery
11. Retention of placental fragments or membranes
12. Improper perineal care

The classic clinical picture predisposing to puerperal infection is one of trauma accompanied by hemorrhage and maternal exhaustion. Contrary to previous and popular thought, it is questionable if anemia actually is a predisposing cause of infection.

Bacterial Organisms

Bacterial organisms in puerperal infections come from two sources:

1. Bacteria that normally exist in the lower genital tract or in the bowel.
2. Bacteria that are in the nasopharynx or on the hands of attending personnel or in the air and dust of the environment.

The former are endogenous sources which become pathogenic only when there is tissue damage or devitalization or when there is contamination of the genital tract from the bowel. The latter are exogenous sources for which scrupulous attention to hand washing is the best preventative. The virulent beta-hemolytic *streptococcus*, group A, which is responsible for epidemic puerperal infection, is an example of a bacterium which gains access to the reproductive tract from an exogenous source, generally an infected individual with some form of direct or indirect contact with the mother. Fortunately such an epidemic is now rare, thanks to antibiotics and emphasis on proper hand washing.

Anaerobic streptococci and enterococci are the most common organisms involved in puerperal infection. Organisms common to the vagina include *Streptococcus viridans*. Organisms common to the lower bowel include *Clostridium welchii, Escherichia coli, Proteus, Aerobacter aerogenes*, enterococci, and *Pseudomonas aeruginosa*. Other offending organisms may include *Staphylococcus, Neisseria*, and *Klebsiella*. Infection more often is due to a combination of pathogens than to only one.

Signs and Symptoms

In general, some signs and symptoms are the same for each site of puerperal infection since all of them are infections — elevated temperature, tachycardia, and pain. The pulse rate is considered the most dependable guide for severity of the illness and its prognosis in infection. A pulse rate greater than 120 beats per minute is considered quite serious. In general, the higher the temperature the more serious the illness, especially if the temperature elevation was sudden rather than a gradual rise and if there are no remissions. Discussion in this chapter of each site of puerperal infection is limited to its signs and symptoms and any helpful related explanatory information that would be useful to the nurse-midwife for screening purposes. Interpretation of laboratory cultures and sensitivities, further investigation, and treatment require collaboration with your consulting physician.

Sites of Puerperal Infection

Puerperal infection consists of inflammatory lesions that actually are bacterial wound infections. Each wound, thus, becomes a potential portal of entry for the pathogenic bacteria. Infections at these sites are localized infections. Such potential portals of entry include wounds of the perineum, vulva, vagina, cervix, and uterine cavity (the decidua/endometrium and/or the placental site). There are also extended infections, which originate from a localized infection and extend via the path of venous circulation or the lymphatics to produce bacterial infection in more distant sites. Extended sites of puerperal infection include pelvic cellulitis, salpingitis, oophoritis, peritonitis, pelvic and/or femoral thrombophlebitis, and bacteremia.

Infected Trauma of the Vulva, Perineum, Vagina, or Cervix
Signs and symptoms of infected episiotomies, lacerations, or other trauma include:

1. Localized pain.
2. Dysuria.
3. Low-grade temperature — seldom above 101°F (38.3°C).
4. Pulse usually below 100 beats per minute.
5. May be acute with sudden chill and spike in temperature to 104°F (40°C).
6. Edema.
7. Repair edges are red and inflamed.
8. Oozing of pus or gray-green exudate.
9. Wound separation or dehiscence (bursting open).
10. Lesion may progress to ulcer if untreated.

Visible episiotomy and laceration repairs should be checked routinely at least twice daily for numbers 6, 7, 8, and 9 above. In addition to episiotomy or lacerations, trauma may be due to bruising, abrasions (skid marks) too small to suture, hematoma formation, or foreign objects inadvertently left in the vagina (e.g., gauze sponge).

Endometritis
Signs and symptoms of endometritis include:

1. Tachycardia — pulse rate between 100 and 140 beats per minute, depending on the severity of the infection
2. Jagged temperature elevation between 101 and 104°F (38.3 and 40°C), depending on the severity of the infection
3. Chills if the infection is severe
4. Uterine tenderness extending laterally
5. Prolonged or recurrent after-birth pains
6. Subinvolution
7. Slight abdominal distention
8. Scanty, odorless lochia or moderately heavy, foul, bloody, seropurulent lochia
9. Onset usually on the third to fifth day postpartum except when the causative organism is beta-hemolytic *Streptococcus*, then the onset is earlier and more precipitous
10. White blood cell count elevated beyond the physiologic leukocytosis of the puerperium

If the infection remains localized to the endometrium or placental site it is often confused in diagnosis with a urinary tract infection. The results of a lochial culture establish a definitive diagnosis regarding endometritis.

Salpingitis and Oophoritis
Signs and symptoms of salpingitis and oophoritis include:

1. Temperature elevation to 103 or 104°F (39.4 to 40°C)
2. Unilateral or bilateral abdominal pain in the lower quadrants
3. Signs and symptoms of pelvic peritonitis (see following)
4. Onset usually between the ninth and fifteenth days postpartum

Salpingitis and oophoritis are rare postpartally. When they occur they are usually a flare-up of a previous gonorrheal infection. Initial gonorrheal infections are even more rare during the puerperium.

Pelvic Cellulitis (Parametritis)

Signs and symptoms of parametritis include:

1. Prolonged and sustained temperature elevation of approximately 102° to 103°F (38.8 to 39.4°C).
2. Nearly always preceded on the third to fifth day postpartum by the signs and symptoms of endometritis (chills, elevated temperature, increased pulse rate, and localized pain); onset is subsequent, generally up to the ninth day postpartum, often beginning with anorexia, nausea, vomiting, and constipation.
3. Subinvolution.
4. Formation of a large abcess which, depending on its location, may be palpated vaginally, rectally, and/or abdominally.
5. Repeated chills and sweats as the temperature fluctuates after formation of a mass of pus later in the course of the infection.
6. Unilateral or bilateral abdominal pain extending laterally.
7. Deep flank pain.
8. Fixation of the uterus.
9. Skin in the inguinal region reddened, edematous, and tender with fluctuation.
10. Usually also has signs of peritonitis, especially local and referred rebound tenderness, involuntary guarding, and decreased bowel sounds.

Pelvic cellulitis is an extended infection site originating from localized infections in either the cervix or the uterus (endometritis). In this instance the bacteria travel via the lymphatics or invade the connective tissue directly, extending through the broad ligament.

Peritonitis

Signs and symptoms of peritonitis include:

1. Severe pain
2. Chills
3. Temperature elevation to 105°F (40.5°C)

4. Weak, rapid pulse rate to 140 beats per minute
5. Rapid, shallow chest breathing
6. Frequent vomiting, often projectile, and, as the woman's condition deteriorates, eventually containing feces
7. Distention of bowel and abdomen with extreme abdominal tenderness and rigidity of the walls and ileus
8. Excessive thirst; dry, brown tongue; and foul breath
9. Anxious expression and restlessness
10. Face first flushed; then pale, gray, cold, and sweaty with sunken eyes
11. Severe reduction in the amount of urinary output
12. Total bodily collapse and death if untreated

Peritonitis is an extended infection site originating from a localized infection in the uterus (endometritis) and spreading to the peritoneum via the lymphatics. Peritonitis is life threatening, ending in death if untreated.

Thrombophlebitis

Signs and symptoms of thrombophlebitis as an extended site of puerperal infection include:

1. Unexplained elevation of pulse (often occurs prior to the development of any other signs and symptoms)
2. Repeated severe chills (a characteristic feature)
3. Extreme swings in temperature, climbing from subnormal to 105°F (40.5°C) and then falling precipitously within an hour's time
4. Hypotension resulting from bacterial shock
5. Pleurisy and pneumonia caused by small pulmonary emboli
6. Preceded by the signs and symptoms of endometritis
7. If a femoral thrombophlebitis, the signs and symptoms of deep venous thrombophlebitis, as listed later in this chapter

Thrombophlebitis reflects extension of the infection via the veins and originates from infected thrombosed veins at the placental site (endometritis). Extension is either into the pelvic veins (e.g., ovarian, renal, inferior vena cava) or into the femoral vein from the uterine veins via the iliac veins. The former is called pelvic thrombophlebitis and the latter is called femoral thrombophlebitis.

Bacteremia

Signs and symptoms of bacteremia include:

1. Severe chills
2. Rapid temperature elevation of 103 to 104°F (39.4 to 40°C)
3. Rapid increase in pulse rate to more than 120 beats per minute
4. Rapid, shallow respirations
5. Pale skin with cyanotic fingers and lips
6. Profuse, foul lochia
7. The signs and symptoms of peritonitis (see above)

Bacteremia arises from two sources: (1) from an endometritis via the lymphatics and/or (2) from a thrombophlebitis yielding vascular bacteremia in which thrombi spread the infection all over the body including the brain, heart, and lungs.

OTHER PUERPERAL COMPLICATIONS

Mastitis

Mastitis is inflammation of the breast. Although it can occur in any woman, it is almost exclusively a complication of the lactating woman, especially the primipara. Mastitis develops as a result of invasion of breast tissue (e.g., glandular, connective, areolar, fat) by bacteria in the presence of breast injury. Injury to the breast may be due to bruising from rough manipulation, breast overdistention, milk stasis in a duct, or cracking or fissures of the nipple. The bacteria may originate from a number of sources: (1) the hands of the mother, (2) the hands of personnel caring for the mother or for

the baby, (3) the baby, who may have been infected in the nursery, (4) the lactiferous ducts, or (5) the circulating blood. The most common causative bacterium in mastitis is *Staphylococcus aureus*.

The best treatment of mastitis is prevention. Prevention is accomplished through meticulous attention to hand washing with antibacterial soap; breast care that includes gentleness, prevention or removal of crusts on the nipple, good support to the breasts, cleanliness, and measures for prevention of nipple cracking (see Chapter 24); daily observation of the baby for skin or cord infection; and no contact with people with a known staphylococcal infection or lesion.

Signs and symptoms of mastitis start with precursory signs, progress to the signs and symptoms of mastitis, and, if treatment is not instituted, end with the signs and symptoms of breast abscesses. Precursory signs and symptoms are:

1. Severe engorgement
2. No signs or symptoms before the end of the first postpartal week, then —
3. Slight fever
4. Mild pain in one segment of the breast, which is exaggerated when the baby nurses
5. Breast fluctuation

Actual signs and symptoms of mastitis include:

1. Rapid elevation in temperature to 103 to 104°F (39.5 to 40°C)
2. Increased pulse rate
3. Chills, general malaise, headache
4. Area of breast reddened, very tender, painful, with hard, sizable lump(s)
5. Culture and sensitivity done on a smear of the breast milk may identify the bacteria

Signs and symptoms of abscesses include:

1. Discharge of pus (suppuration), especially

if high temperature continues for more than 48 hours

2. Remittent fever with chills
3. Breast swollen and extremely painful; a large, hard mass with an area of fluctuation, reddening, and bluish tinge to the skin indicating the location of the pus-filled abscess

There is much conflicting opinion as to whether breast-feeding should be continued, temporarily discontinued, or permanently discontinued in the presence of mastitis. Proponents of continuing breast-feeding state their concern for worsening the condition because of the engorgement and overdistention of the breast that will occur with abrupt cessation of breast-feeding. They further express concern for the benefits to mother and baby to continue breast-feeding or, conversely, the trauma to both mother and baby if breast-feeding is halted abruptly. Proponents of discontinuing breast-feeding believe the infection will be more quickly cured, thereby preventing involvement of further lobes and more abscesses, if there is cessation of stimulation to the breast. They also express concern for the possible reoccurrence of mastitis if breast-feeding is continued.

Between these two extremes is the position of temporary discontinuation. Breast-feeding, with this procedure, is discontinued during the time of high fever and when there may be pus in the milk, so that the baby does not become infected and, in turn, reinfect the mother. In order to avoid engorgement and at the same time to reduce stimulation to the affected breast, heat is applied to the breast to encourage milk flow and the milk is partially removed by hand or electric pump. The milk is not removed by manual massage and expression because of the soreness of the breasts and because such manipulation will exaggerate the already existing breast injury. This milk, collected while the mother has a high fever, contains pus and is discarded.

Treatment of mastitis is geared towards its cure and the prevention of its developing into successive multiple abscesses, each of which will have to be opened and drained and will have a healing process of weeks to months.

Physician collaboration is sought for treatment with antibiotics. The mother, physician, and nurse-midwife need to come to an agreement regarding the management of breast-feeding. Firm, nonconstrictive support should be designed for the breasts. It is important that the mother be fully cognizant of the need to take her full course of antibiotics, usually, continued for 10 days, even though she has a dramatic recovery in a couple of days. If breast-feeding was discontinued temporarily, it may be resumed after the mother is afebrile for 24 hours. Usually breast-feeding is temporarily discontinued for 2 to 3 days.

Thrombophlebitis and Pulmonary Embolism

There is a type of thrombophlebitis that is not an extension or result of puerperal infection, does not have a bacterial origin, and is not septic. Often its etiologic factors are unknown, but it is more common in women with varicosities or who perhaps are genetically susceptible to vein wall relaxation and venous stasis. Pregnancy fosters venous stasis by virtue of vein wall relaxation resulting from the effects of progesterone and pressure on the veins by the uterus. Thrombophlebitis can be superficial or deep, depending on whether it is limited to the superficial veins or involves the deep veins of the lower extremity.

Superficial thrombophlebitis is evidenced by the following signs and symptoms:

1. Slight temperature elevation
2. Slight pulse elevation
3. Leg pain
4. Local heat, extreme tenderness, and redness at the site of the vein inflammation

Deep venous thrombophlebitis is evidenced

by the following signs and symptoms:

1. High fever with tachycardia and chills that may be severe
2. Abrupt onset with severe leg pain (there may have been a precursor of slight leg pain when walking)
3. Edema of the ankle, leg, and thigh
4. Positive Homan's sign (see Chapter 24)
5. Pain with calf pressure
6. Tenderness along the entire course of the involved vessel(s)

The physician is consulted upon eliciting the signs and symptoms of a superficial or deep thrombophlebitis. Treatment includes bed rest, elevation of the affected extremity, hot packs, elastic stockings, and analgesia as needed. A cradle for bedclothes may be needed if the leg is quite tender to touch (more likely with superficial thrombophlebitis). Collaboration with the physician is necessary for decisions concerning anticoagulant therapy and antibiotics (more likely with deep venous thrombophlebitis). Under no circumstances should the leg be massaged.

The greatest danger of thrombophlebitis is pulmonary embolism. This is particularly true with deep venous thrombophlebitis, and unlikely with superficial thrombophlebitis. Signs and symptoms of pulmonary embolism are as follows:

1. Chest pain so sharp that the woman "catches her breath"
2. Shortness of breath, air hunger, and tachypnea; dyspnea
3. Respiratory rales
4. Tachycardia
5. Hemoptysis
6. Apprehension

The physician is notified immediately.

Hematomas

A hematoma is a tissue swelling that contains blood. The dangers of a hematoma are blood loss amounting to a hemorrhage, anemia, and infection. Hematomas arise from spontaneous or traumatic rupture of a blood vessel. In the childbearing cycle this occurs most often during delivery or shortly thereafter as vulvar, vaginal, or broad ligament hematomas. Possible causes include:

1. Forceps
2. Inadvertent nicking of a blood vessel during repair of an episiotomy or laceration or while positioning the needle for a pudendal block
3. Failure to effect complete hemostasis prior to repair of a laceration or episiotomy
4. Unligated vessels above (beyond) the incision opening with failure to start the suture line at that point
5. Rough handling of vaginal tissue at any time or of the uterus during massage

The common sign of a hematoma is extreme pain out of proportion to the expected amount of discomfort and pain for the postpartal period during which this is happening. Other signs and symptoms of a vulvar or vaginal hematoma are as follows:

1. Perineal, vaginal, urethral, bladder, or rectal pressure and severe pain
2. A tense, fluctuant swelling
3. Bluish or blue-black discoloration of tissue

Other signs and symptoms of a broad ligament hematoma are as follows:

1. Lateral uterine pain sensitive to palpation
2. Extension of pain into the flank
3. High rectal examination reveals a painful bulge
4. Ridge of tissue just above the pelvic brim extending laterally (this is the edge of the swollen broad ligament)
5. Abdominal distention

Hematomas of any significant size require

immediate consultation with and referral to the physician. The physician subsequently makes decisions regarding frequency of hematocrit results, need for surgical intervention, need for blood replacement, need for antibiotics, and so forth.

Late (Delayed) Postpartum Hemorrhage

Late (delayed) postpartum hemorrhage is hemorrhage that occurs after the first 24 hours postpartum. Possible causes include the following:

1. Placental site subinvolution resulting from thrombosed blood vessels or endometritis
2. Retained placental fragments
3. Hematoma
4. Reproductive tract laceration previously undiagnosed

Signs and symptoms of late postpartum hemorrhage include obvious external bleeding, signs and symptoms of shock, and signs and symptoms of anemia. The nurse-midwife collaborates with the consulting physician for diagnosis of the cause and appropriate treatment.

Hemorrhage that occurs between that described as fourth stage hemorrhage and late postpartum hemorrhage is managed as discussed for management of immediate postpartum hemorrhage (see Chapter 19). The first step is to diagnose the cause (e.g., uterine atony, reproductive tract laceration), and institute appropriate management while awaiting the arrival of the physician or resolution of the problem.

Subinvolution

Subinvolution is the condition in which the process of involution does not occur as it should and is either prolonged or stopped. Interference with the process of involution may be due to retained placental fragments, myomata, or infection. Retained placental fragments is the most frequent cause.

Subinvolution is most often diagnosed during the 4- to 6-weeks postpartum examination. At that time the woman will give a history of a longer than normal period of lochial discharge for each of the different types of lochia, followed by leukorrhea and irregular, heavy bleeding. Pelvic examination will reveal a soft uterus which is larger than normal for the week postpartum during which the woman is being examined.

Subinvolution early in the puerperium is evidenced by a soft, boggy uterus whose fundal height remains stationary rather than decreasing in size. The lochia is profuse and reddish brown. In this instance a lochial culture should be taken to rule out endometritis. At the 4- to 6-weeks postpartum visit, an infection is not considered unless there is tenderness or pain of the adnexa or upon movement of the uterus.

Treatment of subinvolution is with ergonovine (Ergotrate) or methylergonovine (Methergine) 0.2 milligrams every 3 to 4 hours for 3 days and reevaluation in 2 weeks. If there is also endometritis, antibiotic therapy is prescribed.

Maternal Rejection, Failure to Thrive, and Child Abuse

Definition and Interrelationships

Maternal rejection is an aberration of the maternal attachment and bonding process. The result of this aberration may be child abuse, which in turn may result in serious behavioral disorders of infancy and early childhood. A much higher incidence of abuse during childhood is reported in the criminal population than in the population as a whole. Failure to thrive is a form of child abuse which results from neglected caretaking. Neglected caretaking is a result of maternal rejection. If the mother or caretaker finds the child unrewarding or repulsive and rejects the child, she will not provide care and the child may not survive. The human infant is totally dependent upon the mother or caretaker. The strength of the attachment to this caretaker will determine not only the infant's survival but also whether or not the infant will achieve his or her potential due to optimal circumstances for development.

Characteristics of Potential Child Abusers
The internal and external factors influencing parental attachment behavior were discussed in Chapter 24. Negative variations of these are evident in thus-far identified characteristics of potential child abusers.

1. *A victim of child abuse* — a high percentage of abusive parents were abused children.
2. *Low self-esteem* — this is an almost inevitable outcome if the parent was an abused child. The potential for a vicious generational cycle is obvious.
3. *A lack of trusting and supportive relationships* — this is evidenced by a lack of friends, a poor or nonexistent marital relationship, or a lack of contact with family or relatives. Possibly the parent is unable to establish such a relationship. A higher incidence of abusive parents have unlisted telephone numbers. The result is extreme personal and social isolation.
4. *An expected reversal of parent-child roles* — the parent expects the child to be the source of the parent's own gratification, emotional support, and caretaking. This results in rampant unrealistic expectations for the child's behavior.
5. *Maternal-infant separation at birth* — may result in a bonding delay or failure. Even short periods of separation during the early postpartal hours and days result in fewer maternal attachment behaviors during the first postpartal year than those exhibited by mothers when there is no separation.

There are two categories of factors which may cause bonding delay or failure. One category is problems originating with the baby (e.g., prematurity, congenital anomalies) which delay the bonding process because of necessary hospitalization and grief process. Approximately half of all abused children either were premature or had a serious illness which resulted in prolonged maternal-infant separation during the first weeks of life. A significant incidence of premature babies return to the hospital because of failure to thrive.

The other category of factors which may contribute to bonding delay or failure is problems originating with the mother (e.g., need for cesarean section, serious obstetric or medical complications, experiencing a simultaneous life crisis) which cause some degree of separation after birth. There is a higher incidence of cesarean births in the population of abused children than in the population as a whole. The postsurgical psychologic state of an individual is one of dependence. A postoperative cesarean section mother, thus, is in a state that is less than optimal for bonding. This is of particular concern at a time when the rate of cesarean section has risen so drastically.

Screening for Potential Child Abusers during the Childbearing Cycle
Prenatal Warning Signs. A number of observations which can be made during the prenatal period may be indicative of possible attachment problems and potential child abuse. Observations include:

1. Nonacceptance of the pregnancy into the second and third trimesters
2. Hyperemesis gravidarum
3. Refusal to do those things which would positively affect the well-being of the baby, such as abstain from cigarettes, alcohol, and nonprescribed drugs, and eat a diet adequate in protein and calories
4. Overconcern with the sex of the baby
5. Overconcern with the baby's future performance and meeting of standards
6. Preexisting or current emotional disturbances or depression about this pregnancy
7. Unplanned, unwanted pregnancy for which an abortion was wanted but not done, or there was temporary consideration of carrying the pregnancy to term

and giving the child up for adoption. In either instance, why did the woman or couple change their mind?

8. Lack of supportive friends and family, lack of support from the father of the baby
9. Fears and anxieties that explanations of pregnancy, labor, and delivery do not ease
10. Unlisted telephone number
11. Refusal to plan for the baby and lack of preparations for taking care of the baby
12. History that either parent was abused as a child
13. Overcrowded or unstable living situation to which the addition of a baby is intolerable or "the final straw"

The presence of these warning signs should alert the nurse-midwife to the possibility of maladaptation and potential failure in maternal-infant attachment and bonding. Discussion of feelings towards this baby, past experiences, and the type of birth experiences that will facilitate attachment and bonding are indicated interventions during the prenatal period.

Observations at Birth. Observations at birth focus on the mother's reaction and response to her baby. What does she say? What does she do? How does she look? Is she in a physical condition to be responsive? What is the condition of the baby? Is there physical contact between the mother and baby? When? For how long? With the baby wrapped or unwrapped? What are the specifics (type and content) of the interaction?

Postpartal Assessment of Parenting. Morris identified a number of criteria that can be used to assess the mother's behavior in relation to her infant [1, p. 11]. This behavior reflects the amount and strength of attachment and bonding which has occurred. Other factors, such as her own available physical and mental energy and the support systems available to her, can also affect her behavior [2].

According to Morris, mother-infant unity can be said to be satisfactory when a mother can:

1. Find pleasure in her infant and in tasks for and with her baby
2. Understand her baby's emotional states and comfort her infant
3. Read her baby's cues for new experience; sense his or her fatigue level. Examples: she can receive eye contact from her infant with pleasure; can promote new learnings through use of her face, hands and objects; does not overstimulate her baby for her own pleasure

Specific signs that mothers give when they are not adapting to their infants are as follows [1, 2]:

1. See their infant as ugly or unattractive
2. Perceive the odor of their infant as revolting
3. Are disgusted by their infant's drooling
4. Are disgusted by their infant's sucking sounds
5. Become upset by vomiting, but seem fascinated by it
6. Are revolted by any of their infant's body fluids which touch them, or which they touch
7. Show annoyance at having to clean up their infant's stools
8. Become preoccupied with the odor, consistency, and number of their infant's stools
9. Let their infant's head dangle, without support or concern
10. Hold their infant away from their own body
11. Pick up their infant without warning by touch or speech
12. Jiggle and play with their infant roughly after feeding, even though the infant often vomits at this behavior

13. Think their infant's natural motor activity is unnatural
14. Worry about their infant's relaxation following feeding
15. Avoid eye contact with their infant, or stare fixedly into his or her eyes
16. Do not coo or talk with their infant
17. Think that their infant does not love them
18. Believe that their infant exposes them as an unlovable, unloving parent
19. Think of their infant as judging them and their efforts as an adult would
20. Perceive their infant's natural dependency needs as dangerous
21. Fear their baby will die whenever he or she gets mild diarrhea or a minor cold
22. Are convinced that their infant has defects, in spite of repeated physical examinations which prove negative
23. Often fear that their infant has diseases connected with "eating"; leukemia, or one of the other malignancies; diabetes; cystic fibrosis
24. Constantly demand reassurance that no defect or disease exists but cannot believe relieving facts when they are given
25. Demand that feared defects be found and relieved
26. Cannot find in their infant any physical or psychologic attribute which they value in themselves
27. Cannot discriminate between infant signals of hunger, fatigue, need for soothing or stimulating speech, comforting baby contact, or eye contact
28. Develop inappropriate responses to infant needs: over- or underfeed; over- or underhold; tickle or bounce the baby when the baby is fatigued; talk too much, too little, and at the wrong time; force eye contact or refuse it; leave infant alone in room; leave infant in noisy room and ignore him or her
29. Develop paradoxical attitudes and behaviors. Example: bitterly insist that infant cannot be pleased, no matter what is done, but continue to demand more and better methods for pleasing the baby.

Interventions

When any degree of maladaptation is evident or circumstances such as prematurity predispose to extended early mother-infant separation, immediate intervention is indicated. Intervention includes actions which promote and facilitate attachment. The needs of the mother should be assessed and met. Provision for positive experiences between mother and baby should be made. The following are examples of concrete actions encompassed in the types of intervention indicated:

1. If mother and baby are home:
   a. follow-up telephone calls
   b. follow-up home visits
   c. more frequent return visits
2. If baby remains hospitalized:
   a. 24 hour visiting policy
   b. explanation of frightening equipment and procedures
   c. encouragement of telephone calls and visits
   d. involvement in care of her baby
3. Approach to mother in all circumstances:
   a. concern for her needs
   b. compliments and suggestions rather than criticism
   c. respect for her capabilities
   d. reassurance of availability of self and other resources whenever needed

Assessment of needs and anticipatory guidance range from economic and social concerns, through psychologic aspects, to specific details of caretaking skills and necessary supplies.

REFERENCES

1. Morris, M. G. Psychological miscarriage: An end to mother love, *Trans-Action*. January/February, 1966.

2. Bishop, B. A guide to assessing parenting capabilities, *Am. J. Nurs.* 76:1784, 1976.

BIBLIOGRAPHY

Bishop, B. A guide to assessing parenting capabilities. *Am. J. Nurs.* 76:1784, 1976.

Brecher, R., and Brecher, E. Why some mothers reject their babies. *Redbook* May, 1966.

Ezrati, J. B., and Gordon, H. Puerperal mastitis: Causes, prevention, and management. *J. Nurse-Midwifery* 24(6):3–8 (November/December) 1979.

Funke, J., and Irby, M. An instrument to assess the quality of maternal behavior. *J. Obstet. Gynecol. Neonat. Nurs.* 7(5):19 (September/October) 1978.

Greenhill, J. P., and Friedman, E. A. *Biological Principles and Modern Practice of Obstetrics.* Philadelphia: Saunders, 1974.

Kempe, C. H. Approaches to preventing child abuse. *Am. J. Dis. Child.* 130:941, 1976.

Klaus, M. H., and Kennell, J. H. Mothers separated from their newborn infants. *Pediatr. Clin. North Am.* 17:1015, 1970.

Lynch, M. A., and Roberts, J. Predicting child abuse: Signs of bonding failure in the maternity hospital. *Brit. Med. J.* 1:624–626, March 5, 1977.

Morris, M. G. Detection of high risk parents, Unknown.

Morris, M. G. Psychological miscarriage: An end to mother love. *Trans-Action* (January/February) 1966, p. 8.

Pritchard, J. A., MacDonald, P. C., and Gant, N. F. *Wlliams Obstetrics, 17th.* Norwalk, Conn.: Appleton-Century-Crofts, 1985.

Reid, D. E., Ryan, K. J., and Benirschke, K. *Principles and Management of Human Reproduction.* Philadelphia: Saunders, 1972.

Swanson, J. Nursing intervention to facilitate maternal-infant attachment. *J. Obstet. Gynecol. Neonat. Nurs.* 7(2):35 (March/April) 1978.

Wiedenbach, E. *Family-Centered Maternity Nursing, 2nd.* New York: G. P. Putnam's Sons, 1967.

Ziegel, E. and Cranley, M. *Obstetric Nursing, 7th.* New York: Macmillan, 1979.

VI

Management of the Interconceptional Period

26

Interconceptional Care

Technically the interconceptional period covers the period of time between the delivery of the products of one conception and the occurrence of the next conception, i.e., the period of time between pregnancies. In practice health care during the interconceptional period has come to mean the primary health care of women who are between menarche and menopause as it relates to the reproductive system. Interconceptional care, then, includes women who not only are not pregnant but who may or may not wish to be pregnant.

Nurse-midwives expanded the sphere of their practice into the interconceptional period during the mid to late 1960s when they took on the management of care of individuals and couples desiring family planning. Nurse-midwives quickly became involved in the sexual concerns of women which were expressed to them during family planning visits. The nonpregnant pelvic examination, which encompasses screening for gynecologic problems, became more extensive than previously when it had been limited to the 6-weeks postpartum examination. When it became evident that for

many women the physical examination they received during their annual family planning visit was their only physical examination from year to year, nurse-midwives incorporated into their practice a comprehensive history and physical examination that would screen for abnormality (see Chapter 3). More recently, nurse-midwives have extended the interconceptional period into and past the menopause and expanded the concept of care to that of well-woman gynecology.

Management of interconceptional care by nurse-midwives is based on a comprehensive history and physical examination (see Chapter 3). Special emphasis is given a woman's menstrual history, reproductive history, contraceptive history, douching history, sexual history, and gynecologic history. Additional specific areas of concern include adolescents with their initiating of pelvic health care and first pelvic examination; psychological growth and development; lesbian health care; occupational health hazards and care; and gynecologic and psychologic trauma related to rape and battering. It is also during the interconceptional period that the nurse-midwife may be diagnosing early pregnancy (see Chapter 4); doing abortion counseling (see Chapter 4); and identifying concerns regarding infertility, screening for the need for an infertility workup, and doing related counseling. Components of interconceptional care further include family planning and gynecologic screening. Gynecologic screening encompasses pelvic health care and management of infections; menstrual concerns ranging from the normal physiologic processes involved in menarche and menopause through premenstrual syndrome to amenorrhea or dysfunctional uterine bleeding; differential diagnosis of lower abdominal and pelvic pain; and screening for breast and pelvic malignancies and disease.

This chapter focuses on initial and annual gynecologic screening and the management of the most common findings. The other chapters in this part of the book focus on family planning and its management in caring for individuals who desire family planning and utilize the various contraceptive methods.

INITIAL AND ANNUAL EXAMINATION AND GYNECOLOGIC SCREENING

The initial and annual history and the physical and pelvic examinations for women throughout the interconceptional period are the same as outlined in Chapter 3. If the woman desires family planning, additional history and physical and pelvic findings are elicited and evaluated in relation to the possible presence of any contraindications to any of the available contraceptive methods. If the woman is already using a contraceptive method, then her annual examination must also include additional history and physical and pelvic findings in order to evaluate the possible presence of any untoward side effects to the specific method being used. The contraindications and side effects of each specific method of family planning are presented in subsequent chapters.

The history specific to reproduction for the nonpregnant woman is abbreviated from that given in Chapter 3. This abbreviated obstetric history plus the menstrual history, contraceptive history, douching history, sexual history, and gynecologic history is as follows:

Menstrual History
1. Age at menarche
2. Frequency — range if irregular
3. Duration
4. Amount of flow
5. Characteristics of flow, for example, clots
6. Last menstrual period (LMP) — normal duration and amounts?
7. Dysmenorrhea
8. Dysfunctional uterine bleeding (i.e., intermenstrual spotting or bleeding, menorrhagia, metrorrhagia)
9. Toxic shock syndrome
10. Premenstrual symptoms or premenstrual syndrome (PMS)
11. Perimenopausal symptoms

Douching History
1. Frequency
2. Method (how)
3. Solution used
4. Reasons for douching
5. How long woman has been using douches
6. Last time douched

Contraceptive History
1. Present contraceptive method
   a. type
   b. satisfaction
   c. side effects
   d. consistency of use
   e. length of time using this method
2. Previous contraceptive methods
   a. types
   b. duration of use for each
   c. side effects of each
   d. reasons for discontinuing each

Obstetric History
1. Gravida and para (four-digit system)
2. Date of last baby born

3. Date of last pregnancy termination
4. Blood type (ABO and Rh); RhoGam
5. Any obstetric or medical problems during pregnancy, labor and delivery, or postpartum
6. Any congenital anomalies or neonatal complications

Sexual History
1. Nature of sexual relationship
2. Frequency of sexual relations
3. Satisfaction with sexual frequency
4. Satisfaction with sexual relationship
5. Problems
   a. insufficient foreplay
   b. insufficient lubrication
   c. lack of personal consideration
   d. pain
   e. fear of becoming pregnant
   f. fear of hurting the fetus, if pregnant
   g. problems of partner, for example, impotence, premature ejaculation
6. postcoital bleeding

Gynecologic History
1. Infertility
2. DES exposure
3. Vaginal infections (caused by *Candida, Trichomonas, Gardnerella* [*Hemophilus vaginalis*])
4. Condylomata acuminata
5. Sexually transmitted diseases (STD) (chlamydia, syphilis, gonorrhea, herpes, AIDS)
6. Chronic cervicitis
7. Endometritis
8. Pelvic inflammatory disease (PID)
9. Cysts (Bartholin, ovarian)
10. Endometriosis
11. Myomata
12. Pelvic relaxations (cystocele, rectocele)
13. Polyps
14. Breast masses
15. Abnormal Pap smears
16. Biopsies (cervical, endometrial, breast)
17. Gynecologic cancer
18. Gynecologic surgery

19. Rape, battering

Screening for many of the gynecologic disorders is detailed in Chapters 40 and 44. Screening is done every time you examine a woman's breasts and pelvic organs. Following is a listing of gynecologic disorders and deviations from normal which are screened for by history, physical and pelvic examinations, and laboratory tests:

1. Menstrual/bleeding disorders
   a. primary amenorrhea
   b. secondary amenorrhea
   c. dysfunctional bleeding
   d. premenstrual syndrome
   e. dysmenorrhea
   f. oligomenorrhea
   g. menorrhagia
   h. metrorrhagia
2. Tumors/masses of the reproductive system
   a. breast masses
   b. pelvic masses, including
      (1) ovarian cysts
      (2) hydrosalpinx
      (3) polyps
      (4) myomata
3. Lesions of the reproductive system
   a. pelvic abscess
   b. tubo-ovarian abscess
   c. vaginitis
   d. cervicitis
   e. erosion
   f. eversion
   g. ectropion
   h. endometriosis
   i. adenomyosis
   j. dysplasia
   k. cancer — as determined by Pap smear
4. Gynecologic infections
   a. candidiasis (monilia)
   b. trichomoniasis
   c. *Gardnerella* (*Hemophilus*)
   d. Chlamydia
   e. condylomata acuminata
   f. herpes
   g. syphilis

   h. gonorrhea
   i. skenitis
   j. Bartholin's cysts or bartholinitis
   k. pelvic inflammatory disease (PID)
5. Infestations
   a. pediculosis (lice)
   b. scabies (itch mites)
   c. ascariasis (roundworm)
   d. enterobiasis (pinworm)
6. Fistulas
7. Uterine malpositions
8. Pelvic relaxations — with or without stress incontinence or urge incontinence
   a. cystocele
   b. urethrocele
   c. rectocele
   d. enterocele
   e. uterine descensus (prolapse)
9. Vaginal foreign body
10. Other vaginal or perineal disorder
   a. unrepaired perineal lacerations
   b. vaginismus
   c. vaginal atrophy
   d. incompletely ruptured hymen
   e. vaginal stricture

MANAGEMENT OF THE MOST COMMON GYNECOLOGIC FINDINGS

Management of the most common gynecologic findings involves screening, preventive care, diagnosis, and treatment but not necessarily all of these aspects of management for each disorder or deviation.

There are disease entities which the nurse-midwife detects as an abnormality but does not diagnose. For example, a nurse-midwife may feel a pelvic mass but request a physician to examine the woman for diagnosis. Another example is the management of Pap smear results. In this case the nurse-midwife obtains the specimen needed for cytologic study and subsequently reads and screens the report of the results. Depending on the classification of the results, nurse-midwifery management may range from continuing annual preventive screen-ing for the woman with a normal or negative Pap smear to referral to a gynecologist for a woman with a class III or IV Pap smear. Table 26-1 is a synopsis of this management.

There is controversy as to the frequency of having a Pap smear done. The American Cancer Society currently states that for low-risk women a Pap smear every 3 years after two normal smears done 1 year apart is sufficient and cost-effective screening. The American College of Obstetricians and Gynecologists and Planned Parenthood Federation of America continue to recommend yearly screening Pap smears for all women. Factors that a nurse-midwife should include in considering the frequency of routine Pap smears include the following:

1. The number and type of risk factors associated with an increased incidence of cervical cancer
2. The unknowns and controversies regarding some risk factors
3. The fact that the list of risk factors continues to grow
4. The fact that some cases of cervical cancer can develop and progress to a class III or IV in less than three years

Factors associated with an increased incidence of cervical cancer include:

1. DES exposure
2. Smoking
3. *Trichomonas vaginalis*
4. *Herpesvirus*
5. *Chlamydia*
6. Condylomata acuminata
7. Sexual intercourse before age 20
8. Multiple sexual partners
9. Oral contraception (controversial)
10. Male circumcision (controversial)

This list places the majority of women in an at-risk or high-risk category on the basis of one or more factors. Thus routine annual Pap smear screening is clearly indicated.

TABLE 26-1. Nurse-Midwife Management of Pap Smear Results

Classification	Interpretation	Management
Class I	Normal — minimal or no inflammatory changes present	Repeat Pap smear at annual gynecologic visit
Class II	Inflammatory	Treat any vaginitis or cervicitis
		Decrease preventable risk factors, i.e., multiple sexual partners, smoking
		Have male sexual partner use condoms
		Repeat the Pap smear 8−12 weeks after successful treatment of vaginitis and cervicitis or in 8−12 weeks if there is no vaginitis or cervicitis
		If the repeat Pap smear is again class II, refer to gynecologist for colposcopy and evaluation
Class III	Dysplasia (abnormal tissue in one or more layers of epithelial cells)	Refer to gynecologist for colposcopy, further evaluation and diagnosis, and treatment
	C.I.N.* Grade I — mild dysplasia	
	C.I.N. Grade II — moderate dysplasia	
	C.I.N. Grade III { severe dysplasia	
Class IV	cancer in situ (abnormal tissue the full thickness of epithelium)	Refer to physician, preferably a gynecologic oncologist.

* C.I.N. = cervical intraepithelial neoplasia

The procedure for obtaining a Papanicolaou smear is explained in Chapter 45. Care must be taken when obtaining a Pap smear while a woman is menstruating in order to get an adequate specimen. Gentle blotting of the cervix with a 2 × 2 or 4 × 4 gauze on a sponge stick removes excess blood (which will interfere with the cytologic study) without removing the epithelial cells needed for the specimen.

In other instances the nurse-midwife may diagnose but not treat. For example, a nurse-midwife may diagnose a second degree cystocele with stress incontinence but refer the woman to a physician for decision about and performance of surgical intervention. Students interested in in-depth discussions of the gynecologic disorders included in these two categories are encouraged to read medical textbooks on gynecology. A few are listed in the bibliography to this chapter.

In still other instances the nurse-midwife may both diagnose and treat the condition. This is done, for example, in relation to the common vaginal infections. How to prepare a wet smear slide for microscopic analysis is detailed in Chapter 38. Table 26-2 gives the clinical signs and symptoms, microscopic findings, and treatment for the three most common vaginal infections which are diagnosed microscopically from a wet smear specimen. This side-by-side listing aids in differential diagnosis of vaginal infections. It should be noted that *Gardnerella vaginalis* vaginitis used to be known variously as *Hemophilus vaginalis* vaginitis, nonspecific vaginitis, and *Corynebacterium vaginale* vaginitis. Vontver and Eschenbach detail the history of identifying and classifying this organism [1].

The detection, diagnosis, treatment, and evaluation of gonorrhea, syphilis, herpes,

TABLE 26-2.   Common Vaginal Infections

	Causative Organisms		
	Candida albicans	Trichomonas vaginalis	Gardnerella (Hemophilus) vaginalis
Clinical signs and symptoms	Cheesy, curdy, yellow-white patches on vaginal mucosa and cervix Intense vulvar pruritis Vulvar edema Redness of the vestibule Dyspareunia Discharge may be scant in amount	Frothy, thin, yellow-green/gray discharge Malodorous Vaginal or cervical inflammation ("strawberry vagina") Pruritis More copious in amount of discharge Dyspareunia	Minimal thin, creamy, gray, adherent discharge Malodorous; further, there is a definite "fishy" smell when 10% KOH is added to a specimen of the discharge Discharge has an elevated pH (>4.5; usually between 5.0 and 5.5)
Microscopic findings	Filaments with budding spores (mycelia) Pseudohyphae	Motile, colorless, pyriform, flagellated trichomonads (1 marginal and 4 anterior flagella)	Clue cells (epithelial cells with indistinct border and granular appearance due to attachment of gram-negative bacilli)
Treatment	Miconazole (Monistat) 1 applicatorful or 1 suppository vaginally hs × 7 nights Clotrimazole (Gyne-Lotrimin) 1 applicatorful or 1 suppository vaginally hs × 7 nights or 2 suppositories vaginally hs × 3 nights (not during pregnancy) Nystatin (Mycostatin) 1 applicatorful or 1 suppository vaginally hs × 14 nights Gentian violet 1−2% aqueous solution Mycolog cream external topical application for symptomatic relief	Metronidazole (Flagyl) 2 gm. po stat. or 250 mg. po tid × 7 days (contraindicated during the first half of pregnancy) Clotrimazole (Gyne-Lotrimin) vaginal cream for symptomatic relief Sulfanilamide/amacrine/allantoin (AVC) vaginal cream for symptomatic relief	Metronidazole (Flagyl) 500 mg. po bid × 7 days (contraindicated during the first half of pregnancy) Ampicillin 500 mg. po qid × 7 days Sulfonamide vaginal creams (e.g., Sultrin, Triple Sulfa) 1 applicatorful vaginally hs × 14 nights

and condylomata acuminata is discussed in Chapter 9. Infection by *Chlamydia trachomatis* is now recognized as the most prevalent sexually transmitted disease and a major cause of infertility. It is, however, essentially asymptomatic unless the infection becomes severe enough to cause pelvic inflammatory disease (PID). Then the classical signs of PID cause the woman to seek health care (lower abdominal and pelvic organ pain which is exquisite upon movement of the cervix, chills, and fever). Diagnosis is based on a diagnostic screening test and on a process of elimination of other diagnoses of vaginitis and sexually transmitted diseases, especially gonorrhea, and on finding nongonococcal urethritis in the sexual partner. It is generally assumed that nongonococcal mucopurulent cervical or urethral discharge is due to *Chlamydia trachomatis*. The treatment is tetracycline hydrochloride 500 milligrams orally four times a day for 7 days (500 mg. PO QID × 7 days). Since tetracycline is *contraindicated in pregnancy* an alternate treatment is used for pregnant women with chlamydia: erythromycin 500 milligrams orally four times daily for 7 days (500 mg. PO QID × 7 days). This drug should be taken on an empty stomach. It is essential that the male partner be simultaneously treated with tetracycline.

REFERENCES

1. Vontver, L. A., and D. A. Eschenbach. The role of *Gardnerella vaginalis* in nonspecific vaginitis. *Clin. Ostet. Gynecol.* 4(2):439—460 (June) 1981.

BIBLIOGRAPHY

Beal, M. W. Understanding cervical cytology. *Nurse Pract.* 12(3), March, 1987.

Bensen, R. C. *Current Obstetric and Gynecologic Diagnosis & Treatment, 5th.* Los Altos, Calif.: Lange Medical Publications, 1984.

Centers for Disease Control. Sexually transmitted diseases treatment guidelines, 1982. *Morbidity and Mortality Weekly Report, Supplement.* 31(2s), August 20, 1982.

Cibley, L. J., and Kasdon, S. C. *A New Look at Vulvovaginitis.* Chicago: G. D. Searle & Co., 1971.

Connell, E. B., and Tatum H. J. *Sexually Transmitted Diseases: Diagnosis and Treatment.* Durant, Okla.: Creative Infomatics, 1985.

Danforth, D. N. (Ed.). *Obstetrics and Gynecology, 4th.* Hagerstown, Md.: Harper & Row, 1982.

Glass, R. H. *Office Gynecology, 2nd.* Baltimore: Williams & Wilkins, 1981.

Green, T. H., Jr. *Gynecology: Essentials of Clinical Practice, 3rd.* Boston: Little, Brown, 1977.

Haines, M., and Taylor, C. W. *Gynaecological Pathology, 2nd.* London: Churchill Livingstone, 1975.

Jeffcoate, T. N. A. *Principles of Gynaecology.* New York: Appleton-Century-Crofts, 1975.

Jones, H. W., Jr., and Jones, G. S. *Novak's Textbook of Gynecology, 10th.* Baltimore: Williams & Wilkins, 1981.

Kistner, R. W. *Gynecology: Principles and Practice, 4th.* Chicago: Year Book Medical Publishers, 1985.

Ledger, W. J. *Infection in the Female.* Philadelphia: Lea & Febiger, 1976.

Miles, P. A. Sexually transmitted diseases. *J. Obstet. Gynecol. Neonat. Nurs.* March/April, 1984, pp. 102s—124s (supplement).

Parsons, L., and Sommers, S. C. *Gynecology, 2nd.* Philadelphia: Saunders, 1978.

Pheifer, T. A. et al. Nonspecific vaginitis: Role of *Haemophilus vaginalis* and treatment with metronidazole. *N. Engl. J. Med.* 298(26):1429—1434, June 29, 1978.

Phillip, E. E., Barnes, J., and Newton, M. (Eds.). *Scientific Foundations of Obstetrics & Gynecology.* Chicago: Year Book Medical Publishers, 1977.

Schneierson, S. S. *Atlas of Diagnostic Microbiology.* Chicago: Abbott Laboratories, 1971.

Speroff, L., Glass, R. H., and Kase, N. G. *Clinical Gynecologic Endocrinology and Infertility, 3rd.* Baltimore: Williams & Wilkins, 1983.

Vontver, L. A., and Eschenbach, D. A. The role of *Gardnerella vaginalis* in nonspecific vaginitis. *Clin. Obstet. Gynecol.* 24(2):439—460 (June) 1981.

27

Family Planning

HISTORY AND CONCEPTS OF FAMILY PLANNING

From early time people have attempted by various means to prevent conception. They have tried magic, potions, and the insertion into the vagina or uterus of a variety of items such as stones, shells, coins, bottle caps, buttons, and jewelry. Bottled carbonated beverages have been used as high-pressure douches and various materials, such as transparent kitchen wrap (e.g., Saran Wrap), have been wrapped around the penis in attempts to contain sperm like a condom. These homemade "contraceptives" not only are useless but also are dangerous. Their use can cause mutilation or lead to sterility due to infection. These are not simply examples from antiquity. Many individuals still use such dangerous, nonmedical, and futile methods. Efforts must be made toward finding such persons and guiding them to safe and effective contraceptive methods.

Great strides have been made in the twentieth century in the area of family planning and its related fields. The topics, which once were taboo in public, have evolved into widely discussed and debated subjects. In 1910 a nurse,

Margaret Sanger, began her historical and heroic fight for the right of families to limit their size, the right of women to health and freedom from their biological makeup, and the right of children to the love they may expect through being wanted and planned-for children.

Before the federal government became involved in family planning, the family planning movement in the United States was spearheaded by Planned Parenthood-World Population. This organization was founded in 1916 as Planned Parenthood Federation of America by Margaret Sanger. It is the United States member and major financial support of the International Planned Parenthood Federation, which was also established by Margaret Sanger. Planned Parenthood-World Population is organized through regional offices with hundreds of family planning centers throughout the United States operated by local affiliates. The concern and involvement of prominent citizens and organizations such as the Ford Foundation, the Rockefeller Foundation, and the Pathfinder Fund, greatly facilitated the national and international development and expansion of family planning programs.

National concern has been demonstrated

by the Congress, offices, and departments of the federal government through the provision of support for both domestic and international family planning programs since 1965. The Department of Health, Education and Welfare at that time created the position of Deputy Assistant Secretary for Population and Family Planning, established the National Center for Family Planning Services, and initiated programs through the Office of Economic Opportunities and various antipoverty programs. The United States Agency for International Development (AID) has spearheaded the federal international program and is the largest single source of international population assistance.

The words *birth control, contraception,* and *family planning* are often used interchangeably, although they are not identical in meaning. The term birth control has been attributed to the previously-mentioned Margaret Sanger. It refers to regulation of the number of children that are conceived or born. Contraception refers to the temporary prevention of pregnancy which is accomplished through the use of specific contraceptive, or birth control, methods. Family planning has the broadest connotation. It encompasses the additional considerations of the physical, social, psychological, economic, and theological factors that govern the family's attitudes and influence decisions pertaining to the size of the family, the spacing of children, and the selection and utilization of a contraceptive method.

Family planning is a very broad topic because of its ramifications and implications in all aspects of life. Examples include the population explosion with its subsequent terrifying aspect of overpopulation, involving such dangers as lack of living space and lack of food; the theological acceptability of various contraceptive methods; the reduction of infant mortality resulting from a lack of prenatal care, since those not receiving adequate prenatal care are generally unmarried expectant mothers and those in the lower socio-economic group already overburdened with children; a reduction of parental rejection and child abuse caused by children who

are not wanted; and an avoidance of the physical and physiologic hazards to an individual woman which come with continuous, repeated childbearing. [1, p. 491]

The ability to be maximally effective in helping people with family planning may be enhanced or hindered by the nurse-midwife's feelings and attitudes in each of the following areas as it relates to family planning:

1. Sex and sexuality
2. Religion
3. Race
4. Poverty
5. Marital status

Nurse-midwives, like all personnel in a family planning clinic, need to scrutinize their own feelings and attitudes in these five areas.

The following philosophy of family planning not only averts any accusations of genocide but also focuses on basic rights involved. These beliefs, although phrased differently, reflect those articulated by Margaret Sanger:

1. The right of a woman to have a baby when she wants to have a baby.
2. The right to be a healthy mother bearing a healthy baby.

SELECTION OF A FAMILY PLANNING METHOD

It is well known and undisputed that the ideal contraceptive method has not yet been developed. Research continues in search of a method that would be 100 percent effective, 100 percent safe, free from side effects, easy to use, unrelated to the sexual act, and acceptable to all religions. New contraceptive methods are being explored and already-existing methods are being studied for improvement. Basic in the research are the causes of side effects, the possible relationship with disease (safety), and the mechanisms of action. It is critically important that a means be developed that is able to predict accurately the ovulation time at least 4 days before ovulation.

Before a specific family planning method is chosen, an individual or couple must first decide whether or not to use family planning. A number of factors* may influence this decision, including the following:

1. Sociocultural factors — current trends in family size; effect on an individual of the size of the family in which the individual grew up; stress of a society upon the importance of children; stress any particular society or culture places upon the importance of having a male child to perpetuate the family name; belief in a direct correlation between number of children and proof of virility.

2. Occupational and economic factors — the possibility of lengthy separation until the husband's military obligations have been met; the channeling of economic resources into the individual's or couple's completion of schooling or beginning of a vocation or business; economic ability to provide prospective children with food, clothing, shelter, medical and dental care, and future education.

3. Religious factors — all major religious bodies endorse the principle of family limitation and the basic concept of family planning.

4. Legal factors — since the Connecticut state law which prohibited the use of any device for the purpose of preventing conception was declared by the Supreme Court decision in 1965 to be unconstitutional, there are now no legal barriers to a married couple's being able to obtain contraceptives.

5. Physical factors — conditions requiring that a woman does not become pregnant for health reasons.

6. Marital factors — development of marital relationships and stability of the marriage; the crisis period and innumerable adjustments caused by having a child.

7. Psychological factors — need for a child or "something" to love and to be loved by; pregnancy considered proof of love (these first two factors are common reasons for adolescent pregnancies); erroneous thought that a child will hold together a disintegrating relationship; fear of childbearing or childrearing; threat to present life style.

If the decision of the individual or couple is to utilize family planning, then still other factors might influence their choice of the contraceptive method they want to use. Selection of a family planning method is a matter of choice by the individual or couple as long as the person directly affected has no medical contraindications to the contraceptive method chosen. This is sometimes called the "cafeteria" approach to family planning. It is the individual's or couple's right to know the potential dangers and side effects in making this decision. This information should be included in the general information presented about each contraceptive method. Many private offices and clinics are now requiring that patient consent forms be signed that state that the person signing does understand the risks involved and authorizes receipt of the method, which is specified. Barring medical contraindications, the factors[†] which may influence the individual's or couple's selection of a contraceptive method include the following:

1. Social factors — the current trends with-

---

* These factors have been adapted from a list by the author which appeared in Ziegel, E., and VanBlarcom, C. C. (Eds.). *Obstetric Nursing, 6th.* New York: Macmillan, 1972, p. 492.

[†] These factors have been adapted from a list by the author which appeared in Ziegel, E., and VanBlarcom, C. C. (Eds.). *Obstetric Nursing, 6th.* New York: Macmillan, 1972, pp. 492–493.

in a society as to the contraceptive method most commonly used; family background

2. Religious factors — whether or not a specific contraceptive method is sanctioned by the religious body to which the individual or couple belongs
3. Psychological factors — the feelings of the individual toward any aspects associated with the use of a specific contraceptive method; publicity; unfavorable past experience with a method
4. Technicalities of the various contraceptive methods — the ease of using a particular contraceptive method; the ability of the individual to master the techniques involved in using a specific method
5. Cost of the various contraceptive methods
6. Frequency of sexual intercourse
7. Length of anticipated use of a contraceptive method
8. Possible side effects and questions of safety related to any contraceptive method
9. Effectiveness of a contraceptive method

EFFECTIVENESS OF A CONTRACEPTIVE METHOD

The success or failure of a method is of major importance in family planning. The effectiveness of a contraceptive method is dependent on a number of factors. If a method is ineffective, or fails, the failure may be due to defects in the method itself, to erroneous use of the method, or to a combination of these two factors. The first of these, possible defects in the method, is discussed in the following chapters concerning specific contraceptive methods.

If a contraceptive method fails as a result of human error the failure may be due either to improper use of the technique or to weak motivation. Some users may not have sufficient knowledge of pertinent reproductive anatomy and physiology, may not understand the method and how it works, or may not be able to master the skills needed to perform the technique involved in the method. For one or all of these

reasons, therefore, they do not use the method correctly. Motivation, however, is the dominating factor in human error. How strongly a couple or individual wishes to prevent a pregnancy directly affects the degree of regularity with which a contraceptive is used. Any method will fail without consistent use. A major cause of contraceptive failure due to human error is irregular use of a method. However, influences leading to human error, such as the individual's or couple's lack of acceptance of the procedure involved, may be counterbalanced by their motivation [1, p. 493].

Although often given as percentages, the clinical effectiveness (use effectiveness) of a contraceptive method is usually calculated according to the pregnancy rate per 100 years of exposure (or woman years). This is done by means of a formula developed by Raymond Pearl in the early 1930s. This equation is as follows:

Pregnancy rate (pregnancies per woman years)

$$= \frac{\text{number of pregnancies} \times 1200 \text{ months}}{\text{patients observed} \times \text{months of exposure}}$$

The *number of pregnancies* in the numerator refers to the total of three statistics which are generally available or can be calculated: the number of live births, stillbirths, and abortions. The *1200 months* in the numerator refers to the number of months in 100 years and is obtained by multiplying 100×12 months. The *months of exposure* in the denominator refers to exposure to pregnancy and is determined by deducting those months during which conception was impossible (e.g., physical separation, pregnancy) from the total months the man and woman were together. For example: suppose that 200 couples have used a contraceptive method over an average period of 2 years and that 60 of the couples became pregnant despite its use:

$$\text{Pregnancy rate} = \frac{60 \times 1200}{200 \times 24} = \frac{72,000}{4,800} = 15$$

Thus, the effectiveness this contraceptive method is calculated to have is a pregnancy rate of 15 per 100 woman years.

For all sexually active couples not using a contraceptive method, the average pregnancy rate is 90 per 100 woman years. The effectiveness of a contraceptive method is considered to be high if the pregnancy rate is below 10 per 100 woman years (years of exposure); moderate if between 10 and 20; and low if more than 20. (See Table 27-1.)

The Pearl Pregnancy Index method of calculating the effectiveness of a contraceptive method has been criticized because it treats all data equally for whatever period of time is studied. The problem with this averaging of data is that the risk of pregnancy with any contraceptive method is highest during the first year of use and then declines thereafter. Therefore, some researchers use life-table rates as the statistical methodology instead of the Pearl Index. Life-table rates treat each month of contraceptive use separately, thus controlling for the decreasing risk of pregnancy over time, and then compute these individual months cumulatively up to whatever point is desired (e.g., 12 months). Life-table rates express effectiveness of a contraceptive method as the number of pregnancies per 100 women in the first 12 months of use, in contrast to the Pearl Index, which expresses effectiveness of a contraceptive method as the number of pregnancies per 100 woman years.

How to calculate life-table rates can be found in statistics books. The controversy over the Pearl Index and life-table rates continues as it has now been shown that the Pearl Index rate better predicts long-term life-table rates than do short-term life-table rates when the two sets of calculations are subjected to regression analysis [2]. The Pearl Index also better controls for variables between clinical trials of the same contraceptive method. Effectiveness rates estimated by either method cannot be mathematically translated into the other method. The actual rates calculated by the two methods are not that much different for long-term studies but may be more importantly different regarding the first year of use.

FOLKLORE METHODS

Individuals should be advised against and guided away from using folklore methods of contraception. These are so-called contraceptive methods of long-standing reputation which because of a basic fallacy in concept and low efficacy might as well be labeled as folklore; or are products which, because of misleading advertising, misunderstanding, or ignorance, are thought to be contraceptive in action but are not. Folklore methods include the use of douches, the practice of coitus interruptus, and the use of vaginal cleansing agents.

Douches

One of the most common erroneous ideas is that douching following sexual intercourse is a contraceptive method. The notion is that a woman can flush the semen out of her vagina before the spermatozoa can enter her uterus if she douches immediately following ejaculation. However, the majority of spermatozoa are contained in the first few drops of ejaculate; furthermore, within 90 seconds of the normal deposit of semen at the cervical os, spermatozoa have entered the cervical canal. The fact that it is almost impossible for a woman to douche within this period of time renders the entire supposition invalid.

Various reports have stated a pregnancy rate in excess of 30 per 100 years of exposure for couples using this method. This is better that no contraceptive method at all. However, such low efficacy can scarcely be used to recommend the douche as a reliable method of contraception.

Coitus Interruptus

Coitus interruptus, commonly known as "being

TABLE 27-1. Number of Pregnancies per 100 Woman Years of Exposure

Method	Theoretical Effectiveness*	Use Effectiveness[†]
Condom	3	10
Spermicidal agents	3	18
Foam and condom combined	<1	5
Vaginal contraceptive sponge	?	9−11
Diaphragm	3	19
Cervical cap	3	13
Intrauterine contraceptive device (IUD)	1−2	5−6
Hormonal contraceptives (combined, low-dose)	<0.5	2−3
Natural family planning methods[††]	0.7−8	3.1−28
Coitus interruptus	16	20−25
Douche	?	40
Surgical sterilization (male and female)	<0.20	<0.20

* Theoretical effectiveness means that the method is used perfectly without human error and with perfect consistency.

[†] Use effectiveness means that the method is used both by those who use it perfectly and those who do not and includes the wide range of inconsistency in behavior and in use.

[††] See page 549.

safe," "being careful," or "withdrawal," is based on the fact that the male can feel when he is about to ejaculate. This method depends on the male's withdrawing his penis from the vagina at exactly this moment and ejaculating outside of it. This action relies on split-second timing and idealistic self-control by the male. If the male is late in withdrawing, even by a fraction of a second, the first few drops of semen are deposited in the vagina. The method also may fail if the male ejaculates on the external female genitalia. Another fact which renders this method invalid is that there often are spermatozoa in the drops of penile lubricating coital secretion which precedes and is involved in the insertion of the penis into the vagina.

Many couples have used coitus interruptus at least occasionally, and it is recommended in the absence of an authentic contraceptive method. Some couples have been satisfied with coitus interruptus as a contraceptive method and have used it successfully. However, coitus interruptus has been noted for many family planning failures and has received much criticism. The male may not always be psychologically able to withdraw at the climax of sexual intercourse, and to do so leads to the frequent objection that coitus interruptus limits full sexual gratification. It has a use effectiveness rate of 20 to 25 pregnancies per 100 woman years.

Vaginal Cleansing Agents

These agents are advertised sometimes as being "for feminine protection." This phrase is misunderstood to mean protection from pregnancy when what is meant is protection from "smelling less than pretty." Such agents not only are unnecessary for female hygiene, and may indeed temporarily mask or worsen a vaginitis, but they also do not contain any spermicidal ingredients or even bring about a change in the pH of the vagina which would render it more hostile to spermatozoa.

ALTERNATIVES TO TEMPORARY METHODS

There are several alternatives to the temporary methods of preventing conception. These alternatives are also methods of family planning but differ either in the fact of their permanency in preventing conception or as a means of aborting a conception which has occurred. Abortion counseling is discussed in Chapter 4.

The permanent methods of contraception, or sterilization, include vasectomy, tubal ligation, and hysterectomy. Because these are surgical procedures requiring physician management and performance, they are not discussed in this book. Those interested in the details of these methods are referred to medical textbooks in which these procedures are described. However, the nurse-midwife does become involved with these methods when counseling and educating women about what the individual's or couple's alternatives are for family planning. The permanent methods of contraception should be included in any discussion of family planning as possible options, along with the temporary methods of contraception. In fact, the sterilization methods are the most commonly used family planning method for married couples over the age of 30, and approximately one-sixth of all married couples are sterilized.

Counseling for the permanent methods of contraception requires a knowledge of local resources and medical practices, including the following information:

1. What permanent methods are available? Where? Done by whom? Precisely which procedures are used?
2. How much will each method cost (depending on where, whom, and procedures used)? What financial aid resources are available?
3. What will the surgery really mean in terms of what body structures get touched, changed, or possibly disfigured (depending on procedures used)? Amount of time unable to work? Amount of time too uncomfortable for sex? Reversibility of the procedure? Possible complications?

In addition, counseling should focus on eliciting and talking about the common fears and misconceptions related to sterilization. The most prevalent of these is that of "being changed" — meaning a decrease in sexual desire, functioning, or enjoyment — which is not true except as affected by the psyche.

REFERENCES

1. Williams (idem. Burst), H. V. Family planning. In Ziegel, E., and VanBlarcom, C. C. (Eds.). *Obstetric Nursing*, 6th. New York: Macmillan, 1972.
2. Shelton, J. D., and Taylor, R. N., Jr. The Pearl Pregnancy Index reexamined: Still useful for clinical trials of contraceptives. *Am. J. Obstet. Gynecol.* 139(5):592−596, March 1, 1981.

BIBLIOGRAPHY

Bruce, J. and Schearer, S. B. *Contraceptives and Common Sense: Conventional Methods Reconsidered.* New York: The Population Council, 1979.

Colton, T. *Statistics in Medicine.* Boston: Little, Brown and Co., 1974. Chapter 9. Longitudinal Studies and the Use of the Life Table.

Hatcher, R. A. et al. *Contraceptive Technology, 1984−1985*, 12th. New York: Irvington Publishers, 1984.

International Planned Parenthood Federation. *The History of Contraceptives.* Eighth Conference of the International Planned Parenthood Federation, Santiago, Chile, April 9−15, 1967.

Schirm, A. et al. Contraceptive failure in the United States: The impact of social economic and demographic factors. *Fam. Plann. Perspect.* 14(2):68−75, 1982.

Shelton, J. D., and Taylor, R. N., Jr. The Pearl Pregnancy Index reexamined: Still useful for clinical trials of contraceptives. *Am. J. Obstet. Gynecol.* 139(5):592−596, March 1, 1981.

The Victor Fund for the International Planned Parenthood Federation: Report No. 4. December, 1966.

Tietze, C. Use and effectiveness of contraceptive methods in the United States. In Calderone, M. S. (Ed.). *Manual of Contraceptive Practice.* Baltimore: Williams & Wilkins, 1964.

Williams (idem. Blarcom), H. V. Family planning. In Ziegel, E., and VanBlarcom, C. C. (Eds.). *Obstetric Nursing*, 6th. New York: Macmillan, 1972.

28

Natural Methods of Family Planning

There are four methods of natural family planning. They are:

1. The calendar method
2. The basal body temperature method
3. The ovulation method
4. The sympto-thermal method

The most reliable method of the natural family planning methods theoretically is the sympto-thermal method since it combines the most informative of the other methods, that is, the basal body temperature method, the ovulation method, and other signs and symptoms of impending ovulation or its occurrence. Study reports, however, underline the importance of the basal body temperature method as contributing the most to the effectiveness of natural family planning. See Table 28-1.

What used to be called the rhythm method was either the calender method or the basal body temperature method or a combination of both in the calendar-temperature method. The words *natural family planning, rhythm, safe period, fertility awareness,* and *periodic abstinence* are sometimes used interchangeably as being synonymous. However, the different terms may evoke different philosophic and psychologic responses.

The natural methods of family planning are nonmechanical and nonchemical. They are often vastly misunderstood which, when combined with a lack of commitment to abstinence from coitus during the fertile days, may render them most ineffective. However, when the couple properly understands the method, makes a commitment to each other for abstinence during the fertile days, jointly participates in determining the fertile days and the safe days, and develops alternative methods comfortable to them for expressing their love (ranging from increased use of touching to alternative methods of sexual satisfaction); then the effectiveness rate equals that of the most effective contraceptive methods. This is especially true when the sympto-thermal method is utilized.

Natural family planning is not the most preferred contraceptive method by women for whom all methods of family planning are available. However, there is an increasing number of couples turning to the natural methods of family planning, motivated to do so either out

TABLE 28-1. Effectiveness of Natural Family Planning Methods per 100 Woman Years*

Method	Use Effectiveness
Calendar	14.4−47
Basal body temperature	0.3−8.03
Ovulation	5.3−39.7
Sympto-thermal	4.9−22.1

* Ranges and differences in study results may be the result of variations between populations, health care providers, patient instruction, and statistical methodology.

of religious or philosophic beliefs or out of concern for the potential dangers and unknown long-range effects inherent in other contraceptive methods, especially those which are hormonal. Couples desiring natural family planning need careful education in the methods and strong peer support systems.

THE CALENDAR METHOD

The calendar method can only predict the days in a menstrual cycle during which a woman is more likely to get pregnant. This prediction is based on the preceding 8 months of recorded menstrual cycles. The calendar method of family planning is then based on the concept that abstinence from sexual intercourse during the projected fertile days will prevent conception.

The problem with the calendar method is that it is predicated on the assumption that ovulation occurs 14 days prior to the onset of the next menstrual period. This, however, is only an approximation of when ovulation actually takes place. Ovulation rarely occurs on the same day in a cycle from one cycle to the next, even in the most regular of menstrual cycles, but, rather, occurs on approximately the same day. Some margin of allowance, therefore, must be given for the variations which occur in even the most regular of menstrual cycles. Two days usually are given on either side of the estimated date of ovulation as this margin of allowance. Calculations are then made from the records of the woman's preceding menstrual cycles.

Consider a hypothetical 28-day cycle. Suppose that the woman's estimated date of ovulation is 14 days before her next menstrual period. In a 28-day cycle this is on day 14 of the menstrual cycle. If 2 days are allowed on either side of day 14 for variation of the time of ovulation from month to month, then the basic fertile days are days 12, 13, 14, 15, and 16. Ovum survival must be considered next. Generally it is thought that the ovum survives for a period of 24 hours. In the hypothetical situation, therefore, if a woman ovulates on day 16, she is also fertile on day 17 due to ovum survival. Survival of spermatozoa must be considered also. The generally accepted opinion has been that spermatozoa can survive for 48 hours. Now some medical authorities hypothesize that sperm may survive as long as 72 hours. If the 72-hour figure is used in the hypothetical situation, the woman who ovulates on day 12 is also fertile on days 9, 10, and 11 because of spermatozoa survival. This gives the woman a total of 9 fertile days. Considering 5 days as the length of the average menstrual period, this leaves days 6, 7, and 8 (depending on length of sperm survival) and days 18 through 28 as the days during which sexual intercourse probably will not result in fertilization of an ovum (Fig. 28-1). However, some authorities advocate a 3-day allowance on either side of days 12 and 16 for survival of spermatozoa and ovum; this further extends the fertile period.

Because a fairly regular menstrual cycle is essential to any reliable estimation of the time of ovulation, most authorities recommend that women with the following conditions not depend on the calendar method: women with menstrual cycles of less than 25 days, those who have irregular menstrual cycles, women with menstrual cycles which vary in length by

8 days or more, postpartum women, those who are lactating, and women in menopause. Between eight and twelve previous menstrual cycles must be recorded before reliable calculation of a probable date of ovulation can be made. A record of at least three consecutive menstrual cycles of similar length is necessary postpartally and during lactation if a previous record of cycles has been kept. Otherwise, a record of eight menstrual cycles of similar length is necessary. The range of the cycles is then used in calculating the total number of possible fertile days. This is done to identify the longest and shortest cycles so the total possible fertile days may be projected. See Figure 28-1 for an example of a woman whose menstrual cycles range in length from 26 to

31 days. The Ogino formula quickly makes these calculations as follows:

To calculate the first fertile day subtract 18 days from the total number of days of the shortest cycle. (Subtract 19 days if allowing 72 hours for sperm survival.)
To calculate the last fertile day subtract 11 days from the total number of days of the longest cycle.

It is advantageous, however, to do your calculations as illustrated in Figure 28-1 because it serves as a teaching tool to explain to the couple how you have arrived at your determination of the fertile and infertile days and how they can make these same calculations.

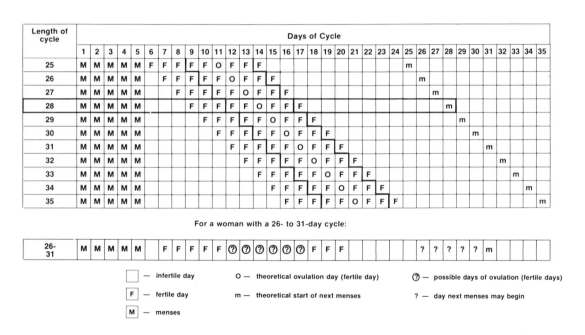

FIGURE 28-1.   An ovulation calendar for 25- to 35-day menstrual cycles based on 9 fertile days per cycle. Theoretically, ovulation occurs 14 days before onset of the next menses, but actually it may occur normally at any time from the twelfth to the sixteenth day before menses (top). For a woman whose menstrual cycles over the preceding 12 months have varied from 26 to 31 days, application of the calendar method would mean a safe period of 1 preovulatory day (discounting the 5 days of the menses) and 5 to 10 postovulatory days, depending on the length of the current cycle. This totals 6 to 11 safe days, and 14 fertile days, which would always fall from day 7 to day 20 of every cycle. (Adapted from Periodic Abstinence (Population Report), Series 1, Number 1, June, 1974. p. 1-4, Fig. 2.)

It is necessary to abstain from coitus throughout the total possible fertile period as mathematically calculated. The calendar method, thus, involves the greatest number of days of abstinence, whereas natural methods that at least identify the time of ovulation, or shortly thereafter, allow for greater preciseness in calculating the number of postovulation fertile days and consequent possible earlier resumption of sexual intercourse.

THE BASAL BODY TEMPERATURE METHOD

The basal body temperature method detects when ovulation actually occurs. This is possible because of the fact that progesterone, released at the time of ovulation, causes an increase of approximately 0.5 to 1.0 degree Fahrenheit in the basal body temperature. Detection of this rise in temperature thus identifies the luteal, or postovulatory, phase of the menstrual cycle. The rise in basal body temperature occurring with ovulation may be abrupt (1 to 2 days), a slow rise extending over several days, in a staircase pattern of sequential steps of slight increases (0.2°F) every 2 to 3 days, or in a zigzag pattern of sequential and progressively higher increase-decrease-increase over a period of several days (e.g., an increase of 0.4°F, decrease of 0.2°F, increase of 0.4°F, etc.). In all varieties of temperature elevation patterns a sustained level of increase is evident. Occasionally a sharp dip in temperature precedes the rise in basal body temperature occurring with ovulation. The pattern of the rise in temperature may vary both from woman to woman and from cycle to cycle for the same woman.

The fertile and safe days from ovulation through the postovulatory phase of the menstrual cycle are determined by considering that the fertile days continue until either there has been a sustained elevation or plateau of the temperature for 3 days or there have been 5 days of temperature recording of progressive increase (e.g., the zigzag, staircase, or slow rise patterns). The safe days follow and continue through the luteal, or postovulatory phase of the menstrual cycle until menstruation.

The instructions for temperature taking are usually found on the back of the graph used for plotting the temperature and must be rigorously followed for greatest usefulness of the record. These instructions include how and when to take the temperature, what data to record, and how to record the data on the temperature record throughout the menstrual cycle. A basal body temperature, or ovulation, thermometer is most useful for detecting temperature change, increasing accuracy, and interpreting records. Such thermometers are calibrated in gradations of 0.1°F rather than the standard gradations of 0.2°F found on regular, or fever, thermometers. Basal body temperature thermometers may be purchased in most drug stores. The daily temperature reading should be recorded on graph paper, preferably also designed for plotting tenths of a degree.

The woman should take her temperature every day, preferably at the same time every day if possible. A basal body temperature should be taken after 5 to 6 hours of uninterrupted sleep. Since any activity may raise the basal body temperature, the woman should take her temperature upon awakening and *before* doing anything else (e.g., talking, eating, drinking, kissing, smoking, getting out of or moving around in bed). The woman may select how she wishes to take her temperature — orally or, for greatest accuracy, rectally. Whichever way she chooses to take her temperature, she should always use the same site thereafter since temperature readings vary from site to site.

Besides the phase of the menstrual cycle, the following factors may affect the basal body temperature and possibly render the month's record invalid.

1. Illness
2. Emotional tension or upset

3. Lack of sleep or irregular sleeping hours
4. Use of electric blankets
5. Sedatives
6. Gastrointestinal disturbances
7. Immunizations
8. Alcohol intake
9. The time of day
10. The climate
11. Those activities identified before as things which should not be done prior to taking the temperature upon awakening

If the woman is aware of these factors, and notes their existence on the temperature graph, she will enable a much more critical analysis and accurate interpretation of the record to be made.

The Basal Body Temperature Method Combined with the Calendar Method

The basal body temperature method is only for determining when ovulation occurs and identifying the subsequent postovulatory fertile and infertile days. This method cannot predict the time of ovulation or determine the preovulatory fertile and infertile days. However, combining the basal body temperature method with the calendar method allows for refinement of the calendar method on the basis of having an accurate record of when ovulation takes place within each menstrual cycle. Greater and greater refinement of this combined method becomes possible as the number of consecutive accurate records increases. The reliability of this method is enhanced by careful calculations of the expected date of ovulation and an understanding of how many days of abstinence are required. A common misconception is that the day of ovulation is the only fertile or "unsafe" day. Nothing could be further from the truth. Careful and complete explanations and extensive patient teaching are necessary to foster the couple's self-confidence in their own ability to keep and interpret their records accurately.

THE OVULATION METHOD

The ovulation method is based on the recognition of changes in the cervical mucus during the menstrual cycle and is often called the *cervical mucus method*. Changes in the cervical mucus during the menstrual cycle are under the influence of estrogen and are as follows:

1. There are a number of "dry days" immediately after menstruation during which there is little to no secretion of mucus. The number of days varies, being more in a long cycle and fewer in a short cycle. These are considered "safe" days.
2. A number of preovulatory days follow. Mucus secretion, which prolongs the life of spermatozoa, has begun. The mucus is a cloudy-white or yellowish secretion with a sticky consistency. These days are considered "unsafe" days.
3. Immediately before and after ovulation are the "wet days," in which the mucus increases in volume and is clear, extremely slippery and lubricating, and stretchy with an egg-white consistency (spinnbarkheit). This is the maximally fertile period. The day these characteristics of the mucus are most pronounced is considered the "peak" day in the ovulation method. The peak day is thought to occur immediately before ovulation. The 3 days after the peak day are counted as unsafe days.
4. The postovulatory days begin on the fourth day after the peak day and continue until menstruation. During this time the mucus again becomes cloudy and sticky and decreases in amount. These are considered safe days.

A woman detects these changes by being aware of a feeling of "wetness" or "dryness" around her vaginal introitus and by tactile examination of the mucus at a time unassociated with or prior to urination. There are record forms available for the ovulation, or cervical mucus, method. These involve sticking color-coded stamps on the record indicating the safe (dry) days, the unsafe (wet) days, and the peak day. During the first month of detecting these changes in cervical mucus, abstinence is necessary in order for the woman to become knowledgeable about her mucus. The woman has to learn to delineate her cervical mucus from semen, normal sexual lubrication, discharge from a vaginal infection, contraceptive foams or jellies, and lubricants. Women who douche cannot use the ovulation method as they eradicate the secretions they need to examine.

THE SYMPTO-THERMAL METHOD

The sympto-thermal method utilizes all the signs and symptoms that ovulation is impending or has occurred. Thus it encompasses both the ovulation method and the basal body temperature method and adds other indicators of ovulation. The other signs and symptoms of impending ovulation or its occurrence, which some women experience, are as follows:

1. Mittelschmerz (midcycle pain) — encompasses a number of signs and symptoms including:
   a. pain located just off center in the lower abdomen and caused by the rupturing follicle
   b. spotting or break-through bleeding
   c. bearing-down or dragging pains
   d. general tenderness in the lower midabdomen and pelvic area
2. Increase in sexual interest (libido) — although this may also occur at other times during the cycle.
3. Mood changes — feelings of depression or mercurial mood swings are more common during the postovulatory (luteal) phase of the cycle.
4. Cervical mucus ferning and spinnbarkheit — this requires microscopic examination of dried cervical mucus.

   A fernlike pattern is observed during the days of the menstrual cycle when estrogen is predominant. Ferning is most pronounced at the time of ovulation. The fern pattern is readily distinguishable and is different from the beadlike pattern which replaces it during the postovulatory (progesterone) phase of the menstrual cycle. Under the influence of estrogen, cervical mucus also exhibits a property known as spinnbarkheit, which was mentioned previously as a distinctive characteristic of the "wet days." Spinnbarkheit is the property of the mucus which allows it to be drawn into long elasticlike strands. It is maximal near the time of ovulation. Because the fern pattern and spinnbarkheit are the result of estrogen stimulation alone, they simply indicate under normal conditions that ovulation is imminent but they do not prove that ovulation has actually occurred.
5. Cervical changes — these changes include a softening of the cervix and slight dilatation of the cervical os, both of which occur near and at the time of ovulation. Under the influence of increased estrogen, the cervix softens and opens slightly. After ovulation the cervix again becomes more firm and closes. These changes can be detected by either the woman or her mate.
6. Breast tenseness and tenderness — occur during the postovulatory (luteal) phase of the cycle under the combined influence of estrogen and progesterone.
7. Other means of determining the time of ovulation — other means are known (e.g., endometrial biopsy, hormonal assay of urine or blood, examination of the ovaries) but practicalities prohibit their use for contraceptive purposes.

BIBLIOGRAPHY

Britt, S. S. Fertility awareness: Four methods of natural family planning, *J. Obstet. Gynecol. Neonat. Nurs.* 6:9, 1977.

Committee on Practice. *Natural Family Planning.* OGN Nursing Practice Resource. Washington, D. C.: Nurses Association of the American College of Obstetricians and Gynecoloists, 1983.

Deibel, P. Natural family planning, different methods. *Am. J. Mat. Child Nsg.* 3:171–177 (May–June) 1978.

Hatcher, R. A. et al. *Contraceptive Technology, 1984–1985, 12th. rev.* New York: Irvington Publishers, 1984.

Hilgers, T. W. Two methods of natural family planning. *Am. J. Obstet. Gynecol.* 136(5):696–697, March 1, 1980.

Hilgers, T. W., and Bailey, A. J. Natural family planning. 2. Basal body temperature and estimated time of ovulation. *Obstet. Gynecol.* 55(3):333–339 (March) 1980.

Hilgers, T. W., Daly, K. D., Prebil, A. M., and Hilgers, S. K. Natural family planning. 3. Intermenstrual symptoms and estimated time of ovulation. *Obstet. Gynecol.* 58(2):152–155 (August) 1981.

Liskin, L. S. Periodic abstinence. *Pop. Rep.* Series I, No. 3 (September) 1981.

Matis, N. Natural family planning: A birth control alternative. *J. Nurse-Midwifery* 28(1):7–16 (January/February) 1983.

Nofziger, M. *A Cooperative Method of Natural Birth Control, 2nd,* rev. Summertown, Tenn.: The Book Publishing Company, 1978.

Ross, C., and Piotrow, P. T. Periodic abstinence. *Population Report* 1:1, 1974.

Wade, M. E. et al. A randomized study of the use-effectiveness of two methods of natural family planning. *Am. J. Obstet. Gynec.* 141:368, 1981.

Williams (idem. Burst), H. V. Family planning. In Ziegel, E. and VanBlarcom, C. C. (Eds.). *Obstetric Nursing, 6th.* New York: Macmillan, 1972.

29

Spermicidal Preparations and Condom Management

SPERMICIDAL PREPARATIONS

Spermicidal preparations contain a spermicidal ingredient that inactivates spermatozoa. The greater part of such a preparation is an inert base which acts as the vehicle. This nonreactive base also serves as a mechanical block to the cervical os. Most spermicidal preparations have an acid pH of 4.5, thus providing the mildly alkaline semen with a hostile vaginal environment. This is particularly important at the external cervical os because the cervical secretions become slightly alkaline at the time of ovulation and therefore receptive to the spermatozoa.

These spermicidal preparations are made, and are so designated in the accompanying literature, to be used with a condom alone and not in conjunction with a diaphragm. There are certain common features that the spermicidal preparations exhibit: ability to immobilize and kill spermatozoa; widespread vaginal distribution of the spermicidal preparation with the initial thrust of the penis; and the formation of a surface film which withstands coital activity. The spermicidal preparation is inserted near the cervix and coital movements distribute it throughout the vagina and over the cervix. However, contraceptive failure due to inadequate distribution is inherent in the method.

In addition to these features, each preparation has its own specific characteristics. These are enumerated with each type of preparation: jellies and creams, aerosol foam, suppositories, and vaginal contraceptive sponge. Two other types of spermicidal preparations, while rarely used and difficult to find in the United States, may be widely used in other countries and are presented here for general information; they are vaginal foam tablets and a sponge and foam method.

Jellies and Creams

The jellies and creams are packaged in tubes. The kits in which they are sold also contain an applicator and instructions. Since these preparations can be diluted by vaginal secretions, an adequate amount of the preparation must be inserted in accord with the instructions. To facilitate depositing the spermicidal preparation near the cervix, it is recommended that the woman, lying in a supine position, insert the applicator in a downward and backward direction the full length of the vagina and then withdraw it about half an inch before pushing the plunger. (See "Patient Instructions for Spermicides," later in this chapter.)

Aerosol Foam

In the aerosol foam, the agent is under pressure in a container with a gas such as Freon. Foam, a variation of the cream spermicidal preparation, is released into the applicator when it is pressed against the container. The remainder of the procedure is the same as that for jellies and creams. (See "Patient Instructions for Spermicides," below.)

Suppositories

Products advertised for feminine hygiene should not be mistaken for contraceptive suppositories. (See "Vaginal Cleansing Agents" in Chapter 27.) Contraceptive suppositories are cone-shaped and contain a spermicidal ingredient incorporated into a cocoa butter or glycerogelatin base. Their melting point is slightly below body temperature. This makes them a poor choice of method in areas where the weather is hot and refrigeration is lacking.

The average melting time of the suppository at body heat is around 10 minutes; therefore the suppository should be inserted into the vagina at least 15 minutes before coitus, and some brands instruct waiting for 30 minutes.

Some couples find this waiting period objectionable. Other couples object to the excessive messiness which may be associated with this method. The suppository is one of the least effective of the spermicidal preparations.

Vaginal Contraceptive Sponge

This contraceptive method doubles as a spermicide and as a barrier method. The vaginal contraceptive sponge is designed to fit against and somewhat over the cervix by virtue of having a concave indentation into which the cervix nestles. It is made of polyurethane and contains 1 gram of nonoxynol-9 spermicide. It is available without presciption in only one size.

Before insertion, the sponge is moistened with tap water. It is then inserted into the vagina, up against the cervix. The sponge provides protection for up to 24 hours, after which time it is removed and discarded. Additional contraceptive measures (e.g., condoms, jellies, creams) are not necessary for repeated sexual intercourse during the 24-hour period.

The effectiveness of the sponge is about the same as that of the diaphragm. The woman should be warned *not* to use the sponge during menstruation for the purpose of absorbing menses or discharge from a vaginal infection, and to be alert for the signs and symptoms of toxic shock syndrome. To date, toxic shock syndrome has not been associated with the vaginal contraceptive sponge but, since the sponge is an absorbent intravaginal foreign object, caution is indicated.

Vaginal Foam Tablets

The 1-gram vaginal foam tablet is round, flat, white, and contains a spermicide, a bacteriostatic agent, and ingredients which, when moistened, produce a carbon dioxide foam. The woman, in a supine position, moistens the tablet with a little water or saliva. She waits to see or hear it fizz. If the tablet does not fizz when moistened, it should be discarded and another tablet used. When the tablet fizzes, she inserts it immediately into her vagina, pushing it in as far as she can with her finger. A 5-minute interval must be allowed between insertion and sexual intercourse for the initial foaming action to occur which distributes foam throughout the vagina. The tablet further dissolves and there is additional foaming action at the time of ejaculation.

Women have complained about an irritative vaginal reaction, and both men and women have complained about a burning sensation felt during the foaming process. Women may also object to this method if they have an aversion to inserting a finger into their vagina.

The vaginal foam tablet is considered one of the least effective of the spermicidal methods. However, it has been accepted by poorly motivated, low-socioeconomic, minimally educated groups because of the simplicity of the technique involved. Because of their greater willingness to use it, the vaginal foam tablet may be used with increased regularity. Thus, for these women, it may be a more effective protection from conception than other contraceptive methods.

Sponge and Foam

In the sponge and foam method, a spermicidal powder or liquid is applied to a small water-moistened sponge. The sponge is squeezed gently to form a foam and then inserted into the vagina with as little loss of content as possible.

An almost total reserve foaming power permits sexual intercourse any time within 6 hours after insertion. Within this period coital movements produce more foam. If more than 6 hours elapse from the time of insertion to the time of sexual intercourse the sponge must be removed and additional spermicidal powder or liquid applied. Then the sponge is reinserted. Removal of the sponge does not take place until at least

6 hours after sexual intercourse. If, before this 6 hours has passed, repeated coitus is desired, then another, but smaller, sponge is inserted in addition to the first sponge.

The sponge and foam method is one of the least effective of the spermicidal contraceptive methods. Nevertheless, it is a simple method, and some women gain confidence that an effective method is being used when they see the sponge filled with foam.

Effectiveness, Complaints, and Management

Except for the vaginal contraceptive sponge, the following principles of use are imperative if the spermicidal preparations are to be an effective method of family planning.

1. Reapplication of the method if the woman gets up, walks around, or goes to the bathroom after insertion but before sexual intercourse.
2. Reapplication of the method if sexual intercourse does not occur within 30 minutes of the time of insertion.
3. Reapplication of the method before each act of sexual intercourse.
4. No douching until at least 6 hours after the last act of sexual intercourse. Douching prior to this time may dilute or remove the spermicidal preparation before complete inactivation of the spermatozoa has occurred, thereby rendering the method ineffective.

These principles may be rephrased and reiterated as patient instructions. (See "Patient Instructions for Spermicides.") These instructions become the most important element of patient management when the choice is for spermicidal preparations with or without condoms.

While spermicidal preparations have a theoretical effectiveness rate equivalent to condoms and diaphragms, they have higher failure rates for use effectiveness than the other contraceptive methods. (See Table 27-1). This may be due to the possibility that the woman using a spermicidal preparation is less well motivated for routine use of a contraceptive method. This, in turn, may be due to infrequent or inconsistent sexual contact. Spermicidal preparations are readily available in drug stores without prescription and they are easy to use. Their cost varies according to type and brand but it generally is not prohibitive.

The messiness of spermicidal preparations has been the major complaint of couples using them. This relates primarily to the postcoital leakage of some degree common to all of the spermicidal preparations except the vaginal contraceptive sponge. By contrast the vaginal contraceptive sponge absorbs secretions and ejaculate, which some users find desirable, while other women using the sponge have complained of vaginal dryness. One of the advantages of the aerosol foam has been a reduction in postcoital leakage because a smaller amount (by weight) of foam is required than of jelly or cream. The least esthetic is the suppository since, when adequately dissolved, it drains freely over the perineum both during coitus and postcoitally. The woman's sexual pleasure may be lessened if she finds postcoital drainage annoying. Postcoital drainage can be controlled by placing a clean towel or tissues between the woman's legs against the perineum. This will absorb moisture and the woman will feel more comfortable.

The other objection has been from couples who enjoy oral-genital sexual activity as part of their lovemaking. Their complaint is that the spermicidal preparations do not taste good. This problem is increased as the amount of drainage increases.

Some couples feel negative about having to watch the clock and time their actions in relation to the action of the spermicidal preparation.

Patient Instructions for Spermicides

Patient instructions are central to counseling

for contraceptive method effectiveness. The following patient instructions are for use of the more common spermicidal preparations: foam, cream, or jelly.

1. Practice filling and inserting the applicator in the dark before actually using it for contraception.
2. If using foam, shake the can fifteen times before filling the applicator.
3. Fill the applicator.
4. Lie down for insertion when and where coitus will occur. If a woman gets up, walks around, goes to the bathroom, and so forth after insertion of the spermicidal preparation but before sexual intercourse, the method is rendered invalid because a large portion of the spermicide will drain out due to positional change. In this circumstance, if contraception is desired, another applicatorful of the spermicidal preparation must be inserted when again lying down before sexual intercourse. For the same reason a woman should not get up and go to the bathroom to insert a spermicidal preparation.
5. Insert the applicator into the vagina as far as it will go. Insert by pressing downward and inward.
6. Withdraw the applicator ½ inch and then push the plunger. This will deposit the spermicidal preparation at the cervical os.
7. If coitus does not take place within 30 minutes of insertion of the spermicidal preparation, another applicatorful must be inserted before sexual intercourse if contraception is desired.
8. Another applicatorful of spermicidal preparation must be inserted prior to each act of repeated sexual intercourse, if contraception throughout is desired.
9. Douching is not necessary or encouraged. However, if douching is going to be done, do *not* douche for at least 6 to 8 hours after the last sexual intercourse. The con-

traceptive protection of the spermicidal preparation may be lost if douching occurs earlier than this.

10. Use a small towel or tissues between the legs to catch drainage and reduce messiness.
11. The spermicidal preparation method of contraception is most effective in protecting against pregnancy when used in conjunction with the condom method of contraception.

CONDOMS

The condom is a sheath of strong, thin, elastic rubber or collagenous material. It is unrolled down over the erect penis to catch the semen during ejaculation and prevent its being deposited in the vagina.

Effectiveness, Complaints, and Management

Three techniques in using the condom will enhance its efficacy:

1. The condom must be in place before the penis approaches the female genitalia because of the possibility that there are spermatozoa in male urethral coital secretions.
2. When using a plain-ended condom, an overlap allowance of ¼ to ½ inch should be made for collection of the semen, thereby decreasing the possibility that the condom might break at the time of ejaculation.
3. Because the penis becomes flaccid following ejaculation, it is important that the male withdraw from the vagina immediately following ejaculation while securely holding the edge of the condom so that there is no leakage of semen out the open end of the condom and to prevent the condom from slipping off into the vagina while withdrawing [1, p. 498].

These three techniques form the major portion of the vital patient instructions. (See "Patient Instructions for Condoms.")

If the condom is used correctly, the only reason for failure is defects in the condom itself. Defects include weakness of material which might allow the condom to break from the force of ejaculation, or minute holes which render its use ineffective. Condoms made in the United States are unlikely to have imperfections because they are manufactured under the supervision and quality control of the Food and Drug Administration of the federal government. While a condom can be tested by overdistending it with water or air and then checking for leakage, testing it in this manner creates the possibility that such stretching may weaken the condom and cause it to break when it is actually used. A condom, if it is given proper care, can be reused, but may be weakened. The best precaution is to use a condom once and throw it away.

There is a large difference between the theoretical effectiveness and the use effectiveness of condoms (see Table 27-1). This discrepancy probably is due to a combination of technique and consistency of usage. Condoms, variously known as "rubbers," "safes," "sheaths," or "prophylactics," are readily available without prescription, generally are lubricated (with wet jelly or dry powder), may or may not have a spermicide on the inside and outside, and may be purchased in different colors or plain. The cost varies with the make but generally is not high.

The condom, as a method of contraception, may be used either by itself or in conjunction with another method, such as the spermicidal preparations. Although it is widely used, many couples have negative feelings about the condom. Some couples feel it dulls sensation; others feel it creates a barrier between them at a time when they desire the feeling of oneness that can be attained during sexual intercourse. The objection that sexual foreplay is interrupted in order to put the condom on the penis can be eliminated if the woman puts the condom on the man as part of their foreplay. In addition, the condom has been associated with prostitutes and disease prevention. Thus, a man may have negative feelings or the woman may feel insulted when a condom is used, especially if not discussed beforehand. This problem requires reeducation of such individuals in order to change mental associations and attitudes.

Patient Instructions for Condoms

1. The condom must be on the penis *before* it approaches the female external genitalia or is inserted into the vagina.
2. Condoms made in the United States do not need to be checked before use.
3. Unroll the condom down over the erect penis.
4. If the condom is plain-ended rather than with a nipple end, an overlap allowance of ½ inch must be made for collection of the semen. This overlap space should be empty, that is, should not have air in it. This space is formed by holding the end in a collapsed state when applying the condom to the penis and starting to roll it down over the penis.
5. Use a spermicidal preparation or K-Y Lubricating Jelly spread over the condom-sheathed penis if additional lubrication is needed for insertion into the vagina. Do not use petroleum jelly; it may rot the rubber.
6. The man must withdraw his penis immediately following ejaculation, before the penis becomes flaccid.
7. As the man withdraws his penis he must hold onto the condom near the base of the penis to prevent its falling off or leaking semen while withdrawing.
8. Condoms are used once and thrown away.
9. The condom method of contraception is most effective in protection against pregnancy when used in conjunction with the spermicidal preparation method of contraception.

SPERMICIDAL PREPARATIONS AND CONDOMS USED TOGETHER

Effectiveness, Contraindications, and Side Effects

When a combination of a spermicidal preparation and a condom is used as the contraceptive method, there is a decrease in the failure rate with fewer pregnancies for both the theoretical effectiveness and use effectiveness of this combined method. (See Table 27-1.) For this reason, the best management of spermicidal preparations and condoms is to encourage their combined use if either one is the individual's method of choice or if there are contraindications to other methods of choice.

Contraindications to the combined method relate to the limited side effects of both spermicidal preparations and condoms — possible perineal or vaginal irritation as an allergic reaction to either the spermicidal preparation, or the lubricant on the condom, or both. If the woman has a known allergic reaction, she will probably not use the method anyway, or at least not very consistently. While this is not a contraindication of life-threatening proportion, it is a contraindication because the method will not be an effective method of contraception due to probable lack of use. However, if the reaction is to the lubrication on the condom, the condom can be washed and lubricated instead with contraceptive foam, jelly, or cream. The use of a spermicidal preparation with a condom also eliminates any problems of insufficient coital secretions.

Management

A spermicidal preparation and condom is the method of choice in the following situations:

1. When other contraceptive methods are contraindicated
2. When it is the method selected by the individual or couple

The individual or couple is encouraged to call for an appointment if there are any problems or side effects. The woman is given an appointment for her annual examination: general screening history, physical and pelvic examinations, Pap smear, and other routine laboratory tests.

A spermicidal preparation and condom may also be used as a backup method "to cover" another primary method at times when it may not be as effective. These include the following circumstances:

1. The first month of initiating oral contraception
2. The first month after insertion of an IUD
3. At the time of presumed ovulation when the primary contraceptive method is an IUD

REFERENCE

1. Williams (idem. Burst), H. V. Family planning. In Ziegel, E., and VanBlarcom, C. C. (Eds.). *Obstetric Nursing*, *6th*. New York: Macmillan, 1972.

BIBLIOGRAPHY

Bruce, J., and Schearer, S. B. *Contraceptives and Common Sense: Conventional Methods Reconsidered*. New York: The Population Council, 1979.

Calderone, M. S. *Manual of Contraceptive Practice*, *2nd*. Baltimore: Williams & Wilkins, 1970.

Connell, E. B. (Moderator). Symposium: A new look at barrier contraceptives, *Contemporary OB/GYN* 10:76, 1977.

Connell, E. B., and Tatum, H. J. *Barrier Methods of Contraception*. Durant, Okla.: Creative Informatics, 1985.

Hatcher, R. A. et al. *Contraceptive Technology, 1984–1985, 12th. rev.* New York: Irvington Publishers, 1984.

Jackson, M., Berger G. S., and Deith, L. G. *Vaginal Contraception*. Boston: G. K. Hall, 1981.

New Developments in Vaginal Contraception. *Pop. Rep.* Series H. No. 7 (January/February) 1984.

Patient Instructions — Guide for Nurses. The University of Mississippi Medical Center Nurse-Midwifery Program, 1970.

Special report: The sponge after one year. *Contraceptive Technology Update.* 5(7):81–87 (July) 1984.

Spermicides — Simplicity and Safety are Major Assets. *Pop. Rep.* Series H, No. 5 (September) 1979.

Update on Condoms — Products, Protection, Promotion. *Pop. Rep.* Series H, No. 6 (September/October) 1982.

Williams (idem. Burst), H. V. Family planning. In Ziegel, E., and VanBlarcom, C. C. (Eds.). *Obstetric Nursing*, *6th*. New York: Macmillan, 1972.

30

Diaphragm and Cervical Cap Management

DIAPHRAGM

Description, Effectiveness, and Patient Response

The diaphragm is a mechanical method of contraception because it provides a mechanical barrier between the spermatozoa and ovum. It is dome-shaped, made of somewhat thicker rubber than the condom, and has a flexible metal spring encased in the rim. The spring permits compression of the diaphragm for insertion, yet allows the diaphragm to regain its shape and fit snugly against the vaginal tissues when in place. When the diaphragm is in proper position, with the dome side down and the rim snug against the anterior and lateral vaginal walls, it completely covers the cervix like a cup into which the cervix is suspended. Thus, the spermatozoa are prevented from access and entry into the cervical os.

The dome of the diaphragm is approximately 1½ inches deep at its apex. Each woman's vaginal size and contour is individual; thus the diameter of a diaphragm may vary from 5½ to 10 centimeters (about 2¼ to 4 inches). Diaphragms are sized in increments of 5 millimeters as measured across the diameter of the rim. They are available in sizes from 55 to 105 millimeters.

There are three types of diaphragms, which differ only in the construction of the metal spring in the rim. They are as follows:

Flat spring — the spring in this diaphragm is a flat band made of lightweight stainless steel.
Coil spring — the spring in this diaphragm is a flexible circular coil of moderate strength.
Arcing spring — the spring in this diaphragm is a combination of the springs in the flat spring and the coil spring diaphragms.

The diaphragm is inserted into the vagina either digitally or with a mechanical inserter.

(A mechanical inserter can be used only with a flat spring or a coil spring diaphragm.) To effectively cover the cervix the diaphragm's position should be as follows: posteriorly, the rim of the diaphragm fits behind the cervix into the posterior vaginal fornix; anteriorly, the rim of the diaphragm rests snugly against the soft tissues posterior to the symphysis pubis; and the diaphragm's entire circumference rests against the vaginal walls. It is important that the woman check to make sure the diaphragm is properly positioned after insertion. Proper positioning is not possible if the diaphragm no longer fits as a result of change in size, shape, or position of the pelvic structures. Therefore a woman should be rechecked for both fit and possible change in size or type of diaphragm (1) a few weeks after her initial sexual experience, (2) after each childbearing experience, and (3) if there is a weight gain or loss in excess of 20 pounds (9.07 kilograms).

The use of a spermicidal jelly or cream applied to the diaphragm greatly enhances its effectiveness because it provides double protection. The spermicidal preparation, which is made specifically for use with a diaphragm, is applied before insertion to the rim and either the inside or the outside of the diaphragm so as to cover the area completely. Approximately 6 hours are needed for the spermicidal preparation or vaginal secretions to immobilize and kill and the spermatozoa; therefore the diaphragm must remain in position for at least 6 hours following coitus. The diaphragm is left in position if sexual intercourse is repeated within 6 to 8 hours, and an additional applicatorful of spermicidal jelly or cream is inserted for each act of intercourse. The woman may douche after 6 hours following the final act of intercourse, but not before if she wants to remain protected. Half of the douche is taken prior to removal of the diaphragm and the remaining half taken after removal, if she so desires.

The woman should check her diaphragm periodically for pinholes, wear, and brittleness of the rubber. It should be usable for at least 2 years if it is properly cared for by washing, thoroughly drying, and dusting with cornstarch after each use.

There are various potential causes of failure of the diaphragm as a contraceptive method. Inherent in the method is the possibility of the diaphragm's becoming dislodged during sexual intercourse. Other major reasons for failure are improper positioning of the diaphragm upon insertion, negligence in using the spermicidal cream or jelly which accompanies the diaphragm, and inconsistent use.

Inconsistent use itself may be due to any one or a combination of objections to the method. Some women have an aversion to the self—intravaginal manipulation the method demands for insertion, checking the position, and removal of the diaphragm. Other women object to what they consider the nuisance of inserting the diaphragm on a nightly or daily basis as is recommended for consistent conception protection, or to the inconvenience of leaving it in for 6 to 8 hours after the last act of sexual intercourse. Although the diaphragm usually is not felt during sexual intercourse, some couples feel it creates a barrier between them. Some women state they lose all feeling of the anterior vaginal wall, which decreases their sexual pleasure. The taste of the spermicidal jelly or cream is objectionable for those who enjoy oral sex during their lovemaking. On the other hand, an advantage of the diaphragm is that it catches menstrual flow, thus making coitus during menstruation less messy than it would be otherwise.

The pregnancy rate for the diaphragm when used in conjunction with a spermicidal preparation is approximately 3 per 100 woman years for consistent users. Without the addition of the spermicidal preparation and in poorly motivated, inconsistent use the pregnancy rate is much higher. This results in a use effectiveness rate of 20 to 25 pregnancies per 100 woman years. (See Table 27-1).

It was thought in the past that some women found the techniques of the diaphragm method too difficult to learn since a good understanding of female reproductive anatomy is beneficial. This idea has been thoroughly discredited with simple, clear instruction; supervision of practice in proper insertion, placement, and removal; and patience, time, and encouragement for this learning.

The cost of the diaphragm may be in addition to the necessary examination for evaluation of pelvic structures and determination of the proper size and type of diaphragm. This cost varies according to the size of the diaphragm but is not high. The diaphragm usually comes in a kit which contains the diaphragm, an instruction pamphlet, a mechanical inserter (this is optional in use), and a tube of spermicidal jelly or cream. Periodic replenishing of the spermicidal preparation adds somewhat to the cost.

Contraindications and Side Effects

The diaphragm is contraindicated in the presence of any of the following:

1. Severe uterine prolapse (descensus) — second or third degree
2. Severe cystocele — second or third degree
3. Severe anteversion or retroversion of the uterus
4. Fistulas — vesicovaginal or rectovaginal
5. Known allergy to the rubber of the diaphragm or to the accompanying spermicidal preparation

The first three conditions are contraindications because they render proper fit of the diaphragm difficult or impossible. Another contraceptive method is better if a good fit cannot be obtained with the diaphragm. The presence or absence of these contraindications is ascertained during the pelvic examination as described in Chapter 44.

The side effects, other than those already discussed as patient responses to the method, are limited to possible allergic reactions to either the rubber of the diaphragm, the spermicidal preparation, or both.

Management Plan for the Diaphragm

Management of the care of the woman or couple selecting a diaphragm as the method of family planning consists of the following components:

1. General history, physical and pelvic examinations, and laboratory tests
2. Screening for any deviations from normal and for contraindications to use of the diaphragm
3. Determination of the type and size of the diaphragm for the individual woman
4. Teaching the woman how to insert, place, and remove the diaphragm
5. Return visits
6. Patient instructions in the use and care of the diaphragm

The first two components have been discussed in previous chapters.

Fitting the Diaphragm

The type of diaphragm to be used depends upon normal or unusual vaginal size or contour, normal position or mild displacements of the uterus, the amount of vaginal muscular support, and the depth of the arch behind the symphysis pubis. The correlations of these characteristics with the types of diaphragm are as follows:

Flat spring — used with normal vaginal size and contour, strong vaginal support, normal uterine position, a shallow arch behind the symphysis pubis.

Coil spring — used with either normal or unusual vaginal size and contour, strong vaginal support, normal uterine position, a deep arch behind the symphysis pubis.

Arcing spring — used with unusual vaginal size and contour, poor vaginal support including first degree uterine prolapse or first degree cystocele; mild displacements of the uterus which may cause the rim of the flat spring or coil spring diaphragm to slide out of the posterior fornix into the anterior fornix, thereby leaving the cervix exposed. An arcing spring diaphragm is indicated for women who have had a vaginal delivery as they will have at least some amount of a first degree cystocele.

The size of the diaphragm has to be determined for each woman since the distance from the posterior fornix to the posterior aspect of the symphysis pubis varies from woman to woman. Generally, a nulligravida will be fitted with size 65, 70, or 75; a multipara with size 75, 80, or 85; and a grand multipara with size 85 or greater.

Fitting a woman for her diaphragm can be done either with fitting rings or with sets of the various sizes of diaphragms for each type of diaphragm. The latter is far superior to fitting rings because the rings are of no use in patient teaching and give no idea of the type of diaphragm appropriate for the woman. In fitting a woman, start with a size in the middle of the probable range of sizes for her parity. With experience your mind will be able to interpret with a fair amount of accuracy what your fingers feel as a size during pelvic examination. Also remember that, as a woman becomes accustomed to a diaphragm in place and the necessary digital manipulation, the resulting relaxation may require refitting her with a larger size diaphragm.

When fitting, lubricate the rim of the diaphragm with the same lubricant you use for performing a pelvic examination. Compress the sides of the diaphragm with the fingers and thumb of one hand and introduce it into the vagina in the same way that you insert a speculum. Be sure to direct it downward and inward, thereby applying pressure against the posterior vaginal wall and avoiding the more sensitive anterior structures. Once the diaphragm is within the vagina, double-check its placement to be sure that the rim of the diaphragm is in the posterior fornix, circumferentially against the lateral vaginal walls, and tucked up behind the symphysis pubis and that the cervix is covered, as can be felt through the rubber of the diaphragm.

To check the fit of the diaphragm, insert the tip of your index finger so that the pad of your finger is facing you between the rim of the diaphragm and the symphysis pubis. Then rub your fingers along the rim, pressing against the lateral vaginal walls. End by running your fingers behind the cervix and feeling the rim in the posterior vaginal fornix. The diaphragm is too small if:

1. There is more space than enough for the flat portion of your fingertip between the rim of the diaphragm and the symphysis pubis.
2. It moves about freely in the vagina.
3. It is not large enough to tuck up behind the symphysis pubis.

The diaphragm is too large if:

1. The rim of the diaphragm fits tightly against the symphysis pubis, thereby not allowing the flat portion of your fingertip to fit between the rim of the diaphragm and the symphysis pubis
2. There is buckling of the rim of the diaphragm forward against the lateral vaginal walls.
3. The edge of the diaphragm bulges out the vaginal introitus.
4. Tucking the rim of the diaphragm up behind the symphysis pubis causes it to buckle forward against the lateral vaginal walls.
5. The woman feels it with discomfort when it is in place.
6. The woman experiences any or all of the following after the diaphragm is in place for an hour or more:
   a. abdominal pain
   b. back pain

c. difficulty in urinating
d. rectal pain
e. cramps in her thighs

The diaphragm is the right size and type if:

1. It fits snugly in the vagina without buckling forward against the lateral vaginal walls.
2. There is just enough room for the flat portion of your fingertip to fit between the rim of the diaphragm and the symphysis pubis.
3. It covers the cervix.
4. It tucks into both the posterior fornix and up behind the symphysis pubis.
5. It is not felt uncomfortably by the woman when in place.
6. It causes no discomfort after it has been in place for an hour or more.
7. It remains tucked up behind the symphysis pubis when the woman bears down or coughs.

Patient Teaching

Once the diaphragm has been fitted for type and size, an essential component of management is to teach the woman how to insert, check for placement, and remove her diaphragm. Whether or not the woman is comfortable with her ability to perform these techniques may well determine whether or not she will actually use her diaphragm.

Pelvic models are invaluable in theoretically teaching a woman the necessary landmarks (i.e., symphysis pubis, cervix, posterior fornix, lateral vaginal walls) and proper placement of the diaphragm. In addition the pelvic models will give her some idea of the depth and direction of the vagina; the proximity of the pelvic organs; and assurance that the vagina is dead-ended and, therefore, a diaphragm can not travel somewhere else inside her body or escape through the cervical opening which obviously is too small. She should practice insertion and removal of the diaphragm in the model until ready to transfer this practice to herself. This portion of teaching the woman using a model can be done prior to the pelvic examination, or prior to fitting the diaphragm but after pelvic examination has ruled out any contraindications to her having a diaphragm, or after the diaphragm has been fitted. It is important when she practices with the model that she hold it so the manipulative techniques will be the same as when she does it on herself and not done from the direction of an outside examiner such as yourself.

The next step is for her to wash her hands and then insert her middle finger into her vagina and explore until she has located and identified her symphysis pubis and cervix. To do this she needs to be supported in an upright sitting position while her feet remain on the same horizontal level as her hips (i.e., on the bed or examining table, or in stirrups). This portion of the teaching may also take place before or after you have fitted the diaphragm. It helps if you have already done your pelvic examination so you can help her locate her cervix if necessary.

Finally the woman practices insertion, placement, and removal of the diaphragm on herself. Wash and dry the fitting diaphragm you used that fit her. Place it on something clean such as a paper towel. Have her hold it, dome side down, with one hand while with the other hand she squeezes from the tube and evenly spreads approximately 1 tablespoon of spermicidal cream or jelly around the inside of the cup, and around the rim, of the diaphragm. Emphasize that the spermicidal cream or jelly is an inherent part of the diaphragm method and the diaphragm should not be used without it. This is because the vaginal vault expands with female orgasm and spermatozoa may escape around the rim of the diaphragm. She would then be without protection unless the spermicidal jelly or cream were there to continue blocking the spermatozoa from entering the cervix. Without the spermicidal cream or jelly the effectiveness of the diaphragm method is reduced.

Have the woman assume the same position she was in when she explored her anatomical structures. Then have her compress the sides of the diaphragm between her thumb and fingers with her hand on top of the diaphragm. With the hand not holding the diaphragm she spreads her labia and introduces the end of the diaphragm in front of her thumb and index finger into her vagina in a downward and inward direction. In order to keep the rims of the diaphragm together during insertion yet be able to push it into the vagina at the same time, she now uses the hand she used for separating the labia for pushing the diaphragm in by placing it behind the hand compressing the diaphragm and pushing until the rim is under the symphysis pubis. She can then tuck the rim up behind her symphysis pubis with a finger of whichever hand she chooses. She then checks the placement of the diaphragm, feeling the rim behind the symphysis pubis and the rubber-covered cervix. You should also check the placement to make sure she is correct in both her placement and checking. The woman removes the diaphragm by inserting a finger into her vagina, bearing down, grasping the upper edge of the diaphragm posterior to the symphysis pubis, and pulling it down and out. She should compress the sides of the diaphragm as it comes out in order to reduce the diameter. This makes the insertion and removal procedures more comfortable. Large doses of encouragement and praise throughout this process are helpful.

Have her practice until both you and she are sure of what she is doing and she is able to correctly prepare, insert, check placement of, and remove the diaphragm without any help from you. Then have her get up and insert the diaphragm in the alternate positions: (1) standing with one foot on a chair, which at home could be with one foot on the edge of the bathtub or on the toilet lid, or (2) while in a squatting position. Check her placement each time. Then have her remove it in the same position in which she inserted it. She may find

one or both of these positions more convenient or easier than the in-bed position.

She is then instructed regarding the use and care of the diaphragm (see "Patient Instructions").

The Return Visits

After being fitted for her diaphragm and having learned the techniques of preparation, insertion, checking, and removal, the woman should leave the clinic or office, with her diaphragm vaginally in place. She should be instructed to leave it in place for several hours. If the diaphragm is too large, she will develop discomfort/pain in her abdomen, back, rectum, or thighs during this time. In this case she should make an appointment to be refitted as soon as possible.

The woman is given an appointment for her first revisit 2 weeks after the time she was fitted. During these 2 weeks she is to practice using her diaphragm daily or nightly whether or not she has sexual intercourse. For contraception during this 2-week practice time she should rely on the combination of a spermicidal preparation and condoms. Ask her to return for her revisit in 2 weeks with her diaphragm in place.

At her 2-week revisit the following history related to the diaphragm should be elicited:

1. How many times she wore it
2. The longest period of time she left it in place
3. Whether or not she had any abdominal pain, back pain, rectal pain, cramps in her thighs, or difficulty in voiding after the diaphragm had been in place for several hours
4. Whether or not she had any difficulties with the techniques of preparation, insertion, checking, or removal
5. What position she is using for insertion and removal
6. Whether or not she likes the method and why or why not
7. What her sexual partner thinks about the method

A pelvic examination is then done to evaluate the following:

1. Proper placement of the diaphragm
2. Fit of the diaphragm and the continuing correctness of the type and size
3. Presence or absence of any pelvic pain
4. Presence or absence of any vaginal irritation

If all is well, the patient instructions are reviewed with her, and the woman is given an appointment for her annual examination: general screening history, physical and pelvic examinations, Pap smear, and other routine laboratory tests.

Patient Instructions
1. Insertion of the diaphragm should be in advance of sexual foreplay so that there is neither interruption nor pressure either to hurry (possibly making insertion difficult) or to neglect using it.

   If coitus always happens at a certain time, then make the insertion of the diaphragm part of your daily routine prior to this time. For example, if coitus occurs only at night, then before going to bed, wash your face, brush your teeth, and insert your diaphragm — every night.

   Preparation, insertion, and checking of the diaphragm can become part of the sexual foreplay prior to approach of the penis to the female external genitalia or insertion into the vagina by teaching your sexual partner how to do these techniques.
2. Empty your bladder and wash your hands with soap and water.
3. Shake excess cornstarch off your diaphragm.
4. Thoroughly spread spermicidal cream or jelly around the inside of the cup of the dome and around the rim of the diaphragm.

   Spermicidal cream and jelly are equally effective. The jelly may be both more lubricating and more messy. Which is used may depend on the need for lubrication.

5. Compress the sides of the diaphragm and insert, dome side down.
6. Tuck the rim of the diaphragm up behind the symphysis pubis and check to be sure that the cervix is covered.
7. You can walk around, bathe, and urinate with your diaphragm in place because it will neither get lost in your body nor fall out. However, if you have a bowel movement, recheck the position of your diaphragm afterwards and reposition it if necessary. It may have slipped out of the posterior fornix, thus leaving the cervix exposed.
8. If more than 2 hours elapse between insertion of your diaphragm and having sexual intercourse, an applicatorful of spermicidal jelly or cream should be inserted, without removing the diaphragm, before intercourse.
9. If coitus is repeated, add another applicatorful of spermicidal jelly or cream, without removing the diaphragm, before each act of sexual intercourse.
10. Leave the diaphragm in place for at least 6 to 8 hours after the last act of sexual intercourse. This is because it takes 6 to 8 hours for either the spermicidal preparation or the hostile vaginal environment, or both, to kill the spermatozoa.
11. Douching is not necessary or encouraged. However, if douching is going to be done, it should be done at the time the diaphragm is removed. Half of a body-temperature, tap water douche is taken prior to removing the diaphragm. The other half of the douche is taken after removing the diaphragm. The douche is divided into these two portions on the outside chance that any semen, containing spermatozoa, remains. Any such semen is thus washed out before the protective barrier is removed. Douching has a tendency to encourage spermatozoa to move inward through the cervical os rather than outward from the vagina.
12. Remove the diaphragm by bearing down,

catching hold of the rim of the diaphragm behind the symphysis pubis, pulling it down and then out, compressing the sides as it comes.

13. Care for your diaphragm as follows:
    a. after each use:
       (1) wash with a mild, nonperfumed soap
       (2) rinse with clear water
       (3) dry thoroughly
       (4) dust with cornstarch — never with talcum powder or any kind of perfumed powder since this will rot the rubber
       (5) store in a dry container away from heat (heat will rot rubber) — use either the case it came in or a clean cardboard box
    b. periodically check for areas of rubber deterioration, weakening, or holes by holding the diaphragm up to light and gently stretching the rubber
    c. replace the diaphragm every 2 years because of deterioration and weakening of the rubber
    d. never use petroleum jelly with a diaphragm as it may rot the rubber
14. Make an appointment to be refitted for a diaphragm in the event of any of the following:
    a. after initiating sexual experience — after approximately twenty to thirty acts of coitus
    b. after having a baby
    c. after having an abortion
    d. after any pelvic surgery
    e. after a weight gain or loss of 20 pounds or more
15. Make an appointment before your annual examination in the event of any of the following:
    a. you lose your diaphragm
    b. your diaphragm is damaged or deteriorating
    c. your diaphragm needs to be refitted
    d. you or your sexual partner are no longer happy with this method of contraception

CERVICAL CAP

Although widely used in Europe, the cervical cap in the United States is classified as a class III "significant risk device" by the Food and Drug Administration (FDA). This necessitates obtaining an FDA Investigational Device Exemption in order to purchase and fit cervical caps. All data collected are sent to the FDA to further the information needed about the effectiveness and safety of the cervical cap. Caps are purchased from England. Two types are currently available: the Prentif Cavity Rim Cap and the Dumas Cap. The Vimule Cap was withdrawn from investigation by the FDA in 1984 due to reports of lacerations and other trauma from its sharp rim.

The round, cone-shaped, rubber cervical cap fits over the cervix and adheres snugly, but not tightly, to either the surface of the cervix (Prentif Cavity Rim Cap) or in the vaginal fornices at the cervicovaginal junction (Dumas Cap). It is kept in place by a partial suction which is created between the dome of the cap and the cervix. The Dumas Cap is a better fitting cap for those women with a short, flat cervix or an irregular-shaped cervix.

Contraindications to use of the cervical cap include:

1. Cervicitis
2. Cervical erosion
3. Pelvic inflammatory disease
4. DES exposure
5. Abnormal Pap smear
6. History of toxic shock syndrome
7. Cervical irregularities that will interfere with cap suction (e.g., multiple Nabothian cysts, deep cervical lacerations, or malformations)

8. Exceptionally long or short cervix
9. Cervix that points posteriorly (this exposes the anterior rim of the cap to penile thrusting and significantly increases the risk of dislodgement)
10. Allergy to rubber
11. Allergy to spermicides

The woman should be at least 6 weeks postpartum or postabortion for a proper fit. In fitting a cervical cap, you first need to note the following during your pelvic examination:

1. Length of cervix
2. Diameter of cervix
3. Which way the cervix points
4. Cervical shape irregularities

This information helps you determine the type and size of the cap. The cap, when properly positioned, should seal 360° around the rim onto the cervix or into the fornices.

For use, the dome is at least one-third filled with a spermicide prior to insertion. Insertion should be at least half an hour before sexual intercourse as there is a better seal from the suction by that period of time. The woman should check herself after insertion to make sure the cap is properly located on and over the cervix. She should also check herself between times of having sexual intercourse as the cervical cap sometimes becomes dislodged from the penile thrusting.

Care of the cervical cap is the same as for a diaphragm. The difference is in the length of time it can stay in before removing. The diaphragm should be removed 6 to 8 hours after the last act of intercourse and no longer than 24 hours after insertion. The cervical cap can be left in for as long as 5 days, although most health care providers advise no more than 3 days. The concern is toxic shock syndrome, which has occurred in a few women who left diaphragms in place for 36 to 48 hours. To date there has not been a reported incidence of toxic shock syndrome with the cervical cap, but caution is indicated.

The cap should not be worn during menstruation. Petroleum jelly should not be used on the cap as it will rot the rubber. If an odor develops, not uncommon if worn for longer than 1 day, the cap should be removed daily for cleaning. The cap can be soaked in vinegar solution (1 teaspoon apple cider vinegar to 1 quart water) to neutralize the odor. This will turn the cap brown.

Follow-up care includes a reappointment in 2 to 4 weeks to check the fit, check the woman's ability to use the cap, and assess her satisfaction with the method. Thereafter the cap should be checked at the time of a woman's annual well-woman gynecology examination.

BIBLIOGRAPHY

Boehm, D. The cervical cap: Effectiveness as a contraceptive. *J. Nurse-Midwifery* 28(1):3−6 (January/February) 1983.

Bruce, J., and Schearer, S. B. *Contraceptives and Common Sense: Conventional Methods Reconsidered.* New York: The Population Council, 1979.

Calderone, M. S. *Manual of Contraceptive Practice,* 2nd. Baltimore: Williams & Wilkins, 1970.

Cappiello, J. D., and Grainger-Harrison, M. The rebirth of the cervical cap. *J. Nurse-Midwifery* 26(5):13−18 (September/October) 1981.

Connell, E. B., and Tatum, H. J. *Barrier Methods of Contraception.* Durant, Okla.: Creative Infomatics, 1985.

Hatcher, R. A., et al. *Contraceptive Technology, 1984−1985, 12th.* New York: Irvington, 1984.

Johnson, M. A. The cervical cap as a contraceptive alternative. *Nurse Pract.* 10(1):37−45 (January) 1985.

King, L. *The Cervical Cap Handbook for Users & Fitters.* Iowa City, Iowa: Emma Goldman Clinic for Women, 1981.

Lehfeldt, H. et al. Spermicidal effectiveness of chemical contraceptives used with the firm cervical cap. *Am. J. Obstet. Gynecol.* 82:446−448, 1961.

Okrent, S. *A Clinical Guide to the Intrauterine Device*

and the Vaginal Diaphragm. New York: Shirley Okrent, 1974.

Patient Instructions — Guide for Nurses. The University of Mississippi Medical Center Nurse-Midwifery Program, 1970.

Swartz, D. P., and Vande Wiele, R. L. *Methods of Conception Control.* Raritan, N. J.: Ortho Pharmaceutical Corporation.

Understanding. Raritan, N. J.: Ortho Pharmaceutical Corporation.

Widhalm, M. V. Vaginal lesion: Etiology — A malfitting diaphragm? *J. Nurse-Midwifery* 24(5):39—40 (September/October) 1979.

Williams (idem. Burst), H. V. Family planning. In Ziegel, E., and VanBlarcom, C. C. (Eds.). *Obstetric Nursing, 6th.* New York: Macmillan, 1972.

31

IUD Management

DESCRIPTION, EFFECTIVENESS, AND PATIENT RESPONSE

Intrauterine contraceptive devices (IUCD or IUD) are made of a variety of materials. Usually the basic material is polyethylene, an inert plastic. The material used must possess the following qualities: (1) noninflammatory in the normal uterus, (2) flexible for insertion and removal, and (3) able to retain its "memory" to resume its shape when in position.

IUDs may be categorized as medicated or nonmedicated. Medicated IUDs are those which have an added chemical feature to the basic design and material for purposes of enhancing effectiveness by decreasing pregnancy rates, decreasing expulsion rates, and minimizing side effects. Current medicated IUDs include the Copper T, the Copper (Cu) 7, and the Progesterone T (Progestasert). The only currently produced nonmedicated IUD is the Lippes Loop. Production of the Saf-T-Coil ceased for economic reasons in 1982.

IUDs are produced in a variety of shapes. Generally the IUD is named after the individual who invented it, or a feature of the IUD, or the shape itself. All current IUDs have a cervical appendage. A cervical appendage to the device in the uterus takes the form of ties or strings. A cervical appendage facilitates removal, enables a woman to check herself periodically to ascertain if the IUD is still in place, and permits an examiner to identify quickly the presence of the IUD.

A number of IUDs are no longer on the market because one problem or another became evident with them. These include the so-called closed devices (e.g., Hall-Stone Ring, Birnberg Bow) because of possible strangulation of a loop of intestine if they perforated the uterus; the Majzlin Spring because of possible imbedding in the endometrium and myometrium; and the Dalkon Shield because of association with spontaneous second trimester septic abortions. A woman who comes for health care with one of these particular devices in her uterus should be informed of the risk now known to be associated with her device. She should be encouraged to select another type of IUD or another method of contraception and to allow you to remove the one she has.

The mechanism of action of the IUD is not

known, although several theories have been suggested. These include possible alterations in the uterine environment with the most popular theory being that the presence of a foreign body creates a local inflammatory reaction that renders the uterine lining temporarily unsuitable for implantation of the fertilized ovum as long as the IUD is in the uterus. The addition of copper or progesterone to the IUD increases the local reaction due to their biochemical reactions with components of the uterine lining. These additional elements of copper and progesterone have thus far been found to be limited to local reactions and not found to be absorbed systemically. Long-term effects are not known.

Research and statistics for evaluation of IUDs generally emphasize pregnancy rates, expulsion rates, removal rates, and continuation rates. The pregnancy rate of the IUDs varies from 1 to 6 per 100 woman years of exposure (excluding size A and B of the Lippes Loop). This variation depends on a multiple of variables ranging from size and shape of the device to unrecognized expulsion of an IUD. The latter probably accounts largely for the difference between the theoretical effectiveness and use effectiveness rates given for the IUD in Table 27-1. An average of approximately 25 percent of women will either expel spontaneously or have the IUD removed during the first year of IUD use.

The cost of IUDs from the manufacturer varies for each device. The device usually comes in a sterile package which includes not only the IUD but also a disposable inserter. Insertion instructions are on the package. Added to this cost is the cost of an examination, lab tests, and IUD insertion.

A favorable patient response to the IUD has been that this method of contraception is quite apart from the sexual act itself. It has the additional advantage of not needing daily or monthly thought and supplies. Women who have an aversion to inserting a finger into their vagina may object to checking for the cervical appendage after each menstrual period. Individuals and couples who are against abortion and believe the IUD to be an abortifacient either decide not to use an IUD for contraception or need to resolve any moral or religious conflict for themselves if seriously considering or, in fact, using an IUD. A number of persons object to the risks and possible side effects associated with IUDs, and some women simply don't like the idea of "something inside of them."

CONTRAINDICATIONS AND SIDE EFFECTS

Contraindications

The following are absolute contraindications to the insertion of an intrauterine contraceptive device in a woman by a nurse-midwife:

1. Pregnancy:
   a. confirmed
   b. suspected
   c. possible (i.e., coitus without a valid contraceptive method since the last normal menstrual period)
2. Pelvic inflammatory disease (PID):
   a. history of chronic PID
   b. presence of acute or subacute PID
   c. history of PID within the past 3 months, including postpartum endometritis or an infected abortion
3. Cervical or uterine carcinoma (known or suspected):
   a. unresolved, abnormal Papanicolaou smears — class III or greater
   b. unexplained or abnormal uterine bleeding
4. History or presence of valvular heart disease (contraindication because of increased susceptibility to subacute bacterial endocarditis)
5. History or presence of blood dyscrasias, including sickle cell disease, leukopenia, leukemia, or any coagulopathy

6. Presence of myomata or congenital malformations that distort the uterine cavity
7. Known or suspected allergy to copper contraindicates the use of the Copper 7 and the Copper T
8. Uterine sound measurements less than 1¾ inches (4½ centimeters)

The following are relative contraindications to the insertion of an intrauterine contraceptive device by a nurse-midwife. The nurse-midwife should consult with the physician in the presence of any of these relative contraindications and a collaborative decision made regarding the insertion of an IUD.

1. Uterine sound measurements between 1¾ and 2½ inches (4½ and 6¼ centimeters) or greater than 4 inches (10 centimeters)
2. Acute cervicitis
3. History of ectopic pregnancy
4. Hemoglobin below 10 grams per 100 milliters
5. Routine corticosteroid medication (corticosteroids both increase susceptibility to, and mask the symptoms of, infection)
6. Uterine abnormalities such as congenital or developmental anomalies, for example, bicornuate uterus

The following are possible contraindications; the nurse-midwife should evaluate them and then make a decision as to whether or not to insert an intrauterine contraceptive device in the presence of any of them:

1. History of dysmenorrhea (painful menstruation)
2. History of menorrhagia (excessive menstrual flow)
3. History of metrorrhagia (bleeding between menstrual periods)
4. Nulligravida (considered because of the increased incidence of PID with IUD use, which may result in sterility)
5. Multiple sexual partners

Side Effects and Complications

The following side effects, some to the extent of being called complications or life-threatening risks, are the ones more commonly identified as being associated with having an intrauterine contraceptive device in utero.

1. Vasovagal syncope with insertion
2. Immediate postinsertion spotting and cramping
3. Cramping, low back pain, or both for several days after insertion
4. Dysmenorrhea, especially for the first 1 to 3 months after insertion
5. Menorrhagia (heavy menses), especially for the first 1 to 3 months after insertion
6. Metrorrhagia (intermenstrual bleeding or spotting), especially for the first several weeks after insertion
7. Severe or prolonged bleeding
8. Continuing severe pain from uterine cramping
9. Expulsion of the IUD
10. Pregnancy, either with the IUD in place or subsequent to unnoticed expulsion of the IUD
11. Ectopic pregnancy
12. Spontaneous septic abortion
13. Cervical or uterine perforation
14. Pelvic inflammatory disease (PID)
15. Death (0.3 to 1 per 100,000 IUD users per year) — usually as a sequela to pelvic infection

There is no evidence that the IUDs are carcinogenic.

MANAGEMENT PLAN FOR THE IUD

Management of the care of the woman with IUD contraception consists of the following components:

1. Informing the woman of the effectiveness

rates and potential side effects and complications and having her sign an informed patient consent form

2. Conducting a general history, physical and pelvic examinations, and laboratory tests including Pap smear, GC culture, and hemoglobin/hematocrit
3. Screening for any deviations from normal and for any contraindications to insertion of an IUD
4. Selecting the IUD appropriate for the individual woman
5. Inserting the IUD
6. Teaching the woman how to check for her IUD
7. Giving the patient instructions (see end of this chapter)
8. Scheduling and managing the return visits
9. Managing the possible side effects and problems related to an IUD
10. Removing the IUD when indicated

The first three components have been discussed previously.

Selection of the Appropriate IUD

The following comments about each IUD are designed to give the clinician information which will be helpful in individualizing the selection of an IUD for the woman. This presupposes availability as well as clinician competence and comfort in inserting and managing any of the IUDs discussed.

Lippes Loop

Lippes Loop sizes A and B should be avoided since they have relatively high pregnancy and expulsion rates. There is little difference in size between sizes C and D. Of these two sizes, the D has a lower failure rate and lower expulsion rate. Lippes Loop D is the standard loop used for the average-sized parous uterus.

Because the Lippes Loop is made of an inert plastic, it can be left in utero indefinitely and does not need periodic replacement. Lippes Loops are the least expensive of the IUDs presently on the market.

Copper 7 200 and Copper T 200

Since both of these are made of polyethylene with 200 square millimeters of copper wound around them, they will be discussed together in this presentation, even though they are manufactured by different companies and have different shapes.

Copper devices need to be replaced every 3 years, as the copper loses its contraceptive effectiveness over time. Therefore they are not the best IUD selection for women who may have difficulty keeping an annual appointment or for women who want long-term contraceptive protection lasting more than 3 years. They are a better selection for child spacing of 2 to 3 years or when a smaller-sized IUD is needed within the range of normal.

The copper devices tend to cause diminution of the menses rather than menorrhagia. Therefore they may be the device of choice for a woman who has heavy menses without an IUD or with another IUD. The copper devices are contraindicated for women who are allergic to copper.

Both the copper devices, but especially the Copper T, have relatively high perforation rates. The Copper T tends to perforate downward through the cervix more than through the uterine wall. The problem seems to be due in some part to the sharp points of these shapes. Because of these sharp points there is also a risk of intestinal perforation if the device is translocated into the peritoneal cavity. Intraperitoneal copper devices irritate the peritoneum and cause dense, tenacious adhesions which make removal more difficult. If copper devices enter the abdominal cavity they must be removed as quickly as possible after diagnosis because of the risk of intestinal perforation and because of adhesion formation. The use of ultrasound to determine the location of a copper device has been questioned because the copper may become hot and damage bowel tissue if located abdominally.

Progestasert-T
This medicated IUD has relatively low pregnancy and expulsion rates. The final design of the device and its inserter has reduced perforations to zero for those thus far studied with this design.

The Progestasert releases approximately 65 micrograms of progesterone per day for 1 year. The device then needs to be removed and replaced by a new Progestasert intrauterine progesterone contraceptive system. The effect of the progesterone is strictly local; there is no systemic hormonal effect.

Procedure for Insertion of the IUD

The insertion of an IUD varies in specific details according to the device and the inserter made for it. The manufacturer's instructions should be studied prior to insertion of an IUD unfamiliar to you. There are, however, some steps in the technique of inserting an IUD that should be followed regardless of which IUD is being inserted. These are as follows:

1. Explain the procedure to the woman (pelvic examination, GC culture, Pap smear, speculum, and the IUD insertion).
2. Do speculum examination and obtain GC culture and Pap smear.
3. Perform bimanual examination. Do not trust anyone else's bimanual examination findings prior to inserting an IUD. Specific findings prior to an IUD insertion are:
   a. rule out pregnancy
   b. rule out acute pelvic inflammatory disease
   c. determine the position, size, and shape of the uterus.
4. Reinsert the speculum and adjust for greatest visualization and exposure.
5. Thoroughly clean the cervix with an anti-

septic solution such as povidone-iodine (Betadine) or benzalkonium chloride (Zephiran) to decrease the risk of infection. Ask first if the woman is allergic to iodine before using an antiseptic solution that contains iodine.

6. Apply a tenaculum to the cervix.
   a. apply a single-tooth tenaculum to the anterior cervix at 10 and 2 o'clock approximately 1½ to 2 centimeters (about ¾ inch) from the level of the external os.
   b. angle the tenaculum from above downward so the bite will not be too shallow and run the danger of tearing out when pulled on nor so deep that the cervical canal is obstructed.
   c. you may find it easier to manipulate the tenaculum if you use both hands with one hand for control of each side of the tenaculum.
   d. close the tenaculum *slowly*, one notch at a time. Forewarn the woman that she may feel a short, sharp pain at this time. If pain occurs, wait until it passes before proceeding to the next step of sounding the uterus.
   e. the tenaculum can also be applied at 8 and 4 o'clock if the posterior cervix is more accessible than the anterior cervix.
   f. the tenaculum should never be applied at 3 or 9 o'clock as the major blood vessels to the cervix are positioned at these locations and excessive bleeding might result.

7. Sound the uterus to confirm the position of the uterus, rule out uterine canal obstructions, and measure the depth of the uterine cavity.
   a. forewarm the woman that she may feel a cramp when the uterine sound passes through the internal cervical os.
   b. hold the sound between your thumb and your first two fingers as you would a pencil or a fork. This gives you more

delicate, sensitive control of the uterine sound.

c. pull steadily and strongly on the tenaculum in order to straighten out the axis of the uterus.

d. using gentle pressure, insert the sterile uterine sound into the cervical canal until you feel the resistance of the internal os. At this time one of three things will happen:

(1) the sound will slip easily right on through the internal os and you will have felt slight to no resistance from the internal os.

(2) the tip of the sound will be resisted by the internal os, requiring the application of steady, mild pressure against the os to cause it to open and admit the sound into the uterine cavity. Care must be taken not to apply too forceful a pressure (i.e., strongly pushing) so that when the os opens the sound does not plunge into, and possibly through, the uterus.

(3) the internal os resists the mild pressure of the tip of the sound against it and does not readily open. It will, but patience is required. This usually occurs in women who are quite nervous and focused in on the procedure.

Position yourself comfortably. While continuing to apply steady, firm (but not forceful) pressure against the internal os, distract the woman by conversing with her on any subject unrelated to health care, IUDs, and so forth. This works best if the woman does the talking. Get her to tell you about her daily routine and ask questions about such things as her home, job, schooling, and children. As she talks, suddenly you will feel the internal os relax and open and the sound will slip into the uterine cavity. This may take from several seconds to a few minutes to accomplish.

You will probably have to repeat this process when inserting the IUD in its inserter through the internal os a little later.

e. let the sound find its own way in the uterine cavity once it has passed the internal os. Do not try to push it in in accord with what you think the uterine position is. Let the sound validate or reject your bimanual findings.

f. once the uterine position is confirmed or determined, then gently push the sound until it meets resistance. This should be the top of the fundus. Tap against it. This should evoke a cramp; ask the woman if she felt one. If not, you may not be at the top of the fundus. Pull hard on the tenaculum to straighten the uterine axis and again guide the sound until it meets resistance. Tap again. You should be at the top of the fundus now.

g. measure the depth of the uterine cavity:

(1) when the tip of the sound is touching the fundus, place a cotton-tipped applicator next to the sound with the applicator tip at the external cervical os.

(2) remove the sound and the applicator from the uterus and vagina at the same time.

(3) measure the depth of the uterine cavity by measuring the length of the sound from the level of the tip of the applicator on the sound to the tip of the sound.

h. If all is within the realm of normal, proceed with the next step.

8. Load the IUD into its inserter. This is a sterile procedure. This step is not done

until now, just prior to inserting the IUD, since plastic devices start to lose their memory (shape retention) as soon as they are loaded. The less time they are in their inserter, the less the memory loss to resume their shape.

9. Insert the IUD into the uterine cavity.

   a. Forewarn the woman that she may feel a cramp at this time.

   b. First pull firmly and steadily on the tenaculum to again straighten the uterine axis. Maintain this traction until the IUD is inserted.

   c. Insert the IUD in its inserter into the cervical canal and through the internal os as described in 7d above.

   d. Insert the IUD into the uterine cavity by removing it from its inserter in accord with proper procedure for the IUD being used. Be sure of which procedure is being used for the device you are inserting; some are pushed into the uterine cavity while others are placed in the fundus and then the sheath of the inserter withdrawn.

   Insertion of the device from its inserter should be done *slowly* in order to reduce the possibility of vasovagal syncope.

   Undue force should never be needed. If such seems to be required, *STOP!* Reevaluate. Never forcibly push an IUD into a uterine cavity — chances are you will be pushing it into the uterine wall instead.

10. Remove the inserter and the plunger in accord with proper procedure for the IUD being used.

11. If there are strings to be cut, cut them no shorter than approximately 2½ inches (6¼ centimeters) from the external cervical os. This allows enough remaining string so that, as the IUD resumes its shape and as the uterus resumes its usual position (both of which will take some of the string up

into the uterus), there will still be enough to be seen and felt. If they are still too long at her first revisit, they can be shortened at that time.

12. Remove the tenaculum. If there is bleeding from the application sites, apply pressure with a sponge stick or with a 4 × 4 gauze on a ring forceps until the bleeding stops. Some clinicians don't do this, believing that with removal of the speculum the vaginal walls will apply sufficient pressure to stop the bleeding.

13. Remove the speculum.

14. Wipe off the woman's perineum.

15. Allow her to rest and recover if she needs to.

16. Teach the woman how to check for her IUD (see next portion of this chapter).

17. Give her a perineal pad to wear and have her get dressed.

18. Chart all findings. Include type and size of the IUD you inserted, whether or not you had any difficulty with the insertion, the depth the uterine cavity measured, and the position of the uterus.

19. Answer any questions and give "Patient Instructions" (see end of this chapter).

There are three safety features in this procedure which, when strictly adhered to, reduce considerably the risk of perforating the uterus during insertion. These are (1) careful bimanual examination, (2) application and use of the tenaculum on the cervix, and (3) careful sounding of the uterus and measurement of its depth. Under no circumstances should a nurse-midwife insert an IUD without using *all* three of these safety features.

Most clinicians prefer to insert an IUD during a woman's menstrual period. This is because the cervical canal is slightly dilated during menstruation, thereby probably making insertion easier, and it eliminates the risk of inserting an IUD into a pregnant uterus. However, a woman may be more susceptible to developing an infection from an IUD insertion during her menses. In fact, IUD insertion can take place on any day of the menstrual cycle. You need, however, to be convinced of the woman's sexual intercourse and contraceptive history since her last normal menstrual period before making a decision to insert an IUD other than during her menses or a few days immediately following. It is best not to be rigid about what day it is but rather to evaluate the sexual and contraceptive history since the woman may never keep an appointment to return again when she is menstruating.

Teaching the Woman How to Check for Her IUD

The following instructions are important for the woman's periodic check of her IUD.

1. Have the woman wash her hands.
2. She can check her IUD in bed, sitting on the toilet or the edge of a chair, or in a squatting position.
3. Have the woman insert her middle finger into her vagina in a downward and inward direction and locate her cervix.
4. Have her feel for the strings of the IUD at the end of her cervix. Caution her not to pull on them.
5. She should check for her IUD at the end of each menstrual period. She may do it as often as she wants.
6. She should immediately call and make an appointment to be seen as soon as possible if she finds either of the following:
   a. no strings
   b. the end or a portion of the device
   In the meantime she is to consider herself unprotected and use a spermicidal preparation and condoms.

The Return Visits

After the woman has her IUD inserted she is instructed to use a spermicidal preparation and condoms for the first month she has her IUD. This more fully protects her from conception while the IUD is rendering the uterus inhospitable for implantation and during the time when the IUD is more likely to be expelled spontaneously. Some clinicians also instruct women with IUDs to use a spermicidal preparation and condoms around the time of anticipated ovulation each month. This provides a double contraceptive method. Studies have shown lower pregnancy rates when these two management regimens are used.

The woman is given an appointment to return for her first revisit in approximately 6 weeks. This is deliberately timed to be after her first postinsertion menstrual period. By this time the first month of higher incidence of spontaneous expulsion will be over and continuing placement of the IUD can be checked, the woman should have had experience with checking herself for her IUD, some of the immediate side effects should have diminished, and the revisit provides for encouragement and reassurance to the woman. This results in an increased user rate. The following history, physical, and pelvic examinations, and laboratory data pertinent to the IUD are elicited at this revisit:

History
1. Menstrual period (compare with pre-IUD menses):
   a. date
   b. length
   c. amount of flow
   d. pain
2. Intermenstrual (compare with pre-IUD):
   a. spotting or bleeding — how long, how much
   b. cramping — how long, how severe
   c. back pain — where, how long, how severe
   d. vaginal discharge — how long
      (1) color
      (2) odor

(3) itching

(4) burning on urination (before or after starting flow)

3. String checks

   a. date of last string check

   b. can sexual partner feel strings during intercourse

4. Satisfaction with method

   a. hers

   b. his

5. Taking any medicines — if yes, what, and what for

6. Been to a doctor or emergency room since IUD inserted — if yes, why

7. Use of spermicidal preparation and condoms

   a. when

   b. any problems

8. Presumptive signs of pregnancy if indicated

Physical examination

1. Abdominal examination for lower abdominal tenderness

2. Check for CVA tenderness if indicated for differential diagnosis

3. Probable signs of pregnancy if indicated

Pelvic examination

1. Speculum examination:

   a. visualization of strings

   b. length of strings — trim if indicated

   c. vaginal discharge — note characteristics and do wet smear if indicated

2. Bimanual examination:

   a. pain with movement of cervix or uterus

   b. uterine tenderness

   c. uterine enlargement

   d. adnexal tenderness

   e. probable signs of pregnancy if indicated

Laboratory

1. Hemoglobin or hematocrit

2. Routine urinalysis if indicated for differential diagnosis

If all is well, the woman is given an appointment for her annual examination, which will include a general screening history, physical and pelvic examinations, Pap smear, GC culture, other routine laboratory tests, and a repetition of the IUD revisit outlined here. Patient instructions for checking her IUD, using a spermicidal preparation and condoms, and when to call for an appointment prior to her annual appointment are reviewed with the woman.

Management of Side Effects and Problems

Vasovagal Syncope (Fainting)

Syncope may occur, infrequently, during or immediately following insertion. The cause is thought to be excessive pain, especially in a woman who is quite nervous, fearful, or emotional at the time of insertion. Gentle manipulation of the instruments and handling of the uterus combined with slow insertion of the IUD may forestall or reduce the incidence of syncope. Abrupt, hurried, rough actions may enhance its occurrence.

In the rare event of syncope, place the woman in as much of a Trendelenburg position as possible (remove pillow from under her head and place instead under her hips, raise her legs), be sure she has an open airway, and keep her warm. If necessary, administer an aromatic (smelling salts). If severe and in an emergency, administer 0.4 to 0.5 milligrams of atropine intramuscularly. Atropine acts as a respiratory and circulatory stimulant.

Immediate Postinsertion Spotting,
Menorrhagia and/or Metrorrhagia for the First
1 to 3 Months Postinsertion

Forewarn the woman about immediate postinsertion spotting and give her a perineal pad to protect her clothes.

Heavier than usual menses and intermenstrual spotting or bleeding are not uncommon during the first 1 to 3 months after insertion. Following insertion, women usually experience a varying amount of spotting or bleeding.

Spotting may continue for a few days and some women have light intermenstrual bleeding during the first menstrual cycle. Two or three longer and heavier menstrual periods are not uncommon. The menstrual periods may gradually return to what a woman had before insertion or remain slightly more heavy. The woman should be forewarned of this possibility. If bleeding seems excessive, check to be sure that the IUD is not partially expelled and into the cervical canal.

Menorrhagia and/or Metrorrhagia, Severe or Prolonged Bleeding after Initial Uterine Adjustment to the IUD

Rule out PID, incomplete abortion, cervical erosion, and partial expulsion of the IUD. Partial expulsion of an IUD is ascertained as follows during speculum examination:

1. Note if the strings of the IUD are longer than expected.
2. Look for protrusion of the IUD from the external cervical os.
3. If unable to see the IUD at the external cervical os:
   a. apply a tenaculum to the cervix as described in the procedure for inserting an IUD, earlier in this chapter.
   b. explore the cervical canal with a uterine sound, seeking contact with the IUD in the canal or at the internal cervical os.

If the IUD is partially expelled, remove it and replace with another if the woman is not pregnant and wants another IUD. If the problem is not the partial expulsion of the IUD, physician consultation is necessary either for treatment of another diagnosed cause or to rule out other forms of pelvic pathology.

A hemoglobin/hematocrit determination should be done and compared with previous findings to see if the blood loss has been such as to affect this parameter of the woman's well-being and she is becoming anemic. A woman may consider that heavy bleeding in the absence of pathology is sufficient reason to request that her IUD be removed and to select another contraceptive method.

Cramping, Low Back Pain, Dysmenorrhea

Women usually experience a varying amount of cramping after IUD insertion. Cramps, which range from light and of brief duration in multiparas to severe and lasting several days in nulligravidas, occur when the uterus contracts in an effort to expel the IUD. The woman should be forewarned of this possibility and advised to take across-the-counter analgesics for the pain. If the insertion was particularly painful and induced continuing painful cramping, a few Darvon capsules may be prescribed.

Dysmenorrhea for the first 1 to 3 months after insertion is not uncommon. It is worse in those already afflicted with dysmenorrhea. The usual comfort measures (e.g., lying down, warm soaks in the bathtub, heat to the lower abdomen or back) and analgesics are in order.

If there is continuing severe pain from uterine cramping, PID must be ruled out. A woman may consider severe, unremitting cramps, without pathology, sufficient reason to request that her IUD be removed and to select another contraceptive method.

Pregnancy

A woman who becomes pregnant with her IUD in situ needs to be informed of the risks involved if the pregnancy continues with the IUD left in place. These risks include intrauterine infection, sepsis, spontaneous abortion, spontaneous septic abortion, placenta previa, and premature labor. The incidence of ectopic pregnancy is higher in women who become pregnant with an IUD in situ.

If the strings of the IUD are not visible at the cervical os or accessible in the cervical canal, the option of a therapeutic abortion should be discussed with the woman or couple. The greatest concern in this circumstance is serious infection, which may lead to death.

Whatever the woman's decision, she is referred to the physician for termination of the pregnancy or for follow-up and closely monitored prenatal care.

If the strings of the IUD are visible, the IUD should be removed whether or not the woman or couple wish to terminate the pregnancy. This is done on the basis that the incidence of spontaneous abortion is lower in those women whose IUDs are removed than in those whose IUDs remain in during the pregnancy and that the risks enumerated before are minimized with removal of the IUD. Approximately 25 percent of women will abort spontaneously following removal of the IUD. The incidence of spontaneous abortion is between 40 and 50 percent for women whose IUDs are left in situ. Those wishing to terminate their pregnancy have their IUD removed and a therapeutic abortion at the same time. Such women are referred to the physician.

Pelvic Inflammatory Disease (PID)

The controversy continues as to whether or not IUDs contribute to the incidence of PID after the first month postinsertion, whether or not the cervical appendage of the IUD is indeed the offending and causative vehicle as a passage for ascending infection resulting in PID, and whether or not the IUD must be removed prior to treatment with antibiotics in order for treatment to be effective. No matter what idea prevails, it is important for the nurse-midwife to follow strict rules of cleanliness in performing pelvic examination; observe strict adherence to sterile technique in the intrauterine procedures involved in insertion, checking for, and removal of IUDs; instruct the woman in hygienic measures related to the perineum and vagina; and to screen for and identify the presence of the signs and symptoms of PID for consultation and collaboration with the physician. Further diagnostic measures may include aerobic and anaerobic bacteriological studies which in turn will identify the appropriate specific antibiotic therapy.

The signs and symptoms of PID include the following:

1. Foul-smelling leukorrhea (vaginal discharge)
2. Vague lower abdominal pain
3. Dyspareunia (painful coitus)
4. Premenstrual bloating
5. Menorrhagia
6. Metrorrhagia
7. Uterine tenderness especially acute with movement of the cervix
8. Tender tubo-ovarian enlargement or mass (indicative of an abscess)
9. Tender, fluctuant pelvic mass (indicative of an abscess)

The current prevalent thought regarding treatment of PID is to remove the IUD. There is concern that if the IUD is left in place the infection will not be adequately treated and a progressively worsening situation may result. Treatment is with antibiotics. Opinion also varies, from 3 months to 1 year, as to how soon to insert another IUD after an episode of PID. The woman should be encouraged to use a different primary contraceptive method.

Missing IUD Strings

IUD strings usually are first noticed to be missing by the woman when she is unable to feel them when checking herself. In such a situation there are four possibilities as to why the strings cannot be felt or, upon speculum examination, seen. These are as follows:

1. The strings were cut too short and retreated fully into the cervical canal as the device assumed its original shape, the uterus resumed its usual position after being pulled down by use of the tenaculum, and the uterine contractions caused the strings to be sucked in.
2. The woman is pregnant.
3. The IUD has perforated through the uterus.
4. The IUD was spontaneously expelled without the woman's being aware of this happening.

When managing a woman whose IUD strings cannot be visualized, you must *first* ascertain whether or not she is pregnant *before* doing any further search for the IUD. This is done by history, physical and pelvic examination for the signs and symptoms of pregnancy, and a pregnancy test (see Chapter 4). Other history you need in addition to that outlined in Chapter 4 is as follows:

1. When IUD was inserted
2. Type of IUD inserted
3. Any previous problems with IUD expulsion
4. Normal pattern of checking herself for IUD strings
5. When she last felt the IUD strings
6. Length of time between when she last felt the IUD strings and when she first was unable to feel them
7. Number of times she had coitus during this period of time and subsequently
8. Use of any other contraceptive method since she was unable to feel the IUD strings

If there is no evidence of pregnancy, you may proceed with your search for the IUD. Position the speculum and apply a tenaculum to the cervix (see procedure for IUD insertion earlier in this chapter). Explore the cervical canal with a narrow sponge forceps for the strings of the IUD. If you find the strings, remove the IUD and replace with another, being careful to leave the strings long.

If no strings can be found, insert a uterine sound into the uterus and feel for the IUD with the sound. If you find the IUD and cannot bring any strings into view to use for removal, remove it with the use of an IUD retriever. Replace with another IUD if the woman so desires, there has been no other problem with the IUD, and there is no reason to suspect a contraindication. Be careful to leave the strings long on the replacement IUD.

If you are unable to feel the IUD with the uterine sound, consult with the physician for further methods of searching for the IUD. These may include ultrasound (possibly contraindicated for copper IUDs) and posteroanterior (PA) and lateral x-ray films. If x-ray films are taken, some means must be used to identify whether the IUD, if visualized, is within the uterus or outside the uterus in the abdominal cavity. This is done in one of the following ways:

1. A marker IUD (an IUD of a different type or shape is inserted into the uterine cavity for purposes of identifying if the missing IUD is in utero, is in the abdominal cavity, or was expelled).
2. A uterine sound or catheter filled with radiopaque dye is inserted into the uterus.
3. A hysterogram is made (an x-ray film is taken immediately after injection of a radiopaque dye into the uterus via the cervical os) — contraindicated if there is intrauterine infection or PID.

If the IUD is found outside the uterine cavity in the abdominal cavity, it should be surgically removed by the physician by laparoscopy, culdoscopy, or laparotomy.

Procedure for Removal of the IUD

The usual reasons for removal of an IUD are desire to become pregnant; replacement of a medicated device; severe, unremitting cramps; and heavy, lengthy menses with or without intermenstrual bleeding. Other reasons include partial expulsion, PID, and pregnancy with visible IUD strings.

After the procedure is explained to the woman and bimanual examination is performed, the speculum is inserted, the cervix cleaned, and the tenaculum applied to the cervix as described in steps 4, 5, and 6 of the procedure for insertion of an IUD detailed earlier in this chapter. Then:

1. Clamp a long-handled forceps or needle-holder on the strings.

2. Pull steadily and strongly on the tenaculum to straighten the uterine axis.
3. Exert a steady, pulling traction on the strings.

or, if using a retriever:

1. Clamp a long-handled forceps or needle-holder on the strings.
2. Pull steadily and strongly on the tenaculum to straighten the uterine axis.
3. Insert the IUD retriever into the uterine cavity (same as step 7, parts *a* through *e* in the IUD insertion procedure for inserting a uterine sound).
4. Hook the retriever onto a part of the IUD so that you meet with resistance when slight traction is applied.
5. Again pull steadily and strongly on the tenaculum to straighten the uterine axis.
6. Exert even, steady, pulling traction on the strings and the retriever simultaneously. If there are no strings, the retriever alone is used.

If you meet with great resistance to removal, *STOP!* Consult with the physician before either breaking the strings off or, if the strings were unavailable to start with, getting into a situation you can't handle such as an imbedded IUD or an IUD partially perforating the uterus.

PATIENT INSTRUCTIONS

Review the following with the woman:

1. A card you give her with the name and size of the type of IUD she has, the date it was inserted, and where to call for help, information, or removal of her IUD
2. How long she can keep the IUD:
   a. if she has a nonmedicated IUD, it can remain in place indefinitely but she should have an annual physical and pelvic examination including a Pap smear
   b. if she has a copper-medicated IUD, it must be replaced every 3 years to remain fully effective
   c. if she has a Progestasert, it must be replaced every year to remain effective
3. How to check herself for the cervical appendage
4. Her first revisit in 6 weeks
5. The effectiveness rate, side effects, and danger signs associated with her IUD, and when to call immediately for an appointment

In addition, the following information and instructions should be given:

1. You may have some spotting or bleeding and cramping after insertion of your IUD for a day or so. Take aspirin or other analgesic every 3 to 4 hours for pain.
2. Avoid sexual intercourse for the first 24 hours after insertion of your IUD.
3. There is an adjustment period to your IUD of approximately 3 months.
   a. during this time your menstrual periods may be longer and heavier than they were before you had an IUD inserted.
   b. the length and amount of menstrual flow you have by your third month after insertion of your IUD will probably be what your normal menstrual period will be like for you with an IUD inside your uterus.
   c. you may have some cramping, especially with your menstrual periods. This is more likely if you have not had a baby. If you did not experience cramps when your IUD was inserted or immediately afterwards, you most likely will not have cramps later. Cramps may be alleviated with aspirin or other analgesia.
4. If your IUD is going to come out spontaneously, it is most likely to do so during a menstrual period. Therefore, in addition to checking yourself for the strings or cervical appendage of your IUD after each menstrual

period, you should do the following:

a. look for your IUD on your sanitary pads or tampons before discarding them (it is alright to use a tampon after the first 48 hours after your IUD was inserted).

b. check yourself for your IUD after any time you have some abdominal cramping.

c. if you find your IUD externally, or if you are unable to feel the strings or cervical appendage, or if you should feel your device coming through your cervix, you should:

    (1) make an appointment to be seen as quickly as possible.

    (2) consider yourself unprotected from becoming pregnant.

    (3) use another contraceptive method until your appointment.

5. Use a spermicidal preparation and condoms for the first month after insertion of your IUD and thereafter around the time you may be ovulating.

6. If you should get pregnant with your IUD still inside, you should have your IUD removed in order to decrease the risk of serious infection. There is half as much chance of spontaneous abortion with the IUD removed than if it is left in. A therapeutic abortion is possible if termination of the pregnancy is desired.

7. The IUD is inserted in accord with the angle of your uterus. Therefore you should obtain medical help to have your IUD removed when desired. You may injure yourself if you or your sexual partner pulls on the IUD strings or cervical appendage.

8. Remember to be seen annually, no matter what type of IUD you have, for a physical and pelvic examination, including a Pap smear.

BIBLIOGRAPHY

Alvior, G. T., Jr. Pregnancy outcome with removal of intrauterine device. *Obstet. Gynecol.* 41:894, 1973.

Cederqvist, L. L., Lindhe, B., and Fuchs, F. Perforation of the uterus by the Copper-T and Copper-7 intrauterine contraceptive devices, *Acta. Obstet. Gynec. Scand.* 54:183, 1975.

Faulkner, W. L., and Ory, H. W. Intrauterine devices and acute pelvic inflammatory disease. *JAMA* 235:1851, 1976.

Hasson, H. M. Copper IUDS, *J. Reprod. Med.* 20:139, 1978.

Hatcher, R. A. et al. *Contraceptive Technology, 1984–1985, 12th.* New York: Irvington, 1984.

Interconceptional Care Module. Georgetown University School of Nursing and the United States Air Force Nurse-Midwifery Educational Programs, 1977.

IUDs: An Appropriate Contraceptive for Many Women. *Pop. Rep.* Series B, No. 4 (July) 1982.

Kahn, H. S., and Tyler, C. W., Jr. IUD-related hospitalizations. *JAMA* 234:54, 1975.

Kahn, H. S., and Tyler, C. W., Jr. Mortality associated with use of IUDs. *JAMA* 234:57, 1975.

Keith, L., Hughey, M. J., and Berger, G. S. Experience with modern inert IUDs to date: A review and comments, *J. Reprod. Med.* 20:125, 1978.

Mishell, D. R., Jr. Historical considerations in the development of modern IUDs: Patient and device selection and the importance of insertion techniques. *J. Reprod. Med.* 20:121, 1978.

Okrent, S. *A Clinical Guide to the Intrauterine Device and the Vaginal Diaphragm.* New York: Shirley Okrent, 1974.

Patient Instructions — Guide for Nurses. The University of Mississippi Medical Center Nurse-Midwifery Education Program, 1970.

Perlmutter, J. F. Pregnancy and the IUD. *J. Reprod. Med.* 20:133, 1978.

Pharriss, B. B. Clinical experience with the intrauterine progesterone contraceptive system. *J. Reprod. Med.* 20:155, 1978.

Piotrow, P. T., Rinehart, W., and Schmidt, J. C. IUDs — Update on safety, effectiveness, and research. *Pop. Rep.* Series B. Baltimore: Johns Hopkins, 1979.

Rybo, G. The IUD and endometrial bleeding. *J. Reprod. Med.* 20:175, 1978.

Second Report on Intrauterine Contraceptive Devices. Medical Device and Drug Advisory Committees on Obstetrics and Gynecology, Federal Drug

Administration, U. S. Department of Health, Education and Welfare. Washington, D. C.: U. S. Government Printing Office, 1978.

Smith, H. M., Smith, W. I., and Edwards, S. J. The detection of intrauterine contraceptive devices by ultrasonic investigation. *Radiography* 43:507, 1977.

Sobrero, A. J., and Goldsmith, A. *Intrauterine Devices: A Manual for Clinical Practice.* Chestnut Hill, Mass.: The Pathfinder Fund, 1973.

Taylor, E. S. et al. The intrauterine device and tubo-ovarian abscess. *Am. J. Obstet. Gynecol.* 123:338, 1975.

The intrauterine device, *ACOG Technical Bulletin.* Number 40. Chicago: The American College of Obstetricians and Gynecologists, 1976.

The Progestasert. Palo Alto, Calif.: Alza Corporation, 1976.

Trobough, G. E. Pelvic pain and the IUD. *J. Reprod. Med.* 20:167, 1978.

Williams (idem. Burst), H. V. Family planning. In Ziegel, E., and VanBlarcom, C. C. (Eds.). *Obstetric Nursing, 6th.* New York: Macmillan, 1972.

32

Hormonal Contraceptive Management

DESCRIPTION, EFFECTIVENESS, AND PATIENT RESPONSE

There are a number of hormonal contraceptive methods. These include the following:

1. The "pill" — a combination of estrogen and progestin taken daily; there are currently three varieties of the pill:
    a. combination — the same amount and type of estrogen and progestin are taken for 20 or 21 days, followed by 7 days of no hormonal intake.
    b. biphasic combination pills — the estrogen dosage and type remain constant, while the progestin level changes midway through the 21-day cycle of pills followed by 7 days of no hormonal intake.
    c. triphasic combination pills — there are three different levels of the progestin during a 21-day cycle of pills followed by 7 days of no hormonal intake. The estrogen level may remain constant or may also change in concert with the progestin.

    Another variety of the pill, called *sequentials*, fell into disfavor and disuse in the mid-1970s. This action was due to the high estrogen content in the sequentials, as they started with 14 to 15 days of estrogen only and ended with 5 to 7 days of a combination of estrogen and progestin.

2. Minipills — progestin only, taken daily
3. The "shot" — injection of a long-acting progestin (e.g., Depo-Provero every 3 months); not available in the United States at the time of this writing (1985)
4. Postcoital combination pills — two Ovral pills, taken within 24 to 72 hours after coitus and repeated 12 hours after the first dose
5. Postcoital progestins — taken after each coitus
6. Postcoital estrogens

7. Male oral contraceptive — still in early stages of research and development

In addition, the following are means of contraception utilizing delivery of hormones via a type of "container" or other contraceptive method:

1. IUDs impregnated with a progestin, such as the Progesterone-T (Progestasert) (see Chapter 31).
2. Vaginal rings impregnated with progestagens placed monthly in the vaginal vault postmenses for 21 days. Being investigated.
3. Silastic capsules filled with progestins — a single capsule placed beneath the skin may last for up to 5 years. Being investigated.

The discussion in this chapter is limited to managing the care of women wanting or taking the combination pill or the progestin-only minipill. It should be recognized, however, that what is said about the contraindications, side effects, and mechanism of action of the pill generally is applicable to the other forms of hormonal contraception.

The combination pill type of hormonal contraception was the first type to be developed. Its name is derived from the fact that each pill consists of a combination of an estrogen and a progestin. The main variations among the different formulations of the combination pill are the dosages, relative proportion of the estrogenic and progestational components, and which estrogenic substance (ethinyl estradiol or mestranol) is used with which of the available progestins. The result is a variety of pills with somewhat different side effects, which allows for a certain amount of changing from pill to pill when necessary in order to best accommodate the individual woman's adjustment to the hormonal therapy.

The mechanism of action of the pill is a combination of the contraceptive action of estrogens and the contraceptive action of progestins. It has been known for some time that any of the sex hormones (progesterone, estrogen, and androgen) can suppress the production of the pituitary gonadotropins (specifically, for contraception, follicle-stimulating hormone [FSH] and luteinizing hormone [LH]). This suppression results from producing a negative feedback action on the hypothalamus, which inhibits secretion of the hypothalamic-releasing factor which in turn suppresses FSH and LH. The administration of synthetic steroid preparations, thus, effectively inhibits the development of a graafian follicle and subsequent ovulation. Without this event there is no ovum to be fertilized.

However, the antifertility effect of steroids is not wholly dependent on the inhibition of ovulation. High doses of estrogen postcoitally inhibit implantation of a fertilized egg due to the effect of estrogen on altering the usual progestational development of the endometrium. Progestins also have the following contraceptive effects:

1. Creation of a hostile cervical mucus that is thick and largely impenetrable by spermatozoa, thus resulting in decreased sperm penetration, transport, and survival.
2. Prohibition of the process of capacitation in the spermatozoa, resulting from changes in the cervical fluid which would normally activate this process, thereby rendering the sperm unable to penetrate the ovum.
3. Production of an atrophic endometrium which will not support implantation.

Other possible mechanisms of action still under investigation include the effect of estrogens and progestins on ovum transport.

The contraceptive steroids in the pill are not naturally occurring hormones but, rather, are pharmacologic drugs which produce a pharmacologic state rather than a physiologic state. In reality, the menstruation of a woman on the pill is a pseudomenstruation which is produced by the administration and then withdrawal of the hormonal pharmacologic drugs. A more precise term is *withdrawal bleeding*. The combined estrogen-progestin pill produces stromal edema, predeciduation, and some degree of glandular involution which, in a few cycles, yields a thin, hypoplastic-appearing endometrium. This accounts for the characteristic shorter duration and scantier flow often noticed by women taking the combination contraceptive pills.

There are two synthetic estrogens presently utilized in the combination contraceptive pills. Each brand name pill contains one or the other. These are ethinyl estradiol and mestranol. Both are pharmacologic drugs different from naturally-occurring estradiol, but they act in the same way. Mestranol is actually a derivative of ethinyl estradiol. The difference between them is that in animal assays ethinyl estradiol has been shown to be 50 percent more potent than mestranol. There is controversy over whether this difference in potency is also true in humans. However, all the pills with less than 50 micrograms of estrogen utilize ethinyl estradiol, whereas both ethinyl estradiol and mestranol are used in pills with 50 micrograms of estrogen and only mestranol is used in pills with more than 50 micrograms of estrogen.

There are six progestins presently utilized in the combination pills. Each brand name of pills contains one. The six progestins actually derive from one of two families of steroids. Nonetheless, each progestin varies in its estrogenic, progestational, and androgenic potency. Each brand name pill thus varies in its estrogenic, androgenic, and progestational potency as determined by which estrogen is combined with which progestin. Table 32-1 lists the six progestins and two estrogens and their comparative biological potency. Table 32-2 lists the progestin and estrogen utilized in the more common combination pills. The importance of this information lies in determining which pill to initiate with an individual woman based on her physical hormonal profile and in alleviating side effects by switching pills.

The theoretical effectiveness of the pills is virtually 100 percent with there being less than 0.5 (0.1 to 0.34) pregnancies per 100 woman years of exposure. However, *method failure can occur*, so women should not be guaranteed "no chance of pregnancy" with the pill. Use effectiveness of the pill is quite different, as these figures are affected by a woman skipping pills for whatever reason — side effects, complications, illness, forgetfulness, anxiety about possible side effects or complications, or a transient desire to become pregnant.

TABLE 32-1. Comparative Biological Potency of the Progestins and Estrogens in the More Common Oral Contraceptive Pills*

Steroid	Estrogenic Activity	Progestational Activity	Androgenic Activity
Estrogens:			
Ethinyl estradiol	100.0	0.0	0.0
Mestranol	67.0	0.0	0.0
Progestins:			
Ethynodiol diacetate	3.44	1.40	0.63
Levonorgestrel	0.0	5.26	9.4
Norethindrone	1.0	1.0	1.0
Norethindrone diacetate	1.52	1.16	1.60
Norethynodrel	8.32	2.63	0.0
Norgestrel	0.0	2.63	4.7

* Adapted from Dickey, R. P. *Managing Contraceptive Pill Patients, 4th.* Durant, Okla.: Creative Informatics, 1984, Table 14-1, pp. 40–41.

TABLE 32-2. Progestin and Estrogen Content of the More Common Oral Contraceptive Pills*

Pill Name	Progestin	mg.		Estrogen	mcg.	
Brevicon	Norethindrone	0.5		Ethinyl estradiol	35	
Demulen 1/35	Ethynodiol diacetate	1.0		Ethinyl estradiol	35	
Demulen 1/50	Ethynodiol diacetate	1.0		Ethinyl estradiol	50	
Enovid E	Norethynodrel	2.5		Mestranol	100	
Loestrin 1.5/30	Norethindrone acetate	1.5		Ethinyl estradiol	30	
Loestrin 1/20	Norethindrone acetate	1.0		Ethinyl estradiol	20	
Lo Ovral	Norgestrel	0.3		Ethinyl estradiol	30	
Micronor	Norethindrone	0.35		None	—	
Modicon	Norethindrone	0.5		Ethinyl estradiol	35	
Nordette	Levonorgestrel	0.15		Ethinyl estradiol	30	
Norinyl 1/35	Norethindrone	1.0		Ethinyl estradiol	35	
Norinyl 1/50	Norethindrone	1.0		Mestranol	50	
Norinyl 1/80	Norethindrone	1.0		Mestranol	80	
Norinyl 2	Norethindrone	2.0		Mestranol	100	
Norlestrin 1/50	Norethindrone acetate	1.0		Ethinyl estradiol	50	
Norlestrin 2.5	Norethindrone acetate	2.5		Ethinyl estradiol	50	
Nor Q.D.	Norethindrone	0.35		None	—	
Ortho-Novum 7−7−7[†]	Norethindrone	0.5	(7)	Ethinyl estradiol	35	(7)
	Norethindrone	0.75	(7)	Ethinyl estradiol	35	(7)
	Norethindrone	1.0	(7)	Ethinyl estradiol	35	(7)
Ortho-Novum 1/35	Norethindrone	1.0		Ethinyl estradiol	35	
Ortho-Novum 1/50	Norethindrone	1.0		Mestranol	50	
Ortho-Novum 1/80	Norethindrone	1.0		Mestranol	80	
Ortho-Novum 2	Norethindrone	2.0		Mestranol	100	
Ortho-Novum 10/11[†]	Norethindrone	0.5	(10)	Ethinyl estradiol	35	(10)
	Norethindrone	1.0	(11)	Ethinyl estradiol	35	(11)
Ovcon 35	Norethindrone	0.4		Ethinyl estradiol	35	
Ovcon 50	Norethindrone	1.0		Ethinyl estradiol	50	
Ovral	Norgestrel	0.5		Ethinyl estradiol	50	
Ovrette	Norgestrel	0.075		None	—	
Ovulen	Ethynodiol diacetate	1.0		Mestranol	100	
Tri-Norinyl[†]	Norethindrone	0.5	(7)	Ethinyl estradiol	35	(7)
	Norethindrone	1.0	(9)	Ethinyl estradiol	35	(7)
	Norethindrone	0.5	(5)	Ethinyl estradiol	35	(7)
Triphasil[†]	Levonorgestrel	0.05	(6)	Ethinyl estradiol	30	(6)
	Levonorgestrel	0.075	(5)	Ethinyl estradiol	40	(5)
	Levonorgestrel	0.125	(10)	Ethinyl estradiol	30	(10)

* Adapted from Dickey, R. P. *Managing Contraceptive Pill Patients, 4th.* Durant, Okla.: Creative Informatics, 1984, Table 13-1, pp. 52−53.

[†] Multiphasic product; the numbers in parentheses are the numbers of days in each phase.

Although the pill is the most popular and effective reversible method of contraception and is used by more than 55 million women all over the world, there is a terribly high attrition or discontinuation rate. Thirty to fifty percent of women who start the pill will not use it for even 1 year. Their reasons for stopping the pill are largely nonmedical. Unfortunately, many women who discontinue taking the pills do so without initiating another contraceptive method even when they do not want to become pregnant. The use effectiveness of the pills is thus around 2 to 3 pregnancies per 100 women years of exposure. (See Table 27-1). Access to pill supply renewal is a major consideration. For this reason many clinicians now (1) initially give women four packages of pills and have them return after 3 months' use rather than giving only two packages of pills and requesting them to return in 6 weeks, (2) give a year's supply (13 packages) at a time if the woman is having no untoward effects rather than having women come back every 6 months, and (3) routinely instruct women about a second method of contraception to use if they stop taking the pill.

There has been diverse patient response to the pill. At one end of the spectrum is fear due to the adverse publicity the pill has periodically received. At the other end of the spectrum, patient response has been very favorable because of the ease of use, its disassociation with the act of sexual intercourse, and its high effectiveness rate.

CONTRAINDICATIONS, SIDE EFFECTS, AND COMPLICATIONS

Contraindications

The following are absolute contraindications to initiating oral contraception for a woman by a nurse-midwife:

1. Pregnancy — known or suspected
2. Thrombophlebitis — existence or history of
3. Thromboembolic disorders — existence or history of
4. Cerebrovascular accident — existence or history of
5. Cerebrovascular disease — existence or history of
6. Coronary occlusion or heart attack — existence or history of
7. Insulin dependent diabetes mellitus
8. Liver damage, impaired liver function, or history of hepatitis within the past 2 years
9. Benign or malignant liver tumor — existence or history of
10. Estrogen dependent neoplasia — known or suspected
11. Carcinoma of the breast — known or suspected
12. Carcinoma of the reproductive system — known or suspected
13. Undiagnosed abnormal genital bleeding

The following are relative contraindications to initiating oral contraception for a woman by a nurse-midwife. The nurse-midwife should consult with the physician in the presence of any of these relative contraindications and a collaborative decision made regarding the initiation of oral contraception for an individual woman on the basis of her total history and physical findings. Preferably, if at all possible, women with any of the following conditions should be given other methods of contraception rather than the pills.

1. Hypertension — blood pressure greater than 140/90
2. History of recurrent toxemia of pregnancy
3. Migraine or other vascular headaches
4. Diabetes
   a. existence of any class of diabetes or prediabetes
   b. history of chemical or gestational diabetes during pregnancy
   c. strong family history of diabetes

d. abnormal glucose tolerance test — present or history of
5. Asthma
6. Epilepsy
7. Cardiac disease — existence or history of
8. Renal disease — existence or history of
9. Gallbladder disease — existence or history of
10. Thyroid disease — existence or history of
11. Uterine fibromyomata
12. Varicose veins
13. Psychic depression — existence or history of — especially if worse premenstrually or postpartum
14. Sickle cell disease
15. Lactation (oral contraception may be initiated with the start of weaning)
16. Acute phase of mononucleosis
17. Lupus erythematosus
18. Arthritis
19. Ulcerative colitis
20. Severe eye problems
21. Profile indicative of subsequent anovulation and infertility problems upon discontinuation of oral contraception (late menarche and very irregular, painless menses)
22. Chloasma
23. Extreme obesity
24. Surgery planned within 4 weeks
25. 45 years of age or older
26. 35 years of age and smokes cigarettes
27. Use of medications or other drugs known to interact with oral contraceptives

The nurse-midwife should evaluate each woman who has any degree of mental retardation, substance abuse, or psychiatric disorder for reliability in pill taking and make a decision whether or not oral contraception is contraindicated on this basis.

Side Effects and Complications

The following side effects, some to the extent of being called complications or life-threatening risks, have been identified as the result of hormonal contraception. The greatest danger associated with use of the oral contraceptive pills is cardiovascular disease. Women at greatest risk for developing cardiovascular complications are 45 years of age or more and women 35 years of age or older who smoke. The risk is even greater if there is a personal or strong family history of cardiovascular disease.

The side effects of pill usage are legion. Approximately 40 percent of women who use the pills have side effects. Experts have categorized these by severity and threat to the woman and by etiology according to the hormonal makeup of the pill. It is helpful to remember that each woman has her own individual hormonal makeup and balance. Therefore the same name brand pill may cause a hormonal excess in one woman and a hormonal deficiency in another woman. Thus both women may have side effects but may differ as to what they are since the underlying hormonal problem is different. Table 32-3 shows the hormonal etiology of a number of the side effects. Following is a simple listing of the known and suspected side effects associated with the pill:

1. Nausea/vomiting
2. Anorexia/loss of appetite
3. Dizziness/syncope
4. Feeling weak
5. Bloating/fluid retention/edema
6. Abdominal or uterine cramps and pains
7. Uterine enlargement
8. Headaches (vascular [migraine] and nonvascular types; cyclic or noncyclic)
9. Leukorrhea/increased cervical secretions
10. Weight change (gain — cyclic or noncyclic — or loss)
11. Increased appetite
12. Tiredness
13. Fatigue
14. Irritability
15. Chloasma
16. Breast tenderness (with or without fluid retention)

17. Breast enlargement (ductal and fatty tissue or alveolar tissue)
18. Leg cramps
19. Cystic breast changes
20. Breast secretion
21. Increased female fat deposition
22. Pelvic congestion syndrome
23. Increase in leiomyoma size
24. Cervical ectropion or erosion
25. Cervicitis
26. Visual changes
27. Epigastric distress
28. Decreased tolerance to contact lenses because of not fitting (due to steepening of the corneal curvature because of fluid retention)
29. Telangiectasia
30. Capillary fragility
31. Menstrual changes (hypermenorrhea, menorrhagia, dysmenorrhea, delayed onset of menses; hypomenorrhea, decreased length of flow; occasional amenorrhea, i.e., no withdrawal bleeding)
32. Nervousness
33. Spotting or bleeding between menses — breakthrough bleeding (early or late cycle)
34. Depression
35. Change in libido (decrease or increase)
36. *Candida* vaginitis (monilia)
37. Skin rash
38. Oily skin and scalp
39. Acne
40. Hirsutism
41. Urinary tract infections
42. Atrophic vaginitis — dyspareunia
43. Pelvic relaxations (uterine prolapse, cystocele, rectocele)
44. Alopecia/loss of hair
45. Allergic rhinitis or chronic nasopharyngitis
46. Hot flushes (vasomotor)
47. Itching/pruritis
48. Neurodermatitis
49. Numbness or tingling of an extremity
50. Venous dilatation and varicose veins
51. Thromboembolic disease (thrombophlebitis, deep vein thrombosis of the leg, cerebral thrombosis, pulmonary embolism)
52. Myocardial infarction/heart attack
53. Cholestatic jaundice (gallbladder disease)
54. Liver tumors/liver disease
55. Hypertension
56. Congenital anomalies if pill taken during early pregnancy
57. Neuro-ocular lesions
58. Breast atrophy
59. Lactation suppression
60. Increase in size of uterine fibromyomata

In addition, altered laboratory results resulting from pill use may include the following:

1. Glucose tolerance test — abnormal results with decreased tolerance for oral glucose. Altered changes are reversible upon discontinuation of the pill.
2. Coagulation tests — increase in prothrombin and in Factors VII, VIII, IX, and X; decrease in antithrombin III.
3. Hepatic function tests — altered results.
4. Thyroid function tests — increase in protein-bound iodine test and in butanol extractable protein-bound iodine. T_3 uptake values are decreased.
5. Serum lipid values — triglycerides and phospholipids are increased.
6. Serum folate values — decreased.

A time framework has been developed by Hatcher and associates for when some of the pill side effects and complications may be expected to occur (Table 32-4).

BENEFITS OF ORAL CONTRACEPTIVES

After a decade of media "pill scares" about pill side effects and complications, the professional literature is now also documenting the benefits which may accrue to women who take the pill. These benefits include the following:

(Text continues on page 606.)

TABLE 32-3. Hormonal Etiology of Contraceptive Pill Side Effects*

Estrogen Excess	Progestin Excess	Androgen/Anabolic Effects	Estrogen Deficiency	Progestin Deficiency
Nausea/vomiting	Tiredness	Increased libido	Irritability	Late cycle spotting and breakthrough bleeding
Abdominal/uterine cramps and pain	Fatigue	Oily skin and scalp	Nervousness	Dysmenorrhea
Epigastric distress	Increased appetite	Acne	Depression	Delayed onset of menses
Vascular-type (migraine) headache	Noncyclic weight gain	Hirsutism	Headache	Hypermenorrhea and menorrhagia
Cyclic headache	Decrease in libido	Skin rash	Decreased libido	Weight loss
Chloasma	Oily scalp	Pruritus	Pelvic relaxations	
Increased female fat deposition	Acne	Increased appetite	Early cycle spotting and breakthrough bleeding	
Bloating/fluid retention/edema	Alopecia/loss of hair	Cholestatic jaundice/ gallbladder disease	Atrophic vaginitis; dyspareunia	
Dysmenorrhea	Feeling weak, faint	Noncyclic weight gain	Hypomenorrhea	
Hypermenorrhea and menorrhagia	Hypoglycemia symptoms		Decreased length of menstrual flow	
Allergic rhinitis	Decreased carbohydrate tolerance		Breast atrophy	
Chronic nasopharyngitis	Breast tenderness without fluid retention		Hot flushes	
Dizziness/syncope	Increase in breast tissue (alveolar tissue)		Occasional amenorrhea	
Leg cramps	Pelvic congestion syndrome			
Uterine enlargement	Depression			
Thrombophlebitis	Neurodermatitis			
Thromboembolic disease	Monilia vaginitis			
Cerebrovascular accident	Venous dilatation, varicose veins			
Hypertension	Hypertension			
Cyclic weight gain	Cholestatic jaundice/ gall bladder disease			
Breast tenderness with fluid retention	Decreased length of menstrual flow			
	Headaches between pill packages			
	Cervicitis			

Lactation suppression
Cystic breast changes
Increase in breast tissue (ductal and fatty tissues)
Irritability
Depression
Telangiectasia
Capillary fragility
Anorexia/appetite loss
Visual changes
Decreased tolerance of contact lenses (poor fit)
Increase in size of uterine fibromyomata
Leukorrhea/increased cervical secretions
Mucorrhea
Myocardial infarction
Urinary tract infections
Cervical ectropion/erosion
Numbness or tingling of an extremity
Increase in leiomyoma size
Hepatic adenoma

* Adapted from Hatcher, R. A. et al. *Contraceptive Technology, 1984–1985, 12th.* New York: Irvington, 1984, Table 4.3, p. 61.

TABLE 32-4. Pill Side Effects and Complications (A Time Framework)*

Worse in First 3 Months	Steady (Constant) over Time	Worse over Time	Worse after Discontinuation
Nausea + dizziness (estrogen excess)	Headaches during 3 weeks pills are being taken (estrogen excess)	Headaches during week pills are not taken (progestin excess)	Infertility, amenorrhea; hypothalamic and endometrial suppression; miscalculation of expected date of delivery[††]
Thrombophlebitis (venous): Leg veins (estrogen excess) Pulmonary emboli[†] Pelvic vein thrombosis[†] Retinal vein thrombosis[†]	Arterial thromboembolic events (estrogen excess), blurred vision, stroke[†]	Weight gain (anabolic progestational-androgenic effect)	One form of acne (progesterone excess)
Cyclic weight gain edema (fluid retention) (estrogen excess)	Anxiety, fatigue, depression (may be due to estrogen excess producing fluid retention, estrogen deficiency, or progestin excess)	Monilial vaginitis (progestin excess or estrogen deficiency)	Hair loss/alopecia (progestin excess)
Breast fullness, tenderness (estrogen excess effect on ductal and fatty tissue; progestin excess effect on alveolar tissue)	Thyroid function studies: Elevated PBI Depressed T_3 resin uptake	Periodic missed menses while on oral contraceptives (estrogen deficiency possibly secondary to progestin dominance)	Depression (in some women)
Breakthrough bleeding (early due to estrogen deficiency; late due to progesterone deficiency)	Susceptibility to amenorrhea after pill discontinuation (combined effect of progestins + estrogens on hypothalamus, pituitary, and also on endometrium)	Chloasma (estrogen excess)[†]	
		Myocardial infarction[†]	
Elevated serum lipid levels even to the extent of pancreatitis[†]	Change in cervical secretions — mucorrhea (estrogen excess)	Spider angiomata (estrogen excess)	
		Growth of myoma (estrogen excess)	

Abnormal glucose tolerance test (estrogen and progestational effect)

Contact lenses fail to fit (estrogen effect via fluid retention)

Abdominal cramping (estrogen effect via fluid retention)

Suppression of lactation (estrogen excess)

Failure to understand correct use of oral contraceptives; pregnancy

Decrease in libido (estrogen deficiency or progesterone excess)

Autophonia, chronic dilatation of eustachian tubes rather than cyclic opening and closing

Acne (androgen excess)

Predisposition to gallbladder disease (estrogen or progestin excess)[†]

Hirsutism (progestin excess)

Decreased menstrual flow (estrogen deficiency)

Small uterus, pelvic relaxation, cystocele, rectocele, atrophic vaginitis (estrogen deficiency)

Cystic breast changes (estrogen excess)

Photodermatitis — sunlight sensitivity with hyperpigmentation (estrogen excess)

One form of hair loss/alopecia (progestin excess)

Hypertension (?) (progestin or estrogen excess)

Focal hyperplasia of the liver and hepatocellular adenomas

* Adapted from Hatcher, R. A. et al. *Contraceptive Technology, 1984–1985, 12th.* New York: Irvington, 1984, Table 4.2, p. 60.
† May be irreversible.
†† To avoid this complication in many patients, advise women desiring to become pregnant to discontinue pills 3 to 6 months before desired pregnancy and use a barrier method of contraception during this period of time.

1. The most effective reversible method of contraception
*2. Protection against pelvic inflammatory disease
*3. Protection against ectopic pregnancy
*4. Protection against endometrial and ovarian cancer
*5. Protection against benign breast disease
6. Relief from menstrual disorders and discomforts

MANAGEMENT PLAN FOR THE HORMONAL CONTRACEPTIVES

Management of the care of the woman taking the pill hormonal contraception consists of the following components:

1. Informing the woman of the effectiveness rates and potential side effects and complications of taking the pill, and having her sign an informed patient consent form
2. Conducting a general history, physical and pelvic examinations, and laboratory tests
3. Screening for any deviations from normal and for any contraindications to initiating the pill for the woman
4. Selecting the pill most appropriate for the individual woman
5. Initiating the pill
6. Giving the patient instructions (see end of this chapter)
7. Scheduling and managing the return visits
8. Managing the possible side effects and complications related to the pill

The first three components have been discussed previously.

---

* *Protection* means that women using the pill have less risk than do either women who use no contraceptive method or women who use a nonhormonal method of contraception.

Selection of the Pill Most Appropriate for the Individual Woman

Selection of the pill most appropriate for the individual woman is based on identification of the woman's hormonal profile, knowledge of the hormonal potency of the pills from which you are selecting, and the best possible matching of these two pieces of information. Table 32-5 summarizes the physical characteristics that reveal each of four possible hormonal profiles and the type of pill thus indicated.

Both the estrogens and progestins have been implicated in physiologic changes which increase the risk of cardiovascular disease. Therefore, the selection of a pill, as a general principle, is best limited to those with only 1 milligram or less of the progestin and 30, 35, or 50 micrograms of the estrogen. Table 32-5 limits itself to this selection. Remember that 30 or 35 micrograms of ethinyl estradiol is thought to be approximately equivalent to 50 micrograms of mestranol. Such a low dose of estrogen increases the incidence of spotting, breakthrough bleeding, and missed menses. Such bleeding irregularities may lead to discontinuation of the pill. However, the triphasic combination pills, which increase the progestin during the middle or latter part of the cycle (or both) and either leave the estrogen constant throughout the cycle or increase it in the middle of the cycle, may counteract these problems.

For some women the most appropriate selection of a pill may be the minipill (progestin only). This is the pill of choice for the immediate postpartum woman, the breast-feeding mother, and the woman between 35 and 45 years of age. The minipill should also be strongly considered for a woman who has a history of hypertensive disorder during pregnancy or a strong family history of hypertension, or who currently has borderline hypertension. The reason for selecting the progestin-only minipill for these women is that it not only does not have any estrogen but also has less progestin than any currently available combination pill.

In 1985, there were three minipills on the market (see Table 32-2).

Initiating the Pill

When to start the woman on the pill depends on where the woman is in relation to any of the following: her menstrual cycle, postabortion, postdelivery, and lactation.

In order to prevent breakthrough bleeding and to be as contraceptively effective as possible, a woman should not start the pills any later than the tenth day in the cycle and preferably on or before the fifth day from the beginning of menstruation and the cycle. So if a woman has her initial visit in midcycle she needs to wait until her next menstrual period to start the pills (either on the fifth day or on the Sunday after she starts to menstruate, depending on the packaging of the pill). For the interim, you give her a spermicidal preparation and condoms to use as a primary method until she is able to start on the pills and then as a secondary method for the first cycle of pill taking. It is possible to start a woman on the pills at any point in the cycle but it practically guarantees breakthrough bleeding and questionable effectiveness until the pills are in "control." Most women will not tolerate this amount of trouble. It is better to synchronize the initiation of the pills with the woman's natural cycle.

Pills may be started immediately after abortion and it is strongly advised to do so. Postabortion women and postdelivery women are *not* physiologically analogous as to hormone levels, reinstitution of ovulation, decidual restoration, and risk of thromboembolic disease.

Pills may be started after delivery between the third and sixth week postpartum without resumption of menses having occurred. Before the third week the risk of thromboembolic disease is increased with the combination pills. The progestin-only minipill is the pill of choice for women who want to start the pill earlier than 4 weeks postpartum. After the sixth week, the risk of pregnancy is increased. Ovulation postdelivery is thought to occur rarely prior to the fourth postpartal week. However, after the sixth postpartal week it is quite possible for ovulation to have occurred and for the woman to be pregnant if she has had unprotected sexual intercourse. Judgment needs to be based on the taking of a careful sexual and contraceptive history since delivery.

As stated before, lactation is a contraindication to starting a woman on the combination pills. However, pills may be initiated when she begins to wean the baby. The reason for this is that breast-feeding may be more difficult to establish since the pills tend to inhibit lactation. Frequent breast stimulation, however, counteracts this inhibition and it is not a problem, especially if the pill is not begun until 4 to 6 weeks postpartum and breast-feeding is well established. The progestin-only minipill does not have the same inhibitory effect on lactation and can be initiated while a mother is breast-feeding if she so desires. The progestin-only pills also minimize the other concern, which stems from the fact that the hormones in the pill have been found in the breast milk of nursing mothers who are on the pill. What effect this may have on the infant has not been determined but many professionals prefer to "play it safe" and advise other methods of contraception until the infant is being weaned.

Regardless of when a woman starts taking the pill, she should be given a spermicidal preparation and condoms "to cover" during the first month of taking the pills. This is an additional protection in case of forgetfulness by the woman in taking the pills until regular pill taking is established; and because not all of the pills may be effective during the first month, depending on their hormonal makeup and when in the menstrual cycle they are started. The most effective approach to these problems is simply to routinely provide the secondary method for coverage. This also enables you to teach her a second contraceptive

(*text continues on page 606*)

TABLE 32-5.   Physical Characteristics of Hormonal Profiles and Type of Pill Indicated*

Trait	High Estrogen	Low Estrogen	Low Androgen	High Androgen
Menses	Regular about every month (cycle 26–32 days); moderate to heavy flow with clots, lasting 6–10 days; moderate to severe dysmenorrhea	Regular about every month (cycle 26–32 days); light to moderate flow without clots, lasting 4–5 days with mild or no dysmenorrhea	Regular about every month (cycle 26–32 days); light to moderate flow without clots, lasting 3–4 days with no dysmenorrhea	Irregular; scant to light flow without clots, lasting 2–3 days; no dysmenorrhea
Premenstrual symptoms	Includes tension, bloating, edema of extremities, nausea, and moderate to severe headaches	Average with little to no premenstrual tension	None	None
Breasts	Full, ample (well-endowed); tender and enlarged before and during menses during menses	Full; mild to no tenderness and enlargement before and during menses	Full to small; no tenderness or enlargement before and during menses	Small to flat-chested; no tenderness or enlargement before and during menses
Figure	Normal female contour	Normal female contour	Slender and angular	Tall, wide shoulders, slim hips, fleshy back
Hair	Normal female hair pattern with no excess anywhere on body	Normal female hair pattern with no excess on face, arms, legs, or body	Mild hirsutism with excess hair on arms, legs, and body	Moderate to severe hirsutism over body, male hair pattern, bitemporal hair loss, may shave face, arms, chest, or legs

Skin	Dry, clear, may be moist	Clear, moist	Oily, mild acne	Oily, moderate to severe acne
Reproductive organs	Large uterus, small clitoris, much leukorrhea	Normal female size, average leukorrhea	Average to small size, minimal leukorrhea	Small uterus, enlarged clitoris, scant leukorrhea, dry
Pregnancy history	Excessive nausea and morning sickness	Some morning sickness	Slight morning sickness	No morning sickness
Type of Pill Indicated and Examples				
	High progestational, high androgenic, and higher intermediate, estrogen potency	Low progestational, low androgenic, and low estrogen potency	Intermediate progestational, intermediate androgenic, and low estrogen potency	Higher intermediate progestational, low androgenic, and intermediate or higher intermediate estrogen potency
For example:	Norlestrin 2.5 Ovral	Brevicon Modicon Ortho-Novum 7–7–7 Ortho-Novum 10/11 Ovcon-35 Tri-Norinyl Triphasil	Norinyl 1/35 Ortho-Novum 1/35 Norinyl 1/50 Ortho-Novum 1/50	Demulen 1/35 Demulen 1/50

* Adapted by permission from Okrent, S. *A Clinical Guide to Oral Contraception*. New York: Shirley Okrent, 1973.

method to use in the event she decides to discontinue the pills.

The Return Visits

The woman is scheduled for her first revisit after three complete pill cycles. This means that you need to give, or prescribe, four packages of pills for her initially. She should be seen sometime in the middle of her fourth package of pills. You can calculate this time on the basis of the date when you are starting her on the pills. The first revisit should consist of the following:

1. Blood pressure
2. Weight
3. History
   a. woman/couple satisfaction with the method
   b. use of spermicidal preparation and condoms
   c. description of how (especially important with 21-day pills) and when she is taking her pills
   d. taking any medications — if yes, what, and what for
   e. been to a doctor or emergency room since starting pills — if yes, why
   f. menses (compare with prepill menses)
      (1) date
      (2) length
      (3) amount of flow
      (4) pain
   g. side effects (see listing earlier in this chapter)
   h. any questions or concerns

If all is well, the woman is given enough pill packages so that she will be in the middle of her last pill package at the time of her next appointment.

The time of the next appointment varies. Some professionals believe that the woman should be seen every 6 months, while others believe that once a year is sufficient. Still others believe in an initial 3-½ month visit followed by a 6-month visit, and then annually thereafter if the woman is exhibiting no problems. Some clinicians who believe in the semiannual visits also believe in Pap smears every 6 months for pill-taking women. Otherwise, the 6-month, or semiannual, revisit consists of the following:

1. Blood pressure
2. Weight
3. History
   a. woman/couple satisfaction with the method
   b. description of how and when she is taking her pills
   c. taking any medications — if yes, what, and what for
   d. been to a doctor or emergency room since last visit — if yes, why
   e. menses (compare with prepill and last record of menses)
      (1) date
      (2) length
      (3) amount of flow
   f. side effects (see listing earlier in this chapter)
   g. any questions or concerns

If all is well, the woman is given enough pill packages so that she will be in the middle of her last pill package at the time of her annual appointment. Yearly visits with 13 packages of pills given to the woman at one time may increase pill continuation rates.

The annual revisit includes that which constitutes a semiannual revisit plus a complete general screening history, physical and pelvic examinations, and Pap smear, GC culture, and other routine laboratory tests as outlined in Chapter 3.

Management of Side Effects and Complications

When a side effect is present you first need to

determine when in the menstrual cycle it occurs, whether it is due to hormone excess or deficiency, and which hormone (the estrogen or the progestin) is involved. Table 32-3 earlier in this chapter listed the side effects resulting from estrogen and progestin excess or deficiency. When the side effect occurs in the cycle may help diagnose the problem. For example, early cycle breakthrough bleeding is due to estrogen deficiency, while late cycle breakthrough bleeding is due to progestin deficiency. The pill you would thus switch the woman to would be quite different in hormonal makeup with higher estrogenic activity for early cycle breakthrough bleeding and higher progestin potency for late cycle breakthrough bleeding.

If pill switching is determined as the course of management, then it becomes a matter of switching to a pill which has the desired direction of hormonal potency to resolve a problem of excess or deficiency. Table 32-1 lists the comparative estrogenic, progestational, and androgenic potency of the progestins and estrogens in the more common oral contraceptive pills. Table 32-2 then lists the dosage of the progestin and estrogen in the more common contraceptive pills.

Pill switching, however, may not be the best course of management. You first have to determine which of the following possible courses the side effect will probably take:

1. Spontaneous remission as the body adjusts to the hormonal effect of the pill (common with side effects occurring during the first three cycles of pill taking).
2. Continuation of the side effect (more likely when the side effect occurs after several cycles of pill taking, but may occur with early cycles of pill taking) necessitating pill switching or discontinuation of the pill and initiation of another contraceptive method.
3. Development into a dangerous complication — some side effects are harbingers of more severe complications. If the side effect is

determined to be such a harbinger, the pills should be stopped immediately and physician consultation obtained.

Because of the possibility of spontaneous remission for side effects occurring during the first one to three cycles of pill taking, women are often encouraged to wait it out through this period of time while the body is adjusting to the hormonal effects of the pill. When the woman is seen again during her fourth cycle of pill taking such spontaneous remission should have occurred by then.

If pill switching is the method of management the following should be remembered:

1. If the switch is to a pill with equal or greater estrogen and progestational potency, the switch can be made any time during the cycle.
2. If the switch is to a pill with less estrogen and progestational potency, the switch must be made only at the beginning of a new pill cycle. Such a switch necessitates longer time for the new pill to achieve hormonal menstrual control, which is why the switch is best made at the beginning of a pill cycle.
3. Depending on the severity of the side effect, it might be less confusing to switch the pill at the beginning of a pill cycle even if the switch is one that can be made in midcycle.
4. The woman should be counseled that her body will again be undergoing adjustment to a different hormonal balance and some temporary side effects may be experienced.

The pill should be discontinued and physician consultation or referral obtained in the presence of any of the following side effects:

1. Severe headaches
2. Visual disturbances, such as:
   a. blurring of vision

b. flashing lights
c. spots before the eyes
d. periods of temporary blindness
3. Unexplained severe chest pain or shortness of breath
4. Unexplained severe abdominal pain
5. Severe calf or thigh pain
6. Temporary numbness or paralysis of any part of the face or body
7. Marked fluid retention and cyclic premenstrual weight gain
8. Marked increase in blood pressure
9. Development of any disease which contraindicates the use of the pill

It is imperative that the woman be provided with another method of family planning when stopping the pills for reason of side effects or complications.

PATIENT INSTRUCTIONS

The following instructions should be given all women taking the pill regardless of whether it is the 21-day or the 28-day pill:

1. Keep your pills in a place safe from children and animals but also where you will be daily reminded to take them. It helps if you place them next to or on something which is part of your daily routine, such as next to your toothbrush or toothpaste, coffee-pot, alarm clock, or so forth.
2. Make your pill taking as much a routine as possible. Taking your pill at approximately the same time every day not only helps make it a routine but also assures a consistent contraceptive hormonal level in your body.
3. Be sure to keep your revisit appointment so you don't run out of pills and so you are examined carefully for any possible side effects.
4. Call for an appointment *immediately* if you are having any of the following symptoms (do not wait to see if they will simply "go away," because these are danger signs):
   a. severe headaches
   b. visual disturbances such as
      (1) blurring of vision
      (2) flashing lights
      (3) spots before your eyés
      (4) temporary moments of blindness
   c. severe chest pain or shortness of breath
   d. severe abdominal pain
   e. severe calf or thigh pain
   f. temporary numbness or paralysis of any part of your body
   g. marked swelling of your fingers, hands, ankles, or face
   h. abnormal hair loss
   i. severe depression
   j. two missed menstrual periods
5. Be sure to tell any doctor or nurse practitioner you see for any medical problems that develop that you are taking birth control pills.
6. Do not ever take another woman's pills or allow another woman to borrow your pills. Most likely they will not be the same strength and hormonal makeup and such pill taking may leave you without contraceptive protection or experiencing side effects you otherwise would not have.
7. Remember to use the spermicidal preparation and condoms during your first cycle of pill taking. You will not need to use this secondary method after this while taking the pills.
8. It is helpful if you keep a menstrual history noting the first and last day of each of your menstrual periods and how heavy the flow is for each day. Be sure to bring your menstrual history with you for your revisits.
9. If you decide to stop taking the pills because of unhappiness with the pills (such as side effects or fear of side effects), *be sure* to call for an appointment and use a spermicidal preparation and condoms for

protection from pregnancy until your appointment.

10. If you have plans for surgery, call for an immediate appointment. Plan on not taking the pills and using an alternative contraceptive method until after the surgery and postoperative period when you are again ambulating well and no extremities are immobilized. This is very important because there is an increased risk of blood clots during this time.

11. If you decide to stop taking the pills because you wish to get pregnant, then stop at the end of a pill cycle and use a spermicidal preparation and condoms or other method of birth control for three months after stopping the pills. When planning conception be sure to allow for these 3 months prior to attempting to get pregnant. There is some evidence of increased congenital malformations and spontaneous abortions in women who get pregnant immediately after stopping the pills. Allowing time for your body to readjust to its own natural hormonal balance and menstrual cycles should resolve this problem.

12. It is necessary to take the pills exactly as instructed if you do not want to become pregnant.

If you miss *one* pill you probably won't get pregnant but you do need to take the forgotten pill. Take the forgotten pill as soon as you remember it and the next pill at the regular time. This may be at the same time.

If you miss *two* pills you may or may not still be protected from pregnancy. To keep your cycle going and to make sure you won't get pregnant, take two pills the day you remember them and two pills the next day. This should catch you up in your pill cycle. *Also,* use a spermicidal preparation and condoms for each act of sex for the remainder of this pill cycle. Do not be surprised or alarmed if you have some midcycle spotting.

If you miss *three or more* pills the chances are good for getting pregnant. Use a spermicidal preparation and condoms for each act of sex until you have your menstrual period and then for the next pill cycle. Throw away the remainder of your old pill package and start a new pill package the Sunday or fifth day after you start your menstrual period. If you do not have a menstrual period, call for an appointment and a pregnancy test. Do *not* take any more pills in this situation.

13. *Specific instructions for taking the 21-day combination pill:* The instructions on the package inserts vary with the pill being taken. The following instructions are safe to use with any of these pills.

a. a pill must be taken every day during the number of days that pills are to be taken. A missed pill equals a chance to become pregnant.

b. no pills are to be taken for 1 week (6 days).

c. start your next package of pills on the same day 1 week (7 days) later from the day you took your last pill. For example, if you take your last pill in your package of pills on a Tuesday, then you should take the first pill of your next package of pills the next Tuesday.

d. you should continue taking pills in this pattern no matter what is happening with your menstrual periods, such as

(1) spotting or bleeding occurring while taking the pills

(2) the menstrual period being over before the week without pills is over

(3) your continuing menstruation when your new package is to be started

14. *Specific instructions for taking the 28-day combination pill:* The only difference in the instructions for the 28-day pill from the 21-day pill is that 28-day pills are

taken every day of the month. For a woman not to take pills for a week between packages of 28-day pills is to assure herself of a pregnancy.

   a. a pill must be taken every day. There is never a day in which a pill is not taken.
   b. when you take the last pill in your package of pills you take the first pill of your next package of pills the very next day. For example, if you take the last pill in your package of pills on a Wednesday you will take the first pill in your next package of pills on the next day, Thursday.
   c. you should continue taking your pills in this pattern no matter what is happening with your menstrual periods, such as
      (1) spotting or bleeding occurring while taking pills
      (2) your continuing menstruation when your new pill package is to be started

Instructions for taking the progestin-only minipill: Include numbers 1, 2, 3, 4, 5, 6, 8, 9, 10, and 11 of the instructions for taking the 21-day or 28-day pill. Additionally,

1. Take one pill at approximately the same time *every* day. Never stop taking a pill every day. When you finish one package of pills on one day start a new package of pills the next day.

2. It is necessary to take the pills exactly as instructed if you do not want to become pregnant.

   If you miss *one* pill, take it as soon as you remember it and take your next pill at the usual time. *Use a second method of contraception along with your pill taking until your next menstrual period.*

   If you miss *two* pills, take one of the missed pills along with your usual pill for the day. Take the other missed pill when you take your usual pill the next day. *Use a second method of contraception along with your pill taking until your next menstrual period.*

3. Call for an appointment immediately if you do not have a menstrual period within 45 days of your last menstrual period. It is not unusual to have irregular or infrequent periods while taking the minipill, but if you go longer than 45 days without a period you need to know whether or not you are pregnant.

4. The effectiveness of the minipill is somewhat less than for the combination pill. Although not essential to do, effectiveness can be improved if you:

   a. use a second contraceptive method such as foam and condoms along with your pill taking for the first 6 months of using the minipill
   b. after the first 6 months, use a second contraceptive method such as foam and condoms during the middle of each menstrual cycle for as long as you take the minipill

BIBLIOGRAPHY

Dickey, R. P. *Managing Contraceptive Pill Patients, 4th.* Durant, Okla.: Creative Informatics, 1984.

Dickey, R. P. The pill. In Tyrer, L. B., Isenman, A. W. and Knox, E. G. (Eds.). *Seminar in Family Planning, Rev.* Chicago: American College of Obstetricians and Gynecologists, 1974.

Hatcher, R. A. et al. *Contraceptive Technology, 1984–1985, 12th.* New York: Irvington, 1984.

Kols, M. A. et al. Oral contraceptives. *Pop. Rep.* Series A, No. 6 (May–June) 1982.

Layde, P. M., Beral, V., and Kay, C. R. Further analyses of mortality in oral contraceptive users. *Lancet* 1:541–546, March 7, 1981.

Nelson, J. H. Clinical evaluation of side effects of current oral contraceptives. *J. Reprod. Med.* 6:43, 1971.

Okrent, S. *A Clinical Guide to Oral Contraception.* New York: Shirley Okrent, 1973.

Oral contraception, *ACOG Technical Bulletin*, No. 41. Chicago: American College of Obstetricians and Gynecologists, 1976.

Patient instructions — Guide for nurses. The University of Mississippi Medical Center Nurse-Midwifery Education Program, 1970.

Rinehart, W., and Piotrow, P. T. OCs — Update on usage, safety, and side effects. *Popul. Rep.* Series A, No. 5. Baltimore: Johns Hopkins, 1979.

Special report: The pill after 25 years. *Contraceptive Technology Update* 6(1):1—24 (January) 1985.

Speroff, L., Glass, R. H., and Kase, N. G. *Clinical Gynecologic Endocrinology and Infertility, 3rd.* Baltimore: Williams & Wilkins, 1983.

Stadel, B. Oral contraceptives and cardiovascular disease, Part 2. *N. Engl. J. Med.* 305(12):672, 1981.

Veninga, K. S. Effects of oral contraceptives on vitamins B_6, B_{12}, C, and folacin. *J. Nurse-Midwifery* 29(6):386—390 (November/December) 1984.

Vessey, M. et al. Mortality in oral contraceptive users. *Lancet* 1:549, March 7, 1981.

Williams (idem. Burst), H. V. Family planning. In Ziegel, E., and VanBlarcom, C. C. *Obstetric Nursing, 6th.* New York: Macmillan, 1972.

VII

Skills

Part VII is a compilation of some of the necessary skills and procedures used in managing the normal childbearing woman and neonate. Some of these are used in obtaining a data base for evaluation; others for implementing the plan of care. Skills which have been incorporated into the management sections in other parts of the book are not repeated here (e.g., timing contractions, Nitrazine test for ruptured membranes, evaluation of dilatation). Conversely, the skills and procedures discussed here are referred to but not repeated in other parts of the book.

As long as a skill or procedure is performed safely, effectively, accurately, and with the minimum possible trauma the variations in the detail of *how* it is done do not matter. The step-by-step procedural and rationale format utilized in this book is based on experience that has shown the described method to be safe, effective, and accurate, with the least possible trauma. However, other approaches may be equally valid. When feasible, alternative methods are given for some skills and procedures, with the advantages and disadvantages of each method stated. Because of the multitudinous variations between hospitals

and supply companies in packaging materials for procedures, a listing of necessary supplies is not given. Basic essentials are self-evident.

The importance of being able to perform essential skills efficiently need not be belabored. Suffice it to say that decisions should never be based on whether or not you are capable of performing the necessary skill or procedure. Since experience and efficiency reduces trauma, the counsel to practice, practice, practice is most germane.

This portion of the book discusses only how to perform a skill or procedure once the decision is made to do it. When and why to use a skill or do a procedure and the factors involved in making these decisions are part of the management process and are discussed in other parts of the book.

In accord with the educational principle of learning theoretical content when it is applicable, relevant anatomy is presented when pertinent. For skills that involve a portion of the physical examination the anatomy may or may not be included. When this content is not presented, references are given for the learner to use for study purposes. Physical and pelvic examination skills also differ in presentation from the other skills and procedures presented in Part VII in that observations and findings elicited by the examination and their significance are included. This is in keeping with the same educational principle.

In addition to performing a skill or procedure in a manner that is safe and effective, will yield accurate results or findings if applicable, and causes the minimum possible trauma, the nurse-midwife should follow a number of general principles and approaches with all procedures; these are as follows:

1. Have the woman's consent and cooperation.
2. Inform the woman of what you will be and are doing throughout the procedure.
3. Use a touch that is gentle, smooth, and firm (*not* jerky, rough, inconsiderate, or with additional nervous movements).
4. Have and demonstrate respect for the woman's body and for her as a person.
5. Do the procedure as quickly as possible.
6. Forewarn the woman immediately prior to any step in a procedure which will be uncomfortable or painful.
7. Be honest—if a procedure is going to hurt, say so.
8. Give the woman reassurance and praise regarding how well she is coping with the procedure.
9. Time the procedure so it is not done at a time when another procedure is being done or when the woman is experiencing temporary pain or other distraction. For example, unless in an emergency, the insertion of an intravenous intracatheter in a woman in labor can wait until it can be performed between contractions.

33

Finger Puncture*

Procedure	Rationale
1. Check and organize materials and equipment, making sure all are present, appropriate, and placed conveniently.	1. Failure to do so may result in the need to restick the woman since hemostasis will occur while you gather missing equipment.
2. Ask the woman if she is left- or right-handed and if she has any preference as to which finger is used.	2. Use a finger on the hand least used because the puncture site will be sore for several hours upon direct pressure.
3. Ask the woman to hold her hand down while you get the materials ready. Do *not* milk the finger as preparation for the puncture.	3. Utilize gravity to aid blood flow to the area. Milking the finger has potential for diluting the specimen with interstitial fluid, thereby possibly yielding inaccurate results.
4. Clean the ball of the selected finger with an alcohol sponge. Air dry or wipe dry with a dry cotton ball or gauze square.	4. Wet alcohol will sting in an open wound such as will be created with the puncture.
5. Grasp the finger firmly in one hand, still holding it down, and tell the woman there will be a short, sharp stick pain and not to jerk her hand away. (See Figure 33-1.)	5. Elicit the woman's cooperation. Jerking her hand may spoil your puncture and necessitate redoing. Your firm grasp of the finger helps to control any tendency to jerk.

*Includes obtaining capillary blood and filling capillary tubes for hematocrit determination.

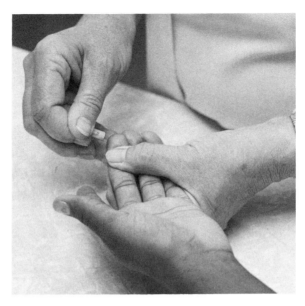

FIGURE 33-1.   Proper positioning for finger puncture.

Procedure	Rationale
6. Make a deep puncture slightly lateral to the center of the ball of the finger. Use a quick down-and-up (in-and-out) movement with deliberate pressure behind the movement to make the lancet go deeper. Some clinicians also twist the lancet a bit at the bottom of their thrust.	6. A puncture from which blood will flow freely is desired. This requires a puncture that cuts enough tissue to obtain this result. Otherwise, excessive pressure and milking of the finger in order to get blood will dilute the specimen with interstitial tissue fluid and render inaccurate test results. A deep puncture is, therefore, preferable to a shallow one that may require a second puncture. One deep puncture is no more painful than two shallow punctures. Don't worry about going too deep as the length of the lancet prohibits this. You should take advantage of the full length of the lancet.
7. Apply slight pressure just above the puncture site with the thumb of the hand holding the finger.	7. This causes the blood to flow freely. More force than a slight pressure will contaminate the specimen with tissue fluid.
8. Wipe off the first drop of blood with a dry gauze square or cotton ball.	8. The first drop of blood usually contains tissue fluid and may be otherwise contaminated. A dry gauze is preferable to a dry cotton ball because the fibers of the cotton ball may stick to the wound or on the finger.

Procedure	Rationale
9. Again apply slight pressure above the puncture site and, when a drop of blood has formed, hold one end of a capillary tube against the blood in as close to a horizontal position as possible.	9. Horizontal position facilitates the flow of blood into the capillary tube, which operates by capillary action. Holding the capillary tube below the blood drop will cause a still faster flow into the tube due to the additional factor of gravity. Holding the tube above the blood drop will inhibit the blood flow.
10. Blood flow into the tube may be controlled by your index finger which is held at the end of the capillary tube opposite the end touching the blood. Blood will not flow in any direction if your finger covers that end. Otherwise, blood will ascend or descend in the tube depending on whether or not the tube is touching blood and the angle of the tube.	10. If air gets into the capillary tube it must be expelled. This is done by covering the end of the tube with your index finger and holding the opposite end over a dry gauze square and releasing your finger. Allow the blood to drop on the gauze square or cotton ball without touching it with the tube. If blood at the end of the tube touches the gauze, more plasma than red cells will be attracted by the gauze and escape from the tube. The blood remaining in the tube will then be a false sample of the proportion of the component parts in the woman's blood. If this happens a new specimen must be collected and the old one discarded. When the air is expelled, cover the end of the tube again with your finger to preserve the remaining blood in the tube and refill the tube with blood from the puncture site.
11. Fill two capillary tubes two-thirds full with no more than one-sixth of the two-thirds being air.	11. A small amount of air will not affect a hematocrit reading so long as the air is not of sufficient quantity to prevent blood from occupying over half of the tube. Two-thirds filling of the tube leaves room for the sealing clay.
12. When each tube is filled, cover the end, move it to a horizontal position, uncover the end, and gently tilt the tube back and forth without letting the blood get too close to either end of the tube.	12. Tilting back and forth mixes the blood with the heparin in the tube. If not mixed immediately with the dried heparin in the tube, the blood will clot and readings will be inaccurately high. A good seal with the sealing clay may be prevented if blood gets in the end of the tube.
13. With sealing clay, close the end of the tube that did not touch the blood, using a	13. Some of the plasma will evaporate if left sitting. This can raise the hematocrit

Procedure	Rationale
pressing and rotary motion. Fill one end of the tube with approximately 5 mm of clay. If the hematocrit is not going to be run immediately, seal both ends of the tube.	reading considerably and erroneously. Evaporation can be prevented for a longer period of time by sealing both ends of the tube. Sealing both ends has no effect on running or obtaining an accurate reading of the hematocrit.
14. Note where the blood is in the tube at the time of sealing and be sure it is not too close to either end.	14. If the blood is too close to the end being sealed an ineffective seal may result and the pad of sealing clay will be smeared. If the blood is too close to the other end it may be pushed out while the first end is sealed and you may be left with too little blood for the test.
15. The tubes can be sealed either with the sealing clay held vertically to a horizontal tube or with the sealing clay on a flat surface and the blood tube held vertically and inserted into it. If done the latter way be sure to cover the upper end of the blood tube with the tip of your index finger. This will keep the blood suspended no matter at what angle you hold the tube, thereby preventing either movement or escape of the blood from the tube.	
16. When you are sure that you have two unbroken, appropriately filled, sealed tubes, clean off the woman's finger and, using an alcohol sponge for antisepsis, apply, or ask the woman to apply, pressure to the puncture site until hemostasis has occurred and there is no further bleeding.	16. Do not apply pressure and effect hemostasis until you are sure you have all the blood you need. Otherwise, you may have to restick the woman.

Regarding the colored ends of the microcapillary tubes:

The purpose of the colored end is color coding. A red-tipped tube is heparinized with dried heparin in it, and a blue-tipped tube is plain with nothing in it. Red-tipped tubes, then, are the capillary tubes to use in doing a finger puncture to obtain capillary blood for a hematocrit.

Since only one end is colored the colored tips can serve an additional function. You can use them for remembering which end has touched the blood drop for filling the tube; use the other end for filling with sealing clay, thereby assuring an effective seal. Form a habit of always using the same end (plain or colored) for the same substance, blood or clay.

34

Venipuncture*

Procedure	Rationale
1. Check and organize materials and equipment, making sure all are present, appropriate, and placed conveniently.	1. Failure to do this may have a number of results, all leading to having to restick the woman. The blood may clot in the syringe prior to transfer to the appropriate test tube; body movements made in trying to reach ill-placed equipment may cause the needle to slip out of or go through the vein wall; you may discover that the syringe is not large enough to collect all the blood needed or that not enough blood tubes are on hand.
2. Apply the tourniquet:	2.
a. tourniquet should be one inch wide.	a. wide tourniquet causes less discomfort than narrow.
b. place tourniquet approximately 3 inches proximal to the intended insertion site.	b. not close enough to interfere with blood drawing; not far enough to prohibit benefit from occlusion and distention of the vein.
c. slip the tourniquet around the arm	c. stretching one end of the tourniquet

---

*Includes applying a tourniquet and drawing venous blood.

Procedure	Rationale
with the ends up; hold one end steady while stretching the other end.	provides the necessary tension on the arm for occlusion of the vein.

d. hold both ends away from the arm while:
  (1) crossing the stretched end in front of the steadied end.
  (2) next cross over the steadied end.
  (3) then create a half loop in the stretched end with your finger.
	d. holding the ends away from the arm avoids pinching the skin of the woman during the formation and anchoring of the loop that creates the slipknot.

e. lower both ends onto the arm with the loop of the stretched end anchored underneath the steadied end of the tourniquet and release your grasp on the tourniquet. (See Figure 34-1.)	e. anchors the slipknot.
f. check if the tourniquet is too tight or too loose, and repeat application if either situation exists.	f. the tourniquet should be tight enough to occlude the vein but not tight enough to occlude arteries. If the tourniquet is too tight the woman usually complains. If the tourniquet is too loose the vein will not become distended.
g. do not leave the tourniquet on an unduly long period of time, as evidenced by the extremity below the tourniquet becoming cyanotic or distended, and the woman complaining of pain.	g. avoid discomfort to the woman resulting from lack of venous circulation below the tourniquet.
3. Distend the vein by one or more of the following methods with the extremity angled downwards: a. have the woman open and close her hand several times. b. rub vigorously with the alcohol sponge while cleaning the area. c. tap or gently slap the vein. d. apply warmth (a warm towel) to the vein.	3. Enlarges the vein, which makes it easier to find and insert the needle into.
4. Select a vein that: a. is well supported by subcutaneous tissue and full-appearing without being prominent.	4. a. vein will not roll or tissue dimple as the needle is inserted; either may happen with a prominent, easily movable vein.
b. is in the forearm — look first at or near the bend of the elbow, in the antecubital fossa (see Fig. 34-2).	b. veins in the forearm are larger than those around the wrist or on the back of the hand. These other veins may

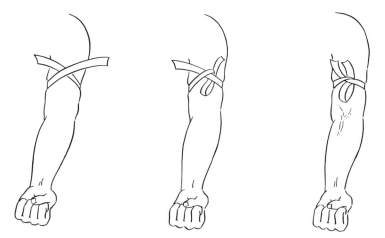

FIGURE 34-1. Applying a tourniquet for venipuncture.

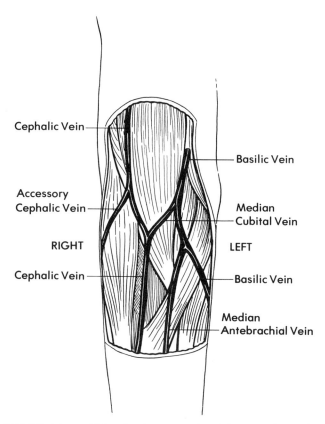

FIGURE 34-2. Veins in the antecubital fossa (right arm).

Procedure	Rationale
	also be used but not as the primary choice since they are smaller and the procedure in this area is more painful to the woman.
c. can be felt and, preferably, also seen.	c. touch is essential to inserting the needle into the vein. Seeing also promotes accuracy in hitting the vein, especially for the inexperienced, but is not absolutely essential. Touch also aids in identifying whether or not the vein will roll when touched by the needle. There should be a feeling of give when the vein is touched but it should not roll.
d. is *not* in the same arm as one receiving an intravenous transfusion. If absolutely mandatory to use the same arm, select a vein which is distal to the IV insertion site.	d. the fluid entering the vein from the intravenous transfusion has chemicals and a diluting effect which cause most laboratory tests to have erroneous results.
e. is *not* anatomically adjacent to a nerve or artery.	e. there is less chance for the inexperienced to puncture a nerve or artery accidentally — the former causing excruciating pain and the latter yielding the wrong blood for lab tests, unless arterial blood is specified.
5. Clean the insertion site with a circular motion, starting at the insertion site and ending peripherally to the insertion site. Use firm pressure and rather vigorous motion. An alcohol sponge is usually used as the antiseptic.	5. Make the area as clean as possible in order to reduce the possibility that the skin will contaminate the needle and cause subsequent infection.
6. Let the area dry.	6. Avoid discomfort of the woman. Wet alcohol stings when it touches tissue such as at the insertion site.
7. If you feel the vein again, reclean the area with another alcohol sponge.	7. You have contaminated the insertion site with your palpating finger.
8. Double-check the needle and syringe to make sure the needle is well attached to the syringe, the barrel of the syringe moves easily, and the syringe is large enough for the amount of blood needed.	8. If the needle is in the vein at the time you notice one of these problems, the subsequent manipulations to resolve them may dislodge the needle.
9. Make sure there is no air in the syringe and the barrel of the syringe fully occupies the syringe.	9. Avoid the danger of inserting air into the vein or of finding that there is no room for blood in the syringe because it is full

Procedure	Rationale
	of air. In the latter situation you have no way of getting rid of the air except to disconnect the syringe from the needle and expel the air; this manipulation may dislodge the needle.
10. Place the thumb of the hand not holding the syringe directly over the vein, approximately 1 to 2 inches below the probable point of entry into the vein, and the rest of your hand on the other side of the arm. Fix the vein by pressing down firmly with your thumb and pulling the skin away from the entry site, thereby making the skin over that area taut.	10. Fixing the vein helps keep the vein from rolling or the skin from dimpling when entered.
11. Align the direction of the needle with the direction of the vein and hold the syringe at approximately a 15-degree angle from the woman's arm. See Figure 34-3.	11. This reduces the chance of going through or missing the vein. A smaller angle may cause the needle to skim along the top of the vein. A wider angle may cause the needle to go through the vein.
12. Enter the vein directly or penetrate the skin and tissue directly adjacent to the side of the vein and then angle the needle into the vein. Either way, use a quick steady motion and control the movement of the needle by holding your index finger against its hub.	12. The users of both methods of entry claim their method decreases the possibility of missing the vein because the vein does not roll. Those who enter the vein directly say they are in and the vein is stabilized before it has a chance to roll. Those who advocate penetration to the side of the vein first and then entry into the vein say that the tissue helps hold the vein in place, keeping it from rolling while the needle pushes against it.

Note: The unending discussion of whether the needle should enter the vein with the bevel up or down, thereby preventing the escape of any blood into the surrounding tissues, which may result from incomplete entry into the vein, seems pointless since the extravasation of blood is possible with the bevel of the needle in either position. Use the method with which you are most comfortable as dictated by your own experience and experimentation.

Procedure	Rationale
13. Hold the barrel steady and withdraw the blood by pulling back on the plunger. Fill the syringe to the amount needed. Some clinicians use their free hand (the hand that set the vein) to do this. Others use that hand to stabilize the needle in the vein by holding the hub or juncture of	13. The syringe is filled by the mechanism of negative pressure.

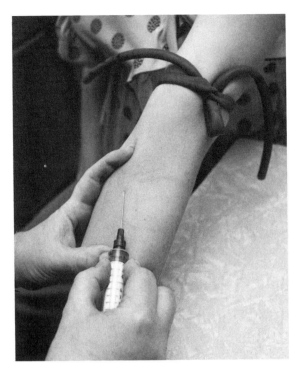

FIGURE 34-3. Prepared to perform a venipuncture: no air in barrel; skin held taut; vein fixed; needle aligned with vein and at a 15° angle.

Procedure	Rationale
the needle and syringe steady while using the hand that had previously held the needle hub and syringe to pull back on the plunger.	
14. Release the tourniquet by pulling on one end of the tourniquet (Fig. 34-4).	14. It is important to release the tourniquet before withdrawing the needle. Otherwise there will be extravasation of blood into the surrounding tissue from the distended vein when the needle is withdrawn. This leaves the woman with a painful blood clot in her tissues to dissolve and absorb.
15. Slowly withdraw the needle as you apply with gentle firmness an alcohol or dry sponge on the puncture site.	15. Slow withdrawal of the needle decreases the risk of injuring any tissue with its point. The alcohol or dry sponge starts the application of pressure instantaneously

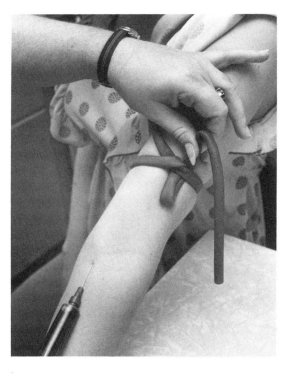

FIGURE 34-4. Releasing the tourniquet before removing the needle.

Procedure	Rationale
	with withdrawal of the needle. A dry sponge hurts less.
16. Apply, or have the woman apply, pressure on the puncture site with the alcohol sponge for 1 to 2 minutes.	16. Pressure facilitates hemostasis.
17. Fill the appropriate test tubes with the appropriate amount of blood by:	17.
a. removing their rubber stoppers. b. removing the needle from the syringe.	a. and b. If the needle is pushed through the rubber stopper, the blood will be drawn into the tube at a rapid rate. The rapidity and force of transfer and the narrow opening of the needle may hemolyze the red blood cells.
c. filling the tubes with blood by slowly pushing the plunger and holding the syringe and test tube at such an angle	c. Forceful transfer of blood to the bottom of the tube may cause it to hemolyze. The appearance of froth on the surface

Procedure	Rationale
that the blood runs down the side of the tube. d. replacing the needle on the syringe and poking a hole through each of the rubber stoppers of the test tubes. e. replacing the rubber stoppers in the test tubes.	of the blood is indicative of hemolysis. d. and e. The rubber stoppers are kept from popping back off the tubes when replaced by releasing the pressure in the tube. Blood is not lost then if the tube subsequently is laid on its side. It doesn't matter if the holes are poked through the rubber stopper before or after they are replaced in the test tube so long as it is done before any blood is lost.
18. If the blood sample was put in a heparinized test tube, then invert the stoppered test tube completely at medium speed approximately 10 times without shaking.	18. The blood needs to be mixed with the heparin in order not to clot; however, shaking the contents can cause hemolysis. Do not use your thumb instead of a stopper to invert the test tube. Besides not being esthetic, this can cause error in laboratory results.
19. Label the test tubes with the woman's name and any other appropriate identifying information and the date and time of collection.	19. Test results may be mixed up if the woman's blood tubes are not properly identified.
20. Check the puncture site before leaving the patient and apply an adhesive bandage or tape and gauze dressing over the site if indicated.	20. Make sure the bleeding has stopped.
21. Dispose of the used needle appropriately.	21. Protect yourself and others from possible infection or disease.

If there is no blood return or if blood enters the syringe and then stops: 1. Rotate the needle so that, if it is simply flush against the vein wall, blood may now enter the needle. If there still is no blood, proceed to the next step. 2. Recognize that the needle is not in the vein. 3. Palpate, with the index finger of the hand that was fixing the vein, for both the location of the vein and the location of the tip of the needle.	4. To identify the location of the tip of the needle, it helps if the hand controlling the needle angles the needle upward toward the surface or skin of the body part so it can be felt more readily by the palpating finger. 5. If the needle simply isn't far enough into the vein, insert it further and withdraw the needed blood. 6. If the needle is not in the vein but rather to the right, left, underneath, or on top of it, then withdraw your needle the necessary amount to reangle and redirect it for inser-

tion into the vein. Do not withdraw any part of the bevel through the puncture site in order to avoid contaminating the needle. Insert into the vein and withdraw the needed blood.

7. If the needle was in the vein but then went on through it (as evidenced by obtaining several drops of blood and then no more blood) *slowly* withdraw the needle while simultaneously pulling back on the plunger of the syringe until the blood flows again into the syringe. Stop the withdrawal of the needle at that point until the needed amount of blood is obtained.

8. If at any time, during this procedure or through manipulations to get the needle into the vein, you touch the needle or scrape it against the woman's skin, the needle is contaminated and must be withdrawn and discarded and the patient restuck with a new sterile needle. Be alert for contamination of the needle; concentration on getting it into the vein may detract from alertness to breaks in sterile technique.

9. If you cannot get the needle into the vein successfully, try again paying particular attention to your vein selection. If you fail twice, ask someone who has a high success rate to do the venipuncture. Do not ask someone inexperienced or try again yourself. Venipuncture is painful and the woman should not have multiple attempts made for a procedure. This is an unwarranted assault on the woman's body.

Thoughts in relation to using Vacutainers in addition to the instructions that accompany the Vacutainer holders, needles, and tubes:

1. The manipulation involved in placing the tube on the Vacutainer needle and removing it again, and this process repeated for several tubes, may cause you to move the needle in the vein, so that when you place a tube on you may go on through the vein or when you take a tube off you may pull out of the vein. This can be prevented by holding the needle firmly in place by stabilizing it at the point of junction with the Vacutainer holder against the body part with one hand while the other hand manipulates the tube and holder.

2. Be sure to put the first tube on the Vacutainer needle to the guideline on the holder so the needle will pierce but not go through the rubber stopper, which would break the vacuum. This preliminary maneuver reduces the sudden jerk in penetrating the rest of the way through the rubber stopper after the needle is in the vein.

35

Spin-Down
Hematocrit*

Procedure	Rationale
1. Obtain the blood specimen. If the blood specimen is in an oxalated blood tube, fill two blue-tipped (plain) capillary tubes as follows:	1. Two tubes are always obtained in order to balance the hematocrit machine and to still have one tube to use in case one gets broken. This avoids sticking the woman again.
a. if the sample has been sitting, mix the blood sample thoroughly by inverting the tube back and forth gently, without shaking, 10 to 15 times.	a. shaking can break down the red blood cells.
b. cover the stopper with gauze. Twist, do not pull, the stopper out.	b. gauze prevents the blood from getting on your fingers. Twisting the stopper out prevents the blood from splattering as might happen if the stopper is pulled out.
c. *slowly* tilt the blood tube until the blood approaches the edge of the tube.	c. tilt slowly because blood moves more rapidly after it begins to flow and might otherwise spill.
d. place the end of the capillary tube in the blood and hold it at an angle as	d. The capillary tubes are filled by capillary action.

---

*Includes filling capillary tubes from a test tube.

Procedure	Rationale
close to the same longitudinal plane of the blood tube as possible.	
e. fill and seal the tubes as described in Steps 10, 11, 13, 14, and 15 in the procedure on finger puncture (Chapter 33).	e.
f. *do not* fill the capillary tubes with blood that has collected in the stopper of the blood tube.	f. such a sample may contain dried red cells and plasma that would yield erroneous results and invalidate the test.
2. Open the microhematocrit centrifuge and remove the cover on the head.	2.
3. Check the rubber lining inside the rim of the head. If there are holes in this lining where you intend to place your capillary tubes, rotate the lining so the capillary tubes will rest against an unbroken surface. The liner should be replaced if it is cracked and brittle.	3. The rubber lining serves two functions: a. it cushions the sealed end of the capillary tube from the metal rim. b. it prevents loss of the specimen that can occur if clay is forced out during centrifuging.
4. Place the capillary tubes in grooves opposite each other.	4. Balance the centrifuge.
5. Make note of the numbers of the grooves you place your specimens in and the woman's name for each set of numbers.	5. Patient specimens will not get mixed up when a number of capillary tubes are centrifuged at the same time.
6. Be sure the sealed end of the capillary tube is resting against the rubber lining.	6. The sealed end is to the outside so blood won't fly out when the centrifuge is spinning. Resting against the rubber lining reduces the chance of breakage which can happen if the capillary tube is not properly in the groove or only partly protruding from the end of the groove.
7. Place the cover on the head and tighten with your hand until there is no give. Do not use a wrench to tighten the cover and do not overtighten it.	7. Hand tightening is sufficient. Repeated overtightening ruins the thread on the screw.
8. Close the microhematocrit centrifuge and lock the lid by closing the latch.	8.
9. Check to see that the centrifuge is firmly attached to the surface on which it rests. If it is attached with suction cups but is loose, put a few drops of oil or water in each cup and force the centrifuge down to create a suction that will hold.	9. Walking of the centrifuge disturbs its balance. Oil is better than water in creating a suction that will hold, but water may be all that is available.

Procedure	Rationale
10. Turn on the centrifuge and set the time by turning the timer dial past 5 minutes and then returning the indicator to 3 minutes.	10. This turns on the centrifuge and sets it to stop automatically after 3 minutes. Red blood cells are completely packed down within 3 minutes of very high speed rotation.
11. The centrifuge will stop by itself. Do not open the lid and try to stop the spinning head with your hand.	11. Trying to stop the spinning head can be dangerous to you. Also, the red cells can become loosened or dislodged if the spinning head is stopped suddenly. This may yield erroneously high readings.
12. Unlock the lid by unlatching it. Open the centrifuge after it has stopped.	12.
13. Loosen the cover and lift it off the head. A wrench comes with the centrifuge to loosen the cover if needed. Place the cover inside the open lid of the centrifuge.	13. The force of the high speed rotation may tighten the cover so that you cannot open it by hand. The cover will not become separated from the centrifuge and get lost if it is routinely placed inside the centrifuge lid.
14. Examine each capillary tube for the following: a. the tube is not in the groove (missing) — probably shattered. Most likely the tube was not properly placed in the groove and became dislodged. b. the tube is empty — the blood has leaked out. The seal was not good or the tube did not rest against the rubber rim of the head. c. the tube is only half full — leakage has probably occurred. d. there is red cell hemolysis. This is indicated by the red color of the plasma layer.	14. a., b., c., and d.: if both tubes are missing, have leaked out, or have hemolyzed, another blood specimen will have to be obtained and the procedure repeated. If this specimen was a finger puncture, the woman will have to be stuck again. If the blood was taken from an oxalated tube, fill two more capillary tubes from the specimen already drawn after checking for hemolysis if this was your problem with the capillary tubes. If the oxalated blood specimen is no good for tests, perform another venipuncture and obtain a fresh specimen. If one capillary tube is not usable but the other one is all right, proceed to read the results on the satisfactory tube.
15. Remove the capillary tubes from the head of the microhematocrit centrifuge.	15.
16. Read the results by using a microhematocrit reader. There are a variety of microhematocrit reader devices. While each has its own way of doing it, they all follow the same basic procedure: a. the junction of the bottom of the red	16. a. and b.: precision in aligning the junc-

Procedure	Rationale
cell layer and the sealing clay is to be aligned with the zero percent reading. Move the tube up and down in whatever slot is provided for it until it is aligned.	tions with the zero percent and 100 percent lines is essential to obtaining an accurate reading.

b. the top of the plasma layer is to be aligned with the 100 percent reading. Do not move the tube to make this alignment because the tube's position was set in the preceding step; move the reader instead.

c. the hematocrit is then read at the junction of the top of the red cell layer and either the bottom of the plasma layer or the bottom of the buffy layer if it is present.

c. the buffy layer of white blood cells and platelets often is visible as a narrow white band between the packed red blood cells and the plasma layer. The buffy layer is not to be included in the reading since the measurement is only for the volume of the packed red blood cells. An unusually large buffy layer generally indicates leukocytosis (increased number of white blood cells).

17. The hematocrit value can also be obtained with the following measurements and formula:

  a. using a ruler calibrated in millimeters, measure:
    (1) the length of the red cell layer
    (2) the length of the entire contents in the tube (red cell, buffy, and plasma layers)

  b. calculate as follows:

$$\frac{\text{length of red cell layer (in mm)}}{\text{length of total contents (in mm)}} \times 100$$

  = hematocrit value

17. This is handy to know in the event your microhematocrit reader gets broken or lost.

18. If two tubes are used the findings should agree within a 1 percent reading value.

18.

19. Record the results and clean up the work area.

19.

36

Inserting an Intravenous Intracatheter

Procedure	Rationale
1. Hang the intravenous infusion bag with tubing attached. Clear the tubing of air in preparation for connection to the intravenous intracatheter.	1. Once the intravenous intracatheter is in place there is an open route into the woman's vein. If the infusion is not ready to connect, blood will be lost if the intracatheter is left open or may clot in the catheter if the system is closed. An open system also increases the chance of infection.
2. Apply a tourniquet and distend the veins in accord with Steps 2 and 3 in the procedure on venipuncture (Chapter 34).	2. Aids in identification and selection of a vein into which to insert the intravenous intracatheter.
3. Select a vein in accord with Steps 4a, c, and e in the procedure on venipuncture. It is preferable to select a vein site that will not have the catheter crossing a joint. Veins in the forearm are first choice with the vein just beside and above the wrist bone a frequent selection. Veins in the back of the hand frequently are used but	3. Insertion of an intravenous intracatheter is more painful in the hand than in the forearm. While one of the ideas behind the flexible catheter was that it would not injure the patient as was possible with a straight needle, it does bend with a patient's flexion of a joint and may occlude the intravenous infusion. This then neces-

Procedure	Rationale
are a second choice to well-defined veins in the forearm. See Figure 36-1.	sitates placing an arm, wrist, or hand board on the woman to immobilize the joint; this is uncomfortable. A board is unnecessary if the catheter does not cross a joint.
4. Place a disposable absorbent pad, such as a Chux, under the limb into which you will be inserting the intravenous intracatheter.	4. This catches any blood or fluid lost during the procedure, thereby avoiding the necessity of changing the bed linen.
5. If blood specimens are going to be collected at the same time, decide which of the following methods you are going to use to collect these specimens:	5. All actions must be preplanned in order not to lose blood, risk blood clotting in the catheter, or have to do manipulations to the point that the catheter comes out of the vein. The procedure should proceed smoothly, quickly and with minimal trauma to the woman.
a. having the blood flow directly from the catheter into the blood tubes.	a. care must be taken not to contaminate the catheter in this method.
b. attaching a syringe (a size large enough for the number of milliliters of blood needed) to the intravenous intracatheter hub.	b. this method may be cleaner than the one described in *a*.
If the latter method is to be used, attach the syringe and make sure there is no air in the syringe.	This eliminates the danger of injecting air into the vein.
If the former method is to be used, have available a paper cup into which you can place the tubes of blood.	The blood tubes need to stand upright after collection since the tops, if replaced, may pop off. It the tubes are on their sides you will lose the blood. After you are through with the procedure you can assure that the tops will stay on the blood tubes if you do one of the following: (1) pierce the rubber top with a needle to release the vaccum. (2) make sure that the rubber top and the part of the blood tube where the top inserts are both dry before replacing the top.
6. Clean the insertion site in accord with Steps 5, 6, and 7 in Chapter 34, Venipuncture.	6.
7. Perform a venipuncture in accord with Steps 9 through 12 in the procedure on venipuncture, Chapter 34.	7. Emphasis should be placed on fixing the vein and holding taut the woman's skin. This facilitates insertion by holding the

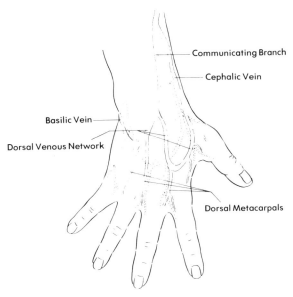

FIGURE 36-1.   Veins of the hand and forearm.

Procedure	Rationale
	vein in place so it doesn't roll and avoids puckering of the skin at the site of puncture. In doing this be careful not to contaminate the catheter against the woman's skin or against your finger.
8. Make sure the tips of the needle and the catheter are in the vein by advancing both approximately ¼ inch once you are getting blood back into the unit.	8. The tip of the needle extends approximately ⅛ inch beyond the tip of the catheter in intravenous intracatheter units. It is possible to get a blood return with just the tip of the needle in the vein. The vein will be lost during the next step if the catheter is not in the vein also.
9. If using a syringe to draw blood for blood specimens, fill the syringe with the number of milliliters of blood needed.	9.
10. Again holding the woman's skin taut with one hand, with the other hand do one of the following:	10. Taut skin will not pucker. Puckered skin causes difficulty in advancing the catheter and creates the need for forceful action which may ram the catheter through the vein.
a. withdraw the needle a short distance, advance the catheter into the vein, and then remove the needle altogether.	a., b., and c.: Whichever method is used, the principle is to cover the needle point, thereby both protecting the vein

Procedure	Rationale

   b. withdraw the needle altogether and advance the catheter into the vein.
   c. leave the needle where it is, advance the catheter into the vein, and then withdraw the needle altogether.

Whichever method is used, never advance the needle inside the catheter once it has been even slightly withdrawn and never move it back and forth within the catheter. If the vein is lost during this step, *do not* reinsert the needle through the catheter. Instead, remove the entire unit, discard, and start again with a new sterile intravenous intracatheter unit. Be careful during this step not to contaminate the catheter by sliding it over the woman's skin while inserting it.

11. If blood is being collected by having it drip directly from the catheter into the blood tubes, press down over the area of the tip of the catheter inside the vein between tubes, between manipulation of materials, and before starting the intravenous infusion.

12. Connect the intravenous infusion tubing to the catheter, release the tourniquet, and start the infusion flow at the desired rate.

from the possibility that the needle might go on through it, and allowing the flexible catheter to be threaded into the vein.

If the needle is not totally removed before advancing the catheter, the needle needs to be immobilized while the catheter is advanced. If the needle is totally removed, blood will drip through the catheter during the threading process.

It is imperative that the needle never be advanced again once the tip of it has been withdrawn inside the catheter. If the needle is advanced again, the sharp tip of it may shear off a fragment of the catheter, which would then be in the bloodstream as a foreign object embolus.

11. Applying pressure stops the woman's blood from flowing since the vein is occluded at the point where blood enters the catheter. This is done briefly so that blood will not clot inside the catheter.

12. It is essential to release the tourniquet before starting the flow of the infusion. Otherwise the vein fills with fluid and ruptures from overdistention. These three steps are listed as one as they must be accomplished quickly, in sequence, in order to have a patent intravenous system.

13. Tape the catheter and IV tubing securely to the limb involved. Following is one way of securely taping (see Fig. 36-2):
   a. First use a narrow (⅛- to ¼-in.) strip of tape underneath the hub of the intravenous intracatheter with its edge against the place where the catheter enters the skin and with its sticky side up. Crisscross it over the insertion site with the ends going at an angle away from it. Attach the tape to the woman's skin so that the catheter is straight and not bent, which would interfere with the flow of the infusion.
   b. Now use a wide (1- to 1½-in.) strip of tape over the crisscross at the insertion site.
   c. Make a loop of the intravenous tubing and tape it down just beside the edge of the catheter hub.
   d. You may need to tape down one or both sides of the loop of the intravenous tubing so it doesn't catch on anything and pull apart from the hub of the catheter.

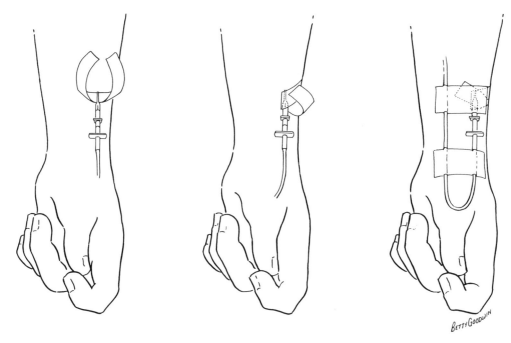

FIGURE 36-2.   Taping an intravenous intracatheter and tubing.

    e. Run the intravenous tubing a few more inches away from the insertion site and tape it to the woman's skin so the strain of the tubing isn't at the site of insertion.
Avoid taping over where the catheter hub and IV tubing join or covering up any connectors or taping over the rubber medication appendage since you may need access to these sites.

    g. Be considerate of people with hairy arms by using a minimal amount of tape.

14. Wipe any blood off the woman with water or soap and water, and dry.

14. This is done for the woman's comfort since blood is sticky. Alcohol sponges will not remove blood.

15. After the procedure is completed, ask the woman to wriggle her fingers, do range of motion at the wrist and elbow, and wave at you. In this way she can learn that it will not hurt her to move her fingers, hand, or arm with the IV in place and she therefore will not hold herself rigid in fear hour after hour.

16. Dispose of all materials appropriately, taking special care in the disposal of the needle.

17. Label the blood tubes in accord with Step 18 in Chapter 34, Venipuncture.

Note: If it is anticipated that the IV will be in place more than 24 hours, the following additional steps should be added to this procedure to decrease the incidence of phlebitis:

1. Use povidone-iodine (Betadine) instead of alcohol for cleaning the insertion site prior to puncture.

2. Apply an antibiotic ointment to, and a sterile dry dressing over, the puncture site.

37

Giving Intravenous Medications

Procedure	Rationale

By Venipuncture

1. Perform venipuncture. (See Chapter 34, "Venipuncture.")

2. Remove the tourniquet when the needle is in the vein but before giving the medication.

3. Aspirate to be sure that the needle is still in the vein.

4. Inject at a rate in accord with the medication, for example, 50 milligrams of meperidine hydrochloride (Demerol) would be injected slowly over a 2-minute period.

1.

2. The tourniquet occludes the vein, which facilitates performance of the venipuncture. However, the vein must be unoccluded for receipt of the medication.

3. Movement during manipulation of removing the tourniquet may have dislodged the needle from the vein.

4. For safety and comfort of the mother and safety of the baby. For example, Demerol given rapidly can induce nausea, vomiting, flushing, dizziness, and a sense of being too warm in the mother—all of which can be avoided by slow injection of the medication.

Procedure	Rationale

By Intravenous Infusion Tubing

Procedure	Rationale
1. Ascertain status of the IV.	1. You must be sure that the IV is patent and that the medication will be going into a vein and not into infiltrated tissue.
2. Wipe off the rubber medication appendage on the IV tubing with an alcohol sponge.	2. Cleanse the site where the entry into the sterile system will be made.
3. Insert the needle of the syringe containing the medication through the rubber medication appendage on the IV tubing.	3. Rubber self-seals, and the appendage is on the IV tubing for the purpose of giving medications. To stick a needle into the IV tubing itself would cause the IV to leak through the resulting hole since the tubing does not self-seal.
4. Pinch off the IV tubing above the rubber medication appendage.	4. Prevents the medication from going up the tubing rather than down the tubing into the body during injection. Occluding the tubing stops the flow of intravenous fluid which allows you to control the amount of medication the mother is receiving and the rate at which it infuses.
5. Inject at a rate in accord with the medication, for example, inject a few milligrams of Demerol, remembering that the entire injection should take 2 minutes for 50 milligrams and 1 minute for 25 milligrams of this drug.	5. 6., 7., 8., and 9.: The drug is injected slowly for the safety and comfort of the mother and safety of the baby (see Step 4 under "By Venipuncture," above). If you follow this procedure you are better able to control how much medication the mother is getting at any one point in time. A full amount of medication hitting the maternal-fetal circulatory system at one time can produce fetal depression. One must remember that the drug injected prior to letting the IV fluid run probably does not even reach the vein as there is insufficient volume to extend the distance of the tubing from the rubber medication appendage to the vein. Running the IV fluid forces the medication on through the tubing in small, controlled amounts.
6. Release the IV tubing, open the IV flow, and let the IV solution run for approximately 15 to 30 seconds.	
7. Pinch off the IV tubing above the rubber medication appendage.	
8. Inject more of the medication, in the present example a few more milligrams of Demerol. If the amount of Demerol is 50 milligrams per milliliter, inject one-quarter of the medication over a period of 15 seconds and then let the IV run for 15 to 30 seconds; within the combined 30- to 45-second period, 12.5 milligrams of Demerol would be administrered.	
9. Repeat steps 6, 7, and 8 until all of the medication is given.	

38

Making a Wet Smear Slide of Vaginal Secretions

Procedure	Rationale
1. Obtain the specimen of vaginal discharge during the speculum examination.	1. The vaginal discharge in the concave posterior blade of the speculum is a good source for a specimen. Plaques of *Candida* on the vaginal walls are exposed during the speculum examination and are a good specimen source.
2. Do one of the following: a. Take a clean microscopic slide and put one drop of normal saline on the middle of the slide. b. Take a clean microscopic slide and put one drop of normal saline on one one-third end of the slide and one drop of potassium hydroxide (KOH) on the other one-third end of the slide. c. Take two clean microscopic slides and put one drop of normal saline on the middle of one slide and one drop of potassium hydroxide on the middle of the second slide.	2. *Candida (Monilia), Trichomonas,* and *Gardnerella* can all be identified microscopically when mixed with a drop of normal saline. Normal saline is used for detection of motile trichomonads. Use of potassium hydroxide facilitates identification of *Candida* because potassium hydroxide dissolves trichomonads, white blood cells, bacteria, and foreign objects. Some clinicians prefer to start with Step 2.a. and, after evaluating the slide for trichomonads and *gardnerella*, add a drop of potassium hydroxide at the edge of the coverslip. This diffuses under the cover-

Procedure	Rationale
	slip, destroys the other organisms, and facilitates identification of *Candida*.
3. Take a cotton-tipped applicator and roll the plain wooden end of the applicator in the specimen of vaginal discharge.	3. The cotton-tipped end is *not* used as cotton filaments may be added to the specimen and be confused with or misidentified as *Candida*.
4. Mix the sample of vaginal discharge on the wooden end of the cotton-tipped applicator with the drop of normal saline on the slide. Repeat Step 3 and mix with the drop of potassium hydroxide if both solutions are being used. Use both a rolling and a stirring motion to mix the vaginal discharge with the drop of solution.	4. Microscopic evaluation of the slide is facilitated if the sample of vaginal discharge is well mixed throughout the drop of solution, thereby avoiding thick areas of sample.
5. Cover the mixture of specimen sample and solution with a coverglass (coverslip) by sliding it onto and over the specimen. This is accomplished by putting the edge of one side of the coverslip into the mixed specimen/solution and drawing it to the longitudinal edge of the slide. When the specimen/solution is under the entire edge of the side of the coverslip, slide the coverslip over the rest of the mixed specimen/solution on the slide.	5. If the coverslip is simply dropped onto the specimen, a number of air bubbles are trapped between the coverslip and the specimen/solution on the slide, making microscopic evaluation difficult.
6. The wet smear slide of vaginal secretion is now ready for microscopic evaluation. (See Chapter 39, Using a Microscope.)	

39

Using a Microscope

Procedure	Rationale
1. Place the slide on the stage of the microscope so that the specimen is over the opening in the stage. Secure it in place with the stage clips.	1. This properly locates the slide for viewing of the specimen.
2. Turn on the light source for the microscope and adjust the light so it reflects evenly throughout the microscopic field.	2. Good visualization is dependent on adequate lighting.
3. Do either of the following: a. Select the low-power objective (10X) and place it over the specimen, making sure it clicks into place. b. Select the high-power objective (40X) and place it over the specimen, making sure it clicks into place.	3. a. or b. Some clinicians feel it is easier to locate the proper plane of visualization by starting with the low-power objective. Other clinicians prefer to start with the low-power objective because they believe it is easier to scan an entire slide under low power and then switch to high power for confirmation of findings (*Candida*, trichomonads) and identification of clue cells, if present. Still other clinicians feel that it saves time to start with the high-power objective.
4. Move the objective and the slide as close to each other as possible with the coarse adjustment knob. Watch from the side so	4. This provides a starting point for locating the proper plane of visualization without breaking the slide in the process. Watch-

643

Procedure	Rationale
you can see if and when the objective touches the slide. Note which way you are turning the coarse adjustment knob.	ing from the side enables you to prevent breaking the slide because you can see when the objective and the slide touch and stop turning the knob. (The objective and the slide usually do not touch when starting with the low-power objective.) Noting which way you are turning the coarse adjustment knob assures that you know which way to turn it (the opposite direction) when you are looking through the eyepiece in order to visualize the specimen and to prevent further pressure of the objective on the slide, which would then break the slide.
5. Look through the eyepiece of the microscope and *slowly* turn the coarse objective knob the other direction until you can see something.	5. If the coarse adjustment knob is turned too quickly the proper plane of visualization will be passed through unnoticed.
6. Check to make sure you are in the right plane of visualization by moving the slide while you look through the eyepiece. Note whether or not what you are looking at changes position or if you see more of the specimen. If so, you are in the proper plane. If not, you are not in the proper plane and should continue with Step 5 above.	6. It is easy to confuse dirt, lint, and grime on the objective and eyepiece for the specimen. Such objects of vision will not change position when you move the slide.
7. When the specimen is in the proper plane of visualization turn the fine adjustment knob back and forth while you look through the eyepiece.	7. The fine adjustment knob brings the specimen into sharper focus.
8. a. If you started with the high-power objective (40X) proceed with Step 10 below.	8. a.
b. If you started with the low-power objective (10X), switch now to the high-power objective. Watch from the side while changing the objective.	b. Switching to the high-power objective after having located the specimen in the proper plane of visualization will further magnify the specimen for ease in identification and diagnosis. If you watch from the side while changing the objective you are assured that you will not hit the slide with the objective. This might either break the slide or

Procedure	Rationale
	knock it out of position, thereby negating your location of the specimen in the proper plane of visualization.
9. Turn the fine adjustment knob back and forth while you look through the eyepiece. Do not use the coarse adjustment knob.	9. Fine adjustment brings the specimen into sharper focus under the high-power objective. If you turn the coarse adjustment knob you will lose the proper plane of visualization you located using the lower-power objective.
10. Systematically move the slide until you have seen the specimen in its entirety or sufficiently to make a diagnosis.	10. Evidence of what you are seeking may not appear in all areas of the slide. Therefore, the entire slide must be evaluated.

11. When finished with your microscopic evaluation of the slide, turn off the light source for the microscope, remove the slide from the stage, and dispose of the slide properly.

Care of a Microscope

1. Keep the microscope covered when not in use.	1. Prevents dirt and lint from collecting in and on the microscope.
2. Routinely clean the microscope of dust and lint and wipe the eyepiece and objectives with optical paper.	2. Facilitates proper functioning of the microscope and ease in looking at the specimens.
3. Carry the microscope with two hands in an upright position or on a movable cart or table.	3. The microscope is a delicate instrument which must be handled carefully to function properly. It must be kept upright to prevent pieces from falling.

40

Breast Examination

RELEVANT HISTORY

RELEVANT HISTORY

1. *Age*
2. *Symptoms*
   a. *tumor* — when found; any change since first discovered if there has been delay in seeking medical consultation; location; any change during menstrual cycle, especially during premenstrual and menstrual phases; and changes in nipples.
      (1) significance — contributes during examination to the differential diagnosis made between normal breast tissue with cyclic physiologic nodularity and breast disease.
   b. *nipple discharge* — spontaneous or elicited; character: serous, bloody, thin and watery without color, thick and yellowish, thick and grayish, greenish, or milky; amount; when noticed; related to pregnancy or non-pregnancy; taking oral contraceptives or not; breast-feeding or not; date of termination of last pregnancy; date of termination of breast-feeding of last

baby; if occurring during menstruation; if occurring during the period of breast growth and development; amount of sexual stimulation and manipulation to the breasts and nipples.
      (1) significance — significant and requiring physician consultation *if* the woman is *not* pregnant, postpartal, breast-feeding, within a year of termination of last baby breast-fed, within 6 months of termination of last pregnancy, taking oral contraceptives, in the period of breast growth and development, having excessive sexual stimulation and manipulation of her breasts and nipples, or making frequent attempts to elicit a discharge.

      Generally an elicited nipple discharge is not of pathological significance. A nipple discharge that is pathologically significant occurs spontaneously. Nipple discharge is especially significant if the woman is amenorrheic and not pregnant or postpartal. A drop of thick, grayish discharge expressed from the nipple of a middle-aged woman is usually normal and comes from terminal ectatic (stretched) ducts. A bloody discharge requires consultation with a physician for further investigation.

c. *pain or tenderness* — in one or both breasts; constant or cyclic with the menstrual cycle; character: dull, sharp, constant, or intermittent.

(1) significance — cyclic character indicates physiologic rather than pathologic origin.

3. *Past history of breast disease* — operations, biopsies, aspirations: date, physician, hospital; location of the disease in the breast(s).

4. *Family history of breast disease* — include woman's female and male relatives; type, if known; age of relative at time of breast disease.

5. *Menstrual history* — age at onset, frequency, duration, amount, regularity, age of onset of menopause.

6. *Pregnancy history* — age at each pregnancy; date of each pregnancy termination; length of each pregnancy.

7. *Lactation history* — whether or not each child was breast-fed; length of time each one was breast-fed; date of termination of last child breast-fed.

8. *Hormonal history* — for contraception, menstrual irregularity, menopausal symptom relief, cosmetics, or medical problems; length of time taking hormones; name and dosage; if still taking or date of termination of last use of hormones.

PHYSICAL EXAMINATION

Inspection of breasts and palpation of lymph node areas

Findings	Significance
1. Have the woman in a sitting position either at the end or the side of the examining table with her legs over the edge so she is facing you.	1. The breasts need to be hanging freely at a level that enables good visualization.
2. The woman should be draped up to her waist with her entire chest area exposed.	2. Exposure of only the area necessary protects the woman's sense of modesty.
3. The room must be well lighted.	3. This is necessary if you are going to be able to see slight changes in breast contour, color, retraction signs, and the nipple epithelium.
4. Inspect the breasts with the woman in each of the following positions: a. with her arms by her side. b. with her arms raised high over her head.	4. a. and b. necessary to see different aspects of the breasts. b. this position elevates the pectoral fascia. If there is a carcinoma, the fibrosis around it may have attached it to the underlying fascia and to the over-

Findings	Significance
	lying skin. Arm elevation will reveal this through the signs of asymmetry (indentation in the contour) or skin retraction.
c. with her hands in either position: (1) pressed against her hips. (2) the palmar surfaces pressed against each other at the level of her chin.	c. either of these maneuvers contracts the pectoral muscles underlying the breasts. A carcinoma may be evidenced by an abnormal elevation of the breast (slight elevation of the breast is normal), resulting from the fibrosis of the carcinoma being fixed to the underlying pectoral fascia, and by retraction signs such as skin dimpling and nipple deviation (Fig. 40-1).
d. have the woman stand and bend forward from her hips with her chin up and her arms and hands extended toward you. You support her with your hands under her outstretched hands as you sit in front of her.	d. the normal breast will fall freely away from the chest wall in this position and be symmetrical. The accompanying fibrosis of a breast lesion will fix the breast to the chest wall, and asymmetry and retraction signs become evident in this position which may not be evident in other positions.

Observations	Significance
1. Breasts unequal in size — usually one breast slightly larger than the other — but perfectly symmetrical in contour with each other.	1. Usually normal; developmental in origin.
2. Size of breasts small, large, or pendulous.	2. Individual variation of no pathologic significance.
3. Accessory breast tissue — alone or any combination of supernumerary nipples, areola, glandular parenchyma.	3. Developmental anomaly; no pathologic significance; usually located along the embryologic milk lines.
4. Asymmetry in breast contour, such as a bulge or indentation in the contour.	4. Abnormal; physician consultation required.
5. Retraction signs, such as skin dimpling, puckering, or furrows (Fig. 40-1).	5. Abnormal; physician consultation required.
6. Nipple deviation (deviation in the direction the nipple is pointing) or nipple retraction with or without broadening and flattening of the nipple (Fig. 40-1).	6. Abnormal; physician consultation required.

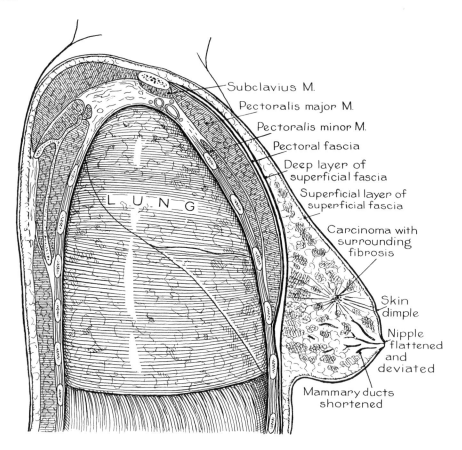

FIGURE 40-1. Diagram of the parasagittal section through the breast and thorax to illustrate the mechanism of retraction in carcinoma of the breasts. (Reproduced by permission from Haagensen. C. D. Diseases of the Breast, 2nd. Philadelphia: Saunders, 1971.)

Procedure		Rationale	
7.	Inverted nipples — not retracted nor deviated.	7.	No pathologic significance.
8.	Shrunken breast.	8.	Abnormal; physician consultation required.
9.	Edema; orange-peel skin.	9.	Abnormal; physician consultation required.
10.	Dilated subcutaneous veins — woman not pregnant.	10.	Abnormal; physician consultation required.
11.	Elevation of skin temperature or redness — woman not postpartal.	11.	Abnormal; physician consultation required.
12.	Ulcerations.	12.	Abnormal; physician consultation required.
13.	Excessive breast elevation and asymmetry with contraction of pectoral muscles.	13.	Abnormal; physician consultation required.

Procedure	Rationale
5. With the woman again sitting on the side of the examining table with her arms by her sides, palpate the supraclavicular region on both sides for nodes.	

Findings	Significance
1. Palpable nodes.	1. Abnormal, usually indicating advanced lymph node involvement; physician consultation required.

Procedure	Rationale
6. Supporting the woman's arm with one of your own, gently palpate the axilla with the fingertips of your other hand. Move the woman's arm through a full range of motion while palpating. Reverse the procedure for the opposite axilla. This procedure may also be done when the woman is lying down.	6. Support of the woman's arm relaxes the pectoral muscles. This relaxation is essential to examination of the axilla. Taking the arm through range of motion may uncover lesions obscured by fat or muscles. Lymph nodes are more easily felt with gentle palpation.

Findings	Significance
1. Palpable nodes. In the absence of breast pathology, inspect the fingers and hand of the affected side for small abrasions and cuts, especially around the cuticles and fingernails.	1. Abnormal; physician consultation required. Infections distal to the nodes may cause inflammation of the lymph nodes and thus yield sizable, soft, palpable axillary nodes. The physician should be consulted for confirmation of this diagnosis.

INSPECTION OF NIPPLE EPITHELIUM AND PALPATION OF BREASTS

Procedure	Rationale
1. Have the woman assume a supine position on the examining table, again draping her so only her chest area is exposed.	1. Inspection of the nipple epithelium requires close observation in a good light. This is more easily accomplished with the woman in a supine position.
2. Inspect the nipple epithelium.	2.

Findings	Significance
1. Erosion, ulceration, thickening, or unusual roughness.	1. Abnormal; physician consultation required.
2. Redness — woman *not* breast-feeding or having nipples sexually manipulated.	2. Abnormal; physician consultation required.
3. Crusting indicating dried discharge — woman *not* pregnant, postpartal, or breast-feeding.	3. Abnormal; physician consultation required.

Procedure	Rationale
3. Have the woman raise her arm above her head on the same side of her body as the breast you are going to palpate. Place a small pillow under her shoulder on the same side if possible, that is, if a pillow is available and there is room for it on the examining table.	3. Raising her arm flattens and more evenly distributes the breast over the chest wall, thereby facilitating palpation of all her breast tissue. The addition of the small pillow under her shoulder distributes the breast tissue more medially toward the thorax, facilitating palpation of the outer lateral breast. The breast tends to fall to the side, especially if large, even with the raising of her arm.
4. Palpate with the flat portion of the fingers of your examining hand (Fig. 40-2), using a gentle to-and-fro or rotary motion which compresses the breast tissue against the chest wall.	4. Gentleness is the key to an informative, accurate examination. Soft breast lesions can be felt only upon extremely gentle palpation. There is no excuse for an examination which traumatizes the woman with pain or causes bruising. It is also possible to cause metastasis of a breast carcinoma by a rough, heavy-handed, or kneading type of examination.
5. If the woman has pointed out to you an area in her breast where she has found a lump or point of tenderness, start your examination by palpating the opposite breast first.	5. To negate the possibility of missing other findings because of concentrating on obvious disease, if present. It also facilitates your differentiating normal from abnormal breast tissue if you have first felt her normal breast tissue.
6. Palpate the breast, using any one of the following methods: a. radial: start on the upper outer margin of the breast and proceed in a circular, clockwise fashion in ever-smaller concentric circles, ending with palpation beneath the nipple (Fig. 40-3).	6. This is an example of different but perfectly acceptable ways of doing the same thing. Certain principles are to be followed regardless of which method is used: (1) every square inch of breast tissue is palpated. This includes beneath the nipple and into the axilla. Which method

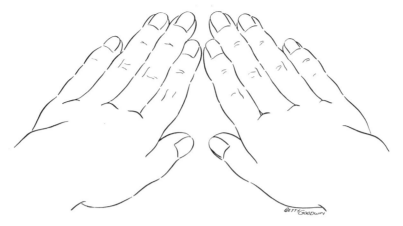

FIGURE 40-2. Position of hands for palpation.

Procedure	Rationale

A variation of this method is to start at the margin of the areola and proceed in a circular, clockwise fashion in ever-larger concentric circles to the outer margin of the breast, returning at the end to palpate beneath the nipple.

b. wheel-spoke: start at the upper outer margin and palpate in to the areola as though following the spoke of a wheel. Move in a clockwise fashion around the breast, repeating the direction of palpation from outer margin to the areola for each spoke of the wheel. End with palpation beneath the nipple (Fig. 40-4).

A variation of this method is to start at the areola and palpate out to the breast margin, again as though following the spoke of a wheel. Repeat around the breast, ending with palpation beneath the nipple.

c. traversing: Divide the breast into its medial and lateral halves, using an imaginary vertical line through the nipple as the dividing line. Start with the medial half at the level of the clavicle

you use to cover the breast doesn't matter as long as you palpate every square inch. The inch you miss may have a lesion.

(2) your palpation is gentle and, therefore, atraumatic.

(3) your palpation compresses the breast tissue against the chest wall. Palpation that compresses breast tissue between your fingers or hands may give the erroneous impression of a mass.

Method *a.* has the advantage of assuring coverage of every square inch of the breast and is particularly useful for beginning practitioners.

Method *b.* has two major drawbacks:

(1) examiners frequently palpate the nipple and areola at the inner end of each "spoke." This means that this area is palpated a number of times in the course of the examination. This is unnecessary; also, repeated palpation can be traumatic.

(2) while the inward ends of the spokes are being repeatedly palpated, areas

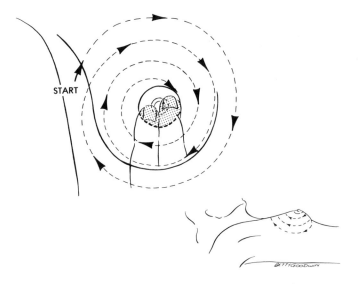

FIGURE 40-3.   Radial method of palpating the breasts.

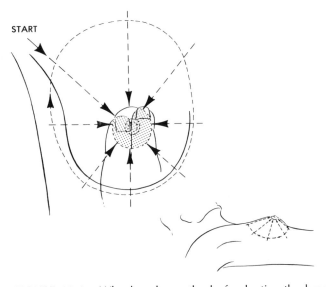

FIGURE 40.4.   Wheel-spoke method of palpating the breasts.

Procedure	Rationale
and palpate in a series of parallel transverse lines from the nipple line to the sternum down to the caudal edge of the breast. Then move to the lateral half of the breast and again palpate in a series of parallel transverse lines this time from the nipple line to the posterior axillary line back up to the level of the clavicle (Fig. 40-5).	between the outer ends of the spokes frequently are missed, especially by learners who are concentrating more on the method than on palpating every square inch of the breast. This problem can be alleviated by adding the maneuver of circularly palpating the outer margin of the breast either at the beginning or at the end of the method. Method *c.* is the most comprehensive coverage of tissue because its borders (clavicle, sternum, caudal breast edge, and posterior axillary line) encompass not only the observable protuberant breast tissue but also the thin layer of breast tissue that extends over a larger area at its outer limits.
7. In all three methods of palpation be sure to palpate the extension of the breast into the axilla. You will need to lower the woman's arm to the level of her shoulder while palpating the axilla.	7. The arm is lowered in order to relax the muscles which may otherwise interfere with your palpation of the axillary area.

8. *Contrary to popular practice*, it is *not* necessary to attempt to express discharge from the nipples as part of a routine breast examination. Unless it is most gently performed it is a traumatic procedure which may of itself cause a discharge from tissue damage. Also, discharge that is elicited by expression from the breast usually has no pathologic significance. If there is a cancerous lesion, traumatic examination and expression run the risk of causing metastasis. Discharge that escapes from the nipple spontaneously during palpation is significant and requires physician consultation.

Findings	Significance
1. A transverse ridge, perhaps slightly tender, at the caudal edge of the breast.	1. Inframammary fold. Normal.
2. Fine nodularity throughout the breast.	2. Normal breast tissue consisting of lobules of glandular tissue.
3. Coarse nodularity generalized throughout the breast, occurring during the premenstrual or menstrual phases of the menstrual cycle.	3. Normal physiologic engorgement. If unsure of normality, consult with the physician.
4. Coarse, granular nodularity in a localized area.	4. Abnormal; physician consultation required.
5. Loss of elasticity of nipples or breast tissue with increased firmness or thickening of the skin texture.	5. Abnormal; physician consultation required.

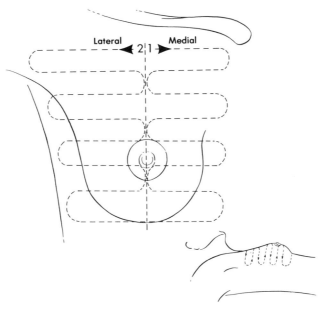

FIGURE 40-5.   Transversing method of palpating the breasts.

Findings	Significance
6. Any mass. Note and chart the following: a. location — locate in accord with a clock face with the woman in a supine position. Note the distance from the nipple. b. size — length and width in centimeters. c. shape or contour, for example, round, nodular, smooth, elongated, irregular. d. consistency, for example, elastic, tense, firm, soft, hard. e. delimitation (demarcation, discreteness, circumscription) — the degree of discreteness or sharpness of the edges or margins of the mass; usually charted as well defined or delimited, or poorly delimited, or difficult to determine boundaries.	6. Abnormal; physician consultation required. All the information to be charted provides baseline data from the first time the mass is noted; especially useful if you have to refer a woman in to a physician from an outlying clinic. The specific observations about the mass aid the physician in making a differential diagnosis and deciding upon a course of action.

Findings	Significance
f. mobility or movability — for example, freely movable, fixed, moderately fixed, movable only in certain directions.	

CHARTING OF FINDINGS

If normal:

1. Breasts symmetrical, soft, and without masses. Nipples symmetrical, clean, and not retracted. No palpable supraclavicular or axillary nodes. History noncontributory.

If abnormal:

1. Describe any findings. If a mass is noted, draw a sketch locating the mass and describe in accord with the observations listed in "Findings" column above. The sketch may be simple, simulating a clock face with the nipple in the center. Note if the sketch is of the left or right breast.
2. Note whether or not there were any palpable supraclavicular or axillary nodes and, if so, the number of them and the size and consistency of each.
3. Describe any asymmetry or retraction signs and where located in what position and maneuver.
4. Note and describe any nipple changes or discharge.
5. Note any relevant history.
6. End your note with the name of the physician with whom you will consult.

VARIATIONS OF BREAST EXAMINATION AND FINDINGS FOR THE PREGNANT WOMAN

The basic breast examination is performed during the initial physical examination of the woman prenatally. Due to physiologic changes occurring because of the pregnancy the fol-lowing breast findings are considered normal in the pregnant woman:

1. Bilateral increase in size — often accompanied with tingling, tenseness, and tenderness. Occurs in the first trimester.
2. Increased generalized coarse nodular and lobular feel of the breast as a result of hypertrophy of the mammary alveoli. Occurs in the first trimester.
3. Escape of colostrum as a nipple discharge. May appear as early as the sixth week of gestation as a clear viscous fluid. May become yellow and less viscous later in the pregnancy. Spontaneous discharge of colostrum during pregnancy may dry and form a crust on the nipples if not carefully cleansed daily with warm water.
4. Montgomery's follicles — hypertrophied sebaceous glands in the areola. Occur in the first trimester.
5. Enlargement and increased erectility of the nipples. Occur in the first trimester.
6. Broadening and increased pigmentation of the areola. Start in the first trimester. Heavier pigmentation of the areola in the first trimester is called primary areola. A darkening of the skin, usually mottled, around and beyond the primary areola during the second trimester is called secondary areola.
7. Dilated subcutaneous veins usually seen beneath the skin as a tracing of bluish veins. Occur in the first trimester.
8. Vascular spiders on the upper chest (also upper arms, neck, and face). Occur in the second trimester.

9. Striae of the breasts. May occur with excessive increase in the size of the breasts.

In subsequent antepartal revisits the woman's breasts are examined for the following:

1. Adequate support with a properly fitting brassiere.
2. Condition of the nipples (e.g., dried or crusted colostrum; duct openings clogged with powder; progress in bringing out flat or inverted nipples in women who plan to breast-feed).

There are certain times when it is of value to attempt to express colostrum from the nipples during pregnancy. These times are as follows:

1. Presence of colostrum is a presumptive sign of pregnancy in primigravidas and in multigravidas who have not had a baby or breast-fed in the past few years. Expression of colostrum is useful in clinically evaluating the possible diagnosis of pregnancy early in the first trimester as it appears by the sixth week of gestation.
2. An anxious woman close to term or immediately postpartum who wants to breast-feed but is deciding against it because she erroneously thinks she has nothing in her breasts to give her baby. Such anxiety is immediately allayed rather dramatically by simply expressing a few drops of colostrum.
3. Women who plan to breast-feed their babies may prepare their breasts for this activity through daily breast massage and manual expression of colostrum during the last month of pregnancy. This technique and its underlying rationale are described in Chapter 48.

VARIATIONS OF BREAST EXAMINATION FOR THE POSTPARTAL WOMAN

The woman has had the basic breast examination during her initial prenatal physical examination and again upon admission to labor and delivery or immediately postpartum. It is important to examine her breasts additionally during each postpartal examination for the following:

1. Adequate support with a properly fitting brassiere or a breast binder
2. Palpation of the breasts to ascertain if they are:
   a. soft
   b. filling — tense, increasing firmness, slightly enlarged
   c. engorged — enlarged, hard, reddened, shiny, skin temperature elevated, painful, dilated veins
3. If the mother is breast-feeding, inspection of the nipple epithelium for:
   a. signs of irritation — reddened, tender
   b. precursory signs of cracking — tiny pinpoint blisters or subepithelial petechiae (best seen with a small magnifying glass)
   c. cracking — sore, possibly bleeding

There are also times during the postpartal period when it is of value to express colostrum or milk from the mother's nipples. These times are as follows:

1. Expression of a drop or two of colostrum or milk helps the baby to learn where to suckle through immediate gratification.
2. When the breasts, and especially the areola, are engorged it will be easier for the baby to "latch on" properly if milk is first expressed to diminish the rigid hardness of the area to the point of being soft enough for compression of the lactiferous sinuses.

TEACHING THE WOMAN BREAST SELF-EXAMINATION

Teaching the woman how to do breast self-examination is an inherent part of performing a breast examination on all women. The experienced clinician often incorporates this teaching while doing her own examination of the woman rather than having a separate time for teaching the woman. This is done in the interest of saving time but still getting the teaching done, which is especially important in a busy clinic situation. There are a number of pamphlets that state the need and illustrate the technique for doing breast self-examination. These are available at no cost from the American Cancer Society.

The woman should first be asked if she knows how to do breast self-examination and if she is doing it. If the answer is affirmative, have her demonstrate her method. Also ascertain the frequency of her examinations. If the answer is affirmative for knowing how but negative for doing it, ascertain why she is not doing it. If her answer is negative for knowing how, ascertain if she wants to learn how and, if not, why not.

The following points should be included when teaching a woman breast self-examination:

1. Why breast self-examination is important.
2. Assurance that a cancer identified early enough can be cured.
3. Not all lumps mean cancer but they must be diagnosed quickly.
4. When to do breast self-examination during the menstrual cycle and why. Instruct the woman to perform breast self-examination on a routine monthly basis a day or so after the end of her menstrual period. The end of the menstrual period serves as a reminder. It also keeps her from doing examinations during the premenstrual or menstrual phases of her menstrual cycle, when physiologic changes may cause her to feel normal changes which may unduly frighten her.
5. The positions to assume for inspection while situated in front of a mirror.
6. What she is looking for during inspection.
7. The position to assume for palpation — supine, the raising and lowering of her arm on the same side of her body as the breast she is palpating, and the placement of a small pillow under her shoulder on the same side.
8. A method of palpation emphasizing proper use of her hand and coverage of every square inch of the breasts and axillae. Women frequently squeeze or mash their breasts rather than palpate gently with compression of the breast tissue against the chest wall.
9. What she is looking for during palpation.
10. Have her feel anatomical structures that she might be unnecessarily frightened by during examination, such as ribs, the inframammary fold, and her normal breast tissue.

In order for breast self-examination to be an effective screening tool for breast lesions for the woman, it is necessary for you to evaluate the effectiveness of your teaching. If your teaching has been effective the woman should be performing monthly breast self-examination and should be able to:

1. State the importance of doing breast self-examination
2. State the proper time of the month for doing breast self-examination
3. Demonstrate the proper positions for inspection in front of a mirror
4. State accurately what she is looking for during inspection
5. Demonstrate the proper position for palpation of her breasts
6. Demonstrate a method of palpation that covers every square inch of each breast, includes palpation of her axillae, and gently compresses the breast tissue against her chest wall
7. State accurately what she is looking for during palpation
8. State what she is going to do if she finds something abnormal during inspection and palpation

REFERENCES

Anatomy and Physiology of the Breasts

Haagensen, C. D. *Diseases of the Breast*, 2nd. Philadelphia: Saunders, 1971. Chapters 1 and 2 are most comprehensive and incorporate clinical significance; see also Chapter 5.

Hibbard, L., Ulene, A., and Christensen, W. Submodule 1: Anatomy and physiology of the breast. *OMNI Module: Breast Examination*. Raritan, N. J.: Ortho Pharmaceutical Corporation, 1974, pp. 1–12.

Netter, F.H. Section XIII: Anatomy and pathology of the mammary gland, *Reproductive System, vol. 2. The Ciba Collection of Medical Illustrations*. Summit, N. J.: Ciba Pharmaceutical Company, 1965, pp. 245–262.

Thorek, P. *Anatomy in Surgery*. Philadelphia: Lippincott, 1962, pp. 256–260.

Townsend, J. Breast lumps. *Clinical Symposia. 32(2)*. Summit, N. J.: CIBA Pharmaceutical Co., 1980.

41

Obstetric Abdominal Examination

The term *obstetric abdominal examination* is used to indicate that this examination pertains only to the manifestations or results of pregnancy as elicited abdominally. The content and procedures contained within this segment of the book make no attempt to include all that would be encompassed in an abdominal examination done during a routine screening physical examination as outlined in Chapter 3.

ANTEPARTAL/INTRAPARTAL ABDOMINAL EXAMINATION

General

As outlined in the first section of Chapter 5, abdominal examination of the pregnant woman includes the following:

1. Noting any scars and obtaining explanation of them
2. Checking for diastasis recti
3. Checking for hernia
4. Observation for linea nigra
5. Observation for striae gravidarum
6. Observation or palpation of fetal movement
7. Measurement of fundal height
8. Determination of lie, presentation, position, and variety
9. Checking for fetal heart tones
10. Estimation of fetal weight

The significance of these findings is also discussed in that portion of Chapter 5. The underlying physiology for findings that are presumptive, probable, or positive signs of pregnancy is discussed in Chapter 4.

The segment here on the antepartal and intrapartal abdominal examination is limited to the methods used in measuring fundal height; indications and procedure for measuring abdominal girth; the procedure for doing abdominal palpation and Leopold's maneuvers for determining abdominal muscle tone and fetal lie, presentation, position, variety, and engagement; and the probable location of the fetal heart tones based on the findings elicited from using Leopold's maneuvers. The skill of estimating fetal weight is discussed in Chapter 5.

Measuring Fundal Height

Fundal height is measured in one of four ways. All have an inherent degree of inaccuracy because each depends on the examiner's identifying the top of the fundus correctly. Unfortunately some unidentifiable point on the anterior slope of the fundus often is mistaken for the top of the fundus. This error can be avoided by doing the following:

Facing the woman's head as she lies supine, place your hands on each lateral side of the uterus approximately midway between the symphysis and the fundus. Ballotte the uterus between your hands with gentle pressure and, being sure to stay on the transverse (lateral) portion of the uterus, palpate up to the fundus. As you near the top your hands will begin to come together and they will meet at the top of the fundus. Staying on the transverse (lateral) portion of the uterus assures reaching the actual top of the fundus and keeping off its anterior slope.

Even when the top of the fundus is identified correctly, sequential recording of fundal height from antepartal visit to antepartal visit will most likely be rendered useless if different examiners using different ways of measuring fundal heights see the woman. If more than one person will be examining a woman during her pregnancy, all the persons involved must agree to measure fundal height the same way in order for this evaluation tool to have any meaning. The discrepancies between ways of measuring fundal height become apparent in comparing the following discussion of each.

1.   The time-honored and most inaccurate way of measuring fundal height combines a knowledge of where to expect the fundal height to be at various weeks of gestation in relation to the woman's symphysis pubis, umbilicus, and tip of the xyphoid process and the use of the examiner's fingerbreadths as the measuring tool.

The inherent inaccuracies of this method are obvious immediately. First, there is considerable variation between women in the distance from their symphysis pubis to their xyphoid process and in the location of the umbilicus between these two points. Second, there is considerable variation between examiners in the width of their fingers. For example, two fingerbreadths of a thick-fingered person can be the same as three fingerbreadths of a thin-fingered person.

Nevertheless, this method is useful if you do not have calipers or a tape measure immediately available as it does enable you to ascertain that growth is occurring. Also, it does provide you with a good guide for establishing general expectations that can be used as a baseline against which to compare actual findings. While, indeed, this may be of somewhat questionable accuracy, it is a rule of thumb accurate enough to identify gross discrepancies between estimated gestational age by dates and by findings and to indicate the need for further investigation to rule out the possible causes for this discrepancy.

Table 41-1 lists the approximate expected location of the fundal height at various weeks of gestation. These are also shown in Figure 41-1.

2.   The caliper method of measuring fundal height is used infrequently, probably because a tape measure is cheaper, more easily portable, easier to read, and less awkward to use. The caliper method is, however, probably the most accurate method of measuring fundal height after the twenty-second to twenty-fourth week of gestation. The calipers are used by placing one tip on the superior border of the symphysis publis and the other tip at the top of the

TABLE 41-1. Approximate Expected Location of the Fundal Height at Various Weeks of Gestation

Weeks of Gestation	Approximate Expected Location of Fundal Height
12	Level of the symphysis pubis
16	Halfway between symphysis pubis and umbilicus
20	1–2 fingerbreadths below umbilicus
24	1–2 fingerbreadths above umbilicus
28–30	⅓ of the way between umbilicus and xyphoid process (3 fingerbreadths above umbilicus)
32	⅔ of the way between umbilicus and xyphoid process (3–4 fingerbreadths below xyphoid process)
36–38	1 fingerbreadth below xyphoid process
40	2–3 fingerbreadths below xyphoid process if lightening occurs

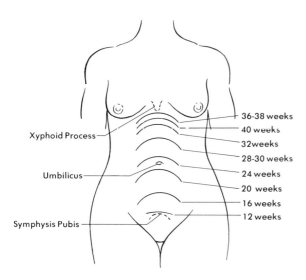

FIGURE 41-1. Approximate expected location of the normal height of the fundus during pregnancy.

fundus. Both placements are in the abdominal midline. Do not confuse the superior edge of the pubic hair line for the superior border of the symphysis pubis. The measurement is then read on a centimeter scale located on an arc close to where the two ends of the calipers come together. The number of centimeters should be equal approximately to the weeks of gestation after about 22 to 24 weeks of gestation.

3. Measuring fundal height with a tape measure is the most frequently used method for obtaining an exact measurement. It is also probably the second most accurate method of measuring fundal height after the twenty-second to twenty-fourth week of gestation. The zero line of the tape measure is placed on the superior border of the symphysis pubis and the tape measure stretched across the contour of the abdomen to the top of the fundus. The abdominal midline is used as the line of measurement. Again, do not confuse the superior edge of the pubic hair line for the superior border of the symphysis pubis. These two *different* landmarks often do *not* coincide. You must palpate for the symphysis pubis in order to locate its superior border. The number of centimeters measured should be approximately equal to the weeks of gestation after about 22 to 24 weeks' gestation.

4. The fourth method of measuring fundal height also utilizes a tape measure. In this method, however, the method of measuring differs. The zero line of the tape measure is again placed on the superior border of the symphysis pubis in the abdominal midline. The hand that is maintaining the identification of the top of the fundus is placed at right angles to the top of the fundus (i.e., the side of the hand with the side of the little finger as the bottom edge is placed at the top of the fundus). The tape measure is then run through the index and middle fingers at the abdominal midline with the centimeter measurement read at the point over the top of the fundus. In effect, then, the tape measure follows the contour of the abdomen only as far as its apex and then is relatively straight to the point held by the fingers, thereby not following the contour of the anterior slope of the fundus. The centimeters lost by the tape measure's not following the contour of the anterior slope of the fundus

are accounted for in the mathematics of this method, which are as follows:

Before the fundus reaches the level of the umbilicus — add 4 centimeters to the number of centimeters measured. The subsequent total number of centimeters should be approximately equal to the weeks of gestation.

After the fundus has reached the level of the umbilicus — add 6 centimeters to the number of centimeters measured. The subsequent total number of centimeters should be approximately equal to the weeks of gestation.

While this method is used by a number of clinicians, there has not been any research done to show its equivalency to (or deviation from) the other methods of obtaining a centimeter measurement or to show its accuracy as to whether the mathematical formula is indeed correct in relation to the weeks of gestation.

The problem is that if one examiner were to use this method and record the actual measurement (without the addition of the centimeters in the formula) and the next examiner were to record a centimeter measurement of the fundal height obtained in accord with the usual method of using the tape measure (method 3), there would be a discrepancy of figures that would cause serious concern about the gestational growth of the fetus. Thus, the plea for communication and uniformity of method among clinicians practicing together is well founded.

Measuring Abdominal Girth

The measurement of abdominal girth is an adjunctive screening tool for deviation from normal after the thirty-fourth week of gestation in women of no more than average size. Specifically, measuring abdominal girth is useful when an oversized uterus is suspected. Of the conditions which may cause an oversized

uterus, two increase the breadth of the uterus as well as the length. These two conditions are multiple gestation and polyhydramnios.

The procedure for measuring abdominal girth is to encircle the woman's body with a tape measure at the level of the umbilicus. Generally, the measurement is normally approximately 2 inches less than the week of gestation. For example, one would expect an approximate measurement of 32 inches (or 81 centimeters) at 34 weeks' gestation; 34 inches (or 86 centimeters) at 36 weeks' gestation, 36 inches (or 91 centimeters) at 38 weeks' gestation, and 38 inches (or 96½ centimeters) at 40 weeks' gestation.

A general rule of thumb is that any measurement more than 100 centimeters (or 39½ inches) is larger than normal at any week of late gestation and requires further investigation to ascertain the reason for this oversized uterus.

Gross obesity will skew the accuracy of abdominal girth findings, which is the reason for limiting the use of this tool to women of no more than average size. Possibly this inaccuracy could be circumvented by obtaining a baseline measurement on obese women prior to the thirty-fourth week of gestation.

Abdominal girth measurement, like fundal height measurement, may be inaccurate due to different body builds. It is, however, still accurate enough to be useful as a gross screening tool, especially when in a situation of limited access to more sophisticated diagnostic tools such as ultrasound.

Abdominal Palpation and Leopold's Maneuvers

The term *abdominal palpation* is often used to mean doing Leopold's maneuvers for determining fetal lie, presentation, position, variety, and engagement. However, this is not precisely accurate. Other information is obtained while doing Leopold's maneuvers, and further abdominal palpation may be involved than that strictly needed for doing Leopold's maneuvers. The following information is obtained from abdominal palpation that includes the performance of Leopold's maneuvers:

Evaluation of uterine irritability, tone, tenderness, consistency, and any present contractility

Evaluation of abdominal muscle tone

Detection of fetal movement

Estimation of fetal weight

Determination of fetal lie, presentation, position, and variety

Determination of whether the head is engaged

Evaluation of abdominal muscle tone is important because muscle tone can influence the pregnancy in a number of ways, ranging from the discomfort of low back pain to the presenting part's overriding the symphysis pubis and having difficulty entering the true pelvis. Abdominal muscle tone becomes progressively more lax with increasing parity, especially if the woman has not done muscle tightening and toning exercises after each delivery. The method for evaluating abdominal muscle tone is presented in the postpartal segment of this discussion on obstetric abdominal examination.

Before performing abdominal palpation and Leopold's maneuvers during the antepartal or intrapartal abdominal examination, several preparatory and general procedures are done:

Preparatory and General Procedures	Rationale
1. The woman's bladder should be empty.	1. A full bladder makes abdominal palpation very uncomfortable for the woman as pressure is applied to it. It also makes it difficult to feel fetal structures beneath the bladder, thereby obscuring findings pertaining to the presenting part.
2. The woman's abdomen is completely exposed from just below the breasts to the symphysis pubis.	2. Exposes no more than that necessary for the examination. Complete exposure of the abdomen at one time is essential for visual observation of the contours of the abdomen.
3. The woman's abdominal muscles should be relaxed. This is accomplished by doing *all* of the following: a. placing a pillow under her head and upper shoulders. b. having her arms by her sides or across her chest. c. explaining what you will be doing. d. helping her with relaxation breathing techniques, if needed. e. having her bend her knees slightly. This is especially important for Leopold's third and fourth maneuvers.	3. Palpation is difficult for both the woman and the examiner if the abdominal muscles are contracted. It is difficult for the examiner to feel the fetus and therefore leads to longer and more forcible palpation. This causes the woman discomfort and she tenses her muscles in bodily self-protection. Thus, a vicious cycle is in operation. All of this is avoided by starting with relaxed abdominal muscles, with warm hands, and with smooth and gentle, but firm, palpation as described in Steps 4 and 6. a., b., and e. These steps reduce stretching

Procedure	Rationale
	and, therefore, tension of the abdominal muscles.
4. Be sure your hands are warm. If not, hold them under warm water, rub them together, or hold them under a light until warm.	4. Cold hands are uncomfortable to the woman. They may also cause muscle contraction.
5. Before palpating, lightly (but not so lightly as to tickle) rest your hand on the woman's abdomen. A good time for this is while you are explaining what you are going to do. (See Fig. 41-2.)	5. This action gives the woman an opportunity to adjust to and become accustomed to your touching her. Since this is not uncomfortable to her, it gives her initial muscle-tightening reaction to being touched time to dissipate.
6. The technique of palpation is as follows:	6. This technique of palpation is designed for the least possible discomfort for the woman and the gathering of the greatest amount of information for the examiner.
a. use the flat palmar surface of your fingers for palpating — *not* your fingertips. b. keep the fingers of your hands together. c. apply smooth deep pressure as firm as is necessary to obtain accurate findings. d. avoid any sudden movement, jabbing, poking, or prodding — you are palpating a woman's abdomen, not kneading bread.	a., b., and c. cover the greatest contiguous area in the shortest amount of time with the greatest degree of tactile sensitivity. d. there is no excuse for a rough abdominal examination. Not only is the woman's cooperation and trust lost but such an examination may also cause abdominal muscle tension and uterine contraction rendering the obtaining of accurate findings difficult if not impossible.

Before actual palpation, the abdomen should be inspected for what its contours can tell you about the fetal lie, presentation, position, and variety. Palpation then gives you further information with which to confirm or rule out this initial impression.

Leopold's maneuvers (Fig. 41-3) consist of four maneuvers starting at the fundus and ending at the pelvic brim. The experienced clinician may be observed starting with any one of the four maneuvers. It is suggested that the learner, however, go through the steps sequentially due to the fact that, in this pattern, they form a thought process and create a mental image for determining fetal position that will most quickly aid you in developing skill and accuracy. Consistently following an orderly sequence will also aid in remembering to include all the maneuvers and gathering all the necessary information. In doing Leopold's maneuvers, stand at the side of the bed most convenient and comfortable for you. Barring contrary room arrangements, right-handed people generally stand on the right side of the woman and left-handed people generally stand on the left side of the woman.

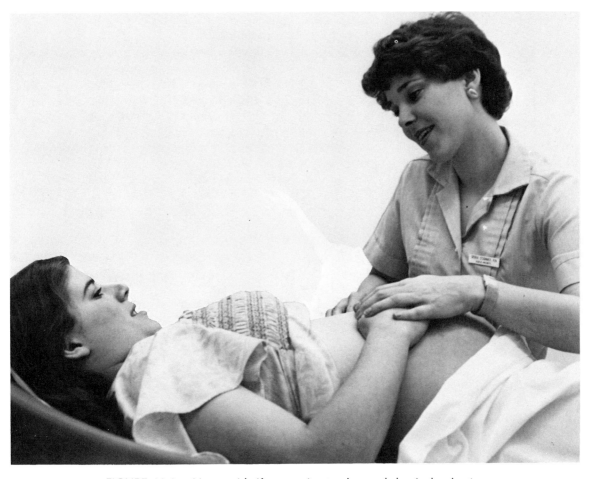

FIGURE 41-2.   Nurse-midwife preparing to do an abdominal palpation.

Observations	Significance
1. A longitudinal ovoid; fundal height as expected for gestational age.	1. Indicative of a longitudinal lie.
2. A transverse ovoid; fundal height lower than expected for gestational age.	2. Indicative of a transverse lie.
3. Long smooth curve prominent on one side of the abdomen.	3. Indicative that the fetal back is on that side of the abdomen.
4. A saucerlike depression just below the umbilicus and a bulge like a full bladder above the symphysis pubis.	4. Indicative of a posterior position.
5. Movement of fetal small parts all over the abdomen.	5. Indicative of a posterior position.

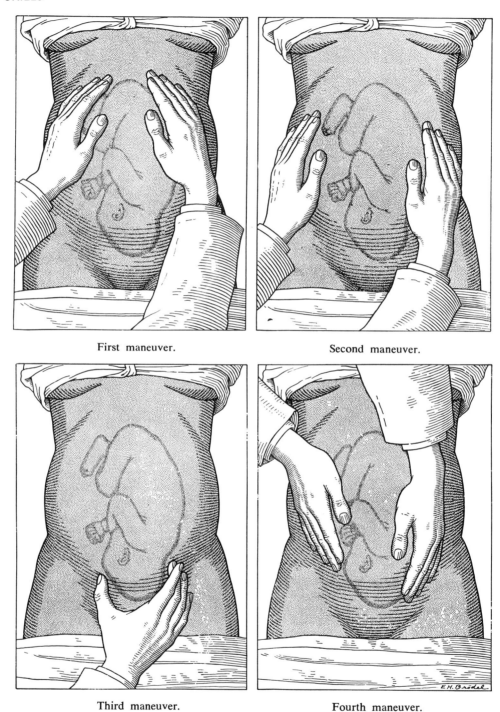

First maneuver.   Second maneuver.

Third maneuver.   Fourth maneuver.

FIGURE 41-3.   Leopold's maneuvers. Palpation in left occiput anterior position. (Reproduced by permission from Pritchard, J. A., and Mac-Donald, P. C. Willams Obstetrics, *15th.* New York: Appleton-Century-Crofts, 1976.)

Procedure	Findings	Significance

1. First maneuver (Fig. 41-3):
  a. face the woman's head.
  b. place your hands on the sides of the fundus and curve your fingers around the top of the fundus.
  c. palpate for shape, size, consistency, and mobility.
  d. ask yourself the question: What is in the fundus?
	1.1 Fetal part feels round and hard; is readily movable; and can be ballotted between the fingers of your two hands or between the thumb and a finger of one hand.
	
	1.2 Fetal part feels irregular, larger or bulkier, and less firm than a head. It cannot be well delineated or readily moved or ballotted.
	1.3 Neither of the above is felt in the fundus.
		1.1 Indicative of a fetal head. The mobility is due to the head's being able to move independently of the trunk. The lie is longitudinal.
		
		1.2 Indicative of the fetal breech. The breech cannot move independently of the trunk. The lie is longitudinal.
		1.3 Indicative of a transverse lie.

2. Second maneuver (Fig. 41-3):
  a. continue to face the woman's head.
  b. place your hands on both side of the uterus about midway between the symphysis pubis and the fundus.
  c. apply pressure with one hand against the side of the uterus, thereby pushing the fetus to the other side of the abdomen and your examining hand, and stabilizing it there. Maintain this pressure while your examining hand palpates the other side of the uterus.
  d. your examining hand palpates the entire area from the abdominal midline to the lateral side and from the symphysis pubis
	2.1 A firm, convex, continuously smooth, and resistant mass extending from the breech to the neck.
	
	2.2 Small, knobby, irregular masses which move when pressed on or may kick or hit your examining hand.
	
	2.3 Small parts all over the abdomen. The back is difficult to feel as it seems to be just out of reach in the posterior portion of the abdomen.
		2.1 Indicative of the fetal back. The location of the back in the left or right side of the woman's abdomen determines the position in a longitudinal lie. The location of the back in the anterior, lateral, or posterior portion of the abdomen determines the variety.
		2.2 Indicative of the fetal small parts — hands, feet, knees, elbows. Should be in opposite side of woman than the side the fetal back is in.
		
		2.3 Indicative of a posterior position.

Procedure	Findings	Significance
to the fundus. Use firm, smooth pressure and rotary movement. e. reverse the procedure for examination of the side of the uterus.		

Some clinicians either add or substitute another procedure for this maneuver. Its name, "walking your fingers over the abdomen," is descriptive of the procedure, which is as follows:

1. Start on one side of the abdomen and apply deep and firm pressure with the fingers of both hands.
2. Then move (walk) your fingers across the abdomen from one lateral side to the other lateral side.

The pressure applied by your fingers will enable you to differentiate the firm back from the knobby small parts, which will ease away from your fingers as you cross over them. The art of this procedure lies in doing it in a way that does not cause discomfort for the woman. This requires fingers experienced and knowledgeable about what they feel. It is, therefore, not suggested for the beginner.

Procedure	Findings	Significance
3. Third maneuver (Fig. 41-3). a. continue to face the woman's head. b. it is essential that the woman have her knees bent in order to avoid discomfort during this maneuver. c. grasp the portion of the lower abdomen immediately above the symphysis pubis between the thumb and middle finger of one of your outstretched hands. It will be necessary to press gently but firmly into the abdomen in order to feel the presenting part below and between your thumb and finger.	3. Same as for the first maneuver except: 3.1 the findings are in the lower pole. 3.2 If the presenting part is the head, it may not be readily movable as will be the situation if the head is engaged. If the head is above the pelvic brim, it is readily movable and ballottable, as described for the first maneuver if it were instead in the fundus.	3. Same as for first maneuver.

The findings from the first and third maneuvers must be compared and final determination made of the lie and presentation.

Procedure	Findings	Significance
d. a movable mass will be felt if the presenting part is not engaged. As in the first maneuver, palpate for shape, size, consistency, and mobility in order to differentiate if it is the breech or head in the lower pole of the abdomen. Ask yourself: What is in the lower pole?		

Leopold's third maneuver is also known as Pawlik's maneuver or Pawlik's grip. An additional procedure to this maneuver is called the combined Pawlik grip, in which Pawlik's grip is done with one hand and the fundus is grasped in the same way with the other hand at the same time. This combination enables you to compare simultaneously what is in the two poles for final determination of the fetal lie and presentation.

Procedure	Findings	Significance

4. Fourth maneuver (Fig. 41-3):
  a. turn and face the woman's feet.
  b. make sure that the woman's knees are bent in order to avoid pain with this maneuver.
  c. place your hands on the sides of the uterus with the palms of your hands just below the level of the umbilicus and your fingers directed towards the symphysis pubis.
  d. press deeply with your fingertips into the lower abdomen and move them toward the pelvic inlet.
	4.1 If the head is the presenting part, one of the following will happen:
	  a. one of your hands will make contact with a hard round mass while your other hand continues on in the direction of the pelvis.
		4.1.
		
		  a. this is the cephalic prominence. If it is on the same side of the woman as is the fetal back the cephalic prominence is the occiput and indicates a face presentation because the head is extended. If the cephalic prominence is on the same side of the woman as are the fetal small parts, it is the sinciput (forehead) and indicates a vertex presentation since the head is well flexed.

Procedure	Rationale
	b. both of your hands will encounter simultaneously a hard round mass which is equally prominent on both sides.	b. indicates a sincipital (or military) presentation. Due to partial flexion of the head your hands are feeling the sinciput and the occiput at the same time.
e. in a breech presentation, or in a head presentation after you have palpated the cephalic prominence, your hands continue their movement toward the pelvic inlet. At the brim of the true pelvis, your hands will be unable to continue in this direction because the symphysis pubis prevents further movement.	4.2 At the brim of the pelvis your hands will either: a. converge around the presenting part with the fingertips of your two hands touching in the abdominal midline. If the presenting part is the head it will be readily movable. If the presenting part is the breech it will have a feeling of give along with the trunk of the fetus.	a. the presenting part is not engaged. Rather, it is floating at or above the pelvic inlet as determined by being at or above the symphysis pubis.
	b. diverge away from the presenting part and the abdominal midline. There will be no give or mobility of the presenting part.	b. this presenting part is either engaged or dipping. Dipping is when the presenting part has entered the pelvic inlet but has not yet descended to the point of engagement. If you are unable to feel the cephalic prominence because it is out of reach in the pelvis, the head is engaged.

5. Share your findings with the woman. Offer to help her feel and identify various fetal parts if she would like.

Location of fetal heart tones

Abdominal palpation determining the lie, presentation, position, and variety of the fetus enables you to locate the fetal heart tones. This is because the sound of the fetal heart is transmitted through the convex portion of the fetus closest to the anterior uterine wall. Therefore the fetal heart tones are best heard through the fetal back in vertex and breech presentations and through the chest in face presentations. Thus, if you know the position of the fetus you can readily locate the fetal heart tones, allowing for some variation depending on the amount of descent of the fetus into the pelvis.

Conversely, location of the fetal heart tones is an additional piece of data that serves to confirm or question your diagnosis of the fetal position. If you find the fetal heart tones loudest in a location different from where you expected to find them, then the question is raised if you were in error in findings or in your interpretation of your findings from abdominal palpation.

In a full-term fetus with an unengaged presenting part, the fetal heart tones are best heard in the following general locations in relation to general presentations, positions, and varieties. Specific locations of the fetal heart tone maximum intensity for specific fetal positions are shown in Figure 41-4 and Table 41-2.

Recording the fetal heart tones consists of two pieces of information: the rate and the location of maximum intensity. The location is identified by dividing the abdomen into four quadrants by drawing imaginary vertical and horizontal lines which bisect each other at the umbilicus as follows:

$$\begin{array}{c|c} RUQ & LUQ \\ \hline RLQ & LLQ \end{array}$$

RUQ = right upper quadrant
RLQ = right lower quadrant

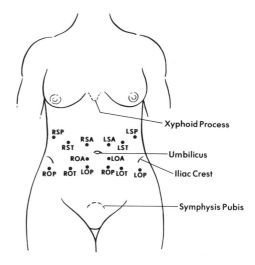

FIGURE 41-4. Location of the point of maximum intensity of the fetal heart tones for specific fetal positions.

TABLE 41-2. Locating Fetal Heart Tones in Various Fetal Presentations and Positional Varieties

Presentations and Positional Varieties	Location
Cephalic	Midway between umbilicus and level of anterior superior iliac spine
Breech	Level with or above umbilicus
Anterior	Close to abdominal midline
Transverse	In lateral abdominal area
Posterior	In flank area or close to abdominal midline on other side of abdomen

LUQ = left upper quadrant
LLQ = left lower quadrant

Charting is then by one of the following three ways:

1. RLQ-140

2. $\dfrac{\quad|\quad}{140\ |}$

3.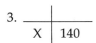

The latter can be the most informative as the X in the quadrant can be placed in accord with the anterior, lateral, or flank position of the fetal heart tones.

POSTPARTAL ABDOMINAL EXAMINATION

The postpartal abdominal examination is that done during the early postpartal period (1 hour to 5 days). It includes the following:

1. Examination of the bladder
2. Examination of the uterus
3. Evaluation of abdominal muscle tone by determination of the degree of diastasis
4. Checking for CVA tenderness (see Chapter 42)

Bladder

Examination of the bladder is specifically for bladder distention due to urinary retention from bladder hypotonicity because of trauma during childbirth. This condition can predispose to bladder infection and be responsible for an increase in uterine bleeding. Evidence of a full bladder, therefore, is looked for during the abdominal examination.

Bladder distention can be seen by observing the abdominal contour as a bulge above the symphysis pubis extending toward the umbilicus. Sometimes the initial indication of a distended bladder is displacement of the uterus upward and to the right side. The full bladder can then be palpated in the lower abdomen.

Uterus

Examination of the uterus includes noting its location, size, and consistency. *Location* of the uterus involves noting if the fundus is above or below the umbilicus and if it is in the abdominal midline or displaced to one side. Location and size overlap, since *size* is determined not only by palpation but also by measuring where the height of the uterine fundus is.

Measuring the fundal height of the postpartum uterus is done by the number of fingerbreadths the top of the fundus is above or below the umbilicus. (See the first part of Chapter 24 for norms.) Like measuring the pregnant uterus, it is essential to accurately identify the top of the fundus. Again, this can be done by placing your hands on the lateral sides of the uterus and ballotting it between your hands as you palpate up to the fundus. Your fingers will come together at the top of the fundus if you stay on the lateral portion of the uterus, thereby avoiding ending on the anterior slope of the uterus and consequently obtaining an erroneous measurement. Within a few days it will be necessary to measure the top of the fundus in relation to the symphysis pubis rather than to the umbilicus; it is not normally palpable after the tenth day postpartum above the symphysis pubis.

The *consistency* of the uterus is evaluated as firm or soft. *Firm* is sometimes qualified as *firms with massage* and *soft* is sometimes elaborated upon as *soft and boggy*. A truly firm uterus feels as hard as a rock. A soft uterus feels indentable, and you can feel it hardening beneath your fingers as you massage it. It is important to observe the perineum while feeling for the consistency of the uterus in order to evaluate the effect of uterine stimulation on the amount of lochial flow. If the uterus is firm initially, there will not be an increase in the flow of lochia or expulsion of clots with palpation. If the uterus is soft initially, uterine palpation will cause contractions which will expel any accumulated blood and clots. After the uterus is emptied of this accumulation, the lochial flow normally will lessen and the uterus become firm.

Findings obtained from examination of the uterus can be recorded in more than one way, as is illustrated in the charting of the two following sets of findings. One way, of course, is to write the findings out. The other three ways utilize types of generally accepted shorthand notations. These notations are further abbreviated by the assumption that the uterus is in the midline unless otherwise noted. They are presented here in the order of their frequency of use.

Findings: The fundus is firm at 2 fingerbreadths below the umbilicus in the midline.

1. ff @ U/2
2. ff @ 2 fb ↓ ⊙
3. ff @ _____
                 ⨯2

Findings: The fundus is soft at 3 fingerbreadths above the umbilicus and displaced to the right side.

1. f soft @ 3/U to the right
2. f soft @ 3 fb ↑ ⊙ to the right
3. f soft @ 3 ⨯|_____

Diastasis

Determination of the amount of diastasis recti is used as an objective means of evaluating abdominal muscle tone. Diastasis is the degree of separation of the abdominal rectus (rectus abdominis) muscles. This separation is measured in terms of fingerbreadths when the abdominal muscles are contracted and again when they are in a state of relaxation.

Measurement of the diastasis is done in the following manner:

1. Position the woman so she is lying on her back without a pillow under her head.

2. Place the tips of the fingers of one of your hands in her abdominal midline with the tip of your index finger just below the umbilicus and the remainder of your fingers lined up longitudinally from there on downward towards the symphysis pubis. The sides of your fingers should be touching each other.

3. Have the woman raise her head and strive to put her chin on her chest in the area between her breasts. (Obviously this is impossible but assures that she will tighten her abdominal muscles, which will not occur if she merely tucks her chin down on the clavicles.) Be sure she is not pressing her hands against the bed or grabbing the mattress to help herself, as this prevents use of her abdominal muscles.

4. As the woman strains to put her chin between her breasts, press your fingertips gently a short distance into her abdomen. You will feel the abdominal muscles, like two bands of rubber, approaching the midline from both sides. If the diastasis is wide, even with the muscles contracted you will need to move your fingers from side to side in order to find the muscles. If the abdominal muscles are in good enough tone to come together in the midline when tightened, you will feel them against your fingers and then underneath your fingers as they push your fingers out of the abdomen.

5. Measure the distance between the two rectus muscles while they are contracted by placing your fingers flat in the longitudinal plane parallel to the rectus muscles and filling in the space between the rectus muscles with your fingerbreadths. Note the number of fingerbreadths between the median edges of the two rectus muscles.

6. Now place the fingertips of one hand longitudinally against the median edge of one abdominal rectus muscle and the

fingertips of your other hand against the median edge of the other rectus abdominis muscle. When properly positioned the backs of your hands should be facing each other in the abdominal midline.

7. Ask the woman to lower her head *slowly* to its original resting position on the bed.

8. As she lowers her head, the rectus muscles will move further apart and become less distinguishable as they relax. With your fingertips follow the rectus muscles as they move apart to their respective lateral sides of the abdomen. This maneuver enables you to still be able to identify them in their relaxed state.

9. Measure the distance between the two rectus muscles while they are relaxed the same way as you did when they were contracted. Note the number of finger-breadths between the median edges of the two rectus muscles.

10. Chart your findings as a fraction with the first or upper number (numerator) the width of the diastasis in fingerbreadths when the muscles were contracted and the second or bottom number (de-nominator) the width of the diastasis in fingerbreadths when the muscles were relaxed. For example, a diastasis that measured 2 fingerbreadths when the muscles were contracted and 5 finger-breadths when the muscles were relaxed would be charted as follows:

diastasis = 2/5 fb.

or, of course, can be written out as:

diastasis = 2 fb. when muscles contracted and 5 fb. when muscles relaxed.

Steps 1, 3, and 7 of the procedure for mea-suring diastasis comprise the chin-chest abdominal muscle tightening exercise. Thus, you have an ideal situation for patient teaching while determining the degree of diastasis.

Unless a woman is in the habit of routine exercising she will need considerable motiva-tion to begin and to continue a program of abdominal muscle tightening exercises. She will exercise only if she experiences a need for it, so you first have to capture her interest. This is done by having her feel "the hole in her stomach" (she's probably already noticed that her abdomen pouches out when she moves around) and then asking her if she wants to know what it is. It is the rare woman who rejects this opportunity. Use the same method for her feeling her abdomen as you did for determining the diastasis.

You now have a listener for your descrip-tion of how the abdominal rectus muscles normally lie side by side, although not con-nected, in the midline; how, as her stomach enlarged with her pregnancy, these muscles became stretched; how, after the baby was born, her muscles collapsed; and how now her abdominal rectus muscles no longer lie side by side but instead are separated and trying to get back together again, as she can feel when she tightens them.

Your next question then is if she wants to know why it is important to get her muscles back together again. Again, it is the rare woman who answers no to this question since this concerns her body. The "whys" total two:

1. To regain her figure. This often is an insuf-ficient motivating factor.

2. To prevent severe backache, especially dur-ing her next pregnancy. Most women will remember having some degree of backache during their pregnancy — frequently, having been miserable with it — and do not want it to an even worse degree the next time.

The motivating factor for many women is an explanation of how it is the abdominal muscles that support the enlarged uterus and baby; how the pregnant uterus will sag for-ward without the support of the abdominal muscles; and a demonstration by you of the effect this will have on the back in the form of an exaggerated lordosis, which is what causes backache during pregnancy.

Your final question then becomes if she wants to know how to get her abdominal muscles back together again. In the vast majority of cases she is now experiencing a need for this information. This is your entree for teaching her the postpartal abdominal tightening exercises, starting with the chin-chest exercise she has already done. Women respond positively to your reminding them that they now know how to check their own progress and that they have reached their goal when they can no longer feel the "hole in their stomach" but can instead feel the muscles lying side by side again.

42

Checking for Costovertebral Angle Tenderness

ANATOMY

The costovertebral angle (CVA) is formed by the junction of the twelfth, or lowermost rib with the paravertebral muscles which run parallel to and on both sides of the vertebral column. The kidney is posteriorly closest to the skin surface in this area and pain is transmitted through the tenth, eleventh, and twelfth thoracic nerves. Ureter pain is transmitted through the twelfth thoracic nerve and the first three lumbar nerves.

SIGNIFICANCE AND CHARTING

Pain elicited in the area of the costovertebral angle is indicative of renal disease. In addition to being a routine part of the physical examination, CVA tenderness is always checked whenever a woman gives a history suggestive of a urinary tract infection after her initial examination.

If there is no CVA tenderness, this is noted under the examination of the abdomen as "No CVAT."

If there is CVA tenderness, this is noted under the examination of the abdomen with its location: "right CVAT," "left CVAT," or "bilateral CVAT."

PROCEDURE AND RATIONALE FOR EXAMINATION

There are several methods for eliciting CVA tenderness. All involve deep pressure or a mild blow to the area. It is important that this not be too vigorous because pain will be experienced if trauma is caused. The point is to identify already existing pain.

Procedure	Rationale

Method A

1. Have the woman in a sitting position with her entire back and trunk exposed.
2. Make a fist out of your examining hand. Use the fleshy side (ulnar surface) of your fist, which is the same side as your little finger, for gently hitting the woman. Forewarn her that this is what you are going to do.
3. Gently pound down one side of the woman's back from the midportion of the woman's scapular area to the midportion of her buttock area just lateral to her paravertebral muscles. Be sure that you hit the costovertebral angle as you move down. Repeat for the other side.

4. Note if the woman winces, jumps, or otherwise evinces pain when you hit the costovertebral angle.

1. This provides exposure of the area to be used in this method of examination.
2. The thumb side of your fist is painful for hitting because of the projection of the knuckle or the thumb on this side of your fist.

3. By starting and ending in areas other than the costovertebral angle, the woman is not conditioned to concentrate on whether or not she feels pain in any one area. It does condition her to feel slight jars or thuds so she is not jumping from being startled by the time you arrive at the costovertebral angle.

4.

Method B

1. The woman is in a sitting position with the area of the costovertebral angle exposed.
2. Place the palm of one hand over the costovertebral angle on one side.
3. Make a fist out of your other hand. Use the ulnar surface of your fist for striking.
4. Strike the back of your hand placed over the costovertebral angle with the fist of your other hand.
5. Note if the woman winces, jumps, or otherwise evinces pain. If so, ascertain if her response was due to pain or to being startled by feeling a mild blow, jar, or thud in this area.
6. Repeat for the costovertebral angle on the other side.

1. Exposure of the area to be examined.
2. through 6. This method is less extensive in performance than Method A and would be better for thin or emaciated women who would feel discomfort wherever hit in Method A.

    Method B requires closer differentiation between actual pain and being startled by the blow — both of which might cause the woman to jump — since she has not been conditioned to being jarred as is true in Method A.

    Method B, however, is useful for double-checking a positive finding elicited by Method A to make sure the pain was indeed elicited at the costovertebral angle. Method A is necessarily less precise in hitting the costovertebral angle.

Procedure	Rationale

Method C

1. The woman is in a supine position, looking up.	1. through 4. Method C is particularly useful when examining a woman who is lying in bed, for example, as a routine part of the postpartal examinations in the hospital.
2. Encircling the woman's waist, locate by palpation the costovertebral angles with the flat part of your index and middle fingers on each hand.	
3. Alternately strike each costovertebral angle with your fingers by a sudden, upward motion of your hand.	Method C requires close differentiation between actual pain or the woman being startled by the blow. This differentiation can be facilitated by telling the woman what you are going to do.
4. Note if the woman winces, jumps, or otherwise evinces pain. If so, ascertain if her response was due to pain or to being startled by feeling a mild blow, jar, or thud in this area.	

A good way to double-check a positive finding elicited by any of the above methods is by deep palpation and pressure in the costovertebral angle. This may be done with the woman either sitting or lying down. Such careful palpation in the precise area aids	differentiation of CVA tenderness from pain in the immediately adjacent back muscles caused by muscle spasm. Deep palpation over these muscles will elicit any existing muscle pain.

43

Checking for Deep Tendon Reflexes and Clonus

DEEP TENDON REFLEXES

Anatomy

Deep tendon reflexes (DTR) are also known as stretch reflexes because they are elicited by briefly stretching a muscle by tapping its tendon briskly. The brisk tap stimulates a sensory nerve impulse that travels through the reflex arc and ends with stimulation of the muscle in a brief contraction. This brief contraction causes a corresponding brief movement, or jerk, of the anatomical body part affected by the contraction of the muscle. Therefore it is necessary, for each reflex tested, to know the name and location of the tendon to tap, the muscle in which to feel the contraction, and the anatomical body part in which to observe the jerk. Table 43-1 supplies this information for the most commonly tested reflexes.

Significance and Charting

Hyperactive deep tendon reflexes are indicative of disease of the upper motor neuron or pyramidal tract and require physician consultation. Hypoactive or absent deep tendon reflexes are indicative of a number of diseases and require physician consultation.

Reflexes are evaluated on a scale of 0 to 4+ as follows:

0 = absent; no response
1+ = decreased; diminished; sluggish
2+ = normal; average
3+ = brisk
4+ = very brisk; hyperactive (usually associated with clonus)

Reflexes designated 1+ are low-normal reflexes; 3+ reflexes are more brisk than the average reflex response and indicate the possible but not absolute presence of disease; 0

TABLE 43-1.   Anatomy of Deep Tendon Reflexes

Reflex	Tendon	Muscle	Body Part That Jerks
Quadriceps (knee-jerk)	Ligamentum patellae — from the apex of the patella to the tuberosity of the tibia	Quadriceps femoris — the anterior thigh muscles consisting of four muscles covering the front and sides of the femur and comprising the front of the thigh; the extensor muscle of the leg	Knee extension and leg jerk
Gastrocnemius-soleus (ankle-jerk)	Tendo calcaneus — (Achilles tendon) — from the middle of the posterior lower leg to the heel	Gastrocnemius and soleus muscles — the posterior leg (calf) muscles	Plantar flexion of the foot at the ankle (points the toes)
Biceps	Tendon of the biceps brachii — crosses the bend of the elbow and inserts in the posterior portion of the tuberosity of the radius	Biceps brachii — the anterior muscle of the upper arm	Flexion of the elbow, arm, and forearm; supinates the hand
Triceps	Tendon of the triceps brachii — from the middle of the posterior upper arm to the elbow	Triceps brachii — the posterior muscle of the upper arm	Extension of the elbow and the forearm; adducts the arm (towards the body)
Brachioradialis	Tendon of the brachioradialis — from the middle of the forearm to the wrist, inserting in the lateral side of the base of the styloid process of the radius	Brachioradialis — the superficial muscle on the radial (thumb) side of the forearm	Flexes the elbow and the forearm

and 4+ reflexes are definitely abnormal and indicative of disease requiring physician consultation. Reflexes should be symmetrical for homologous muscles and so noted in the charting.

In a routine physical examination in which all five deep tendon reflexes are evaluated, a stick figure is frequently used to designate the reflex findings. The figure is marked for its right and left sides. It visually tells the response

evaluation and symmetry of each reflex by location (Fig. 43-1).

If only one or two of the reflexes are evaluated bilaterally then the charting would reflect which ones. For example:

Quadriceps and biceps deep tendon reflexes (DTR) — 2+ and symmetrical

or

Quadriceps DTR — 3+, no clonus, symmetrical

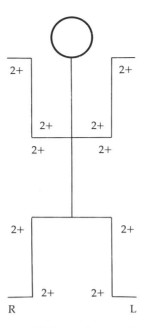

FIGURE 43-1.   Stick-figure for charting that all five deep tendon reflexes are normal (2+) and bilaterally symmetrical.

Procedure	Rationale
1. General:	1.
a. symmetry is determined by comparing the reflex response on one side with the same reflex response on the other side; *not* by comparing the response of different reflexes on the same or opposite sides.	a. different tendons may vary considerably in reflex amplitude, so only the same reflexes on both sides of the body can be compared.
b. in testing reflexes, you should if possible palpate the muscle of the reflex being tested while tapping its tendon.	b. enables evaluation of the vigor of the muscle contraction and the time taken for the muscle to relax after contraction. Slow relaxation of a muscle after contraction is indicative of hypothyroidism.
c. the limb to be tested should be in a flexed or semiflexed position.	c. this places slight tension on the muscle to be tested by mildly stretching it and aids in eliciting the reflex.
d. the woman should be as relaxed as possible. If necessary, in the event the	d. adequate relaxation of the woman is necessary in order for a deep tendon

Procedure	Rationale
woman's reflexes appear absent or symmetrically diminished, use the technique of reinforcement. The technique of reinforcement involves isometric contraction of muscles other than those being tested. For example, while testing leg reflexes ask the woman to interlock her fingers and pull in opposite directions with her eyes closed; or when testing arm reflexes have the woman clench her teeth or squeeze her thigh with the opposite hand, again with her eyes closed.	reflex to be elicited. Reinforcement works in two ways: (1) it distracts the woman and, thereby, causes relaxation. (2) the deliberate contraction of different muscles than those being tested may increase reflex activity. A reflex is not considered absent unless it cannot be elicited while using the technique of reinforcement.
e. tap the tendon briskly. A reflex hammer is most useful for this purpose. If a reflex hammer is not available the edge of your stethoscope or, for the quadriceps reflex, even the tips of your fingers suddenly striking the tendon may suffice.	e. a brisk tap produces a sudden additional stretch of the tendon. The reflex hammer, when held loosely and swung in an arc using wrist action, provides just the tap with the force and briskness necessary. Use of objects other than a reflex hammer is a make-shift way of striking the tendon that may or may not be successful, depending on a number of factors including patient obesity and your ability to really give a brisk tap with either of these alternatives.
f. position the woman so her limbs are symmetrical.	f. this facilitates comparison of sides for each reflex.

2. Eliciting the biceps reflex:
   a. feel for the tendon of the biceps brachii muscle in the bend of the elbow. This can be identified by bending the woman's arm up and down at the elbow.
   b. place the thumb of one of your hands firmly on the tendon.
   c. position the woman's arm so it is partially flexed at the elbow and resting either in her lap or supported on your arm (the same arm as the thumb you are using).
   d. tap the tendon indirectly by striking your thumb with the pointed end of the reflex hammer.

Procedure	Rationale

3. Eliciting the triceps reflex:
   a. position the woman's arm so it is flexed at the elbow and resting across her chest with the palm of her hand of that arm towards her body. Lightly hold the woman's arm in this position with your hand around her wrist.
   b. palpate for the tendon of the triceps brachii muscle on the back of her upper arm above the elbow.
   c. directly strike the tendon just above (approximately 2 inches, or about 5 centimeters) her elbow with either the pointed or the broad end of the reflex hammer.
4. Eliciting the brachioradialis reflex:
   a. position the woman's forearm so it is resting on her lap or abdomen with her arm slightly flexed at the elbow and hand slightly bent at the wrist.
   b. palpate for the radius. Since the brachioradialis tendon inserts directly into the radius it is sufficient to strike the bone itself to elicit this reflex.
   c. tap the radius with either the pointed or broad end of the reflex hammer approximately 1 to 2 inches (2½ to 5 centimeters) above the wrist.
5. Eliciting the quadriceps (knee-jerk) reflex:
   a. position the woman so that her knees are somewhat flexed. If the woman is lying down, support her knees in the flexed position with your hand under her knees so her lower leg is relaxed. It is not, however, necessary to have the woman's foot off of the bed. If the woman is sitting, be sure that her legs dangle over the edge of the examining table or bed with her weight on her buttocks and thighs, and her feet not resting on any object or the floor.
   b. palpate for the patella and then identify the patellar tendon just below it.

Procedure	Rationale

c. tap the patellar tendon with the pointed end of the reflex hammer.
6. Eliciting the gastrocnemius-soleus (ankle-jerk) reflex:
    a. position the woman's leg so it is somewhat flexed at the knee.
    b. with one hand, dorsiflex the ankle by holding the foot in a position approximating the dorsiflexion it would be in if the woman were standing.
    c. palpate for the Achilles tendon above the woman's heel.
    d. tap the Achilles tendon approximately 2 to 3 inches (5 to 7½ centimeters) above the heel.	

CLONUS

Clonus ranges from one or two beats to a sustained beating.

Definition

Clonus is involuntary, rapid, repetitive, rhythmical contractions and relaxations of a muscle when it is sharply stretched and the stretch is maintained in either flexion or extension.

Procedure for Eliciting Clonus

Clonus may be elicited at a number of sites such as the wrist, knee, big toe, and ankle. The most commonly used site in obstetric care, however, is the ankle. For this reason, only the procedure for eliciting ankle clonus will be given.

Significance and Evaluation

Clonus should always be checked for in the presence of hyperreflexia since extremely hyperactive reflexes are a precursor of clonus.

Clonus is indicative of upper motor neuron disease and is never present except when there is disease of the central nervous system. Physician consultation is required when there clonus.

Clonus is evaluated not only by its presence but also by counting the number of times the muscle contracts and relaxes while stretched. The sequential contractions are felt as jerks and are frequently called the number of beats.

1. Position the woman so her knee is partially flexed. Support this position with one of your hands underneath the bend in her knee.
2. With your other hand grasping her foot, sharply dorsiflex her foot and maintain pressure to keep it in dorsiflexion.
3. Any existing beats of clonus may be both felt and seen as the muscle contractions and relaxations would cause rhythmical alteration between dorsiflexion and plantar flexion. The muscles being stretched are the same as for the ankle-jerk reflex—the gastrocnemius and soleus muscles.

44

Pelvic Examination

PROCEDURES, OBSERVATIONS OR FINDINGS, AND SIGNIFICANCE

Preparatory and General Procedures

Procedure	Rationale
1. In general terms explain what you will be doing during the pelvic examination. If this is a woman's first pelvic examination, show her the equipment you will be using and explain its purpose. Ask the woman if she would like to learn about her own body, if not already familiar. If so, provide a mirror in order to identify her external genitalia and hymenal ring. Use the mirror and a flashlight to enable her to see her own cervix and vaginal walls during the speculum examination. During the different parts of the examination keep the woman informed a half-jump ahead of what you are doing. Forewarn her when you are about to touch her or insert the speculum, or when something may be uncomfortable or hurt.	1. To elicit the woman's cooperation. An informed woman is more relaxed than an uninformed woman. Explanations of what you are doing and the equipment you are using is in keeping with the philosophy of a woman's right to know what you are doing in relationship to her body.
2. Be sure the woman's bladder is empty before starting the examination.	2. Bimanual examination is extremely uncomfortable for a woman if her bladder is

Procedure	Rationale
	full. A full bladder also makes it difficult for you to palpate the pelvic organs.
3. Position the woman in the lithotomy position on an examining table. Be sure that her buttocks are slightly beyond the edge of the table. Help her to know how far to move down the table by telling her to move until she touches your hand (which is just beyond the edge of the table). Her arms should be down beside her or across her abdomen. Place a pillow under her head. In the absence of a pillow and in the presence of a thin covering mat on the table, roll up the mat behind her as she moves down to the end of the table and use the rolled mat as a pillow.	3. If the woman is not properly positioned with her buttocks just beyond the edge of the table, it will be in the way of the handle of the speculum and you will have difficulty positioning the speculum. Many women automatically put their hands behind their head when in the lithotomy position. Raising her arms stretches and tightens the abdominal muscles, making the bimanual examination more difficult and uncomfortable. This is circumvented by having the woman put her arms down (explain why) and putting something else under her head to increase comfort and relaxation.
4. Drape the woman in such a way that she feels the minimal possible exposure and so that your view of her face is not blocked in either the sitting or standing positions you will assume during the examination.	4. To protect her modesty and privacy, which facilitates relaxation. You must be able to see her face at all times in order to maintain personal contact with the woman and notice any facial expressions indicative of discomfort, pain, embarrassment, or fear so you can help her. In other words, you must maintain active awareness that there is a person involved above the waist.
5. Wash your hands and put on a glove or gloves.	5. It does not matter whether you use the one-glove or two-glove method as long as your technique of use is such that: a. you do not bring any disease to the woman by touching her with an ungloved hand or touching her with a gloved hand that has touched something else. b. you do not risk contracting any disease from the woman by virtue of touching her with an ungloved hand. c. you keep clean, clean and you keep dirty, dirty. For instance, you need to be able to turn on and off the gooseneck lamp and manipulate it for visualization without touching the woman either before or afterwards with the same glove or hand.

Procedure	Rationale
	Some clinicians use a combination of the methods by positioning the lighted lamp first, then putting on two gloves for inspection of the external genitalia and insertion of the speculum, and then removing one glove for further manipulation of the lamp and turning it off.
6. Ask the woman to separate or spread her legs. Do not try to spread the woman's legs forcibly or even gently.	6. Pelvic examination is an intrusive procedure and should proceed only as the woman is ready for it. This act signals her readiness and cooperation.
7. Help the woman throughout the examination to be as relaxed as possible. This is *not* done by telling her to relax. It *is* accomplished by telling her *how* to relax: a. if she is familiar with breathing and relaxation techniques used in labor, have her utilize these. If not, have her concentrate on slow abdominal or chest breathing — whichever she can do most easily. b. ask her to think of herself as a rag doll or wet washcloth or anything else you can think of that connotes the idea of limpness. It is vital that her legs remain well separated as she relaxes and that this point and its rationale are emphasized to the woman.	7. Relaxation is essential to a pelvic examination. It makes the examination of the least possible discomfort to the woman; facilitates your ability to adequately feel and evaluate the pelvic organs; and shortens the length of time of the examination by virtue of your not having difficulty in the conduct of the examination. It is next to impossible to conduct an adequate and accurately informative pelvic examination if the woman clamps her legs around your examining hand. You simply cannot maneuver your hand in this situation to feel and evaluate the pelvic organs and structures.
8. Your approach to the woman should be super gentle, both verbally and physically. Your touch and manipulation of the speculum should be firm but gentle (i.e., firm enough not to tickle but not so firm as to traumatize). Remember that the woman's whole attitude toward necessary future pelvic examinations, her self-concept of her sexuality, her sex life, and her willingness to cooperate with any therapeutic regimen you suggest may be positively or negatively	8. There is no excuse for a rough pelvic examination. There is considerable difference between gently doing something that may be uncomfortable or even hurt, such as clinical pelvimetry, and being rough. The woman knows the difference. Pelvic examination is an intrusive procedure and women are acutely alert to your attitude of respect — or lack of respect — to their bodies. They can tolerate and cope with any necessary discomfort or pain

Procedure	Rationale
influenced by your conduct of her pelvic examination.	if forewarned and told why it is necessary, and if it is done in a supportive, caring manner that expresses regret for its necessity and facilitates the woman's efforts to relax throughout.
9. If the woman gets uptight, tense, or generally upset during your examination, immediately stop whatever you are doing. This means holding your fingers, hand, or speculum still — do not remove your hand or the speculum. Ascertain what the problem is. If the complaint is pain, have the woman differentiate between feeling discomfort as a result of pressure, feeling actual pain, or not feeling any discomfort or pain but being fearful and tense in anticipation of feeling pain. Tell the woman that you will not proceed further until she is again in control, relaxed, and ready. Help the woman with relaxation techniques and anything else she identifies that will be helpful to her in coping with this procedure.	9. The rationale is the same as for 6, 7, and 8 above.

Inspection of the External Genitalia

Procedure	Observations	Significance
1. Seat yourself on a stool at the end of the examining table so you are at eye level with the woman's perineum. Your light should already be adjusted for good visualization of the woman's perineum and your gloves should be on. Tell the woman that you are going to examine her external genitalia ("privates," "the outside down here") and that she will feel your fingers touching this area.	1. a. observe the mons pubis (mons veneris) for: (1) pattern of hair growth (2) pediculosis (lice)	1. a. (1) secondary sex characteristic. Useful information in determining which oral contraceptive to prescribe for a woman (2) if present. Treatment indicated will vary, depending on whether or not the woman is pregnant

Procedure	Observations	Significance
	b. inspect the labia majora and perineum for: (1) normal appearance in size and shape (2) localized labial swelling, edema, or small cysts	b. (1) may vary from individual to individual (2) localized labial swelling may be caused by a Bartholin's abscess or cyst; labial edema may be due to an allergic reaction; small cysts may be sebaceous cysts
	(3) inflammation, dermatitis, irritation	(3) may be indicative of a vaginal infection. Ask the woman if she has been itching or scratching in the area.
	(4) discoloration and tenderness (5) varicosities	(4) traumatic bruising (5) useful information in planning delivery techniques for a pregnant woman
	(6) lesions, vesicles, ulcerations, crusting (7) condylomata (lata or acuminata, wart-like growths)	(6) may be syphilitic chancre, herpes (7) condylomata lata — usually syphilitic; condylomata acuminata — nonveneral in origin, they are often stimulated by increased vaginal secretions during pregnancy
	(8) old episiotomy scar or scars of repaired or unrepaired perineal lacerations	(8) useful information in planning delivery techniques for a pregnant woman
2. Separate the labia majora, inspect the labia minora. Then separate the labia	2. a. inspect the labia minora and vestibula for: (1) normal appearance	2. a. (1) this may vary great-

Procedure	Observations	Significance
minora and inspect the clitoris, the inside of the labia minora, vestibule, urethral orifice, and vaginal introitus.	in size and shape	ly within the realm of normal
	(2) inflammation, dermatitis, irritation, or caking of discharge in the fold between the labia majora and the labia minora	(2) may be indicative of a vaginal infection or of poor hygiene
	(3) discoloration and tenderness	(3) traumatic bruising
	(4) fistulas	(4) physician consultation required
	(5) fissures	(5) physician consultation required
	(6) herpetic vesicles	(6) physician consultation required
	(7) chancre — syphilitic lesion	(7) physician consultation required
	b. inspect the clitoris for:	b.
	(1) adhesions with the labia minora	(1) ascertain if problematic or not
	(2) enlargement	(2) possible masculinizing condition
	c. inspect the urethral orifice for:	c.
	(1) growths — polyps, caruncles	(1) physician consultation required
	(2) irritation, dilatation	(2) may be indicative of repeated urinary tract infections or insertion of foreign objects. Question the woman accordingly
	(3) fistulas	(3) requires physician consultation
	d. inspect the vaginal introitus for:	d.
	(1) the hymen or its remnants (myrtiform caruncles)	(1) normal unless tight and rigid or imperforate

Procedure	Observations	Significance
	(2) vaginal discharge	(2) may be indicative of a vaginal infection
	(3) discoloration and tenderness	(3) traumatic bruising
	(4) scars of old lacerations	(4) useful information in planning delivery techniques for pregnant women
	(5) abnormal growths	(5) physician consultation required
	(6) fistulas	(6) physician consultation required
	(7) fissures	(7) physician consultation required
	(8) uterine prolapse	(8) physician consultation required
	(9) note if the introitus is nulliparous, parous, or gaping	(9) helpful in determining what size speculum to use

Examination of the Urethra and
Skenes's and Bartholin's Glands

Examination of the urethra and Skene's and Bartholin's glands is done by some clinicians prior to the speculum examination. Other clinicians examine these after the speculum examination as the first part of their bimanual examination.

The advantage to examination of the urethra and Skene's and Bartholin's glands before the speculum examination is four-fold:

1. It can be incorporated into the total pelvic examination during the inspection of the external genitalia.

2. It allows for immediate palpation of a suspicious labial swelling, cyst, or growth.
3. The pressure of the speculum may cause discharge from the urethra or Skene's glands, which may go unnoticed during the procedure and yield a false negative result when they are stripped afterwards.
4. It allows the clinician to also identify the position of the cervix. This information is useful to have prior to insertion of the speculum.

The disadvantage to examination at this time is that no lubrication (other than water) can be used on the examining fingers as it may interfere with the Pap smear obtained during the speculum examination.

Procedure	Findings	Significance
1. The labia are separated with the thumb and index finger of one hand. Tell the woman that you are going to insert one finger into her vagina (birth canal) and that she will feel you pressing forward with it. With your palm up, gently insert the index finger of your examining hand as far as the second joint into the vagina. Exerting upward pressure, strip (or milk) the Skene's gland on one side of the urethra by moving your finger alongside the urethra from inside to outside. Repeat for the Skene's gland on the other side. Then strip the urethra by again inserting your index finger and exerting upward pressure directly on the urethra itself as you move your finger from inside to outside.	1. Identify the urethral meatus. While stripping the Skene's glands look for discharge either from the vestibule on either side of the urethra or from the urethra itself. Sometimes the ducts of the Skene's glands open on the posterior wall of the urethra just inside the meatus. If a discharge is obtained while stripping the Skene's glands or the urethra, note its color, consistency, and odor.	1. Discharge from the Skene's glands or urethra is indicative of an inflammation of one or all these structures (e.g., urethritis). Usually such an inflammation is due to gonorrhea. A specimen of any discharge present from stripping the Skene's glands and urethra is obtained immediately and cultured.
2. Tell the woman that she will now feel you pressing around the entrance to her vagina (birth canal). From the position you used in examining the Skene's glands and urethra, sweep your finger laterally, palpating between it on the inside of the vagina and your thumb on the outside of the labia majora. Palpate the entire area, paying particular attention to the posterolateral portion of the labia majora, behind	2. Palpate for: a. tenderness b. swelling c. masses d. heat e. fluctuation Observe for any discharge from the opening of the Batholin's gland duct just outside the posterolateral margin of the vaginal introitus on the side of the vestibule. Palpation and observation are bilateral because each gland is separate.	2. Painful swelling, hot to touch and fluctuant, is indicative of an abscess of the Bartholin's gland. Such an abscess usually is gonococcal in origin and contains pus. A specimen of any discharge expressed from a Bartholin's gland duct is obtained for culturing. A nontender mass of variable size is indicative of a Bartholin's cyst, which is the result of chronic inflammation of the gland. The usual, although not

Procedure	Findings	Significance
which the Bartholin's glands are located. Continue the sweep of your finger and thumb across the perineum and palpate the same area on the other side. Your hand will have turned 270° by the time you are finished. Some clinicians prefer to switch hands for palpating the opposite side for the Bartholin's gland.	If there is a discharge, note its color, consistency, and odor. Also note any erythema of the duct opening.	only, cause of bartholinitis is gonorrhea since the Bartholin's glands are a site that harbors the gonococci.

The Speculum Examination

Description of a Speculum
The speculum consists of two blades and a handle. A thumb-piece on the side is attached to the anterior blade. The posterior blade of the speculum is fixed. The anterior blade is hinged and movable as controlled by the thumb-piece attached to it. A thumbscrew on the thumb-piece, when tightened, holds the anterior blade in the position desired and attained by use of the thumb-piece for intravaginal visualization. The posterior and anterior blades of the speculum are together at the distal end when the speculum is closed. From this point the anterior blade slants slightly upward away from the posterior blade and curves sharply upward at the proximal end to a distance of approximately 1 inch from the posterior blade.

When the speculum is opened by use of the thumb-piece, a tubelike space between the blades is created from the proximal to the distal end. Through this tubelike space intravaginal observations are made and instruments are passed for any intravaginal procedures. The blades may be further separated by manipulating the thumbscrew on the handle of the speculum. Ordinarily, and always during insertion, this is adjusted for the closest possi-

ble approximation of the two blades. Once the speculum is in place and opened by use of the thumb-piece and its thumbscrew, the entire anterior blade may be elevated from the posterior blade, if needed, by sliding the anterior blade away from the posterior blade and tightening it in this position with the thumbscrew on the handle.

It is important that the inexperienced examiner practice manipulation of the speculum and become intimately familiar with how it is put together and how it operates before attempting insertion into a woman. Such practice will eliminate the possibility of hurting the woman due to mishandling the speculum during examination. Also, it is not uncommon for a speculum to come apart or become malaligned during storage and the examiner needs to know how to get it ready for use.

Types of Specula
There are three types of specula. The variations between the three are useful because they enable the examiner to select for use a speculum that is appropriate for the individual woman.

The smallest speculum is the *virginal speculum*. It has short, narrow, and flat blades. It is used in young girls and in women who have had little or no coitus.

The *Graves speculum* is both the standard and largest speculum as it comes in these two sizes. The standard size is most commonly used since it is most appropriate for women who are sexually active or have had a baby. The large size is used with women who have collapsing vaginal walls, generally grand multiparas or very obese women. The Graves speculum varies in length from 3½ to 5 inches (8¾ to 12¾ centimeters) and in width from ¾ to 1¼ inches (about 2 to 3¼ centimeters). The blades are curved, forming a concave space between the two blades. The posterior blade is approximately ¼ inch longer than the anterior blade to conform with the longer posterior vaginal wall and aid in visualization of the cervix.

The *Pederson speculum* is as long as the Graves speculum but has more narrow blades. Also, its blades are flat rather than curved. It is used in women who may be sexually active but tight and have never had a baby. It is also useful for women who may have a vagina contracted by scars, radiation, or senescence.

Procedure for Speculum Examination

Procedure	Rationale
1. The woman has been properly positioned, draped, and informed as to the procedure and has her bladder empty and her legs apart for the examination. You have already positioned the lighted gooseneck lamp, washed your hands, and put on your glove(s).	1. See Steps 1 through 6 under "Preparatory and General procedures" for the pelvic examination.
2. Select the appropriate speculum for the woman on the basis of her sexual and obstetric history and your observations during inspection.	2. The appropriate speculum is one which will cause the least discomfort to the woman while providing adequate intravaginal and cervical visualization.
3. Lubricate the speculum with only water if you plan to obtain cytologic or other studies. If no studies are planned you may lubricate the speculum with any lubricating jelly used for the purpose of a vaginal examination. However, some unplanned studies may be indicated after you have visualized the vaginal walls and the cervix. For this reason most clinicians never lubricate the speculum with anything but water.	3. Lubricating jellies or creams may interfere with cytologic or other studies, rendering them invalid.
4. Warm the speculum by: a. using *warm* water to lubricate it b. holding it in your hands until warm c. holding it under the gooseneck lamp until warm	4. For comfort. This has a great effect on what the woman thinks of you and about the examination. Using warm water is the quickest and most effective method. The other variations are useful in the event warm water is not available.

Procedure	Rationale
5. Touch the woman with the warmed speculum on the inner aspect of her thigh close to the external genitalia. Ask her if the temperature of the speculum is comfortable.	5. Reassures yourself and the woman that you will neither burn nor freeze her when you insert the speculum. This also involves the woman in the procedure.
6. Help the woman to relax and tell her she will feel you touching her on the outside and then will feel the speculum going inside her vagina (birth canal).	6. See Steps 1, 7, and 8 under ''Preparatory and General Procedures'' for the pelvic examination.
7. Separate the woman's labia with a gloved hand. (See alternative method at end of this procedure.)	7. Done to expose the vaginal orifice.
8. Hold the speculum in your other hand with your index finger over the top of the proximal end of the anterior blade and your other fingers around the handle.	8. This assures that the blades will stay closed.
9. Insert the speculum into the vagina at an oblique angle past the hymenal ring.	9. Pressure on and trauma to the urethra and periurethral structures is avoided with the speculum inserted at an oblique angle.
10. Rotate the speculum to a horizontal angle and while pressing firmly downward, insert the speculum the length of the vaginal canal. Avoid catching pubic hair or pinching or pushing in the labia by virtue of not having spread the labia enough during this insertion procedure.	10. Downward pressure again avoids trauma to the urethra. The anatomical angle of the vagina when the woman is in the lithotomy position is approximately 45° downward toward the lumbar area. If the speculum is inserted straight in, the anterior vaginal wall and urethra are traumatized and the woman feels pain.
11. Maintaining downward pressure, open the speculum by pressing on the thumbpiece. Downward pressure can be maintained either by exerting downward and outward pressure on the lower end of the speculum handle or by putting your thumb or a finger on the proximal end of the posterior blade and exerting downward pressure. Adjust your light source as needed.	11. and 12. For intravaginal visualization. If the speculum was directed downward firmly during insertion and this position was maintained, you are assured of finding the cervix during your sweep upward, regardless of whether the cervix is located in a posterior, midline, or anterior position. This eliminates a hunt, seek, and find method of locating the cervix, which would entail much maneuvering of the speculum up and down and in and out to the discomfort of the woman and the distress of both the woman and the examiner.
12. Sweep the speculum slowly upward from its posterior downward position until the cervix comes into view.	
13. Manipulate the speculum a little further into the vagina so the cervix is well ex-	13. Adequate visualization is needed for observation and exposure of the cervical

Procedure	Rationale
posed between the anterior and posterior blades.	os for obtaining the Papanicolaou smear and gonoccocal culture specimens.
14. Tighten the thumbscrew on the thumb-piece. If further exposure is needed, elevate the anterior blade by manipulating the slide and thumbscrew located on the speculum handle. Remember the comfort of the woman and do not open the speculum any wider than is absolutely necessary.	14. To free your hand for handling other equipment. Watch that the woman does not involuntarily push the speculum back out. This is possible even with the speculum in an open position. If it looks like this may happen keep one hand on the speculum at all times to sense and prevent this from occurring.
15. If the cervix is covered with a copious amount of discharge, put a gauze 2 × 2 or 4 × 4 on a sponge stick and blot or gently wipe off the cervix.	15. Too much discharge will prevent obtaining a Pap smear representative of the tissue being scraped. Do not use a cotton ball because the cotton fibers will interfere with the wet smear microscopic examination you will want to make of the discharge.

16. Specimens for Papanicolaou smears and gonococcal cultures and specimens for wet smears of vaginal discharge are obtained at this time, as well as any other indicated tests or treatments. The procedures for obtaining these specimens are found as separate procedures in Chapters 38, 45, and 46.

Procedure	Rationale
17. Before removing the speculum, gently rotate it 90° while again exerting downward pressure on the speculum. This will most likely be uncomfortable to the woman so forewarn her of this manipulation before doing it.	17. To visualize the anterior and posterior walls of the vagina as well as the lateral vaginal walls.
18. Return the speculum to its horizontal position. Release the thumbscrew on the thumb-piece (and on the speculum handle, if used). While holding the blades apart with pressure on the thumb-piece, begin withdrawal of the speculum until the cervix is released from between the blades of the speculum.	18. To avoid pinching or pulling on the cervix during removal of the speculum.
19. Release your pressure on the thumbpiece, thereby closing the blades. Avoid pinching the vaginal mucosa or catching pubic hair when the blades close. Again avoid pressure on or trauma to the urethra and periurethral structures by exerting downward pressure, rotating the speculum to	19. For the woman's comfort.

Procedure	Rationale
the oblique angle, and making sure the blades are closed by hooking your index finger over the anterior blade as the speculum is withdrawn. Some clinicians ask the woman to bear down to ease the speculum out, serving only to guide its removal.	
20. Note the odor of any vaginal discharge pooled in the posterior blade and obtain a specimen for making a wet smear if indicated and not already obtained.	20.
21. Deposit the speculum in the proper container.	21. For sanitary purposes.
22. Wipe any discharge from the genitalia and perineum if a bimanual examination is not being done.	22. For the woman's comfort.

Note: An alternate method of inserting the speculum is to insert one to two fingers of one hand just inside the vagina (to the first joint on the fingers). These fingers then gently but	firmly depress the perineal body while the other hand guides the entry of the speculum over and past your fingers.

Observations	Significance
1. Cervix. Observe for: a. color b. growth, nodules, masses c. polyps d. lesions, erosions, ulcerations e. position of the cervix f. size (hypertrophy, atrophy) and shape g. edema h. nabothian cysts i. inflammation (cervicitis) j. discharge — color, amount, character, consistency, odor k. friability (bleeding) l. eversion m. ectopy n. size and shape of os and any lacerations o. patulousness and dilatation	1. *Color* is significant in aiding in clinical diagnosis of pregnancy. A bluish color to the cervix is due to increased vascularity to the cervix and is known as Chadwick's sign, a presumptive sign of pregnancy. A nonpregnant cervix is pink. *Growths, nodules, masses, polyps, lesions, erosions, ulcerations, and infected nabothian cysts* are all abnormal findings requiring physician consultation. It is useful to note the *position of the cervix* based on where you locate it with the speculum. This information serves to identify or give confirming evidence as to the position of the uterus during the bimanual examination. A cervix located anteriorly is indicative of a retroverted uterus, while a posterior cervix indicates an anteverted uterus and a cervix in the horizontal midline indicates a uterus in

Observations	Significance
	midposition. Deviations of the cervix to the right or left of the vertical midline indicate the possibility of pelvic masses or uterine adhesions; these need to be carefully ruled out during the bimanual examination.
	Variations in the *size* and *shape* of the cervix give different information. The normal cervix in a woman of childbearing age is 2 to 3 centimeters (about ¾ to 1¼ inches) in diameter with the exception of the larger patulous cervix of the grand multipara. A *small cervix* is seen in the postmenopausal woman concomitant with the endometrial and myometrial atrophy of the rest of the uterus. Normal cervical size should match the size of the nonpregnant uterus. A *hypertrophied, large,* or *edematous cervix* is generally an indication of cervical infection and may be observed along with the other signs of *cervicitis*. An *irregularly shaped cervix* may indicate the presence of an *infected nabothian cyst* swollen with fluid.
	Nabothian cysts may be observed as white or yellow pinpoints on the cervix. *Infected nabothian cysts* distort the shape of a portion of the cervix since it is swollen with fluid. Nabothian cysts are retention cysts arising from the occlusion of the ducts of endocervical glands extending near the surface of the vaginal portion of the cervix. They most frequently occur in the presence of chronic cervicitis.
	Cervicitis is an inflammation of the cervix usually caused by an infection (e.g., *Trichomonas vaginalis*, gonorrhea) but which may also be caused by irritation from injury, obstetric lacerations, mechanical devices, foreign objects, or allergic reactions.
	Careful note must be taken as to whether any *discharge* is merely a continuation of a

Observations

Significance

vaginal infection deposited on the cervix (e.g., the plaques of a *Candida* [monilial] infection) or originates from the endocervix itself as seen in the pus of gonorrhea exuding from the external cervical os.

Friability of the cervix, as evidenced by its bleeding easily after obtaining the Pap smear or sponging for purposes of observation, frequently accompanies cervicitis.

Eversion of the cervix, due to too much pressure in the vaginal fornices by the tips of the blades of the speculum, exposes the rougher and redder looking columnar epithelium of the cervical canal. Usually it is circumoral, showing the line of demarcation between the continuation of the stratified squamous epithelium of the vagina that covers the vaginal portion of the cervix and extends a short distance into the cervical canal, and the columnar epithelium. It is differentiated from erosions or ectopy by simply withdrawing the speculum slightly and watching the columnar epithelium disappear from view as the cervical canal returns to its correct noneverted position.

Ectopy, by definition meaning *out of place*, is when the columnar epithelium of the cervical canal has grown downward and outward and competes for territorial space with the squamous epithelium on the vaginal surface of the cervix. Again, the rougher, redder-looking columnar epithelium is visible. Unlike eversion, however, it may be quite irregular in its line of demarcation with the squamous epithelium. This is sometimes observed in the multiparous cervix, especially if the cervix has been lacerated. Usually ectopy is also present in women who use oral contraceptives.

Size and shape of the os is largely dependent on the woman's childbearing experience. A nulligravid os is small and

Observations	Significance
	round or oval, while the typical parous os is a horizontal slit. Trauma due to induced abortion results in a change in the shape of the external os. Trauma due to difficult removal of an intrauterine contraceptive may change the shape of a nulligravid os to a slit os. *Cervical lacerations* as a result of trauma during childbirth are clearly observable. Severe cervical lacerations may result in subsequent difficulty in carrying a pregnancy to term due to an incompetent cervix (see Chapter 9). Observation of the shape of the os is important as confirmatory evidence of the woman's obstetric history. Infrequently a woman will attempt to conceal a previous pregnancy. In so doing she unknowingly also conceals information vital to the management of another pregnancy. An os which does not match the obstetric history or family planning history needs explanation.
	The nulligravid cervix is closed, whereas the multiparous os is *patulous*, the degree depending on the woman's parity. The higher the parity the more patulous the os, possibly permanently open 2 to 3 centimeters at the external os. *Dilatation* of the os is also observable upon speculum examination, making the fetal membranes visible when examining a pregnant woman, if they have not ruptured. Determination of the amount of dilatation is done by manual vaginal examination.

2. Vagina. Observe for:
  a. color
  b. inflammation/vaginitis
  c. discharge — color, odor, character, consistency, amount
  d. plaques
  e. bleeding/friability
  f. lesions and ulcerations
  g. growths or masses
  h. cysts
	2. *Color* in the vagina has the same significance as color of the cervix. The nonpregnant vagina is pink, while the vagina of pregnancy is bluish. This color change in pregnancy is known as Chadwick's sign.
	    Growths, masses, lesions, ulcerations, cysts, and fistulas are all abnormal findings requiring physician consultation.
	    Inflammation and *discharge* go hand in hand as signs of *vaginitis*. Vaginitis caused

Observations	Significance
i. fistulas j. vaginal wall muscle tone	by *Trichomonas vaginalis* additionally may cause red petechiae. Vaginitis due to candidiasis (monilial infection) also exhibits whitish or grayish patches or *plaques* which adhere to the vaginal wall and may *bleed* when scraped off. Severe vaginitis causes *friability* of the vaginal mucosa. *Blood* in the vagina must always be investigated for its source. If it is not obviously due to menstruation, a friable cervix or vagina, or trauma in these areas, physician consultation is required.

The Bimanual Examination

When clinical pelvimetry is indicated, clinicians include it while doing the bimanual examination. The procedure and findings for clinical pelvimetry are described separately in this part of the book. Whether or not clinical pelvimetry is performed during the bimanual examination, it is important that the clinician develop a procedure of doing the bimanual examination that (1) is the same each time, as a routine aids in not forgetting any part of it (if clinical pelvimetry is included it should be incorporated and a routine established for the combined skills) and (2) moves smoothly *once* from outside to inside and back out again, which is most comfortable for the woman, without repeatedly going back and forth.

The woman is already properly positioned, draped, informed as to the procedure and has her bladder empty and her legs apart for the examination. You have already positioned the gooseneck lamp, washed your hands, and put on your glove(s). If you have done a speculum examination, it is not necessary to rewash your hands or change your glove(s).

Be sure that the woman's arms are down by her sides or across her abdomen to aid relaxation of her abdominal muscles. Remember to use firm but gentle touch and to be alert to any indication of discomfort or tenseness on the part of the woman throughout the examination causing her to tighten up or move away from you. See Steps 1 through 9 under "Preparatory and General Procedures."

Procedure and Rationale	Observations and Findings	Significance
1. Lubricate generously the index and middle fingers of your examining hand. 2. Separate the labia and insert your lubricated fin-		

Procedure and Rationale	Observations and Findings	Significance
gers gently into the vagina at least to their second joint, palm side down, pressing downward as you insert your fingers as you did with the speculum to avoid the anterior urethral and periurethral structures. If the introitus is small, insert only one finger.		
3. Sitting so you can easily visualize the vagina, firmly exert pressure with your fingers posteriorly against the vaginal musculature. Ask the woman to bear down or cough. (It is wise to first ask the woman if she ever urinates accidentally when she laughs, coughs, or sneezes unexpectedly. If so, position yourself accordingly.)	3. a. observe the anterior vaginal wall for evidence of a cystocele or urethrocele. A urethrocele will evidence itself as the distal (vulvar) end of the anterior vaginal wall bulging downward into the vagina and outward towards the introitus. Observe for involuntary loss of urine (stress incontinence) while the patient is bearing down or coughing. A cystocele is evidenced by bulging of the upper (cervical) end of the anterior vaginal wall.	3. a. a first degree cystocele is a condition in which there is bulging of the anterior wall. In second degree cystocele the bulging reaches the vaginal orifice or introitus. A third degree cystocele is present when the bulging extends beyond the introitus. Nearly every woman who has borne a child has a first degree cystocele. It is so common that if it is not accompanied by stress incontinence it is considered a normal finding. Its significance lies in making a proper selection of the type of diaphragm to prescribe for a woman if she desires this method of family planning. A second degree cystocele without stress incontinence and not causing any sexual difficulties is considered asymptomatic and noth-

Procedure and Rationale	Observations and Findings	Significance
		ing is done except to note it. A symptomatic second degree cystocele, a third degree cystocele, or a urethrocele requires physician consultation for evaluation and possible surgical repair.
	b. observe for descensus of the uterus (uterine prolapse).	b. frequently cystocele accompanies uterine prolapse. A first degree uterine prolapse is any minor degree of descent with the cervix remaining inside the vagina. In second degree uterine prolapse the cervix protrudes through the vaginal introitus. A third degree uterine prolapse comprises prolapse of the entire uterus outside the vulva. A second or third degree uterine prolapse or symptomatic first degree uterine prolapse requires physician consultation.
4. Continuing to press posteriorly with your fingers, now spread your fingers and again ask the woman to bear down.	4. Observe the posterior vaginal wall for rectocele or enterocele. A rectocele evidences itself at the lower (vulvar) end of the posterior vaginal wall by bulging upward into the vagina and outward toward the introitus. If the rectocele is severe (second or third degree) ask if the woman has difficulty in	4. A severe rectocele requires physician consultation. Rectoceles are graded in degrees the same as cystoceles. An enterocele is almost always associated with herniation of the cul-de-sac of Douglas, which will probably contain loops of bowel. Physician consultation is required.

Procedure and Rationale	Observations and Findings	Significance
	bowel elimination necessitating digital holding back of the rectocele. An enterocele is evidenced by prolapse of the upper (cervical) end of the posterior vaginal wall.	
5. Put your fingers together again and ask the woman to tighten her muscles around your fingers.	5. Assess the tone of the perineal muscles. Now is a good time to teach the woman perineal tightening (Kegel) exercise (see page 512).	5. Muscle tone may affect the length of the second stage of labor, sexual satisfaction, urinary continence, and support of the pelvic organs.
6. Sweep the vagina with your fingers as you insert them the full length of the woman's vagina.	6. Feel for cysts, nodules, masses, or growths.	6. All are abnormal findings requiring physician consultation.

Be careful where your thumb is during the bimanual examination. Some authorities suggest that it be tucked into the palm of your hand with your fourth and fifth fingers. However, this will cut down on the distance you can insert the length of your index finger. The principle to remember is to keep your thumb off the woman's clitoris; pressure on the clitoris is most uncomfortable.

7. Locate the cervix with your fingers and run your fingers around it circumferentially and across its vaginal end.	7. Feel for: a. size (length and width) and shape	7. a. the *size* of the nonpregnant cervix should correspond with the size of the nonpregnant uterus. The *length* of the cervix is important in assessing effacement during labor. See discussion of the significance of the *size* and *shape* of the cervix under "The Speculum Examination," above.
	b. consistency	b. the *consistency* of the cervix is noticeably different when the woman is nonpregnant (firm — the tip of a nose is

Procedure and Rationale	Observations and Findings	Significance
		often given as an analogy) from when she is pregnant (soft —the lips are often given as an analogy). A ripe cervix, a sign of approaching labor, is softer still—pudding would be an analogy.
	c. smoothness	c. normally the cervix is *smooth*. The *roughness* of ectopy or erosions and bumps caused by nabothian cysts can be felt. Since roughness may be an indication of abnormality, if a speculum examination was not done for some reason as part of the pelvic examination, it should be done after completion of the bimanual and rectovaginal examination to visualize the cause of the roughness.
	d. position of the cervix	d. see the significance of the *position* of the cervix discussed under "The Speculum Examination." The position of the cervix is additionally important when evaluating the possibility that a woman is in labor.
	e. dilatation of the os	e. dilatation of the os generally is a phenomenon of labor and is discussed in Chapter 10. Painless dilatation

Procedure and Rationale	Observations and Findings	Significance
		of the os without bleeding during the second trimester may indicate an incompetent cervix. The os also dilates with inevitable abortion (see Chapter 9).
8. Grasp the cervix gently between your fingers and move it from side to side.	8. Observe the woman for expression of pain or tenderness with movement of the cervix.	8. Painful cervical movement is indicative of a pelvic inflammatory process such as acute PID (pelvic inflammatory disease). It is also a sign of a ruptured tubal pregnancy.
9. Palpate the uterus in the following manner: (1) place your abdominal hand midway between the umbilicus and the symphysis pubis. Use the flats of the palmar surface of the first joints of your fingers to press downward and forward toward the symphysis pubis and your vaginal fingers. (2) with your palm upward place your two vaginal examining fingers on either side of the cervix. Bring them together on top of the cervix as you push downward on the cervix with the back of your fingers and in and upward with the tips of your fingers toward your	9. Palpate the uterus for: a. size, shape, and contour	9. a. the *size* of the nonpregnant uterus in a woman of childbearing age varies according to parity. A multiparous uterus is larger in all dimensions than the nulliparous uterus, being from 1 to 4 centimeters (about ½ to 1½ inches) larger in length, 1½ to 2½ centimeters (about ⅔ to 1 inch) wider, and ½ to 1½ centimeters (about ¼ to ⅔ inch) thicker. The normal nulliparous uterus ranges in size from 5½ to 8 centimeters (about 2 to 3 inches) long, 3½ to 4 centimeters (about 1½ inches) wide, and 2 to 2½ centimeters (about 1 inch) thick. The uterus decreases

Procedure and Rationale	Observations and Findings	Significance

abdominal hand. The sensation is one of trying to bring your hands together as you push down on the cervix. If the uterus is anterior or anteflexed it will slip between the fingers of your two hands as they come toward each other.

(3) If you do not feel the uterus with the maneuver described in (2) above, then return your fingers to the position of having them on both sides of the cervix. Place your abdominal hand immediately above the symphysis pubis and press firmly downward. Bring your vaginal examining fingers together under the cervix and pressing against it follow it inward and wherever it leads. If the uterus is retroverted or retroflexed you will feel it with this maneuver.

(4) If you still are unable to feel the uterus with either of the maneuvers in (2) and (3) above, then return your fingers to the position of having one on either side of the cervix. Maintaining contact

b. location

in size with the menopause, during which there is atrophy of the endometrium and the myometrium.

The dimensions of the uterus give it its *shape*, which is frequently compared with a somewhat flattened pear. A uterus larger than expected in a woman of childbearing age is indicative of pregnancy or benign or malignant tumors. As the pregnant uterus enlarges, its shape changes, becoming first globular and then an ovoid of increasingly larger size.

The normally smooth and symmetrical *contour* of the uterus is disrupted in the presence of a growth or a mass. Uterine myomata are felt as irregular masses on the surface of the uterus. Piskacek's sign of early pregnancy is felt as an irregularity in one of the cornual areas, causing uterine asymmetry.

b. the *location* of the uterus is normally in the midline. Deviation of the entire corpus of the uterus to the right or left is

Procedure and Rationale	Observations and Findings	Significance
with the cervix, press straight inward and feel as far as you can. Then slide your fingers around the uterus until one finger is on top of the cervix and one finger is underneath the cervix. Continue your inward pressure while moving your fingers in order to feel as much of the uterus as is possible when it is in the middle (military) position.	c. position (1) anteverted (2) anteflexed (3) military (midposition) (4) retroverted (5) retroflexed The prefixes *ante-* and *retro-* mean *forward* and *backward*, respectively. The suffix *-verted* indicates that the entire uterus *tilts*, either forward or backward. The suffix *-flexed* means that the uterus *bends at the isthmus* (at the level of the internal os) forward or backward. In the *military position* the uterus is perfectly straight in a midposition, neither tilting nor bending forward or backward. d. consistency	indicative of possible adhesions or pelvic masses. c. knowing the *position* of the uterus is imperative prior to inserting an intrauterine contraceptive device or performing any other intrauterine procedure. The position of the uterus may be a cause of dyspareunia unless counteracted by appropriate positions during sexual intercourse. While the uterus is usually in a position of slight anteflexion, the variations of anteversion, retroversion, and retroflexion are all considered normal. Slight retroversion of the uterus and the so-called military position place the fundus out of reach for palpation by many examiners. d. the normal nonpregnant uterus is firm in *consistency*. It is somewhat softer during early pregnancy and postpartal involution when it is a pelvic organ. Hegar's sign of early pregnancy is a marked

Procedure and Rationale	Observations and Findings	Significance
		softening of the isthmus of the uterus.
	e. mobility	e. the normal uterus is *mobile* above the cervix in the anteroposterior plane. It is laterally held in place by the broad, uterosacral, and cardinal ligaments. Lack of anteroposterior mobility indicates adhesions possibly due to infection or previous surgery.
	f. tenderness or pain	f. *tenderness or pain* on movement of the uterus is indicative of a pelvic inflammatory process in the nonpregnant woman and of endometritis and other puerperal infections in the postpartum woman.
10. Examine the adnexal areas in the following way: (1) place your abdominal hand in the area between the iliac crest of the innominate bone (hip) and the abdominal midline midway between the level of the umbilicus and the symphysis pubis. Use the flats of the palmar surface of the first joints of your fingers to press deeply downward and obliquely toward the	10. Palpate the adnexal areas for: a. size, shape, and any tenderness or pain in the adnexae b. consistency, size, shape, and tenderness or pain of any adnexal masses The adnexae are frequently difficult for even an experienced clinician to feel, depending on the position of the uterus and concomitant location of the adnexae and the amount of adipose tissue. If you are unable to feel anything in the adnexal areas after	10. a. the *size* of the normal ovary in a woman during the childbearing years ranges from 2½ to 5 centimeters (1 to 2 inches) long, 1½ to 3 centimeters (about ⅔ to 1¼ inches) wide, and ½ to 1½ centimeters (¼ to ⅔ inches) thick. This gives it the *shape* of a small almond, with which it is often compared. The size of the ovaries diminish markedly after menopause, frequently being

Procedure and Rationale	Observations and Findings	Significance
symphysis pubis and your vaginal fingers. (2) with your palm upward, place both of your vaginal examining fingers in the lateral vaginal fornix corresponding to the side (right or left) that your abdominal hand is positioned to examine. Press your fingers deeply inward and upward toward your abdominal hand as far as possible. (3) palpate the entire area between the uterus and the walls of the hip bone with a sliding, gentle but firm "pressing together" movement of your two hands as they synchronously move from the highest to the lowest level as visualized abdominally. (4) reverse and repeat the manuevers in (1), (2), and (3) above for examination of the other adnexal area. (5) it helps to have formed a mental picture of the location of the adnexae in relationship to the position of the uterus before starting this part of the examination. 11. Withdraw your vaginal	thorough palpation, normality has to be assumed in the absence of any clinical signs and symptoms and this portion of the examination is charted as "not felt." The adnexal areas should always be palpated in doing the non-pregnant pelvic examination. It is also done on the initial prenatal examination if this takes place during the first trimester. However, as the pregnant uterus become an abdominal organ, it is futile to palpate for the adnexae. By virtue of their location and attachment in the broad ligament, the adnexae also enter the abdominal cavity along with the uterine fundus as the pregnancy progresses.	a mere ½ centimeter (less than ¼ inch) in any of the aforementioned diameters. The normal ovary is *tender* when touched, which aids in identifying the ovary when you palpate it. The fallopian tubes are rarely felt when normal due to the smallness of their width, which varies from 2 to 3 millimeters at the most narrow portion to 5 to 8 millimeters at the widest portion. b. any *adnexal masses* are abnormal and require physician consultation. Their size, shape, location, consistency, and any areas of pain should be noted. Ovarian cysts and tumors usually are not tender. Generalized pain in the adnexal area may prohibit outlining of an adnexal mass and is indicative of pelvic inflammatory disease when bilateral. If unilateral, a ruptured tubal pregnancy is a possibility. In either case, such findings require physician consultation.

Procedure and Rationale	Observations and Findings	Significance
examining fingers to just inside the introitus preparatory for the rectovaginal examination if you are doing one. If not, smoothly withdraw your fingers from the woman's vagina.		
12. If this ends your pelvic examination, proceed with Steps 12 to 16 under "The Rectovaginal Examination," which follows.		

The Rectovaginal Examination

The rectovaginal examination is an inherent part of the total pelvic examination. The only time it is eliminated is when only a partial pelvic examination is being done for a specific reason (e.g., speculum examination for checking the strings of an intrauterine contraceptive device, vaginal examinations for evaluating labor status, speculum examination for evaluation of treatment of a vaginal infection).

Because it is an uncomfortable examination for many women, it is not uncommon to be asked by a woman if it can just be skipped. The answer is no, followed by an appropriate explanation of why not. The request usually stems from the woman's lack of understanding that there is more to the rectovaginal examination than just confirming the findings of the vaginal bimanual examination. This needs to be explained to the woman. Rectovaginal examination enables many examiners to reach almost 1 inch higher into the pelvis, an invaluable aid in evaluating pelvic organs and structures.

Procedure and Rationale	Observations and Findings	Significance
1. The bimanual vaginal examination ended with the withdrawal of your examining fingers to just inside the vaginal introitus. Keep your index finger inside of the woman's vagina while removing completely your middle examining finger.		

Procedure and Rationale	Observations and Findings	Significance

Note: If there has been any indication of gonorrhea during the vaginal examination (observation of the cervix and palpation of the urethra and Bartholin's and Skene's glands), it is necessary for you to completely remove your examining fingers and change your gloves. Some clinicians routinely change gloves anyway to avoid the possibility of spreading asymptomatic gonorrhea of the urinary or genital tracts to the rectum. Other clinicians wash their gloves before proceeding with the rectal examination. Still others will proceed as outlined in Steps 1 and 2 in this procedure.

2. Generously relubricate your middle examining finger to aid in sliding your finger gently into the rectum.

3. Tell the woman that your examination may be uncomfortable and that she might feel as though she is having a bowel movement. Assure her that she will not pass stool and help her with breathing techniques to relax. Tightening her sphincter, rectum, and buttocks will make the examination more uncomfortable and hinder your ability to examine her.

4. After observing the anus, place your middle examining finger against the anus and ask the woman to bear down and push against your finger. As she does this, slide the tip of your finger into the rectum just past the sphincter.

4. Observe the anus for:
   a. external hemorrhoids
   b. anorectal fistula
   c. sentinel tag or anal fissure
   d. rectal prolapse
   e. lesions

4. *Thrombosed external hemorrhoids, anorectal fistula, anal fissure, lesions,* and *rectal prolapse* are all abnormalities requiring physician consultation.

5. Palpate the area of the anorectal junction and just above it. Ask her to tighten and relax her rectal sphincter.

5. Palpate for:
   a. internal hemorrhoids

5. a. *internal hemorrhoids* are difficult to feel because they are soft. History of problems with constipation,

Procedure and Rationale	Observations and Findings	Significance
		straining with bowel movements, and impactions is important. Consultation with the physician is indicated if the problem is severe. Otherwise, the woman should be instructed in all the measures for preventing constipation. Prescription of a laxative may be indicated.
	b. sphincter tone	b. an extremely tight sphincter may be indicative of spasticity caused by a fissure, lesion, or inflammatory process; may be due to scarring; or may be due to extreme anxiety about the examination. A lax sphincter, unless attributable to frequent anal intercourse, which causes sphincter laxity, may indicate neurological disease requiring physician consultation. An absent sphincter may be the result of an unrepaired or improperly repaired third degree perineal laceration most likely occurring during childbirth. A history of fecal incontinence should have alerted you to the possibility of this finding. Physician consultation is required.

Procedure and Rationale	Observations and Findings	Significance
6. (1) as you slide both your vaginal and rectal examining fingers as far as they will reach, palpate half of the rectal wall, sweeping your finger back and forth as you methodically cover the distance. (Decide which half you will cover as a routine based on the face of a clock — for example, between 6 and 12 o'clock or between 3 and 9 o'clock. Slightly extend the half-clock you choose so no area is missed in dividing it up, e.g., 5:30 to 12:30.) You will examine the remainder of the rectal wall when you remove your finger. (2) ask the woman to bear down when you have reached as far as you can as this will bring an additional centimeter or so within your reach.	6. Palpate for: a. polyps/masses b. nodules/irregularities c. strictures d. rectovaginal musculature	6. a. polyps, if felt, may be benign or malignant. *Masses* may be polyps, bowel herniation, or pelvic masses such as ovarian cysts or tumors, adnexal masses, and so forth located more posteriorly and not felt during the vaginal bimanual examination. Physician consultation is required in the presence of any of these conditions. b. *nodules* and *irregularities* may indicate the presence of an ulcerated malignancy. Physician consultation is required. c. *strictures* which are causing problems with bowel evacuation require physician consultation. d. evaluation of the thickness and tone of the *rectovaginal musculature* provides useful information in anticipating difficulties during the second stage of labor if it is too thin (or too thick and muscularly overdeveloped, as may be found in some female athletes).
7. With your abdominal hand pressing firmly and deeply downward just above the symphysis	7. Palpate for confirmation of vaginal findings regarding the size, location, position, consistency, shape,	7. Same as for vaginal palpation of the uterus. See Step 9 under "The Bimanual Examination."

Procedure and Rationale	Observations and Findings	Significance
pubis and your vaginal examining finger located in the posterior vaginal fornix and pressing strongly upward against the posterior side of the cervix (this will move the uterus posteriorly), palpate as much of the posterior side of the uterus as possible with your rectal examining finger. This is particularly useful in evaluating a retroverted uterus.	contour, and any tenderness or pain of the uterus.	
8. If you were unable to evaluate the adnexal areas thoroughly or had any questionable findings in this area during the vaginal bimanual examination, then palpate the adnexal areas using the same maneuvers as in Step 10 of "The Bimanual Examination."	8. Same as in Step 10 of "The Bimanual Examination."	8. Same as Step 10 of "The Bimanual Examination."

9. If you are doing clinical pelvimetry during your pelvic examination, you may wish to reevaluate the shape of the sacrum, the ischial spines, the sacrospinous ligaments, the sacroiliac notch, and the coccyx during your rectovaginal examination since these structures may be more readily felt through the rectum. See the procedure for clinical pelvimetry in Chapter 47.

10. As you remove your fingers, repeat the maneuver in Step 6. (1) of the "Rectovaginal Examination," covering the remaining half of the rectal wall. For example, if you covered between 5:30 and 12:30 o'clock on your way in, cover the area between 11:30 and 6:30 o'clock on your way out.	10. Same as for 6. a, b, and c above.	10. Same as for 6. a, b, and c above.

Procedure and Rationale	Observations and Findings	Significance

11. Gently remove your examining fingers.
12. Wipe off any secretions, discharge, and lubricating jelly from the perineum and external genitalia. Use a single front-to-back motion and use fresh tissue for each front-to-back stroke in order to avoid contamination from the rectum.
13. Remove your glove(s) and discard appropriately.
14. Be sure that the woman is helped back up on the table and aided into a sitting position. Some women, usually either young women having their first pelvic examination or older women, may need to sit several minutes to regain their equilibrium and composure.
15. Be sure that the woman is given a sanitary pad if she is menstruating or spotting from any procedure so she will not soil her clothes. If bleeding is not expected by the woman, tell her to expect it, for how long, and why there is spotting.
16. If not already done, either now or after she is dressed, share your findings from the examination with the woman.

45

Obtaining a Papanicolaou (Pap) Smear

Procedure	Rationale
1. Before starting the actual procedure be sure that the slide is labeled *in pencil* with the date and the woman's name and number.	1. Ink may smear or wash off during fixation of the slide, thus making it difficult to read. The fixative also makes it difficult to label the slide after it has been sprayed.
2. Insert the appropriate size speculum, visualize the cervix, and fix the speculum for appropriate exposure. (See "Preparatory and General Procedures" and "The Speculum Examination" in Chapter 44.) Be sure to gently remove any material that obscures visualization of the cervix or may interfere with the cytological study (e.g., mucous, discharge, blood) with a 2 × 2 or 4 × 4 gauze on a sponge stick.	2. If a total pelvic examination is being done, inspection of the external genitalia and checking of the urethra and the Bartholin's and Skene's glands precedes the speculum examination. The bimanual examination follows the speculum examination. It is imperative that no lubricating material except water be used prior to obtaining the Pap smear because it may render this cytological study invalid. Cleaning of the cervix that is too vigorous will remove the epithelium.
3. Place the longer portion of the slightly notched end of the wooden spatula or plastic scraper against and into the exter-	3. Pressing inserts the tip of the spatula a short distance into the cervical canal; how far depends on the patulousness of the

Procedure	Rationale
nal os of the cervix and press. Scrape the cervical canal by turning the spatula firmly a full circle. Be sure that, if the squamocolumnar junction is visible, it is included and scraped throughout the full circle.	cervix. Cells from the squamocolumnar junction are needed for cytological study for the Papanicolaou smear. Cervical cancer most frequently begins at the squamo-columnar junction.
4. If the squamocolumnar junction is not visible or it is not possible to reach it with the spatula, then do this step instead of Step 3. This most likely will be the situation if the woman is postmenopausal. Lightly moisten the cotton end of a cotton-tipped applicator and insert it into the cervical canal 2 to 3 centimeters. Roll the applicator back and forth between your thumb and index finger.	4. Atrophy of the uterus during the menopause causes the squamocolumnar junction to retreat within the cervical canal. Cells from the squamocolumnar junction are vital for a valid Pap smear (see 3). The cotton-tipped applicator is lightly moistened with saline in order to prevent absorption of the endo-cervical cells and secretions by the cotton and to prevent cotton fibers from getting on the slide.
6. Spread the cells on the labeled slide. If the cells were collected on a wooden spatula, place one flat side next to the label on the top half of the slide and stroke once to the end of the slide. Then turn the spatula over and place the other flat side next to the label on the bottom half of the slide and stroke once to the end of the slide. Do not stir in circles, repeatedly stroke, or stroke one side of the spatula on top of cells already spread from the other side of the spatula. If the specimen is too thick, then take the edge of the spatula and, with a single light stroke down the slide, remove the excess. If the cells were collected on a cotton-tipped applicator, gently roll the cotton end down the upper half of the slide from the label to the end of the slide. Repeat, rolling the cotton end down the lower half of the slide. Do not stir in circles or rub back and forth.	6. This procedure for spreading the cells is designed to avoid breaking and destroying the cells, a condition which will render the Pap smear useless.
7. Immediately spray the slide generously with the fixative or place it in a jar of fixative solution. Speed is of essence. Avoid waving the slide in the air or placing under a lighted gooseneck lamp prior to its being fixed.	7. Drying of the cells by air or light distorts the cells.

Procedure	Rationale
8. Appropriately dispose of the spatula or cotton-tipped applicator. 9. Proceed with the remainder of the speculum examination, making the necessary observations. Remove the speculum and deposit it in the proper container.	

There are individual and institutional variations in the procedure of obtaining a Papanicolaou smear. The variations from the above procedure relate to the number of slides made with specimens from the different locations. Some make two slides: one made from a specimen taken with the wooden spatula swept circumferentially at the os, and the second made from a specimen taken with the cotton-tipped applicator inserted into the cervical canal. Still others make a third slide from a specimen taken from the posterior vaginal fornix or vaginal vault either by aspiration or with a cotton-tipped applicator.

46

Obtaining A Gonococcal (GC) Culture

Procedure	Rationale
1. Insert the appropriate size speculum, visualize the cervix, and fix the speculum for appropriate exposure. (See "Preparatory and General Procedures" and "The Speculum Examination" in Chapter 44.) Remove any material (mucus, blood, discharge) obscuring the cervix with a 2 × 2 or 4 × 4 gauze on a sponge stick or ring forceps.	1. The cervical canal is considered the best site to culture for diagnosis of gonorrhea in the female since in 85 percent of cases the gonococcus will be harbored at this site. If a total pelvic examination is being done, inspection of the external genitalia and checking of the urethra and the Bartholin's and Skene's glands precedes the speculum examination. The bimanual examination follows the speculum examination.
2. Insert a dry sterile cotton-tipped applicator (swab) 1 to 2 centimeters (about ⅓ to ¾ inch) into the cervical canal and gently rotate it, being sure to move it against the sides of the canal. Leave it in place for approximately 30 to 60 seconds.	2. Time is needed for the organisms to be absorbed on the cotton swab.
3. Streak a Thayer-Martin (T-M) medium culture plate by rolling the cotton swab	3. T-M medium contains several antibiotics that discourage growth of the many other

on the medium in a large Z pattern which covers at least three-quarters of the plate.

organisms found in the vagina and cervix, which would otherwise overgrow the *Neisseria gonorrhoeae*. Rolling the cotton swab in a large Z pattern allows the swab to be adequately exposed to the culture for maximum transfer of organisms. This also allows for easier morphological study by spacing out the colonies.

4. Cover the culture plate with its cover and turn it upside down.

4. Avoid contamination from airborne organisms.

5. Appropriately dispose of the cotton swab.

5.

6. Many clinicians also obtain a second specimen from the cervical canal to make a slide for Gram's stain. Except as an adjunct to the culture, smears are not recommended either for an absolute diagnosis or as a test of cure of gonorrhea in the female. The presence of gram-negative intracellular diplococci is considered sufficient evidence to initiate treatment in sexually active individuals.

If a second specimen is obtained, a second sterile cotton-tipped applicator (swab) should be used and the specimen collected in the same manner from the cervical canal. Roll the cotton swab down the upper half of the slide from the label to the end of the slide. Repeat, rolling the cotton end down the lower half of the slide. Do not stir in circles or rub back and forth as this will damage the leukocytes.

7. As soon as you complete the remainder of the speculum examination place the culture plate in a candle jar, light the candle, and replace the lid on the jar.

Be sure the culture plate is properly labeled with the date, where the specimen was obtained, and the woman's name and number before placing in the candle jar.

7. The candle jar provides an atmosphere of 3% carbon dioxide, which is favorable for the partially anaerobic *N. gonorrhoeae*.

The candle jar holds a number of culture plates from different patients, so correct labelling is crucial.

8. Obtain another specimen for a second culture from the rectum:
   a. insert a dry sterile cotton-tipped applicator (swab) into the rectum approximately 1 inch (2½ centimeters).

8. Not all individuals and institutions routinely obtain a specimen from the rectum. However, it is recommended by the Centers for Disease Control of the Department of Health and Human Services that cultures be obtained from both the cervical canal and the rectum. In about 10 percent of cases of female gonorrhea, positive results will be obtained only from the rectal culture. It is the site most likely to be positive for gonorrhea when the cervical results are negative.

b. gently rotate the swab around the rectal wall for approximately 30 to 60 seconds.

c. remove the swab. Discard it if it is contaminated with feces. Take another cotton-tipped applicator and obtain another specimen from the rectum.

b. time is needed for the organisms to be absorbed on the cotton swab.

c. organisms from feces impede the growth of the *N. gonorrhoeae* on the culture medium. If fecal contamination is unavoidable, the special antibiotic composition of the T-M medium may help suppress the fecal organisms.

d. roll the uncontaminated cotton swab on a T-M medium culture plate in the same manner as the specimen taken from the cervical canal.

d. same as for 3 above.

e. replace the cover on the culture plate, place the properly labeled plate in the candle jar, light the candle, and replace the lid on the jar.

e. same as for 7 above.

f. appropriately dispose of the cotton-tipped swab.

9. Some clinicians think that the throat should also be routinely cultured.
10. *Note:* A gonococcal culture should always be obtained of any discharge elicited during examination of the urethra and Bartholin's and Skene's glands. The specimen is obtained with a dry sterile cotton-tipped applicator and handled in the same manner as a specimen obtained from the cervical canal or rectum.

Note: Many clinics and institutions now have culturettes. These consist of a container with one or two cotton-tipped applicators and a transfer medium. The specimen is taken and then inserted into the transfer medium for transfer to the laboratory for plating. If there are two cotton-tipped applicators they can both be used and transferred at the same time, with one for gonococcal culture and the other for culturing beta Streptococci if the site being cultured is the same (i.e., cervix).

47

Anatomy of the Pelvis, Pelvic Types, Evaluation of the Bony Pelvis, and Clinical Pelvimetry

Anatomy

Pelvimetry refers to measurement of diameters of the pelvis. These diameters are most accurately measured by roentgenographic study called x-ray pelvimetry. However, x-ray pelvimetry today is rarely done in order not to expose the mother and baby to the potential hazards of radiation unless absolutely necessary. It is possible to measure some of the critical diameters clinically using either your hands or a pelvimeter such as Thom's pelvimeter. In addition, it is possible to evaluate the general structure (size and shape) of the pelvis by feeling certain bony landmarks of the pelvis. The combined information of pelvic diameters and structure obtained clinically is compared with the estimated size of the baby.

Determination is then made as to the adequacy of the pelvis for passage of that particular baby or, earlier in pregnancy, of a certain-sized baby. Generally, a trial of labor has replaced x-ray pelvimetry when there is a question of the adequacy of the pelvis, which may indicate the need for cesarean section because of cephalopelvic or fetopelvic disproportion. Many physicians, however, will obtain x-ray pelvimetry on women who are primigravidas in labor with a breech presentation that they plan to deliver vaginally in order to confirm their clinical impressions of the adequacy of the pelvis, especially the inlet. X-ray pelvimetry is not performed until labor has begun and the pelvis has been evaluated in relationship to the estimated actual size of the baby about to be born.

Therefore a thorough knowledge of the anatomy of the bony pelvis is an essential prerequisite not only to the performance of clinical pelvimetry and accurate interpretation of these findings but also for evaluation of the total pelvis and its adequacy to accommodate the passage of the baby.

The pelvis is comprised of four bones: two innominate bones, the sacrum, and the coccyx. See Figure 47-1. Each *innominate bone* is comprised of three parts: the pubis, the ischium, and the ilium. The *ilium* is the posterior and upper portion of the innominate bone. The two ilia form the false pelvis, share with the sacrum the important bony landmark of the sacroiliac notch, and join the sacrum at either side at the *sacroiliac synchondroses*. The *ischium* is the medial and lower portion of the innominate bone and has such important bony landmarks as the ischial spine, the ischial tuberosity, and the pelvic side-wall. The *pubis* is the anterior portion of the innominate bone. The two pubic bones join each other in the front at the *symphysis pubis* and their inferior

angles from the descending rami form the important bony landmark of the pubic arch.

The sacrum and the coccyx form the posterior portion of the pelvis. The *sacrum* is formed by the fusion of the five sacral vertebrae, includes the important bony landmark of the *sacral promontory*, and joins the coccyx at the *sacrococcygeal symphysis.* The *coccyx* is formed by the fusion of four (sometimes three or five) rudimentary vertebrae, is usually movable, and is itself an important bony landmark.

The sacrococcygeal symphysis, symphysis pubis, and the two sacroiliac synchondroses (or sacroiliac articulations) are all amphiarthrodial *joints* consisting of a network of cartilage and ligaments that join the bones of the pelvis.

The pelvis is divided by the linea terminalis into the false pelvis above this demarcation and the true pelvis below it (Fig. 47-2). The *false pelvis* has little obstetric significance relevant to the passage of the fetus through the pelvis. The true pelvis constitutes the bony passageway through which the fetus must

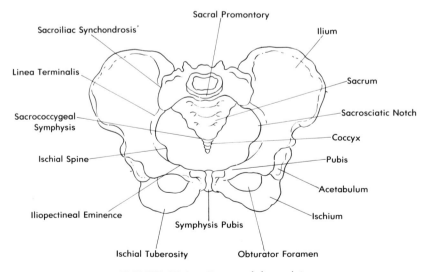

FIGURE 47-1. Bones of the pelvis.

maneuver to be born vaginally. Therefore, its construction, planes, and diameters are of utmost obstetric importance.

The true pelvis has the following as its boundaries:

superiorly: the sacral promontory, linea terminalis, the upper margins of the pubic bones
inferiorly: the inferior margins of the ischial tuberosities and the tip of the coccyx
posteriorly: the anterior surface of the sacrum and coccyx
laterally: the sacroiliac notches and ligaments, and the inner surface of the ischial bones
anteriorly: the obturator foramina, and the posterior surfaces of the symphysis pubis, pubic bones and ascending rami of the ischial bones

The *true pelvis* has three planes of obstetric significance: the inlet, the midplane, and the outlet. For each plane there are theoretically six diameters. However, not all diameters are used in measuring or discussing each of the planes or in discussion of pelvic types. Table 47-1 shows which diameters are pertinent to which planes. Those with an asterisk are considered critical to evaluation of pelvic adequacy. The sagittals (anterior and posterior) measure the distance from the midpoint of the transverse diameter to the points used in measuring the anteroposterior diameter.

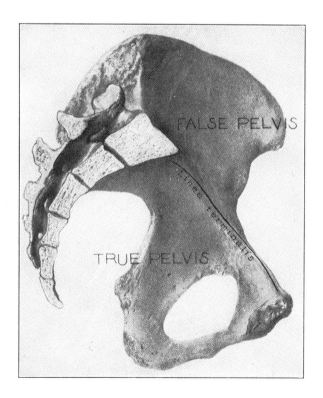

FIGURE 47-2.   Sagittal section of pelvis showing false and true pelvis. (Reproduced by permission from Pritchard, J. A., and MacDonald, P. C. *Williams Obstetrics, 15th.* New York: Appleton-Century-Crofts, 1976.)

TABLE 47-1.   Diameters of the Three Pelvic Planes of Obstetric Significance

Diameters	Inlet	Midplane	Outlet
Anteroposterior	X*	X*	X*
Right oblique	X		
Left oblique	X		
Transverse	X*	X*	X*
Anterior sagittal	X		
Posterior sagittal	X	X*	X*

* Critical to evaluation of pelvic adequacy.

The pelvic *inlet* (superior strait) is the upper entry into the true pelvis. Its boundaries are the sacral promontory posteriorly, the linea terminalis laterally, and the upper portion of the symphysis pubis and horizontal rami of the pubic bones anteriorly. The diameters of the inlet which are frequently referred to follow (see Figs. 47-3 and 47-4):

anteroposterior — actually there are three antero-posterior diameters of the inlet:

1. *conjugata vera* — the true conjugate of the inlet; extends from the middle of the sacral promontory to the middle of the upper margin of the symphysis pubis; normally measures 11 centimeters or more.
2. *obstetric conjugate* of the inlet — extends from the middle of the sacral promontory to the middle of the symphysis pubis on its inner surface a short distance (several millimeters) below its upper margin. The minimum measurement of this diameter before the pelvis is considered contracted is 10 centimeters. This is the shortest anteroposterior diameter because the symphysis pubis is slightly thicker at this point than at its upper or lower margin.
3. *diagonal conjugate* of the inlet — extends from the middle of the sacral promontory to the middle of the inferior (lower) margin of the symphysis pubis. The diagonal conjugate is the only diameter of the pelvic inlet that can be measured clinically. A normal clinical measurement is considered to be at least 11.5 centimeters.

transverse — the transverse diameter of the pelvic inlet measures the greatest distance between the linea terminalis on either side of the pelvis; this distance is approximately 13.5 centimeters or a little less, depending on the shape of the pelvis.

oblique — the oblique diameters of the pelvic inlet measure the distance between the sacroiliac synchondrosis on one side of the pelvis and the iliopectineal eminence on the opposite side of the pelvis. The location of the sacroiliac synchondrosis on the right or left of the pelvis determines whether the diameter is the right oblique diameter or the left oblique diameter. For example, if the diameter extends from the right sacroiliac synchondrosis to the left iliopectineal eminence it is the right oblique diameter. The oblique diameters average slightly under 13 (12.75) centimeters each.

The *midplane* of the pelvis is the plane of least dimensions because it is the narrowest portion of the pelvis the fetus has to navigate. The transverse diameter measures the distance between the ischial spines. Called the *inter-spinous diameter*, it normally measures about 10 centimeters. This measurement is critical as

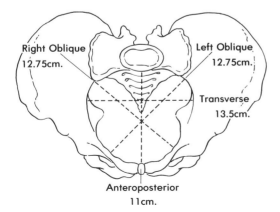

FIGURE 47-3.   Diameters of the pelvic inlet.

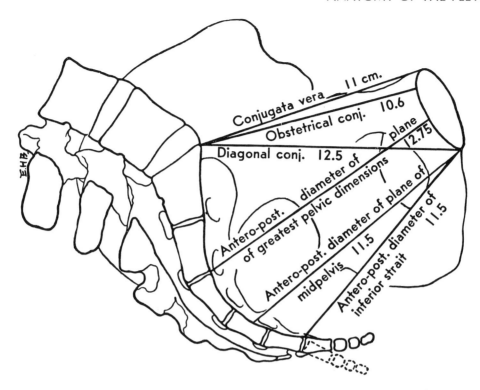

Conjugata vera — 11 cm.
Obstetrical conj. 10.6
Diagonal conj. 12.5
plane 12.75
Antero-post. diameter of greatest pelvic dimensions
Antero-post. diameter of plane of midpelvis 11.5
Antero-post. diameter of plane of inferior strait 11.5

FIGURE 47-4.   Pelvic planes and diameters. (Reproduced by permission from Pritchard, J. A., and MacDonald, P. C. *Williams Obstetrics, 15th*. New York: Appleton-Century-Crofts, 1976.)

the smallest diameter of the pelvis to which the fetus has to accommodate itself. If the ischial spines are prominent or sharp or the sidewalls converge so that the ischial spines protrude to the extent of encroaching on the space of the pelvic cavity, the interspinous measurement is diminished and pelvic adequacy for vaginal delivery of an average-sized baby is highly questionable. A contracted midplane is very often associated with a contracted outlet.

The anteroposterior diameter extends from the middle of the inferior margin of the symphysis pubis through the middle of the transverse diameter to the point on the sacrum dictated by this angle. This normally measures a minimum of 11.5 centimeters. The posterior sagittal diameter of the midplane is usually a minimum of 4.5 centimeters.

It is not clinically feasible to measure the diameters of the midplane. However, its ade-

quacy may be estimated by noting whether or not the ischial spines are prominent or encroaching rather than blunt, the sidewalls are convergent rather than straight, the sacrum is flat or shallow rather than hollow, and the outlet is contracted rather than measuring within normal limits.

The pelvic *outlet* is conceptualized as being composed of two triangles with the transverse diameter of the outlet serving as the common base of these two triangles. The transverse diameter of the outlet is the distance between the inner aspect of the lowermost part of the ischial tuberosities (*intertuberous* or *biischial diameter*), which usually measures approximately 10 centimeters. The posterior triangle has the tip of the sacrum as its apex and the anterior triangle has the middle of the inferior margin of the symphysis pubis as its apex. The anteroposterior diameter of the outlet extends from the middle of the inferior margin of the symphysis pubis to the tip of the sacrum. Unlike the anteroposterior diameter of the midplane, it does not transect the transverse diameter. It generally measures 11.5 centimeters. The posterior sagittal diameter of the outlet usually measures 7.5 centimeters. When these measurements are done clinically a rule of thumb is that the sum of the transverse diameter and the posterior sagittal measurements must equal at least 15 centimeters for pelvic adequacy of the outlet.

Other anatomic features of the pelvis considered in evaluation of pelvic adequacy include the following:

inclination of the symphysis pubis (Fig. 47-5). The longitudinal axis of the symphysis pubis is normally parallel to the longitudinal axis of the sacrum. If the symphysis pubis is not at least approximately parallel to the sacrum, the anteroposterior diameter of the inlet can be changed significantly. Tilting of the superior margin of the symphysis pubis towards the sacral promontory and of the inferior margin away from the sacrum is called *anterior inclination*. Tilting of the inferior margin of the symphysis pubis towards the sacrum and the superior margin away from the sacral promontory is called *posterior inclination*.

angle of the pubic arch. The descending rami of the pubic bones and the inferior margin of the symphysis pubis form what is known as the *pubic arch*. The angle of this arch should be at least 90° as determined just below the symphysis pubis. An arch that is 90° a few centimeters below the symphysis pubis but narrow above that (just below the symphysis pubis) decreases the available space in the anteroposterior diameter and may indicate an inadequate outlet.

general structure of the forepelvis. The inner aspect of the forepelvis (the anterior portion of the pelvis) should be rounded. A forepelvis that is not rounded but instead angles sharply toward the lateral portion of the pelvis decreases the oblique diameters of the inlet.

angle of the pelvic sidewalls. The pelvic sidewalls extend from the upper anterior angle of the sacrosciatic notch at the point of the widest transverse diameter of the pelvic inlet in a downward and forward line to the ischial tuberosities at the point of the widest transverse diameter of the pelvic outlet. They are normally slightly convergent in that, if the lines of their angles were extended beyond the pelvis, they would meet at about the level of the knees. However, when felt on pelvic examination they feel generally straight. Their importance is in whether or not the width of the pelvis at the inlet remains the

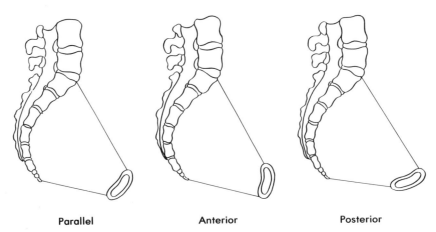

Parallel   Anterior   Posterior

FIGURE 47-5. Inclination of the symphysis pubis.

same throughout the pelvis. Divergence or convergence is based on whether the point of origin at the inlet and the ending point at the ischial tuberosities are essentially equidistant from the anteroposterior diameter of the pelvis. Convergent sidewalls usually decrease the angle of the pubic arch and may be accompanied by more prominent ischial spines. Divergent sidewalls always means a very wide angle of the pubic arch.

sacrosciatic notch. The shape and width of the sacrosciatic notch is important because it affects the posterior sagittal diameter of the inlet, which combines with the shape and rotation of the sacrum to determine the amount of room in the posterior portion of the pelvis for passage of the fetus.

TYPES OF PELVES

There are four basic pelvic types according to the Caldwell-Moloy classification: gynecoid, android, anthropoid, and platypelloid (Fig. 47-6). These are determined by certain characteristics of the pelvis and classified in accord with the characteristics of the posterior segment of the inlet. Anatomical portions of the pelvis used in evaluation of pelvic types are inlet, sacrum, sacrosciatic notch, sidewalls, ischial spines, and pubic arch.

Many pelves are not pure types but, rather, a mixture of types. For example, a gynecoid pelvis may be said to have an android tendency. This means that the posterior segment is gynecoid while the anterior segment is android or that the pelvis has certain android characteristics.

The importance of being familiar with pelvic types lies in the fact that many of the characteristics used in determining pelvic types affect the obstetric capacity of the pelvis, that is, the adequacy of the pelvis for accommodating passage of the baby. So while a pelvic type, in and of itself, may not seem too important, the characteristics of the pelvis that are being evaluated are extremely valuable when combined with clinical pelvimetry for evaluation of pelvic adequacy. This is especially true of the inlet, sacrum, ischial spines, and pubic arch.

Gynecoid Pelvis

The gynecoid pelvis is commonly known as the "female pelvis" because it is the type that occurs most frequently in women; 41 to 42 percent of women's pelves are gynecoid. This shape is ideal for childbearing. Its identifying characteristics are as follows:

inlet — the anterior, lateral, and posterior segments of the pelvis are well rounded, with the transverse diameter about the same or slightly greater than the anteroposterior diameter. The posterior sagittal diameter is only a little shorter than the anterior sagittal diameter.

sacrum — parallel with the symphysis pubis.

sacrosciatic notch — well rounded with an approximate distance of 2½ to 3 fingerbreadths along the sacrospinous ligament which runs between the ischial spine and the sacrum.

sidewalls — the pelvic sidewalls are straight.

ischial spines — blunt and neither prominent nor encroaching.

pubic arch — the pubic arch is wide (90° angle or more).

Android Pelvis

The android pelvis is commonly known as the "male pelvis" because it occurs more frequently in men. However, it does occur in 32.5 percent of white women and in 15.7 percent of nonwhite women. The android pelvis is a heavy pelvis which poses difficulty for vaginal delivery and increases the incidence of posterior position, forceps delivery, and stillbirth. The midplane and outlet contracture of the android pelvis increases the incidence of fetopelvic disproportion and cesarean sec-

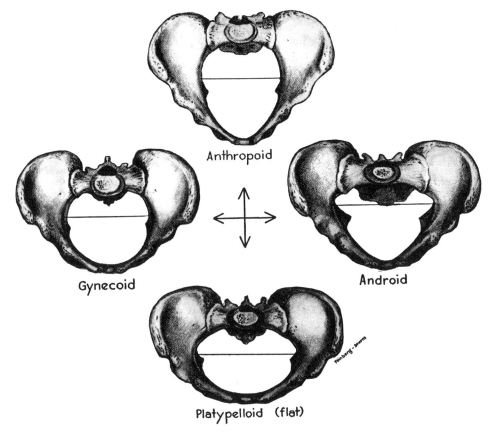

Anthropoid

Gynecoid

Android

Platypelloid (flat)

FIGURE 47-6.   Four pelvic types. A line passing through the widest transverse diameter divides the inlet into anterior and posterior segments. (Reproduced by permission from Pritchard, J. A., and MacDonald, P. C. *Williams Obstetrics, 15th.* New York: Appleton-Century-Crofts, 1976.)

tions. Characteristics of the android pelvis are as follows:

inlet — often referred to as heart-shaped; the posterior segment is wedge-shaped and the anterior segment (forepelvis) narrow and triangular. The posterior sagittal diameter is quite short in comparison to the anterior sagittal diameter. This means that there is very limited space in the posterior portion of the pelvis for accommodating the fetal head.

sacrum — anteriorly inclined and flat, thereby contributing to the shortness of the posterior

sagittal diameters throughout the pelvis.

sacrosciatic notch — has a high arch and is narrow with an approximate distance of 1½ to 2 fingerbreadths along the sacrospinous ligament between the ischial spine and the sacrum.

sidewalls — the pelvic sidewalls usually are convergent.

ischial spines — usually prominent and frequently encroaching, thereby decreasing the transverse (interspinous) diameter of the midplane.

pubic arch — narrow, with an acute angle of much less than 90°.

Anthropoid Pelvis

The anthropoid pelvis is most common in the nonwhite races, with occurrence in nonwhite women at 40.5 percent as compared to white women at 23.5 percent. The shape of the anthropoid pelvis favors a posterior position of the fetus. It is adequate for vaginal delivery if on the large size.

inlet — characteristically oval with an antero- posterior diameter much larger than the transverse diameter. The anterior segment (forepelvis) of the pelvis is somewhat pointed and more narrow than the posterior segment.

sacrum — the sacrum is posteriorly inclined and so, although flat, the posterior sagittals are long throughout the pelvis. Therefore the space in the posterior portion of the pelvis is increased for accommodating the fetal head. The anthropoid pelvis has the longest sacrum of the four types of pelves, and hence, is the deepest pelvis.

sacrosciatic notch — of average height but quite wide; has an approximate distance of 4 finger- breadths along the sacrospinous ligament between the ischial spine and the sacrum.

sidewalls — frequently somewhat convergent.

ischial spines — usually prominent but not encroaching, so the transverse (interspinous) diameter of the midplane is generally less than that of the gynecoid pelvis but not as contracted as the android pelvis.

pubic arch — may be somewhat narrow, but the potential problem of outlet contracture generally is counterbalanced by the lengthy anteroposterior diameter's having a long posterior sagittal, thus providing room in the posterior portion of the pelvis for the baby.

Platypelloid Pelvis

Fortunately the platypelloid pelvis is rare, be- cause it is not particularly conducive to vaginal

delivery. It occurs less than 3 percent of the time in both white and nonwhite women.

inlet — has been likened to a flat gynecoid pelvis. It is the opposite of the anthropoid pelvis, having instead a short anteroposterior diameter and a wide transverse diameter. The anterior segment (forepelvis) of the pelvis is quite wide.

sacrum — inclined posteriorly and quite hollow, thereby creating a short sacrum and shallow pelvis.

sacrosciatic notch — wide and flat with an acute angle between the ischial spines and the sacrum. *sidewalls* — slightly convergent.

ischial spines — the ischial spines are some- what prominent but, because of the flattened character of the pelvis and wide transverse diameters throughout the pelvis, this pro- minence has no effect. The transverse dia- meter of the midplane of a platypelloid pelvis is the widest of all the pelves.

pubic arch — quite wide; this pelvis is the widest of all the pelvic types.

PROCEDURE, RATIONALE, AND DESCRIPTION OF FINDINGS

Before doing clinical pelvimetry it is important that you measure your fingers and your fist because they will become your instruments of measurement. Specifically you should measure the length of the reach of your examining fingers, that is, from the tip of your longest finger to the juncture of your first finger (palm) with your thumb. This length should be mea- sured both with the measurer just resting against this juncture and with the measurer pressed into this junction with the same degree of force you use against the perineum when reaching for the diagonal conjugate. This latter pressing usually adds ½ to 1 centimeter to your reach.

Even if you have access in your setting to a Thom's pelvimeter for measuring the diameters of the outlet, it is wise to have measured your fist as you may not always be in a setting with a Thom's pelvimeter. Measurement of your fist is done from the outer (ulnar) aspect to the outer (radial) aspect of the collective group of knuckles of your fingers where they attach to your hand. If this does not measure at least 8 centimeters, then position your thumb in a way that you will position it each time and add the joint or knuckle of your thumb into the measurement.

Clinical evaluation of the pelvis and pelvimetry are usually included as part of the initial antepartal examination and, depending on circumstances, repeated again either late in the third trimester or at the time of the initial intrapartal bimanual pelvic examination. (See "The Bimanual Examination" in Chapter 44.) It is important to develop a routine procedure

for performing clinical evaluation of the bony pelvis so that all aspects are remembered and included, and so the procedure progresses as smoothly and comfortably for the woman as possible.

The woman is prepared for this procedure as for the pelvic examination: empty bladder, lithotomy position, careful draping, and instruction about both the procedure and relaxation techniques to help her cope with the examination. (See "Preparatory and General Procedures" in Chapter 44.)

One useful explanation of how it will feel to the woman to have you pressing against her pelvic bones is to hold one of her arms and press firmly with your thumb against her wrist bone while explaining that any discomfort she will feel will be like this and will be due to pressure.

Procedure and Rationale	Description of Findings
1. Insert your two vaginal examining fingers palmar surface up just inside the woman's vagina. Slightly separate your fingers and gently palpate the inner surface of the symphysis pubis. This separation of your fingers places them on either side of the urethra, thus sparing it any trauma and the woman any additional discomfort while palpating.	1. Note any abnormal thickening of the symphysis pubis that would decrease the obstetric conjugate diameter of the pelvic inlet. Note if there is any separation of the symphysis pubis. Also note the position of the symphysis pubis so that after palpating the sacrum you can determine if the symphysis pubis is parallel with the sacrum or if it has anterior inclination or posterior inclination.
2. Move your fingers to either side of the symphysis pubis, palpating the horizontal rami of the pubic bones toward the lateral portion of the pelvis.	2. Evaluate the curvature of the upper portion of the forepelvis for round and roomy or angular structure which would decrease the oblique diameters of the inlet.
3. Follow the horizontal rami of the pubic bone on one side of the pelvis to the lateral portion of the pelvic inlet. Then palpate down the pelvic sidewall to the ischial spine. Be sure to get to the lateral portion of the pelvis before beginning your descent from the inlet to the midpelvis. Otherwise, by starting your descent too early, you will end up at the ischial tuberosity rather than at the ischial spine.	3. Evaluate the pelvic sidewall and determine if it is straight, convergent, or divergent.

Procedure and Rationale	Description of Findings
This maneuver is used not only for evaluation of the pelvic sidewalls but also as a means of locating the ischial spine.	
4. Palpate the ischial spine.	4. Evaluate the ischial spine for its protuberance and determine if it is blunt (or flat), prominent (or sharp), or encroaching.
5. Sweep your fingers across the pelvic cavity to the ischial spine on the opposite side of the pelvis, palpate it, and sweep your fingers back to the first spine.	5. This is done to estimate the distance between the ischial spines. While the interspinous (transverse) diameter cannot be clinically measured, you can get an impression of its adequacy. This impression improves in accuracy with experience, comparing clinical findings with x-ray pelvimetry whenever circumstances provide this opportunity, and practicing on objects whose diameters you can measure.
6. Starting at the ischial spine outline the sacrosciatic notch and return to the ischial spine.	6. Note the shape and height of the sacrosciatic notch.
7. Now palpate across the sacrosciatic notch, following the sacrospinous ligament from the ischial spine to the sacrum.	7. Measure the width of the sacrosciatic notch, which is the same as the length of the sacrospinous ligament, in terms of fingerbreadths.
8. From where you ended on the sacrum from following the sacrospinous ligament over, move down the sacrum to the coccyx. Press firmly on the coccyx. (See Step 17 if not sure of mobility.)	8. Note whether or not the coccyx is mobile. This is described as movable or fixed.
9. Now walk your fingers up the sacrum (palpating its width as you go) as far as you can reach.	9. Determine the shape of the sacrum as hollow, flat (or straight), or J-shaped (Fig. 47-7). Note if the sacrum is in alignment with the sacral promontory or instead either anteriorly or posteriorly inclined. Also note the longitudinal axis of the sacrum and correlate it with the position of the symphysis pubis you have already felt in order to determine if the symphysis is parallel with or has anterior or posterior inclination in relation to the sacrum.
10. The diagonal conjugate is measured next. The sacral promontory is reached in one of two ways. The first is a continuation of the preceding step where you walk your	10. If you felt the sacral promontory then you chart the measurement of the diagonal conjugate as whatever you measure it to be. If you did not feel the sacral promon-

Procedure and Rationale	Description of Findings

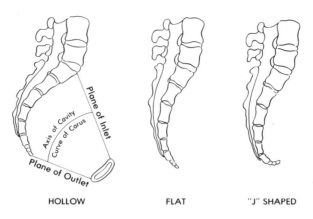

HOLLOW   FLAT   "J" SHAPED

FIGURE 47-7.   Sacral shapes.

fingers up the sacrum to the sacral pro-montory. However, if the sacrum is hollow it is possible that you might lose contact with the sacrum as it may become too far away for you to reach. It is possible to extend the normal reach of your fingers by depressing the perineum by exerting pressure against it. This also exerts pres-sure on the juncture of your first finger (palm) with your thumb, which addition-ally extends your reach. Maximal pressure is exerted against the perineum by sup-porting the elbow of your examining hand against either your hip or your thigh (which is elevated horizontally by placing your foot on a stool) and using this as a brace to further exert pressure against the perineum.

Reaching for the sacral promontory in-volves having your examining hand at the proper angle and in the proper location. It helps to visualize mentally where the sacral promontory is in relation to the vaginal introitus. The tips of your exam-ining fingers should be in the posterior fornix of the vagina. Then drop your wrist

tory then chart the diagonal conjugate as being greater than whatever you have measured the length of your examining fingers to be.

Procedure and Rationale	Description of Findings

(it helps to lower your elbow) and press against the perineal body with the knuckles of your last two fingers. Dropping your wrist changes the direction of your fingers from horizontal to an angle upwards. This angle needs to be approximately 45°.

If you feel the sacral promontory, maintain contact with it while raising your wrist until your hand touches the inferior margin of the symphysis pubis. With your other hand mark on your examining hand the point which is touching the symphysis pubis. After your hand is removed from the vagina, measure the distance from the tip of your finger which was touching the sacral promontory to the mark on your hand which was touching the symphysis pubis.

If you are unable to feel the sacral promontory, you know that the diagonal conjugate is greater than the length of your examining fingers, which you have already measured.

Measurement of the diagonal conjugate is the last of the internal evaluations of the bony pelvis to be done, as it is the most uncomfortable. The woman should be forewarned that this maneuver may be uncomfortable for her.

11. As you withdraw your fingers from the woman's vagina turn them horizontally and place them against the inferior margin of the symphysis pubis.

12. With the thumbs of both of your hands palpate the pubic arch by following it down the descending rami of the pubic bones.

13. Continue your palpation down the pubic rami to the ischial tuberosities. Measure

11. If your fingers fit comfortably in this location the pubic arch is probably at least a 90° angle. If you cannot fit your two fingers in this location the pubic arch is probably less than a 90° angle.

12. The arch should become progressively wider from a rounded apex. Visualize the angle of the arch immediately below the symphysis pubis as you palpate and combine these findings with those of Step 11 to finalize your determination of the angle of the pubic arch.

13. Chart your measurement of the intertuberous diameter either as what it mea-

Procedure and Rationale	Description of Findings
the transverse diameter of the outlet (intertuberous diameter; biischial diameter) either by using a Thom's pelvimeter or by placing your premeasured fist between the tuberosities.	sured if you used a Thom's pelvimeter or as greater or lesser than the measured width of your fist. If you use your fist it is important to recognize that the thickness of the tissue between your bones and the woman's bones will make the actual bony measurement approximately 1 centimeter greater. This centimeter, however, is not added to your measurement but should be considered in evaluating the adequacy of the intertuberous diameter.
14. If you have a Thom's pelvimeter, measure the posterior sagittal diameter. The anterior sagittal diameter is not generally measured. It is not possible to measure either of these diameters with your hands.	14. The posterior sagittal diameter of the pelvic outlet should measure 7.5 centimeters.

15. It is possible, although not usually done, to measure the anteroposterior diameter of the pelvic outlet with your hands. If this measurement is done it should be done after doing the diagonal conjugate and before removing your examining hand from the vagina. Simply come down the sacrum from the promontory until you locate the tip of the sacrum and place the tip of one of your examining fingers on the tip of the sacrum (at the sacrococcygeal junction); then raise your examining hand until it touches the inferior margin of the symphysis pubis, while maintaining contact with the tip of the sacrum with the tip of your finger. With your other hand mark on your examining hand the point which is touching the symphysis pubis and measure the distance between it and the tip of the finger which was on the tip of the sacrum.

16. If you have had difficulty evaluating middle and lower pelvic structures vaginally, end your examination of the pelvis during the rectovaginal examination to confirm your vaginal findings, as it is easier to feel these structures through the rectum. This includes palpation of the coccyx, ischial spines, sacrospinous ligament, and the lower sacrum.

17. If you are unsure of coccyx mobility, test for it during the rectovaginal examination by holding the coccyx between your rectal finger and your thumb which is positioned externally. Now attempt to move it back and forth between your finger and your thumb.

18. Some clinicians believe that it is necessary to palpate and evaluate completely both sides of the bony pelvis. Other clinicians believe that, with the exception of sweeping across the pelvic cavity to feel the opposite ischial spine and estimate the transverse diameter of the midplane, it is sufficient to actually feel only one side of the bony pelvis unless there is obvious pelvic deformity as observed during the physical examination from the woman's posture, stance, and position of the lower spinal column. In such rare cases both sides of the bony pelvis should be evaluated. Otherwise, one can assume that the two sides of the pelvis are equilateral and thus reduce the amount of discomfort to the woman by palpating only one side.

Procedure and Rationale   Description of Findings

    The procedure described above is in accord with the latter viewpoint. Those who believe in complete examination of both sides of the pelvis can do so either by turning their examining hand over or by switching hands for palpation of the second side.

19. If evaluation of the bony pelvis was incorporated as part of the total pelvic examination, one now proceeds with the remainder of the pelvic examination. If clinical pelvimetry was done as an isolated procedure, then the procedure ends with wiping the woman off and sharing your findings with her as outlined in Steps 12 to 16 in "The Rectovaginal Examination" in Chapter 44.

EVALUATION OF FINDINGS

Following is a listing of generally accepted findings that indicate pelvic adequacy upon clinical evaluation of the bony pelvis:

Forepelvis: rounded
Sidewalls: straight
Ischial spines: blunt
Sacrospinous ligament: 2½ to 3 fingerbreadths
Coccyx: movable
Sacrum: hollow
Diagonal conjugate: 11.5 centimeters or greater
Pubic arch: 90° or greater (2 fingerbreadths)
Intertuberous diameter: 8 centimeters or greater

There may be variations of the above findings which in and of themselves would not indicate pelvic inadequacy. It is well to remember that these rather precise findings must be combined with the other findings regarding inclination of the symphysis pubis, depth and angle of the sacrosciatic notch, alignment of the sacrum, and roominess of the posterior portion of the pelvis. The sum of all these findings is then put into a composite mental image of the total pelvis and its general type.

    The individual pelvic architecture is then weighed against the estimated size of the fetus at term, the type of presenting part, and its position. A determination of pelvic adequacy is made from these findings. When evaluation of the bony pelvis is done early in pregnancy it is often evaluated as adequate for a certain size baby. This specificity is helpful if there is a question of adequacy when the baby ends gestation larger than that which is felt could be accommodated. For example, charting may include a summary statement such as "adequate for a 7½-pound baby"; at term, if the estimated fetal weight is 8 pounds one is alerted to a potential problem requiring re-evaluation of the pelvis and evaluation of labor status with this concern in mind.

48

Breast Preparation: Massage, Manual Expression, and Nipple Rolling

Breast preparation for breast-feeding involves a number of components: examination, care (e.g., support, cleansing), and specific techniques of preparation. The preparation presented here concentrates on techniques and includes breast massage, manual expression, and nipple rolling.

This method of breast preparation for breast-feeding serves several purposes:

1. Promotion of the flow of breast milk post-partally by clearing the lactiferous sinuses and ducts of the early viscid colostrum and establishing the free flow of the later, less viscid, colostrum during the antepartal period
2. Strengthening of the erector muscles of the nipples prior to the birth of the baby, thereby providing an erect nipple for the baby to latch on to

3. Preparation of the mother with skills, massage, and manual expression, which will be useful to her in many ways while initiating breast-feeding and during the entire period of time during which she breast-feeds her baby
4. Increasing familiarity, comfort, and naturalness in touching and caring for her breasts

Breast massage, manual expression, and nipple rolling should not begin before the thirty-sixth week of gestation. This is because of the possibility that antepartal breast stimulation might cause the release of oxytocin, which may in turn cause the initiation of labor. Although this reasoning is hypothetical, of questionable validity, and both theoretically and clinically unproven, it has been the basis for some objection against the method of breast preparation presented here. Usually this objection is overcome by not starting preparation until the thirty-sixth week of gestation. This compromise diminishes the potential for preterm delivery, yet it allows enough time for all purposes of this breast preparation to be fulfilled.

Breast massage, manual expression, and nipple rolling are done in that sequence because massage increases circulation and facilitates the flow of milk through the ductal system of the lactiferous sinuses. Manual expression then expresses the milk out of the sinuses through the ducts in the nipple to the outside. All three techniques should be done daily, preferably immediately after bathing to take advantage of the increased circulation resulting from the warmth of the water.

Before starting this breast preparation, the woman should first do the following:

1. Wash her hands
2. Be comfortably seated
3. Remove clothing covering her breasts
4. Protect her other clothes by covering them and her lap with a bath towel
5. Lubricate her hands with some form of lubricant, such as hand lotion or cream, mineral oil, baby oil, cocoa butter

PROCEDURE FOR BREAST MASSAGE

The following is the procedure for breast massage:

1. Visualizing a total breast as the face of a clock, place one hand, palmar side down, at 12 o'clock just above the upper margin of the breast. Place the other hand, palmar side down, on top of the first hand.
2. Apply firm, even pressure while drawing the two hands apart laterally, one hand then going down each side of the breast.
3. As the hands go down the sides of the breasts, keep the thumbs on the upper portion of the breast as the fingers again meet and cover each other under the breast, thereby cupping the breast in the hands.
4. Continuing the firm, even pressure, draw the breast upward and forward as the fingers press up toward the areolae and nipple and the thumbs press down toward the areolae and nipple.
5. Without touching the areolae and nipple, allow the breast to slip between the fingers and thumbs as they slide off of the breast.
6. Repeat steps 1 to 5 in sequence 10 to 15 times, relubricating the hands as needed.

PROCEDURE FOR MANUAL EXPRESSION

The following steps are used for manual expression:

1. Support a breast with one hand.
2. Use the thumb and index or middle finger of the other hand and place them across from each other on opposite sides of the nipple at the outer margin of the areola. (The lactiferous sinuses are located in the area beneath the outer edge of the areola.)
3. a. in a milking motion, press backward (away from the areola), then inward (down into the tissue), then forward (toward the nipple), and then release the pressure.
   b. the pressure applied must be of gentle-firm quality. Undue pressure could undesirably traumatize the tissue, yet the pressure must be firm enough to actually compress the sinuses.
4. Observe for beads of colostrum on the nipple surface where the duct openings are. Beads of colostrum may not be observed for each placement of the fingers when first doing manual expression. However, with daily expression, all of the ducts will

soon become free-flowing and colostrum beads not only will be seen but will become little squirts or streams for each milking motion performed.

5. Gently wipe or blot the colostrum off the nipple surface with a clean washcloth.
6. Methodically move the thumb and finger around the areolae, repeating steps 2 to 5 for each location. There are 15 to 20 lactiferous sinuses, all of which should be emptied. This means 8 to 10 thumb and finger placements with the thumb having covered half of the areola and the finger of the other half of the areola by the end of all the placements.
7. When first doing manual expression, perform the milking motion no more than twice for each location in order not to traumatize tissue while the technique is being learned. After all ducts have become free-flowing and the woman has facility with the technique, manual expression can be done until the flow of colostrum ceases.

PROCEDURE FOR NIPPLE ROLLING

The procedure for nipple rolling follows:

1. Support a breast with one hand.
2. Place the opposite sides of the nipple between the sides of the thumb and the index finger of the other hand. Proper placement of the thumb and index finger on the nipple avoids the nipple surface (end) where the ducts open and includes the entire side of the nipple down onto the adjacent aspect of the areola.
3. Apply gentle pressure and roll the nipple back and forth as far as it will go between the thumb and finger without moving the placement of either on the nipple.
4. Roll the nipple for approximately 30 seconds.
5. Repeat steps 1 to 4 for the other breast.
6. Avoid skin friction with light lubrication on the thumb and index finger, yet not so much lubrication that the nipple becomes too slippery to manipulate.

49

Second Stage Pushing

There are two reasons why it is important that a woman know how to push effectively during the second stage of labor. First, while maternal pushing effort is normally a natural response to a reflex mechanism, it is at times necessary for the woman to push without the benefit of the stimulating reflex mechanism. Secondly, a woman may feel like pushing but pushes so ineffectually that progress is inhibited. There are a number of techniques which enhance the maternal pushing effort and which when utilized can change ineffectual pushing into effective maternal pushing.

Breath Control

The usual instruction has been for the woman to take one or two cleansing breaths (a deep breath in and out) when she feels the start of the contraction and while the contraction is building. Then she was to take a deep breath and hold it while she pushed for as l—o—n—g as she could. Two or three good pushes were usual during a contraction.

However, it is possible that this kind of breath holding, combined with prolonged bearing down, may produce fetal hypoxia and acidosis because the breath holding closes the glottis while the bearing down increases the intrathoracic pressure. This combination results in a drop in arterial pressure caused by decreased cardiac output due to diminished venous return to the heart. Decreased arterial pressure has two effects, decreased blood flow to the placenta and decreased oxygen content in the blood that does circulate to the placenta. Fetal hypoxia may be prevented with different pushing instructions to the woman.

These different instructions are for the woman to push after expiration, as a forced exhalation, for short periods of time (5 to 6 seconds). This often will be accompanied by a grunt. In such an effort the glottis is at least partially open, the abdominal muscles are shortened and contracted against the uterus, and the intrathoracic pressure doesn't increase to interfere with the venous return to the heart and produce its resulting effect on cardiac output and arterial pressure.

Body Position

A woman can push in any position — on her back, on her side, on her hands and knees, kneeling, or squatting. Her position depends on her preference or her own or the baby's condition or situation. Squatting has the advantage of adding the effect of gravity to the bearing down effort. Upright positions (squatting, sitting, standing) may shorten the total length of labor. Second stage is facilitated because of the increased pressure of the fetal head on the pelvic floor and the improved alignment of the fetus with the pelvis.

The woman should be encouraged to be on her back if pushing is ineffectual in other positions and her condition or the baby's condition does not contraindicate it. Several techniques for effective pushing can be instituted best or only with her on her back. The following instructions are to be used when the woman is on her back. All of them must be done in order to enhance pushing effectiveness. Using one alone will not accomplish the desired effect.

When the woman starts her breathing for pushing she brings her legs up and apart. She raises up and curves her back, tucks her chin down onto her chest, and grasps either her knees or behind her thighs with her hands. Pillows, backrests designed for this purpose, or an arm placed underneath her shoulders helps her get into the raised, curved-back position. The importance of this position is that it directs her pushing effort in the right direction. Many women arch their backs rather than curve their backs. This wastes their pushing effort because it decreases the force they could get behind the push if they were properly positioned.

Many women spoil their effort by letting their heads hang back. This posture diverts some of the pushing effort to the throat as well as being distracting since this is an uncomfortable position. If the woman starts a contraction with her head back and is unable to change and tuck her chin onto her chest, lift and support her head with a hand behind her head.

The woman's grasping either her knees or behind her thighs with her hands serves two purposes: (1) it helps her get into and maintain the curved position of her back and (2) it provides her with something to pull back on as she pushes down.

Arm Position and Action

The maternal pushing effort is greatly facilitated if the woman has something to pull back on while she pushes down; this gives her a counterforce to push against. There are other means of providing a counterforce besides having her grasp her knees or behind her thighs if either of these positions is not feasible. The handlebars on the delivery room table serve this purpose. The bars on the siderails of her hospital bed can be used. The best alternative is to have someone on both sides of the bed, standing below the level of her hips, facing her, and each extending a hand to her underneath her leg to grasp. As she pulls against these hands the individuals also pull sufficiently to maintain their position and provide a counterbalance to her pulling.

How the woman pulls back is also important. Pulling straight back tends to throw her body out of its curved position and may cause her to arch her back. Therefore, her elbows should be bent and out from her sides as though she were rowing a boat. This will maintain her proper body position.

Pubic Pressure

This technique is done by someone other than the woman. It is used if the woman seems to be having some difficulty in pushing in the right place. The admonition to "bear down as if you were having a bowel movement" not only lacks in aesthetic quality but also misdirects the pushing effort more posteriorly than is optimal.

With the edge of your slightly cupped hand, mild pressure is applied immediately above the symphysis pubis and the woman is instructed to push against your hand. This directs her pushing effort more properly anteriorly and involves the maximum use of her abdominal muscles.

Vaginal Stimulation

This technique is also done by someone other than the woman. In instances where it is mandatory for the woman to push but she does not feel the urge to push, it is possible to stimulate the perineal floor reflex mechanism by simulating the pressure of the presenting part with your fingers. As the woman pushes, you insert two or three fingers into the vagina and forcefully press down on the posterior vaginal wall. In keeping with the philosophy of nonintervention in normal processes and the principle of as little vaginal manipulation and examination as possible in order to reduce the possible introduction of infection, this technique is used only when absolutely indicated. Generally it is quite effective.

50

Perineal Prep (Cleaning)

The perineal cleansing prep is a procedure for making the perineum and surrounding region as clean as possible. The same basic procedure is followed regardless of when it is done for whatever reason (e.g., delivery, sterile vaginal examination).

The principle followed in this procedure is the one of going from inside to outside (from a central point to the periphery) with inside being the area desired clean and outside being periphery or adjoining region. The inside therefore becomes the point of emphasis for both cleansing and avoiding contamination.

The purpose of this procedure is to clean, and the mere motions of passing lightly over the skin surface with cotton balls or 4 × 4s thwart this purpose. Scrubbing, not so vigorous as to be painful but vigorous enough to cleanse, is called for.

The solutions used for the perineal cleansing prep vary and therefore are eliminated from this discussion, which deals only with the mechanics of the actual cleaning itself. The use of cotton balls or gauze 4 × 4s also varies from setting to setting. To facilitate presentation, 4 × 4s will be used in this procedure with the understanding that cotton balls can be used instead.

The following procedure (Fig. 50-1) is actually a listing of steps to be gone through in the sequence presented. The sequence is important in order to avoid contamination of the perineal area. Dry 4 × 4s are held over the introitus during the first three series of scrubbing strokes.

1. The first series of scrubbing strokes begins at the level of the clitoris and moves back and forth across the mons pubis upward onto the lower abdomen.
2. The second series of scrubbing strokes begins in the crease of the groin between the thigh and the lateral edge of the labia majora on one side and moves back and forth across the width of the inner thigh to midway up to the knee.
3. The third series of scrubbing strokes is the same as for the second series only for the opposite side.

These first three series of scrubbing strokes direct any excess cleansing fluid to the outside

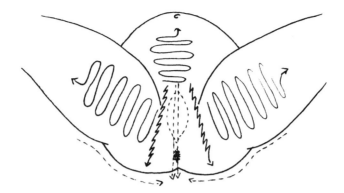

FIGURE 50-1. Cleaning the perineal area. (Adapted from Ziegel, E., and VanBlarcom, C. C. *Obstetric Nursing, 5th.* New York: Macmillan, 1963.)

and also are directed so contamination from the outside is not brought to the inside.

4. With very short back-and-forth motions (approximately 1 inch in length) the labia majora on one side is scrubbed from the level of the clitoris downward past the level of the anus to the level of the bed or table.
5. The same is done for the labia majora on the opposite side.
6. With a single downward motion from front to back (or top to bottom) the vulva, perineum, and anus are cleansed.
7. Step 6 is repeated with unused 4 × 4s. This is the one area cleansed twice.

Steps 4, 5, 6, and 7 are designed to avoid any contamination of the perineum or vulva from the anal area. In all of the above steps more than one 4 × 4 may be used at a time but none are reused. They are used once for a step and then discarded.

8. If any remaining solution is poured over the area it should be poured at the level of the vulva downward in order to avoid the contamination which would occur if poured higher over surrounding skin surfaces.
9. The wet pad underneath the woman is removed and replaced with a dry sterile pad.

51

Pudendal Block

Pudendal block is a regional anesthesia in which the pudendal nerve is blocked, or anesthetized. Pudendal block has these advantages: (1) anesthetizes the perineum and vulva including the clitoris, labia majora, labia minora, perineal body, and rectal area; (2) has no effect on the uterus or its contractions; (3) poses minimal potential danger to the mother provided that the proper medication is used in proper amounts, and (4) poses minimal potential danger to the baby if care is taken not to inadvertently give the anesthetic agent intravenously. With the exception of local infiltration of the perineal body as described in Chapter 52, pudendal block is by far the safest obstetric anesthesia known.

The anesthetic agent usually used in pudendal block is 1% lidocaine hydrochloride (Xylocaine) — 10 milligrams per milliliter — although a number of other local anesthetics can be used. The length of effect of the anesthesia depends on the success of the pudendal block and on the medication. An effective block with lidocaine will last approximately 1½ hours. It has the advantage of being fast-acting. The amount used is 10 milliliters (100 milligrams) per side. The maximum safe total dosage of lidocaine is 500 milligrams. If you use 200 milligrams for the pudendal block you will be able to use another 100 milligrams for a quick local infiltration of the perineal body if the pudendal block failed and still have some, if needed, for further local infiltration for repair of the episiotomy or lacerations.

The pudendal nerve arises from the pudendal plexus, which is formed by branches of the second, third, and fourth sacral nerves. The pudendal nerve is the largest branch of the pudendal plexus and leaves it as a single nerve trunk. The pudendal nerve passes across the posterior surface of the sacrospinous ligament just as this ligament attaches to, or within 0.5 to 1.0 centimeter of, the ischial spine as the nerve momentarily leaves the pelvic cavity from the greater sciatic foramen and reenters the pelvic cavity in the lesser sciatic foramen (Fig. 51-1). It is helpful to remember that it is the projection of the ischial spine that divides these two foramina. As the pudendal nerve enters the lesser sciatic foramen it enters Alcock's canal, which directs the pudendal nerve anteriorly to the inferior ramus of the ischium and pubis. As it courses through Alcock's canal the pudendal nerve divides into

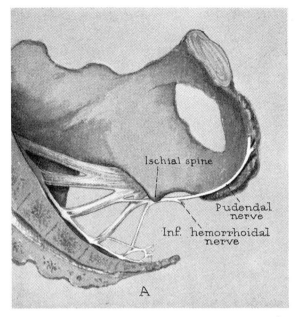
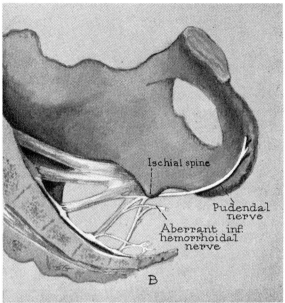

FIGURE 51-1.   Relationship between the pudendal nerve and the bones of the pelvis. (Reproduced by permission from Bonica, J. J. *Principles and Practice of Obstetric Analgesia and Anesthesia, Volume 1.* Philadelphia: Davis, 1967.)

three main branches: (1) the inferior, hemorrhoidal nerve, (2) the perineal nerve, and (3) the dorsal nerve of the clitoris. Each of these branches further subdivide to become the primary nerve supply of the perineum.

Thus, the art of successfully performing a pudendal block lies in:

1. Knowing the pertinent anatomy
2. Identifying accurately, by palpation, the ischial spine and also, ideally, the sacrospinous ligament
3. Placing the anesthetic agent properly in relation to the ischial spine

The technique of pudendal block described here is the transvaginal route. While it is possible to perform a pudendal block by using a transperineal route, which was the original route for pudendal blocks, it no longer is commonly done. The transperineal route is much more uncomfortable and painful for the woman, and more difficult to perform. Even the idea of doing a transperineal pudendal block in the event that the fetal head is too far down to do a transvaginal pudendal block has given way to doing a local infiltration of the perineal body instead.

A long, 12- to 15-centimeter (5- to 6-inch), 20- or 22-gauge needle is used with or without a needle guide. See Figure 51-2. If available, a needle guide is usually used; most often it is an Iowa trumpet. Whatever is used, the needle guide should allow for the needle to protrude 1.5 centimeters beyond the end of the needle guide. A 10-milliliter syringe with a Luer-Lok attachment completes the necessary equipment in addition to the medication (poured into a medicine glass).

If there is no needle guide the needle point can be protected from catching on the vaginal mucosa during insertion by holding it parallel

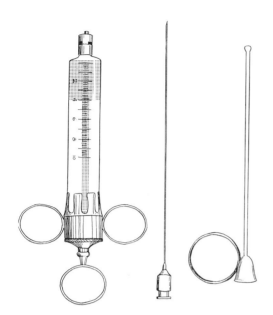

FIGURE 51-2.   Equipment used for pudendal block, consisting of 10-milliliter syringe; 6-inch, 20-gauge needle; and Iowa trumpet needle guide. (Reproduced by permission from Bonica, J. J. *Principles and Practice of Obstetric Analgesia and Anesthesia, Volume 1.* Philadelphia: Davis, 1967.)

in the groove between your two examining fingers with the point between your fingertips. If an Iowa trumpet is used it is inserted first, once your examining fingers have located the ischial spine, positioned, and then the needle with the syringe attached is inserted through this needle guide.

You use your left hand as the vaginal hand when palpating the woman's left ischial spine and your right hand as the vaginal hand when palpating the woman's right ischial spine. First you palpate the ischial spine. Then you insert the needle guide and position the end of it immediately beneath and medial to the inferior, medial border of the ischial spine (see Fig. 51-3). Palpate the sacrospinous ligament. The insertion of the protrusion of the needle is then directed posterior to the ischial spine, through the sacrospinous ligament to the space occupied by the pudendal nerve and vessels.

You will feel a slight give as the needle exits from the sacrospinous ligament and enters this space. This is a distance of approximately 1 to 1½ centimeters (around ½ inch) from the end of the needle guide.

Aspirate. Turn the needle 180° and aspirate again in order to assure yourself that the needle is not in a blood vessel and that the lack of blood return on the first aspiration was not merely due to the bevel being snug against the inner wall of the vessel. This careful aspiration is a safeguard to ensure the safety of the procedure and must be deliberately performed as part of the procedure. This precaution is necessary because the internal pudendal artery and internal pudendal vein are immediately adjacent to the pudendal nerve, with the pudendal nerve actually lying between the posterior surface of the sacrospinous ligament and the internal pudendal vessels.

Intravenous injection of any of the local anesthetics will most probably cause maternal toxic reactions (including the hazard of possible respiratory depression, convulsions, and death) and fetal distress or neonatal depression. Great care must be taken to prevent inadvertent intravenous administration of the local anesthetic while performing a pudendal block. After assuring yourself that you do not have the needle point in a blood vessel, inject 10 milliliters of 1% lidocaine (100 mg.).

Repeat the entire procedure for the other side. After injecting both sides and waiting a few minutes, test the effectiveness of the block by using a sharp object, such as a needle, and scratching along each side of the perineal area (both sides need to be evaluated). Validation of effectiveness for each side is from two sources: (1) the woman's lack of verbal complaint even when asked and (2) visual observation of a lack of anal sphincter or vaginal orifice contraction.

If the pudendal block is ineffective, and you plan to cut an episiotomy, do a local infiltration as described in Chapter 52.

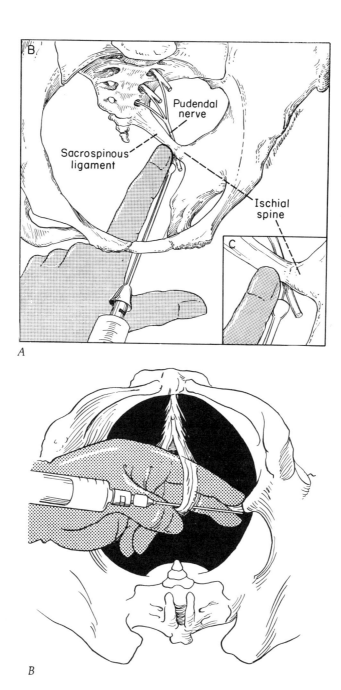

FIGURE 51-3.   Position of the needle for pudendal nerve block using the transvaginal approach: A. superior view of the pelvis showing how index finger is used to direct needle point as it approaches ischial spine. The use of the Iowa trumpet guide for needle is shown; B. the syringe is directed downward and laterally to pierce the vagina just below the projection of the ischial spine. In the final position the needle is parallel with the longitudinal axis of the mother. (Reproduced by permission from Bonica, J. J. *Principles and Practice of Obstetric Analgesia and Anesthesia, Volume 1.* Philadelphia: Davis, 1967.)

52

Local Infiltration

Perineal local infiltration done before delivery is for the purpose of anesthetizing the area to be cut for an episiotomy and its subsequent repair. Local infiltration done after delivery but before or during repair of an episiotomy or lacerations is for the purpose of anesthetizing the area to be repaired. At times the effects of a local infiltration done before delivery may last throughout any repair work to be done. At other times the effects may have worn off before the repair is completed or even begun, or the laceration may extend beyond the area originally anesthetized. Local infiltration of the unanesthetized area is then in order.

LOCAL INFILTRATION BEFORE DELIVERY

Local infiltration prior to delivery is usually chosen as the method of anesthetizing the perineal body in the following circumstances:

1. When administration of a pudendal block has failed
2. When second stage has been so rapid as not to allow time for performance of a pudendal block

3. When the decision to perform an episiotomy is a last-minute decision, reversing an earlier decision not to do an episiotomy, and the fetal head is too low to do a pudendal block
4. When the woman has stated a preference for this mode of anesthesia if any anesthetic is indicated at all

Local infiltration is secondary in choice to a pudendal block. The primary reason is that a pudendal block anesthetizes a larger area (including the lower vaginal tract as well as the perineum) and provides an anesthesia that does not distort the tissues for repair. Since neither mode affects the baby these considerations can be given priority.

There are two techniques for doing local infiltration of the perineal body. In both techniques a 22-gauge, 1½-inch (4-centimeter) needle attached to a syringe that holds at least 10 milliliters is used. Longer needles and larger syringes can be used but the gauge should not be any larger. The medication is usually 1% lidocaine hydrochloride (Xylocaine), 10 milligrams per milliliter, although a number of other local anesthetics can be used.

The standard, but not necessarily always the most efficacious, technique is to insert the needle point at the center of the fourchet and then fan the injection centrally, to both sides of center, and in both the anterior and posterior planes of the perineal body. The disadvantage of this technique, when compared with the other possible technique, is that it takes more time to perform, is more awkward for learners, and entails considerable relocating of the needle, which involves much backing up and repositioning of the needle and enhances the chance of necessitating multiple sticks.

The second technique is simply to insert the needle at the center of the fourchet and direct the needle straight down the midplane towards the rectum without puncturing into that orifice. Then, after aspirating, up to a maximum of 10 milliliters (100 milligrams) of lidocaine is injected as the needle is slowly withdrawn. The desired effect is to create a large, visible and palpable perpendicular wheal approximately 3/4 to 1 inch wide and extending from top to bottom in the center of the perineal body. If the plan is to cut a mediolateral episiotomy, then the direction of the needle and resultant wheal are in accord with the path this cut will take. This technique is very quickly performed and involves just one needle thrust.

The second technique is ideal because in the majority of cases when local infiltration is used it is done just shortly before delivery, when the perineal body has thinned and flattened considerably. This allows for ready development of a broad wheal since there is little anteroposterior tissue and only one plane. In fact, this poses the one difficulty with performing a local infiltration: the perineal body is so flattened that it is easy to pierce the posterior wall and insert the local anesthetic uselessly into the vagina. This problem can be avoided by being very observant, both visually and with a finger posterior to the insertion line to detect this happening. To rectify the problem, merely withdraw the point of the needle until it is again within tissue and redirect it so it will stay within the tissue of the perineal body.

LOCAL INFILTRATION FOR REPAIR AFTER DELIVERY

Local infiltration is used when anesthesia is needed for repair of a laceration or episiotomy and (1) predelivery anesthesia has worn off, (2) a postdelivery pudendal block has failed, or (3) local infiltration is the mode of choice. The primary disadvantage of local infiltration for repair is that it distorts the tissue, thereby making tissue approximation and judgment of the tightness of the sutures more difficult.

Selection of the gauge and length of the needle and amount of anesthetic agent used is dependent on the laceration. A 22-gauge, 1½-inch needle is fine for infiltrating an episiotomy cut, a lacerated extension of one, or a vaginal sulcus tear. However, a smaller gauge needle should be used for smaller lacerations in more sensitive areas. For example, a 25-gauge, 1-inch needle would be the needle of choice for anesthetizing a clitoral laceration. Judgment needs to be exercised in making this selection.

The technique of local infiltration is to insert the needle point at the end or corner of the laceration or cut and run it the length of the wound along the line where the suture needle will be either entering or exiting. Then, after aspirating, the anesthetic agent is injected as the needle is withdrawn to the point of insertion. Medication injection is stopped while the needle is redirected along another line of projected suturing, and the process is repeated until the entire area of possible pain is anesthetized.

53 Hand Maneuvers for Delivery of the Baby in an Occipital Anterior Position with the Mother in Lithotomy Position

Hand maneuvers for delivery of the baby in the most common delivery position of occiput anterior (OA) when the mother is in lithotomy position are designed to (1) effect a safe, atraumatic delivery for the baby, (2) facilitate the mother's efforts in delivering her baby with minimum possible trauma to herself, and (3) give you a feeling of absolute security and control of the baby and confidence in what you are doing, free from fears of the baby's slipping out of your hands, during every moment of the delivery.

The following pages and Figure 53-1 describe in detail what to do with your hands every moment of the actual delivery of the baby. It is strongly suggested that, before you deliver a baby, you practice these hand maneuvers until you are comfortable with them, can readily adjust them to whichever way the head rotates during restitution and external rotation, and can smoothly use them no matter how fast the baby might come. For practice you need someone else to serve as the power to manipulate a doll through a pelvis or anything with a hole large enough to accommodate the doll. Have this person vary the rate of speed of delivery and the direction of restitution and external rotation.

These same hand maneuvers are applicable for babies who deliver in the occiput posterior position with the exception of the direction of pressure exerted for control of the delivery of the head. This is also true for babies who deliver with a face presentation; once the head is out the remaining hand maneuvers are the same.

The hand maneuvers differ after birth of the baby's head if the mother is in a dorsal position. These are detailed in Chapter 54.

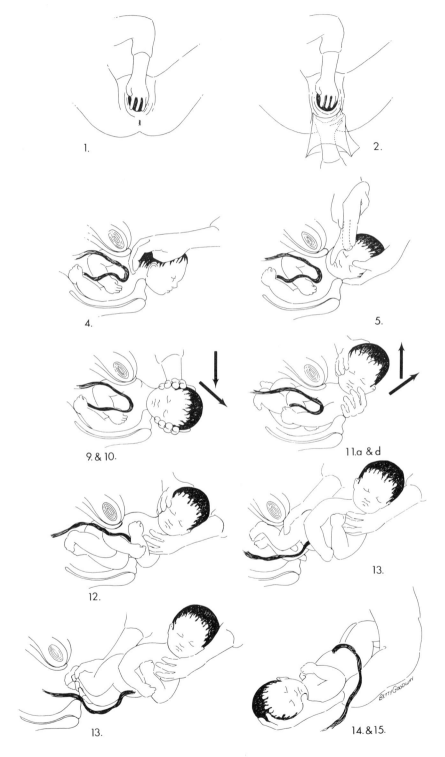

FIGURE 53-1. Hand maneuvers for delivery of the baby in occipital anterior position with the mother in lithotomy position. Numbers correspond with the narrative text.

Hand Maneuver	Rationale
1. For control of the baby's head place the pads of your fingertips on the portion of the vertex showing at the vaginal introitus. Be careful not to let your fingers slip inside the vagina alongside the head. As more of the head is accessible at the vaginal introitus, spread your fingers over the vertex of the baby's head with your fingertips pointing towards the as yet unseen face and your elbow pointing upward towards the mother. Allow the head gradually to extend beneath your hand by exerting a controlling, but not prohibitive, pressure with your hand. Use the length of your fingers in doing this and not just your fingertips.	1. Letting your fingers slip inside the vagina increases the possibility of introducing infection. Spreading your fingers over the vertex evenly distributes the pressure you are exerting, thereby avoiding any possibility of intracranial injury. Pressure applied at this time keeps the head flexed until the suboccipital region impinges under the symphysis pubis and extension begins. If the head is allowed to extend too soon, the frequent result is periurethral lacerations. Gradual extension of the head as the diameter changes from the suboccipital-bregmatic diameter of 9.5 centimeters to the suboccipital-mental diameter of 13.5 centimeters does the following: a. prevents popping of the baby's head, which can cause intracranial injury b. reduces the possibility of trauma (lacerations) to the mother Using the length of your fingers rather than just your fingertips again more evenly distributes the pressure and also enables you to have better control as you are in contact with more of the head and you can better adjust the pressure as needed.
For head control, use the hand most comfortable for you. Most practitioners use their minor hand leaving their dominant hand to handle any equipment or supplies that may be suddenly and quickly needed. For example, a right-handed person would use the left hand on the head, thereby leaving the right hand free for other actions.	
2. Some clinicians believe that proper control of the head will preserve the perineum and result in delivery over an intact perineum. Others believe that it is necessary to support the perineum in addition to proper control of the head in order to achieve this result.	2. See b., c., and d. below.

Hand Maneuver	Rationale

If you want to try supporting the perineum in order to make up your own mind about its efficacy, it is most important that you do it correctly. It is incorrect simply to place your hand against the perineum and press. The correct method is as follows:

a. cover the hand not being used on the baby's head with a towel.

b. place your thumb in the crease of the groin midway on one side of the perineum.

c. place your middle finger in the crease of the groin midway on the other side of the perineum.

d. apply pressure with the thumb and finger downward and then inward toward each other and the middle of the perineum (perineal body).

e. while doing this be sure to keep your hand parallel to the perineum in order to be able to observe the perineum in the space between your thumb and middle finger and your hand.

3. Watch the perineum while the head extends and is born.

4. As soon as the head is born place the fingertips of one of your hands on the occiput and then slide them down the curve of the baby's head to the baby's back at the level of the top of the shoulders

(Rationale column)

This serves only to place additional stress on the perineum and to obliterate your view of the perineum.

a. to prevent your hand from being contaminated by accidentally brushing it against the rectal orifice.

b., c., and d. the placement of your thumb and middle finger in the crease of the groin on either side of the perineum (perineal body) avoids placing stress on the perineum itself. The downward pressure adds more tissue to the action and the inward motion distributes any additional tissue towards the crucial midpart of the perineum, thereby providing a little give to relieve the strain there.

e. see 3 below.

3. Watch, so you can observe the final stretching of the perineum. The appearance of thin white lines occurs immediately prior to the perineum tearing. If these lines are seen, a last-moment episiotomy, or extension of one if already cut, may be possible. Watching the perineum also keeps your other hand away from the perineum if you're not supporting the perineum, thereby preventing the possibility of contaminating it on the anal opening and causing subsequent infection.

4. This maneuver is done to determine if there is an umbilical cord around the baby's neck and, if there is, to make a judgment as to how tight it is as a basis for deciding how to manage the situation.

Hand Maneuver	Rationale
and sweep them in both directions, feeling for the umbilical cord. Most clinicians use their dominant hand for this maneuver as it is the hand most accustomed to and sensitive for touching.	Starting at the occiput helps locate where you are on the baby as it is easy for inexperienced fingers to get confused and have difficulty identifying what they are feeling during this maneuver because the neck of a baby is short. Sliding your fingers down from the occiput to the top of the back assures your feeling a nuchal cord if one is present. Sweeping your fingers from side to side picks up a cord over a shoulder.
Management of a nuchal cord is as follows:	
a. if the cord is loose, slip it over the baby's head. b. if the cord is too tight to slip over the baby's head but not tight around the neck, slip it back over the shoulders as the baby's body is born.	a. and b. a loose cord may tighten as the baby's body is born unless it is slipped away from around the baby's neck.
c. if the cord is tight, immediately clamp and cut the cord at the neck before the baby's body is born. Tell the mother to pant while you are clamping, cutting, and unwinding the cord.	c. a tight cord may cause hypoxia or anoxia. Having the mother pant will keep her from pushing the remainder of the baby out before you are through clamping, cutting, and unwinding the cord, thereby defeating your effort; and before your hands are in position for the next maneuver.
5. Wipe the baby's face and head and wipe off fluid from the nose and mouth with a soft, absorbent cloth. 6. Suction the nasal and oral passages of the baby with a soft rubber bulb syringe.	5. and 6. Drying the baby's face and head prevents loss of body heat from these surfaces. Wiping away fluid from the nose and mouth and aspirating the nasal and oral passages clear the airway, thereby preventing aspiration of fluid into the lungs with the baby's first breath.
7. Wait for a contraction and watch the head return to anatomical alignment with the body (restitution) and external rotation.	7. Watching may inhibit any inclination to interfere, gives the shoulders time to rotate internally to the anteroposterior diameter of the pelvic outlet, confirms or refutes your prebirth judgment regarding the fetal position, and prepares you for placement of your hands for the subsequent hand maneuver.

Hand Maneuver	Rationale
Place a hand underneath the upper half of the baby's head while watching.	This provides support to the head. Limiting yourself to having your hand under just the upper half of the head keeps your fingers away from the rectum, thereby avoiding contamination.
Unless the cord has been cut there is no need for hurry or interference by rotating the shoulders manually. If the cord has been cut and external rotation is not yet completed by that time, then assist rotation of the shoulders into the anteroposterior diameter of the pelvis as described in the management of shoulder dystocia on page 344–348.	
8. Adjust your body position by shifting it a little to the right or left as indicated. If the head rotates to the LOT, then shift your body position toward the mother's left. If the head rotates to the ROT, then shift your body position toward the mother's right.	8. This shift in your position enables you to place your hands correctly and comfortably for the next hand maneuver.
9. Place one hand on each side of the baby's head so that your fingers point toward the baby's face and the side of each hand (the side of your little finger) is closest to the mother's perineum. This means that for a baby in the LOT position, your left hand will be the bottom hand underneath the baby's head and your right hand will be the hand on top of the baby's head; and that for a baby in the ROT position, your right hand will be the bottom hand underneath and baby's head and your left hand will be the hand on top of the baby's head.	9. This places your hands in a position to avoid contamination from the rectum. The natural inclination is to place the bottom hand so the fingers are pointing towards the rectum, but invariably in so doing, the fingers inadvertently touch the anus or even slip inside slightly while concentration is placed on the delivery of the baby. Deliberate placement of the hands sideways prevents this possibility. This placement of your hands also provides for the correct hand to be in the correct location for the hand maneuvers in 11 d., 12, and 13 below.
10. Exert downward and outward pressure on the side of the baby's head with your top hand until the anterior shoulder has impinged beneath the symphysis pubis and can be seen.	10. Placement of the hands on the sides of the baby's head keeps the fingers away from pulling anywhere under the mandible or pressing in or on the neck, thereby avoiding injury to the cervical or brachial nerve plexus. (Steps 10 and 11 constitute the mechanism of labor called *birth of the shoulders and body by lateral flexion via the curve of Carus*.)

Hand Maneuver	Rationale
11. a. apply upward and outward pressure on the side of the baby's head with your bottom hand, and with both hands lift the baby's head toward the ceiling.	11. a. same as for 10. The direction of this maneuver follows the curve of Carus.
b. while doing this, bend over sufficiently to watch the perineum during the birth of the posterior shoulder.	b. observe the perineum for rapidity of delivery and to see if there is a hand of the baby's to be controlled alongside the shoulder.
c. if the baby is coming too rapidly, you can slow it down by telling the mother to pant and by applying controlling pressure with the side of your bottom hand to the top of the posterior shoulder.	c. you want the shoulders to ease out over the perineum and to have control of the upper arm, elbow, and hand as described in d. below in order to prevent perineal laceration.
d. as the baby is being born, slide your bottom hand under the baby's head from the side of the baby's head, across the neck and onto the shoulder and upper arm of the baby as it clears the perineum. In effect, you slide your hand down until the side of it rests against the top of the perineum at the fourchet. Then as the shoulder is born the upper arm is actually born into the palm of your hand while your ring finger, little finger, and the edge of your hand control the baby's elbow and hand as they clear the perineum.	d. this hand maneuver is absolutely essential for control of the upper arm, elbow, and hand of the posterior shoulder as they are being born. Otherwise, the hand or elbow can flip out and cause a perineal laceration. Perineal laceration is prevented if your hand keeps the upper arm pressed against the body until the elbow and hand have cleared the perineum.
12. As the upper half of the baby's body is born and the elbow and hand have cleared the perineum, "shake hands" with the baby's body with your bottom hand by having your thumb on the baby's back, your fingers across the baby's chest, the baby's neck in the V created between your thumb and fingers, and the baby's head supported on your wrist.	12. This gives you a hold on the baby that gives you complete control of the remainder of the delivery of the body and places the baby securely in your grasp without any possibility of the baby slipping past you or through your hands or fingers.

Note: Control of the baby's delivery has gone from your top hand for delivery of the head and the anterior shoulder to your bottom hand for delivery of the posterior shoulder and body. This latter has been accomplished with one smooth movement of your bottom hand from the side of the head in 9, down to the perineum in 11 d., and into the "hand" shake in 12 above.

13. As the baby's body is being born, slide	13. This hand maneuver, combined with 12

Hand Maneuver	Rationale
your top hand down the baby's back, slip your index finger between the baby's legs as the buttocks clear the perineum, curve your middle finger and thumb around the legs, and continue running your hand down the legs until you can grasp the baby around the ankles. At this point, close your thumb and middle finger onto your index finger thus totally encircling and enclosing the legs in your grasp. The baby's feet will thus be caught with one foot resting in the *V* created between your thumb and index finger, and the other foot resting in the *V* created between your index and middle fingers.	above, gives you an absolute hold on the baby. No baby, no matter how slippery with fluid and vernix, can slip out of this hold. The baby is securely held in your two hands and there is no chance of the baby's "falling in the bucket," which is the primary fear of the inexperienced student delivering a baby with the mother in lithotomy position.

14. Move the baby in a smooth arc into the football hold by:

    a. letting the baby's head and shoulders pivot in your bottom hand so that the head is now supported by the palmar surface of your outstretched index and middle fingers, the suboccipital region and back of the neck are in the palm of your hand, and your thumb and remaining fingers are *resting*, not pressing, against the sides of the neck. Your top hand continues its grasp around the ankles during this maneuver.

    b. place the baby's legs between the elbow and upper arm of your bottom hand and your body at waist level and remove your top hand from around the baby's ankles. This means that the baby's back is supported on your lower arm and the bottom part of the baby's body is tucked securely between your elbow/upper arm and your body.

14. The football hold is known as a safety hold in nurseries. Putting the baby into a football hold keeps the baby at the same level as the placenta.

    a. the thumb and fingers resting against the neck serve as a barrier to movement between the mandible and the shoulders. If the baby slides either way it will go no further than the fingers. *Do not* close your thumb and fingers around the baby's neck. The baby's head is supported and you have control over the position of the baby's head for suctioning. Your continued grasp on the ankles assures absolute safety from the baby's falling.

    b. this completes getting the baby into the football hold and frees one hand for subsequent actions of suctioning, drying the baby, clamping and cutting the cord, and so forth.

Hand Maneuver	Rationale
15. *Be sure* as the baby is born in 11 d. and 12, and placed in a safety hold in 13, that you: a. keep the head of the baby in a downward, dependent position, and turned somewhat to the side. b. have no tension on the umbilical cord. c. keep the baby well supported at all times.	15. a. for drainage of fluid from the oral and nasal air passageways. b. to prevent tearing of the cord from its insertion in either the placenta or the baby. c. so the baby does not feel a frightening loss of support.

The hand maneuvers for the actual delivery of the baby end with the baby's being held securely in the football hold. If the baby was born from a LOT position, the baby will end up under your left arm. If the baby was born from a ROT position, the baby will end up under your right arm. If you are unable to use your minor hand for the necessary subsequent actions then you will need to switch the baby from under one arm to under the other arm. If you are inexperienced in handling babies and do not know how to get a baby into a football hold or how to transfer football holds from one side to the other, go to a normal newborn nursery and practice until you are comfortable.

You will see many other methods, or variations of this method, used in delivering a baby with the mother in lithotomy position. Before trying variations or alternatives, the inexperienced student needs to learn one method, whatever it is, that is guaranteed safe and atraumatic and that will foster self-confidence. This one is recommended. Consideration of another method, or variations of this one, should involve scrutiny and analysis of the method for valid rationale and for safety and security features.

54 Hand Maneuvers for Delivery of the Baby in an Occipital Anterior Position with the Mother in Dorsal Position

If you have been accustomed to delivering a baby with the mother in the lithotomy position and are now preparing yourself for delivering a baby with the mother in the dorsal position, the most important thing for you to realize is that the hand maneuvers you used for delivery in the lithotomy position, as described in Chapter 53, will not work with the mother in the dorsal position. There are certain similarities but it is unsafe even to think of running from one side of the table or bed to the other side depending on the direction of restitution and external rotation of the head at the very time your hands should be facilitating and controlling the delivery of the baby's shoulders and body. If you are learning delivery of babies and are learning with the mother in the dorsal position the above is not your problem. However, when you later learn delivery in the lithotomy position you must realize that in order to do it safely you will need to learn a different set of hand maneuvers.

The hand maneuvers described below and illustrated in Figure 54-1 describe in detail what to do with your hands every moment of the actual delivery of the baby. While there is no danger of dropping the baby any great distance when the mother is in the dorsal position, it is still important to practice these maneuvers before actually delivering a baby in order to effect an atraumatic delivery for both the baby and the mother. For practice you need someone else to serve as the power to manipulate a doll through a pelvis or anything with a hole large enough to accommodate the doll. Have this person vary the rate of speed of delivery.

These same hand maneuvers are applicable for all babies who deliver from a cephalic presentation once the head is born. Prior to that time the hand maneuvers vary in accord with the indicated direction of pressure exerted for control of the delivery of the baby's head.

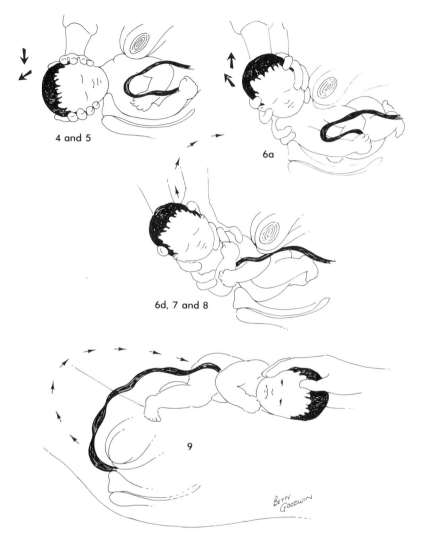

4 and 5

6a

6d, 7 and 8

9

BETTY GOODWIN

FIGURE 54-1. Hand maneuvers for the delivery of the baby in occipital anterior position with the mother in dorsal position. Numbers correspond with the narrative text.

Hand Maneuver	Rationale
1. Position yourself on one side of the table or bed. If you are right-handed you will be positioned on the mother's right side. If you are left-handed, you will be positioned on the mother's left side.	1. Proper positioning in accord with your dominant hand is important for your own comfort and for your facility in doing examinations and in managing the situation and relevant supplies and equipment.
2. With the mother's knees flexed and well separated out to the sides, you should be positioned just below the level of her knee. From this position you function from within her leg, reaching upward	2. Working inside her leg keeps the mother's knee from getting in your way; gives you an element of control, if necessary, of the mother's legs; and positions you in a way that guarantees access to both the baby

Hand Maneuver	Rationale
toward the perineum for assisting the mother with delivery of her baby and downward toward the foot of the table or bed to where your supplies and equipment are located.	and the necessary supplies and equipment.
3. The hand maneuvers involved in control of the delivery of the baby's head, checking for a nuchal cord, wiping the baby's head, suctioning, and watching of the mechanisms of labor of restitution and external rotation are the same as the hand maneuvers for delivery of the baby with the mother in lithotomy position (Steps 1 to 7) described in Chapter 53.	3. See the rationale for Steps 1 to 7 described in Chapter 53.
4. Place one hand on each side of the baby's head. If you are standing on the right side of the mother, your left hand will be on top of the baby's head and your right hand will be the bottom hand underneath the baby's head. If you are standing on the left side of the mother, your right hand will be on top of the baby's head and your left hand will be the bottom hand underneath the baby's head. This positioning of your hands will be true regardless of which direction restitution and external rotation take. Be sure that the palms of your hands are on the baby's head with your fingers pointing toward the opposite leg of the mother. This places the sides of your hands at right angles to the perineum.	4. This placement of your hands is designed to: a. prevent contamination of your bottom hand in or from the rectum. b. prevent grasping the baby under the mandible or around the neck for delivery of the shoulders and body. c. prevent damage to the cervical or brachial nerve plexus.
5. Exert downward and outward pressure on the *side* of the baby's head with your top hand until the anterior shoulder has impinged beneath the symphysis pubis and can be seen.	5. Same as for 4 b. and c. above. (Steps 5 and 6 constitute the mechanisms of labor called *birth of the shoulders and body by lateral flexion via the curve of Carus.*)
6. a. apply upward and outward pressure on the *side* of the baby's head with your bottom hand and with both hands lift the baby's head towards the ceiling. b. watch the perineum during the birth of the posterior shoulder.	6. a. same as for 4 b. and c. above. The direction of this maneuver follows the curve of Carus. b. observe the perineum for rapidity of delivery and to see if there is a hand to

Hand Maneuver	Rationale
	be controlled alongside the posterior shoulder.
c. if the baby is coming too rapidly, you can slow it down by telling the mother to pant and by applying controlling pressure with the side of your bottom hand to the top of the posterior shoulder.	c. you want to ease the shoulders over the perineum and to have control of the posterior upper arm, elbow, and hand in order to prevent perineal lacerations.
d. as the baby is being born slide both your top and bottom hands, with the exception of your index fingers, down from the sides of the baby's head and onto the shoulders and upper arms of the baby as they clear the perineum and are born. The index fingers of both of your hands remain on the parietal bones on either side of the baby's head. During this maneuver your bottom hand slides down until the side of it rests against the top of the perineum at the fourchet. Then as the posterior shoulder is born the upper arm is actually born into the palm of your hand while your ring finger, little finger, and edge of your hand control the baby's elbow and hand as they clear the perineum.	d. this positions your hands for the next hand maneuver, described in Step 7. Your index fingers on the parietal bones steady and support the baby's head between them. This action of your bottom hand is essential for control of the upper arm, elbow, and hand of the posterior shoulder as they are being born. Otherwise, the hand or elbow can flip out and cause a perineal laceration. If your hand keeps the upper arm pressed against the body until the elbow and hand have cleared the perineum, then perineal laceration is prevented.
7. As the upper half of the baby's body is born, grasp the baby's body around the upper arms, upper chest, and upper back. Your thumbs will be on one side of the baby's body, your index fingers will be on the parietal bones, and your remaining fingers will be on the other side of the baby's body.	7. This provides you with a secure hold of the baby's body which also enables you to guide the direction of the remainder of the birth of the body via the curve of Carus.
8. Guide the baby's body upward and outward in a smooth arc for the birth of the lower half of the baby's body.	8. Follows the curve of Carus.
9. Continue your arc and place the baby on the mother's abdomen.	9. Placement on the mother's abdomen causes the uterus to contract, gives the mother immediate contact with her baby, and keeps the baby out of the fluids which have now accumulated on the table or bed in the area between her legs.

Hand Maneuver	Rationale
Be sure as you place the baby on the mother's abdomen that: a. the baby's head is lower than the baby's body. b. the baby's head is turned to the side if in a prone position, or the baby is placed on his or her side. c. there is no tension on the umbilical cord.	a. for drainage of fluid from the oral and nasal air passageways. b. to maintain a patent oropharyngeal airway. c. to prevent tearing of the cord from its insertion in either the placenta or the baby.
10. Keep one hand on the baby as you use your other hand for securing necessary supplies and equipment for the subsequent actions of suctioning, drying the baby, clamping and cutting the cord, and so forth.	10. This is a safety measure that protects the baby from sliding, falling, or flipping off the mother's abdomen.

The hand maneuvers for the actual delivery of the baby end with the placing of the baby on the mother's abdomen.

55

Inspection of the Placenta, Membranes, and Cord

The inspection of the placenta, membranes, and cord is for the purpose of diagnosing normality of the placenta, umbilical cord insertion, and cord; screening for abnormality; and ascertaining whether or not the placenta and membranes have been completely delivered.

In order to diagnose normality of the placenta and cord insertion, the parameters of normal must be known. Screening for abnormality then encompasses anything not within the parameters of normal; however, it is useful to know and be able to recognize the more common deviations from normal. The causes of these deviations are not always known, and their significance may lie not in pointing to a diagnostic cause but instead in pointing to potential problems their existence may have created. All of this information makes up the necessary data base for inspection of the placenta and membranes.

DATA BASE

Normal Placenta, Cord Insertion, and Cord

The normal term placenta weighs approximately 500 grams (just under 1 pound 2 ounces), which is roughly one-sixth of the weight of the newborn. It varies in shape, usually being discoid (flattened and circular) with an average diameter of 15 to 20 centimeters (roughly 6 to 8 inches) and an average thickness of 1.5 to 3 centimeters (about ⅔ to 1¼ inches).

The maternal surface of the placenta is the side of the placenta that was attached to the uterine wall. Normally it is dark red (primarily as a result of fetal hemoglobin), covered with a grayish film of decidua basalis, soft, and friable if torn. It evidences a variable number of cotyledons separated by decidual septa composed of fibrous tissue and interwoven with innumerable blood vessels (see Chapter 6).

The fetal surface of the placenta is the side that was next to the fetus and thus is covered with the shiny fetal membranes that extend beyond the placenta to form the two-layered membranous sac in which the fetus was enclosed. The outer layer, or chorion, and the inner layer, or amnion, are separable up to the insertion of the umbilical cord. It is difficult to impossible to separate the chorion from the fetal surface of the placenta. The chorion is more easily torn, more opaque, and thicker than the inner, glistening, transparent amnion. The fetal surface of the placenta is irregular because of the branching of the placental blood vessels from the umbilical cord. While the color is grayish, the redness of the placenta can be seen through the membranes except where there are infarcts.

Degenerative changes in the placenta are normally observed as infarcts. These are hard, nodular, whitish areas which may be found on either the maternal or fetal surface or both. They vary in size from a few millimeters to several centimeters. Frequently small calcifications are also observed on the maternal surface of the placenta. These feel gritty to touch and normally may be spread all over the maternal surface to a moderate degree. Developing a reasonable amount of these degenerative changes (infarct formation and small calcifications) is a normal part of the aging process of the placenta.

Insertion of the umbilical cord into the placenta occurs on the fetal surface and is usually somewhat eccentric (inserts somewhere between the center and the margin). A central cord insertion is normal but much less common. The umbilical cord normally averages approximately 55 centimeters (22 inches) in length and thus is slightly longer than the total length of the average term newborn. The amount of Wharton's jelly supporting and protecting the blood vessels in the cord varies considerably but the cord is normally full and firm to touch. The number of blood vessels in the umbilical cord is normally three: two arteries and one vein. Although these vessels collapse after the cord is cut they can be easily identified because the vein has a larger aperture than either of the two arteries.

Placental Variations, Anomalies, and Abnormalities

All abnormal placentas indicative of a disease process require consultation with a physician and should be sent to pathology for detailed examination. A list of placental variations, anomalies, and abnormalities follows:

1. Larger and heavier than normal placentas — may occur with excessively large fetuses, fetal syphilis, or erythroblastosis.
2. Smaller and lighter than normal placentas — may occur with general systemic diseases or local uterine conditions causing undernourishment of the placenta and usually resulting in intrauterine growth retardation.
3. Color of placental tissue obviously lighter than normal — caused by fetal anemia such as is found in erythroblastosis.
4. Extensive infarct formation — infarction of entire cotyledons is abnormal and usually is due to disease processes such as severe chronic maternal hypertension or severe preeclampsia or eclampsia. Such extensive infarcting reduces effective placental functioning which may result in intrauterine growth retardation or, if a substantial portion of the placenta is infarcted, may result in fetal death.
5. Cysts — most frequently observed on the fetal surface. The smaller cysts, a few millimeters in size, are more common than the very uncommon larger cysts of up to 8 to 10 centimeters in diameter. Usually not significant except in the occasional instance in which the cyst contains a blighted twin.
6. Edema of the placenta — placenta is mushy,

thick, and pale, and fluid can be squeezed from it. May be caused by severe maternal heart disease, diabetes, or nephritis, and by severe erythroblastosis. The fetus usually dies in utero either as a stillbirth or earlier as an abortion.

7. Tumors — may be found in association with prematurity and polyhydramnios. Perinatal mortality and maternal hemorrhage are both increased.

8. Syphilitic placenta — abnormally large, pale yellowish-gray placenta; syphilitic fetus.

9. Lobulated placenta — there appear to be multiple placentas for a single baby. In fact, it is one placenta which is divided into two or more parts either completely separated or joined in part. Either way, the lobes are held together by the one set of membranes and by the blood vessels (which may extend from one lobe to another or may be separate and distinct, uniting just before entering the cord, which is not inserted into any lobe). The number of lobes determines the name, for example, placenta duplex (two), placenta triplex (three). This anomaly is thought to be due to abnormalities in the blood supply to the decidua. Its main significance is that you need to be alert to make sure that all lobes have been expelled from the uterus.

10. Succenturiate placenta (placenta succenturiata) — a not uncommon placental anomaly in which one or more separate accessory lobes are in the membranes a variable distance away from the main placental mass. These accessory lobes are usually connected to the main placental mass by blood vessels extending out from the main placental mass. When there are no connecting blood vessels, the anomaly is called *placenta spuria*.

The primary significance of a succenturiate placenta lies in the possibility that the succenturiate lobe(s) will be retained in the uterus after expulsion of the main placental mass. Retained succenturiate lobes may cause severe postpartal hemorrhage.

The retention of succenturiate lobes can be detected during inspection of the placenta and membranes by:

a. noting torn blood vessels at the margin of the maternal surface of the placenta with the fetal membranes, or the extension of blood vessels into the membranes (this may also be noted from the margin of the fetal surface of the placenta).

b. noting rough or torn roundish defects in the membranes a short distance from the placenta; occasionally these may have a fragment of decidua attached on the periphery of the defect.

Manual exploration of the uterus and removal of the succenturiate lobe(s) is indicated if retention has occurred.

11. Extrachorial placentas — a placental anomaly observed on the fetal surface as a thick, white ring which gives the impression that the central portion of the placenta is somewhat depressed. Within this depression the fetal surface looks as usual with the insertion of the umbilical cord. However, all the large blood vessels pass into the depths of the placenta before reaching the ring instead of their usual coursing over the totality of the fetal surface.

There are two varieties of extrachorial placentas which are determined by the location of the ring. Both may be complete or incomplete as dictated by whether or not the ring circumscribes a full circle:

a. placenta circumvallata (circumvallate placenta) — the ring is situated a variable distance between the margin and the middle of the placenta. The ring is formed by a double fold of both the chorion and amnion doubling back on themselves, with fibrin and degenerated decidua interposed between the folds of the membranes. This gives it its raised effect.

b. placenta marginata (circummarginate placenta) — the ring is located at the edge, or margin, of the placenta and is raised by the presence of degenerated decidua and fibrin interposed between the membranes and the placenta at the edge of the placenta; the membranes do not fold back on themselves.

The etiology of extrachorial placentas is not known. Their incidence and significance are controversial in the literature. At any rate, any significance occurs prior to the time of delivery of the placenta (e.g., antepartal hemorrhage) so at the time you note that it is an extrachorial placenta it may answer some diagnostic questions but there is no indication for clinical action.

Variations, Anomalies, and Abnormalities of the Umbilical Cord and Its Insertion

1. Battledore placenta — the variation in which the umbilical cord inserts in the edge or margin of the placenta. Although considered a normal cord insertion, marginal insertion of the cord occurs in less than 10 percent of placentas.

2. Velamentous insertion — the blood vessels in the umbilical cord separate and leave the cord prior to insertion into the surface of the placenta (the three vessels course between the chorion and amnion for a variable distance before each enters the placenta surrounded by only amnion). Velamentous insertion occurs approximately 1 percent of the time, with an increased incidence in the event of multiple gestation.

A velamentous insertion of the cord is fraught with danger for the fetus. Rupture of the membranes may also rupture a fetal blood vessel because their protection is flimsy since they are covered only with amnion. A ruptured vessel may cause hemorrhage in, and exsanguination of, the fetus. The vessels are also liable to compression, which would cause fetal anoxia.

At the time you note such an insertion upon inspection of the placenta after its delivery, any disaster that might have happened will have already happened. In such an event, noting of a velamentous insertion would be of diagnostic value. Fortunately such circumstances are rare.

3. Vasa previa — a dangerous anomaly with a high perinatal mortality if rupture occurs. Vasa previa consists of unprotected blood vessels, covered only with amnion and coursing between the chorion and the amnion, which present first at the cervical os by crossing the os ahead of the fetal presenting part. With fetal descent and rupture of the membranes, the vessels are subject to compression and rupture with resulting exsanguination and anoxia of the fetus.

Vasa previa usually occurs in conjunction with a velamentous insertion of the cord. However, vasa previa may also occur when there is a succenturiate placenta since the vascular connections to the succenturiate lobe are also unprotected vessels coursing between the chorion and amnion.

Vasa previa occurs in less than 0.2 percent of pregnancies. While extremely rare, it should be thought of as a possibility any time you are not positive of what you feel presenting at the cervical os. Your examination should include feeling for pulsations synchronous with the fetal heart rate in the questionable presenting entity. Consultation with the physician is mandatory whenever you cannot identify the presenting part or believe it to be abnormal.

4. Abnormal number of blood vessels in the umbilical cord — has a high correlation with fetal anomalies. About one-third of infants born with only one umbilical artery will have multiple, severe malformations.

5. Short cord (relative or absolute) — an absolute short cord is one that is short in length; a relative short cord is one of average length (or, more likely, excessively long) which has become looped around the body or neck of the fetus so that it is short in terms of reaching from its placental insertion to the newborn's umbilicus outside the maternal vulva as is necessary for normal delivery.

   A short cord, although unusual, may be the causative factor in failure of the fetus to descend. In such an event, it might additionally cause abruptio placentae, umbilical hernia, fetal distress, rupture of the cord, shoulder dystocia, or a combination of these.

   Recognition of a short cord usually does not take place until there is evidence of a problem. Therefore, it should be considered as a possibility whenever descent is not normally occurring in the presence of an adequate pelvis and good contractions. Fetal distress enhances the accuracy of the diagnosis and compounds the urgency for action, which will require a physician.

6. Excessively long cord — more common than a short cord. Of itself, it has no significance. However, a long cord is of great clinical significance if it becomes looped around the fetal body or neck, thus causing a relative short cord. It can also become knotted or prolapse in front of the presenting part.

7. Cord looping — usually the result of a cord that is longer than average (50 to 55 centimeters, or about 20 to 22 inches). A vast majority of cords longer than 100 centimeters (39 inches) will be looped. Looping occurs in approximately 20 percent of all pregnancies. Single or multiple looping may cause a short cord with all its possible complications. In addition, looping of the cord around the neck may cause fetal distress (although rarely death) as a result of either compression of the cord between the clavicle and the mandible during flexion, or tightening of the cord around the neck during descent, especially if the distance is short between the loop and the placental insertion. Therefore it is important to check for a cord around the neck as soon as the baby's head is born.

8. Cord knotting — true knotting must be differentiated from false knotting. False knotting of the cord occurs when the cord appears to be knotted but instead has kinking of the blood vessels within the cord. A true knot occurs when the fetus has passed through a loop in the cord and a real knot has been created. True knotting is most apt to occur in one of two situations:

   a. small fetus, long cord, and large amount of amniotic fluid. The higher ratio of amniotic fluid to fetal size in early pregnancy makes this the time of greatest incidence. These knots are usually benign because they are kept from tightening by pulsations in the blood vessels.

   b. multiple gestation within a single amnion. All sorts of cord entanglements and knots are possible because the fetuses have greater freedom of movement within the fetal sac thereby increasing both the chance of a knot forming and of its tightening. Mortality rate is high.

9. Markedly decreased amount of Wharton's jelly — may be seen in malnourished and postmature newborns.

10. Rarities — Other conditions that may occur in the umbilical cord are hematomas, tumors, cysts, and edema. Hematomas usually are the result of rupturing of the

umbilical vein. Edema is not uncommon with an edematous or macerated fetus.

PROCEDURE

A gross inspection can be done as the placenta is delivered. Obvious immediately is whether or not the membranes trail, with or without tearing; the general appearance and characteristics of the cord; the general size, wholeness, health, and characteristics of the placenta; and the type of cord insertion. A thorough inspection is done as follows.

1. *Umbilical cord*:
   a. count the number of cord vessels. In order to do this, take a gauze 4 × 4 and wipe off the cut end. Apply pressure and the apertures of the vessels will be visible. If for some reason time has passed and the vessels have collapsed beyond your being able to identify them, reclamp and recut the cord and look for them at the site of the new cut, where they will be readily visible.
   b. measure the length of the cord. Measuring the cord usually is dictated by institutional policy and is not always done. Regardless of policy, if the cord appears abnormally long or short it should be measured. Remember to include the length of cord cut off the baby's end when the baby's cord was finally clamped and cut.
   c. Inspect the cord for knots, hematomas, tumors, cysts, edema, and the amount of Wharton's jelly.
2. *Cord insertion* — inspection of the cord insertion includes the following:
   a. location of normal cord insertion, that is, eccentric, central, or marginal (Battledore placenta).
   b. abnormal cord insertion (velamentous cord insertion).

3. *Membranes* — inspect the membranes for the following:
   a. completeness; this is done by placing the placenta maternal side down, then placing a hand inside the membranes on the fetal surface of the placenta and holding the membranes up to simulate the sac they once were. If unable to form a sac, the membranes are incomplete and most likely ragged. Your hand will have gone inside the membranes in the opening created when the membranes ruptured. This is also the opening the placenta will have come through if delivered via the Schultz mechanism of expulsion. If so delivered, the sac will have been inverted and will need to be turned right side in again for this inspection.
   b. succenturiate lobes, defects, or blood vessels.
4. *Placenta* — Several steps are involved in inspecting the placenta, as follows:
   a. inspect the placenta for meconium staining and areas of calcification.
   b. inspect the fetal side for cysts and for being an extrachorial placenta (either a placenta circumvallata or a placenta marginata). If necessary, tear or invert the membranes in order to see the entire fetal surface. The fetal surface should also be examined closely for torn or intact blood vessels leading into the membranes in order to identify a missing or intact succenturiate lobe.
   c. inspect the maternal side for cysts, tumors, edema, abnormal color, and multiple placentas.
   d. inspect the maternal side for infarcts and the extensiveness of the infarct formation.
   e. examine the maternal side for intactness. To do this, place the placenta on a flat surface, maternal side up. Use a 4 × 4 gauze to wipe off blood and extraneous

material in order to clearly visualize the placental surface.

To identify a cotyledon missing from the margin of the placenta or a missing accessory lobe, wipe off the margin of the placenta and run your finger around the edge of the placenta. It should feel smooth. Any area of roughness should be investigated thoroughly because roughness is indicative of torn placental tissue. Examine closely the placental margin for torn or intact blood vessels leading into the membranes in order to identify a missing or intact succenturiate lobe. Compare this with your findings for the same from the fetal surface.

A cotyledon missing from the main placental mass is identified by a defect with a rough surface where it tore away. This must be differentiated from a simple tear in the placenta without loss of tissue, which also leaves a rough surface. Differentiation is made by holding the placenta in your hands, maternal surface up, so that the cotyledons fall into place against each other. A missing cotyledon is then readily evident because the surrounding pieces, like a jigsaw puzzle, won't fit together.

f. measure and weigh the placenta. This usually is dictated by institutional policy and is not always done. Regardless of policy, if it appears to be of abnormal size, measuring and weighing the placenta are indicated. This information is then recorded on the baby's chart.

56

Postdelivery Inspection of the Cervix and Upper Vaginal Vault

This discussion concentrates just on the postdelivery inspection of the cervix and upper vaginal vault since these are not, generally speaking, routinely done and since they involve skills beyond those used in the routine inspection of the vulva, perineum, and lower vaginal tract. This latter inspection is merely a matter of separating the labia and looking, and inserting two fingers into the vagina, applying pressure in different directions, and again looking.

The following considerations and key points apply to both cervical inspection and inspection of the upper vaginal vault:

1. These are uncomfortable, possibly painful, procedures. Therefore you need to:
   a. forewarn the woman of discomfort or pain and give a brief explanation of why the examination is necessary
   b. perform the procedure as quickly as possible
   c. provide some form of pain relief if the situation permits and the woman's threshold of pain warrants it

2. The key to performing an inspection that will indeed allow you to inspect (i.e., visualize the area) in order to obtain accurate information is to insert three or four of your fingers the full length of the vagina and exert strong pressure to compress the vaginal tissue in a direction away from the area you want to inspect. Otherwise, the just distended vaginal walls literally collapse around two fingers and an instrument and obstruct your path of vision. Being able to readily visualize the area also reduces considerably the amount of time it takes to perform the procedure and assures access to accurate information.

PROCEDURE FOR CERVICAL INSPECTION

The following are steps taken in inspecting the cervix:

1. Insert three or four of your fingers, palmar side down, the length of the vagina to just in front of the cervix and exert strong pressure downward on the posterior vaginal wall.
2. Insert a long-length ring forceps and grasp the anterior lip of the cervix with it. Be careful not to mistake a fold of redundant bladder or lax vaginal wall for the anterior lip of the cervix.
3. Now move your fingers the full length of the posterior vaginal wall (i.e., into the posterior fornix) and again exert strong pressure downward on the posterior vaginal wall.
4. Insert a second long-length ring forceps and grasp the posterior lip of the cervix with it.
5. Hold the handles of the two ring forceps in your hand. Pull, if necessary, to bring the cervix more into view. Move the forceps toward one side of the perineum, thus slightly pulling the cervix so that one lateral side of it can be visualized.
6. Visually inspect the area of the cervix between the two ring forceps on one side.
7. If necessary, confirm your visual inspection by using the index finger of your vaginal hand to feel the edge of the cervix while continuing to exert vaginal pressure with your remaining fingers.
8. Repeat Steps 5, 6, and 7 above, reversing the direction of moving the handles of the ring forceps in order to visualize and inspect the other lateral side of the cervix.
9. If there are no cervical lacerations, remove the ring forceps and your vaginal hand.
10. If there is a cervical laceration move the ring forceps to appropriate placements for repair of the laceration.

Hints and Alternatives

1. Maintain firm contact with the posterior vaginal wall as you insert your fingers. This helps you know precisely where you are, thereby aiding you in correct identification of the multitudinous folds of tissue and keeping your fingers from inadvertently entering a patulous cervix.
2. Be sure to insert your fingers the *full* length of the posterior vaginal wall and press *firmly* downward in order to bring the posterior cervical lip into view. Visualization and grasping of the posterior cervical lip seems to be the most troublesome aspect of the procedure of cervical inspection for the student. Utilizing this technique with your vaginal hand will minimize this problem.
3. If the cervix is very patulous, such as is found in a grand multipara, you may not be able to visualize adequately all of the cervix between the ring forceps placed on the anterior and posterior lips of the cervix. In such an event, you can assure yourself of having inspected the entire circumference of the cervix by walking the ring forceps around the cervix. This is done by placing one ring forceps on the anterior lip of the cervix and the second forceps next to it. Release the first forceps and place it on the other side of the second. Continue to leap-frog the ring forceps around the cervix. This technique can also be used if you are unable to locate the posterior lip of the cervix.

PROCEDURE FOR INSPECTION OF THE UPPER VAGINAL VAULT

The procedure for inspection of the upper vaginal vault includes the following steps:

1. Fold a 4 × 4 gauze square in fourths and clamp a long-length ring forceps on it.

2. Insert three or four of your fingers, palmar side down, the full length of the posterior vaginal wall.

3. Exert strong downward pressure on the posterior vaginal wall with your fingers.

4. Insert the ring forceps with the gauze on it by sliding it down the top of your vaginal fingers. This helps you avoid the tender anterior structures and keep as much of the gauze as possible away from the vaginal walls since it is abrasive to them.

5. a. locate both your fingertips and the end of the ring forceps in the posterior fornix.

   b. press with the ring forceps against the cervix and with your fingers against the vaginal wall.

   c. as you press, move your fingertips and the ring forceps away from each other and inspect the area you visualize between them.

   d. Repeat b. and c. after sequentially locating your fingertips and the tip of the ring forceps in each of the lateral fornices and in the anterior fornix.

Hint

The gauze serves as a sponge to blot the area being exposed of blood and other fluids in order to facilitate visualization. If the gauze becomes saturated, remove the ring forceps, dispose of the saturated gauze, clamp on another gauze, and reinsert the ring forceps.

57

Manual Removal of the Placenta

Manual removal of the placenta is one of several actions to take in the management of a third stage hemorrhage (see Chapter 17). If at all possible the woman should have a patent IV and some form of analgesia or anesthesia as this is an extremely painful procedure.

The woman should be catheterized unless you are sure she has an empty bladder. A full bladder not only impedes your performing a manual removal of the placenta but may also impede resolution of the problem by preventing proper contraction and position of the uterus. An empty bladder also reduces trauma to the bladder during this procedure.

While ideally a gauntlet glove should be put on the hand doing the manual removal, the reality is that most hospitals do not have these gloves readily available. If at all possible to do so quickly, you should at least change the glove on the hand you are going to insert into the uterus. As time is of the essence, however, most clinicians proceed with the gloves they have on.

The *whole* hand (including the thumb) is placed inside the uterus by following the cord to the placenta.

Once you have inserted your hand into the uterus, do not bring your hand out until you have separated the placenta from the uterine wall and are bringing out the placenta. Do not go in and out, in and out, as this increases the risk of infection.

Your other hand grasps the uterus (fundus) externally through the abdominal wall. This accomplishes three purposes:

1. Controls the mobility of the uterus
2. Keeps the fundus as contracted and thick as possible, which both facilitates separation and reduces the risk that the internal hand might perforate the uterus
3. Serves as a specific counterforce to your internal hand, which better enables you to feel what you are doing between your two hands

Once the placenta is located, the entire fetal surface of the placenta is quickly felt to obtain an anatomical perception of the size of the placenta and where the cord is inserted in order to get a sense of what needs to be done. At the same time, the margin of the placenta is swept to find any area of separation which will give you a starting point in the right plane for separating the placenta from the uterus.

The back of your hand is placed against the uterine wall, as this slight cupping of the hand parallels the curve of the intrauterine cavity. Insinuate your fingers between the placenta and the uterus to establish a line of cleavage. Your hand then sweeps back and forth from side to side, cutting through the decidua with the outer edge of your little finger, finger tips, and first finger. You will perceive a spongy feeling with a definite give to it as the placenta separates from the uterus. You may need to turn your hand over in order to separate the anterior portion of the placenta. This leaves the back of your hand still against the uterine wall.

The entire placenta should be in the palm of your hand before you bring it out. If you are unsure that the placenta is totally separated, sweep the uterine wall with your hand, keeping the back of your hand in contact with the uterine wall, feeling for and separating any remaining areas of attachment. Make sure the placenta is totally separated before bringing it out so as not to invert the uterus when you remove your hand (and the placenta).

The whole placenta should be in your hand in order to bring it out. Don't pull on just a piece, as that piece will simply tear from the rest of the placenta and make assessment of the placenta difficult and potentially inaccurate. Bring the placenta out slowly as your external hand continues to provide contraction of the uterus behind the emptying uterus. The membranes may need to be teased out, which is done the same way as for any delivery of the placenta and membranes (see page 369).

Make sure the uterus is contracted and immediately do an inspection of the placenta, membranes, and cord (see Chapter 55). The placenta should be intact with complete membranes.

Clinicians disagree on the question of whether the uterus should be explored routinely after manual removal of the placenta. Those who argue in favor of routine intrauterine exploration after manual removal of the placenta state that they do it to be sure that all the placenta and membranes have indeed been removed. Those who argue against routine intrauterine exploration after manual removal of the placenta state that such action increases the risks of infection, trauma, and uterine rupture. All clinicians agree that intrauterine exploration is mandatory if the placenta comes out in pieces or is not intact upon inspection. See Chapter 58 for the technique of fourth stage intrauterine exploration.

The administration of oxytocin is the last step in manual removal of the placenta. It is given after intrauterine exploration of the uterus (if this is done) to assure contraction of a now traumatized and possibly exhausted uterus. Further follow-up with an ergotrate series postpartally is done if there is any question of possible retained placental fragments or incomplete trailing membranes.

58

Fourth Stage Intrauterine Exploration

Intrauterine exploration is one of the several actions to take in the management of an immediate (fourth stage) postpartum hemorrhage. If done, intrauteruine exploration should be performed as quickly and smoothly as possible, as it is a painful procedure. It is performed when you think there might be placental fragments, cotyledons, or membranes retained in the uterus after the placenta has been expelled. The debate between clinicians as to whether the uterus should routinely be explored after manual removal of the placenta is discussed in Chapter 57.

The woman should be catheterized unless you are sure she has an empty bladder. This will reduce trauma to the bladder during this procedure. It also assures that a full bladder will not be displacing the uterus, thereby decreasing the ability of the uterus to contract properly.

Wrap one 4 × 4 gauze around two (or four) fingers. A gauze is used because it provides a rougher surface than your gloved hand. A rougher surface helps pick up any placental fragments or ragged membranes which your uncovered gloved hand would just slip by. *One* gauze is used as a routine in order to best keep track of the gauze to be sure no gauze is left inside the uterus or vagina. Your thumb holds the end of the gauze against the side of your first finger.

The *whole* hand (including your thumb) is placed inside the uterus. Your other hand grasps the uterus externally through the woman's abdominal wall for the same reasons this is done during manual removal of the placenta (see Chapter 57).

Once you have inserted your hand in the uterus, keep it there until you have explored the entire inner surface of the uterus. Do not repeatedly go in and out, in and out, as this increases the risk of infection.

Use the back of your hand to sweep the inside of the uterus. The cupping of your hand inside the uterus will cause the outer surface (back) of your hand to conform with the inner contour of the uterus.

Sweep the entire uterus. You will need to turn your hand over in order to do this and keep the back of your hand in contact with the uterine wall. Carefully use the tips of your fingers to separate any cotyledons. Such action should be well counterbalanced by your external hand in the precise area in order to better feel what you are doing and reduce the risk of perforating the uterus.

When you have explored the entire intrauterine cavity, slowly withdraw your hand. Look at what you bring out and identify everything as blood clots, placental tissue, or membranes. If *unsure* that you got everything out in the process of bringing out your hand, unwrap and discard the gauze on your hand, wrap *one* fresh gauze around your hand as before and go back in *once*. Quickly sweep the uterus, bring your hand out slowly, and identify whatever you bring out.

Unwrap and discard the gauze from around your fingers. Mentally note that you have done this so you will have no question later of having left this gauze in the uterus or vagina.

Massage the uterus with your external hand. The uterus should be well contracted.

The administration of oxytocin is done after fourth stage intrauterine exploration to ensure continuing contraction of the uterus. Some clinicians will also follow-up with a postpartal series of ergotrate.

59

Bimanual Compression

Bimanual compression is one action used for controlling immediate postpartum hemorrhage. (See Chapter 19.) It is well named because it literally involves the clinician's compressing the uterus between his or her two hands. As can be seen in Figure 59-1, this is accomplished as described in the following paragraphs.

One hand is inserted into the vagina and then doubled up into a fist. The fist is placed into the anterior fornix, palmar side up. It is important that the fist be positioned palmar side up because this position provides the proper directional thrust and allows for greater power behind the fist for use in compression. Pressure and massage are then applied inward and upward against the anterior wall of the uterus, largely in the area of the lower uterine segment and the corpus (body) of the uterus.

At the same time, the other hand presses deeply into the abdomen behind the uterus. The open abdominal hand, palmar side against the uterus, then applies pressure and massage in an in-and-downward direction against the posterior wall of the uterus, largely in the area of the fundus and the corpus of the uterus.

The in-and-upward directional thrust of the vaginal fist and the in-and-downward directional thrust of the abdominal hand compresses the uterus between the two hands. This compression of the uterus places direct pressure on the bleeding uterine vessels as well as providing stimulus for the uterus to contract, which will also compress the vessels by virtue of the uterine musculature arrangement through which the arteries and veins course.

Bimanual compression is continued until uterine contraction is assured and bleeding is diminished. This can be tested for by momentarily releasing the pressure on the uterus and then evaluating the uterine consistency and amount of bleeding.

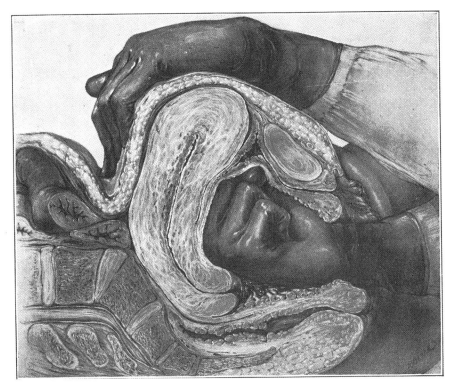

FIGURE 59-1. Bimanual compression of the uterus. Note the position of the hands. (Reproduced by permission from Pritchard, J. A., and MacDonald, P. C. *Williams Obstetrics, 15th.* New York: Appleton-Century-Crofts, 1976.)

60

Cutting an Episiotomy and Repairing Episiotomies and Lacerations

An episiotomy is a surgical incision of the perineal body. The factors to be considered in making the decision of whether or not to cut an episiotomy are discussed in the chapter dealing with management of the second stage of labor (Chapter 13). The discussion here pertains to knowledge and skills necessary for performing the cutting and repair of episiotomies and the repair of various lacerations, and to specific techniques involved in these skills.

RELEVANT ANATOMY

A thorough knowledge of pelvic muscles and structures is essential to proper cutting and repair of episiotomies and repair of lacerations.

Structures of the perineum are discussed in Chapter 44. Pertinent pelvic muscles and their location are as follows and as illustrated in Figure 60-1.

The muscles of the perineum include the bulbocavernosus, ischiocavernosus, superficial transverse perineal, deep transverse perineal, sphincter of the membranous urethra, and external anal sphincter. The central tendinous point of the perineum is also a part of the perineum. Table 60-1 gives the boundaries and functions of each.

The urogenital diaphragm is located between the inferior rami of the pubis and the ischium (ischiopubic ramus) which, with the symphysis pubis, comprises the anterior triangle of the pelvic outlet. It is a musculomembranous sheath that serves as the anterior portion of

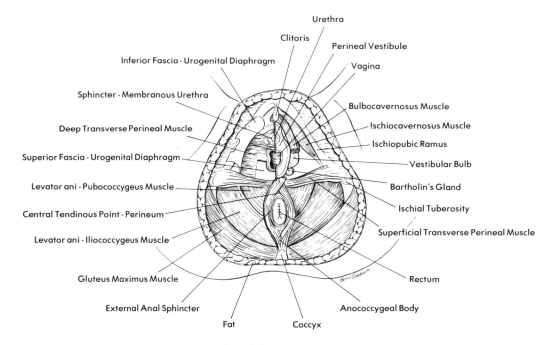

FIGURE 60-1. Muscles of the perineum and related structures.

the pelvic floor musculature. Muscles of the perineum that are superficial to the urogenital diaphragm are the bulbocavernosus, ischiocavernosus, and superficial transverse perineal.

The urogenital diaphragm consists of the inferior fascia (which lies immediately beneath the superficial muscles) and the superior fascia (which is the posterior fascia of the urogenital diaphragm). Between these two layers of fascia, and therefore within the urogenital diaphragm, are the following muscles of the perineum: deep transverse perineal and sphincter of the membranous urethra. The urethra and the vagina are openings through the urogenital diaphragm.

The pelvic diaphragm consists of the levator ani and coccygeus muscles and their fascia (see Fig. 60-2). These combine with the piriformis and obturator internus muscles to comprise the muscles within the pelvis. Together they serve as the most inferior portion of the body wall. As such they give support to the pelvic viscera, confine the contents of the abdo-

men, and close the abdominopelvic cavity. They also affect the vagina and rectum by having a sphincteric action on them. The coccygeus, piriformis, and obturator muscles are much too far posterior and lateral to be involved in either episiotomies or lacerations of the vagina or perineum, and so are not described here.

The muscle comprising the largest portion of the pelvic floor is the levator ani. Because it is a broad muscle and because of its attachments, it is often described as a hammock of muscle. Its superior attachments are anterior to the pelvic brim on the pelvic surface of the superior ramus of the pubis, medial to the medial surface of the ischial spine, and more posterior to the fascia of the obturator muscles. The muscle fibers sweep across the pelvic cavity at varying degrees of direction with some crossing the sides of the urethra and vagina and others sheathing the rectum between the external and internal sphincter. They are separated from each other anteriorly by the

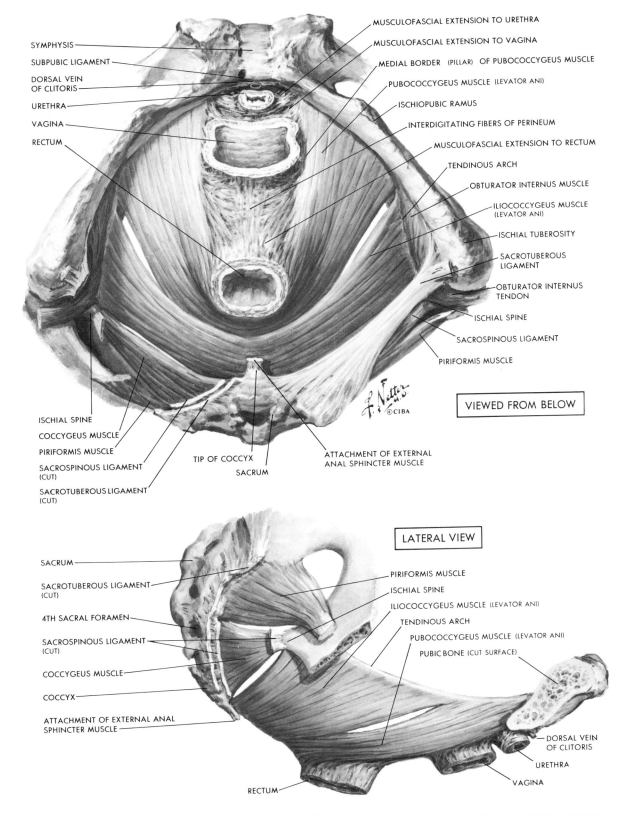

FIGURE 60-2. Pelvic diaphragm. (© Coypright 1965 CIBA Pharmaceutical Company, Division of CIBA-GEIGY Corporation. Reprinted with permission from *The CIBA Collection of Medical Illustrations* by Frank H. Netter, M.D. All rights reserved.)

TABLE 60-1. Muscles of the Perineum

Muscle	Boundaries	Function
Bulbocavernosus	There are two bulbocavernosus muscles, one on either side of the vaginal orifice; posteriorly they attach to the central tendinous point of the perineum and the inferior fascia of the urogenital diaphragm; anteriorly they insert into the corpora cavernosa clitoridis; laterally they surround the orifice of the vagina, covering the vestibular bulbs and Bartholin's glands on either side	Known as the sphincter vaginae, their contraction reduces the size of the vaginal orifice The anterior muscle fibers contribute to clitoral erection
Ischiocavernosus	There are two ischiocavernosus muscles, one on either lateral boundary of the perineum; posteriorly they arise from the inner surface of the ischial tuberosities; anteriorly they cover and insert into the sides and posterior surface of the crus clitoridis; laterally they extend from the clitoris to the ischial tuberosities along the ischial ramus, from which they derive some of their fibers	Maintains clitoral erection
Superficial transverse perineal (transversus perinei superficialis)	There are two superficial transverse perineal muscles, which generally follow the transverse diameter of the pelvic outlet; they arise from the inner and anterior surface of the ischial tuberosity of the superior ramus of the ischium by a small tendon; they insert into the central tendinous point of the perineum	Fixes the location of the central tendinous point of the perineum
Deep transverse perineal (transversus perinei profundus)	There are two deep transverse perineal muscles, which are broader than the superficial transverse perineal muscles; they arise from the inferior ramus of the ischium; they insert into the sides of the vagina	Helps to fix the vagina
Sphincter of the membranous urethra (sphincter urethrae membranaceae)	There are two sphincters of the membranous urethra muscles, consisting of external and innermost fibers; they arise from the margin of the inferior ramus	Urethral sphincter

Muscle	Boundaries	Function
	of the pubis on either side; they cross the space of the pubic arch, pass around all sides and encircle the urethra, and unite with the muscle fibers from the other side by blending with them	
External anal sphincter (sphincter ani externus)	The external anal sphincter consists of two strata of fibers (superficial and deep); which together form one flat plane of muscular fibers; it arises from the anococcygeal body, which is a tendinous band extending from the tip of the coccyx to the posterior margin of the anus; it passes around, encircles, and surrounds the anal canal; it inserts in the central tendinous point of the perineum	Anal sphincter Helps to fix the location of the central tendinous point of the perineum
Central tendinous point of the perineum	A fibromuscular structure in the midline between the vagina and the anus and at the base of the urogenital diaphragm; the tissue is fibrous because it is the point of fusion of both the superior and inferior fascia of the urogenital diaphragm and of the external perineal fascia and Colles' fasica; it has muscular fibers because it is a common point of attachment for a number of muscles whose fibers blend together into the central tendinous point of the perineum: bulbocavernosus superficial transverse perineal some fibers of the deep transverse perineal external anal sphincter levator ani-pubococcygeus	Common point of attachment for a number of layers of fascia and muscles

passage between them of the urethra, vagina, and rectum. Posteriorly most of the muscle fibers simply become continuous with their counterparts from the other side in the area between the rectum and the coccyx, while some blend with muscle fibers of the rectum, and others insert posteriorly into the anococcygeal body and the coccyx.

The levator ani has two major groupings of muscle fibers: (1) the pubococcygeus and (2) the iliococcygeus. Of these two, the iliococcygeus, arising in part from the ischial spine and inserting in the anococcygeal body and the coccyx, is too far posterior and lateral to be involved in either episiotomies or lacerations of the vagina or perineum.

The pubococcygeus group of muscle fibers arise from the pelvic surface of the superior ramus of the pubis on either side of the pelvis. The muscle fibers extend posteriorly as they descend in the pelvis on either side of the urethra, vagina, and rectum and sheath these structures. They are separated by the interlevator cleft (genital hiatus), which accommodates the passage of the urethra, vagina, and rectum. The anterior, or medial, muscle fibers of the pubococcygeus form musculofascial extensions which support these organs and insert into the posterior aspect of the urogenital diaphragm and the central point of the perineum. The majority of the muscle fibers pass horizontally posterior around the rectum with the lesser number of superficial, anterior fibers inserting into the anococcygeal body and the greater number of deep, more posterior, fibers forming a sling in the space between the rectum and the coccyx by joining and blending with the muscle fibers from the other side.

In effect, then, there are three layers of muscles from outside to inside starting at the perineal body and vaginal introitus and following an imaginary pathway paralleling the posterior and lateral walls of the vagina. These three layers are as follows:

Layer 1: bulbocavernosus and superficial transverse perineal

Layer 2: deep transverse perineal
Layer 3: pubococcygeus of the levator ani

Layer 1 contributes with other muscles to the makeup of the central point of the perineum. Layers 2 and 3 have muscle and fascial fibers which extend to the posterior aspect of the central point of the perineum.

CUTTING AN EPISIOTOMY

There are two types of episiotomies: (1) the midline (medial) and (2) the mediolateral, which may be to the left or to the right (see Fig. 60-3). The following principles should be observed, regardless of which type is cut:

1. The presenting part of the fetus is protected from injury.
2. A single cut in any direction is far preferable to repeated snipping because the latter will leave jagged edges.
3. The episiotomy should be large enough to meet the purpose for deciding to cut it.
4. The timing of the cut should be such that lacerations are prevented (too late) and unnecessary blood loss avoided (too soon). The perineum should be bulging, the vaginal orifice distended by approximately a 3-centimeter diameter of fetal presenting part between contractions, and delivery of the presenting part should be expected to occur within the next two to four contractions.

Midline Episiotomy

The midline episiotomy, cut into the central tendinous point of the perineum, separates the two sides of the bulbocavernosus and superficial transverse perineal muscles. Depending on the depth of the cut, the two sides of the deep transverse perineal muscle may also be separated.

The technique for cutting a midline episiotomy follows.

Procedure	Rationale
1. Place your index and middle fingers into the vagina, palmar side down and facing you. Separate them slightly and exert outward pressure on the perineal body (Fig. 60-3).	1. This provides protection to the presenting part in two ways: a. your fingers are against the fetal presenting part and are thick enough so that scissors properly placed between them will not touch the baby. b. the outward pressure directs the perineal body away from the baby. The pressure also flattens the perineal body a bit more, making it easier to incise in a single cut.
2. The blades of the scissors are placed in a straight up-and-down position so that one blade is against the posterior vaginal wall and the other blade is against the skin of the perineal body, with the point where the blades cross at the midline of the posterior fourchette.	2. A midline episiotomy is cut in the middle of the central tendinous point of the perineum from the posterior fourchette down to the external anal sphincter.
3. a. with your vaginal fingers and with your thumb of the same hand on the outside of the perineal body, palpate for and locate the external anal sphincter.	3. a. a midline episiotomy cuts to, but not into or through, the external anal sphincter. Knowing the location of the external anal sphincter removes any hesitation in cutting an adequate episiotomy due to fear of accidentally cutting through the sphincter.
b. adjust the length of the blades of the scissors on the perineal body and the projected length of the incision accordingly.	b. the length of the incision should be adequate to meet the purpose for deciding to cut it. Knowing the location of the external anal sphincter informs you as to the maximum length possible.
4. Cut.	4.
5. Sponge, observe, and palpate again for the external sphincter. Evaluate if another cut in this plane is needed.	5. The sharpness or dullness of the scissors may effect the efficiency of the first cut.
6. Cut again, if needed.	6. Avoid snipping. Two cuts should accomplish the incision in this plane even if the scissors are dull.
7. Evaluate the extent of the incision into the vagina. Feel for a band of tight, restricting vaginal tissue shortly inside the introitus.	7. This band is frequently felt in primigravidas and may be a vestige of the hymenal ring.
8. Extend the vaginal side of the incision, if needed, or if the band of tissue is there and needs to be incised. Extension is accomplished by now pressing downward	8. The vaginal side of the incision usually needs extending since the cut on that side usually does not go as far as on the skin side when the perineal body is incised.

Procedure	Rationale
with your two vaginal fingers, holding them apart to splint the incision line and in far enough to extend beyond the projected lengthening of the incision line. The scissors now come from above the back side of the hand to slide between the fingers and make the cut.	To protect the fetal presenting part.
9. Apply pressure with 4 × 4 sponges to the incision.	9. To staunch any bleeding.

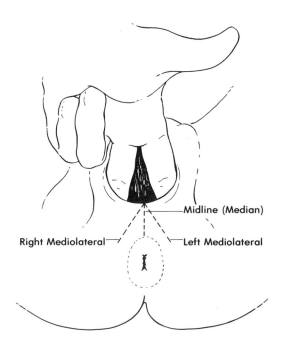

FIGURE 60-3.   Cutting an episiotomy.

Mediolateral Episiotomy

The technique of cutting a mediolateral episiotomy is the same as that for cutting a midline episiotomy with the exception of the direction of the cut and, therefore, the placement of the scissors for cutting. It does not matter if a mediolateral episiotomy is cut to the left or to the right. It is easier for a learner to repair a left mediolateral episiotomy if right-handed and a right mediolateral episiotomy if left-handed. A mediolateral episiotomy is cut at a slant starting at the midline of the posterior fourchette with the points of the scissors directed toward the ischial tuberosity on the same side as the incision. Care must be taken to palpate for the external anal sphincter, to direct the cut far enough laterally to avoid the sphincter, and, preferably, to leave approximately 1 centimeter of levator ani muscle between the incision and the sphincter for repair. Care must be taken also not to start the cut on the lateral aspect of the fourchette or direct the cut too far laterally, in order to avoid the Bartholin's gland on that side.

A mediolateral episiotomy cuts into the central tendinous point of the perineum, through the bulbocavernosus and the superficial and deep transverse perineal muscles, and into the pubococcygeus (levator ani) muscle. How much of the pubococcygeus muscle is cut is dependent on the length and depth of the incision. Usually it is a larger cut than the midline episiotomy because it usually is performed when more space is needed than that which is available between the posterior fourchette and the external anal sphincter.

AIDS TO WOUND HEALING

Wound healing is facilitated by actions taken at different times in the maternity cycle. These are as follows.

Antepartally:
1. Prevention of nutritional deficiencies
2. Prevention of anemia

Intrapartally:
1. Prevention of maternal exhaustion and dehydration
2. Strict adherence to aseptic technique
3. Prevention of unnecessary further trauma to the incisional tissues, such as:
   a. use of an eyed needle pulling a double strand of suture through the tissue when eyeless or swaged-on needles (atraumatic suture) pulling a single strand of suture are available
   b. use of suture with suture gauge and needle size larger than needed
   c. inappropriate use of a traumatic cutting needle rather than an atraumatic round needle
   d. misplacement of stitches requiring removal and replacement
   e. placement of stitches too close together
   f. tissue strangulation resulting from too tight stitches
   g. repeated unnecessary sponging, prodding, and probing of the wound
   h. use of instruments that crush tissue
4. Removal of blood clots and debris before closure
5. Visible hemostasis before closure to avoid formation of hematomas
6. Precise approximation of tissues
7. Closure which obliterates all dead space

Postpartally:
1. Diet high in protein and vitamin C
2. Perineal cleanliness
3. Warm sitz baths

These actions are aimed at the prevention of infection, tissue devitalization, and tissue trauma; minimizing of inflammatory reaction; provision of tissue building and healing nutrients; and increased circulation to the area.

MANIPULATION OF EQUIPMENT

These are hints which may ease some of the awkwardness and mistakes experienced when first learning how to suture.

Suture:
The following are hints about sutures:

1. Use suture with a swaged-on needle.
2. This suture may come with a curved cutting needle swaged on to one end and a curved, circular, non-cutting needle swaged on to the other end. While holding the two needles in one hand, gently straighten the suture and cut it in half. Remove the half with the cutting needle on it from your immediate working area.
3. In order to prevent the length of suture from dangling or dragging across areas of contamination, keep the excess suture gathered up into the palm of the hand holding the needleholder.
4. Never place a clamp or the needle holder on the junction of the needle with the suture, or on the suture itself, except for an end that is to be cut off after tying a knot with an instrument tie. Such an action weakens the suture.

Needle:
The following hints apply to the needle:

1. The needle is held by clamping the needleholder on the portion of the needle closest to the suture without being on the junction of the two.
2. The needle is clamped by the tip of the needleholder.

3. The needle is clamped so that its curve is at a 90° right angle to the needleholder.

Needleholder:
The following hints are about holding the needleholder:

1. When taking a stitch you have the most control of the needleholder and most latitude for wrist action by holding it so that the thumb holes are in the palm of your hand (hold them there with your ring and little fingers), your thumb and middle fingers are on either lateral side of the shaft, and your index finger is on one side (usually the upper) of the broad side of the shaft.

2. The same hand position on the needleholder is used for pulling the needle through the tissue after reclamping the needleholder on the tip (point) of the needle for this purpose.

3. When doing an instrument tie, the needleholder is held by inserting your thumb and middle finger in the holes provided for this at the hand end of the needleholder, and placing your index finger on the broad side of the shaft. Your two remaining fingers help hold the excess suture in the palm of your hand.

Stitching with a Curved Needle:
Wrist action, combined with entry into tissue with the point of the needle, is the key to success for stitching with a curved needle. This is done as follows:

1. Be sure to use the point of the needle in inserting it into tissue, even though this seems to direct the needle in a direction opposite from where you wish to bring the needle out. A common mistake is to try to insert the needle by holding and pointing it in the direction and shape of the stitch to be taken. In so doing, one tries to insert the needle with the side of its tip and then wonders why the skin is so tough or the needle is so dull.

2. Start the stitch by having the needle with its curved midportion up and then turn it even further until entry will be made with the point of the needle. This means that your hand will be holding the needleholder shaft so that the back of your hand is up and then further pronated as the needle point is positioned for entry.

   As the needle enters the tissue you rotate your wrist and hand approximately 180° so that the needle follows the necessary directional path for exit and making of the stitch.

3. In pulling a curved needle through tissue the principle of following the curve of the needle is used. If, after reclamping the needleholder on the tip of the needle, you pull straight up you will meet resistance and traumatize the tissue. Instead, again using wrist action, simply draw the needle through in the direction of the curve of the needle and it slips through the tissue with ease. One caution with this maneuver: be careful not to poke the woman with the point of the needle which is now directed for entry again with this completion of the circle.

KNOTS AND SUTURE STITCHES

Knots

An essential skill in repairing episiotomies and lacerations is knowing how to tie knots, whether used for starting and ending a series of suture stitches or for interrupted stitches.

The knot used is the square knot. This is accomplished by either hand ties or an instrument tie or both. Which method is used for tying a knot does not matter as long as you become proficient in doing it that way. There are advocates of each. Those who know how to do both hand ties and an instrument tie have the advantage of being able to use whichever will be easier for any given location.

Skill in tying knots is a matter of much

patient and repetitive practice. The learner is encouraged to study the *Manual of Surgical Knots* [1], which clearly illustrates both methods of how to tie a square knot. Use the practice board which accompanies this monograph; both are put out by Ethicon, Inc. Pay particular attention to the rules for tying knots, on page 7 of the manual.

Suture Stitches

There are four basic suture stitches used in repairing an episiotomy: (1) blanket (continuous locked), (2) interrupted, (3) continuous, and (4) continuous mattress (Fig. 60-4). In addition, a crown suture may be used to repair the bulbocavernosus muscle. Knowledge of and skill in these various suture stitches will also enable you to repair any perineal, vaginal, cervical, periurethral, and clitoral lacerations, including third and fourth degree perineal lacerations. Following is a description of each of these suture stitches as done by a right-handed person. If you are left-handed, simply reverse the direction of the horizontal stitching. This description is only of the mechanics of doing these sutures and is not of how these stitches are done in relation to the repair of an episiotomy or laceration. The latter is described later in this section.

Blanket (Continuous Locked)
The blanket, or continuous locked, suture stitch is used for closing the vaginal mucosa. After placing an anchoring stitch and knot (one end of the suture in the knot is cut short, the other end continues for the suture stitches), proceed with the following (see Fig. 60-4):

1. Move the anchoring knot to the left side of the anchoring stitch
2. Hold the suture down along the left side of the incision line
3. Make sure the entry and exit point of this stitch are precisely across from each other
4. Take a bite on the right side of the incision

5. Feel the point of the needle just beneath the tissue surface in the midline of the incision
6. Continue the bite to the left of the incision
7. Exit the needle between the incision and the suture to the left of it (this locks the stitch)
8. Pull the needle and suture through
9. Repeat steps 2 through 8 for as many stitches as are needed of this suture

Interrupted
Interrupted stitches are used for deep muscle repair. An interrupted stitch is a single stitch with a knot (both ends cut short). It is taken from right to left, with the entry and exit points directly across from each other (see Fig. 60-4).

Continuous
A continuous suture is used for closure of the subcutaneous layer. The continuous suture is exactly like the blanket suture except that it is *not* a locked stitch (see Fig. 60-4). Therefore, instead of holding the suture down along the left side of the incision line (step 2 of the blanket suture stitch), hold it up alongside the stitches already taken and above where the stitch is being taken.

Continuous Mattress
A continuous mattress suture stitch is used for the subcuticular closure of an episiotomy or laceration. Therefore, it is described here as an ascending line of subcuticular suture stitches because this is their placement in an episiotomy or laceration repair in closure of the perineal skin (see Fig. 60-4). The stitches can, of course, go in either direction and can be used as the final layer of stitches in repairing deeper periurethral lacerations. From the anchoring point:

1. Take a shallow bite on the left side of the incision line, inserting and exiting the needle approximately "one cell layer" beneath the skin layer, in a perpendicular

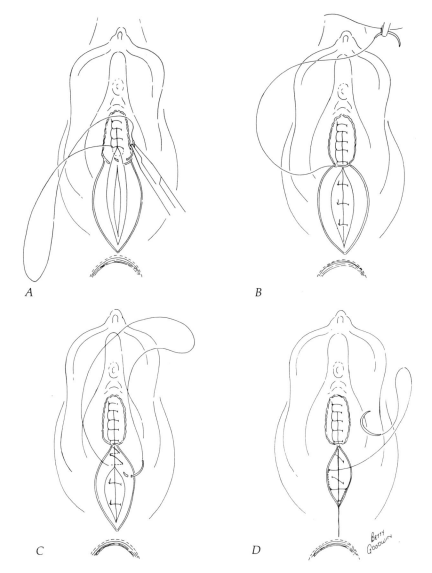

FIGURE 60-4.   Suture stitches. A. blanket (continuous locked); B. deep interrupted; C. continuous unlocked; D. mattress.

line on the same side of the incision. The depth of the bite between the entry and exit points can be greater than the one cell layer.

2. Pull the needle and suture through.
3. Take a shallow bite on the right side of the incision line. The entry point should be directly across from the exit point of the

preceding stitch on the left side of the incision line. Again, the entire stitch is on the same side of the incision in a perpendicular line. And again, the entry and exit points are approximately one cell layer beneath the skin layer with the depth in between being somewhat greater.

4. Pull the needle and suture through.

5. Return to the left side of the incision line and repeat step 1. The entry point should be directly across from the exit point of the preceding stitch on the right side of the incision line.

6. Repeat steps 2 through 5 for as many stitches as are needed of this suture.

While it may be easier for some to use a straight needle to do a subcuticular closure with the mattress stitch, it is not suggested. Doing so means cutting off the swaged-on curved needle and using an eyed straight needle. This means an unnecessary double strand of suture going through the tissue, which violates an aforestated aid to wound healing. With practice, it is possible to learn to become proficient and comfortable in doing this stitching with the curved needle.

Crown Stitch
The crown stitch is used to reunite the cut bulbocavernosus muscle. Its purpose is to reduce gaping of the vaginal introitus and to facilitate the return of good muscle tone by deliberate approximation of this muscle. This, in turn, facilitates enjoyable sexual relations by both the female and the male. Care must be taken, however, only to closely approximate the muscle for its repair, since pulling and stitching the two sides together tightly may have the reverse and adverse effect of causing dyspareunia. Study the following steps in relation to Figure 60-5.

1. Enter the tissue at the upper left side of the perineal incisional line. Be sure to enter (start this stitch) sufficiently far enough away from the skin edge to allow for both subcutaneous and subcuticular closure over the completed crown stitch.

   Direct your needle so that after entry it follows a sequence of swinging up, laterally, down, and medially to where it exits in the same plane, only further down, as it entered.

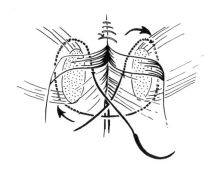

FIGURE 60-5. Crown stitch. Reuniting the divided bulbocavernosus muscle. (Reproduced by permission from Oxorn, H., and Foote, W. H. Human Labor and Birth, *3rd* New York: Appleton-Century-Crofts, 1975.)

The amount of lateral thrust must be carefully judged. It must be enough to catch the retracted cut end of the bulbocavernosus muscle but no more than this. The further lateral you go, the more vascular the area you are getting into and the greater the risk of unknowingly nicking a blood vessel. Subsequent slow seepage will result in a hematoma which may evidence itself approximately an hour later. This is a rare happening that can be avoided by simply going only as far lateral as needed and not exaggerating this part of the stitch.

2. Check that you have indeed included this side of the bulbocavernosus muscle in this half of your stitch. This is done by grasping the two ends of the suture a short distance from the tissue and pulling down on them. If you have the bulbocavernosus muscle you should see the entire left side of the perineum from the clitoris to your stitch pull down as you pull on the suture ends. If this does not happen, pull the suture on through and try again or get someone more experienced to put the stitch in. If you do see the pulling and know that you have the bulbocavernosus muscle on the left side, then proceed to the next step.

3. Enter the tissue at the upper right side of the perineal incisional line directly across

from your exit point on the left side of the incisional line.

Direct your needle so that after entry it follows a sequence of swinging laterally in, up, down, and medially to where it exits in the same plane, only further up, as it entered, and directly across from the entry point on the left side of the perineal incisional line.

Again judge carefully the amount of lateral thrust as explained in Step 1.

4. Check that you have caught the right side of the bulbocavernosus muscle using the same technique as described in Step 2. You should see the entire right side of the perineum from the clitoris to the right half of your stitch pull down as you pull on the suture.

5. Tie your knot so that the cut ends of the bulbocavernosus muscle are closely joined, but not too tightly. The placement of the two halves of the stitch assures the approximation of the muscle.

6. Cut both of the suture ends close to the knot.

PRINCIPLES OF AND THOUGHTS ABOUT EPISIOTOMY AND LACERATION REPAIR

The repair of an episiotomy or laceration should be as artistic as is within the capability of the individual. By artistic is meant that the repair is done with special care taken for a result that not only serves the woman well functionally but is cosmetic as well.

All repairs should, of course, have good functional results. Specifically, the repair should restore the structure of the pelvic musculature and its support to the pelvic organs. Such action provides for prophylactic gynecology, particularly in years to come, against cystoceles, rectoceles, and uterine prolapse. It also promotes sexual satisfaction by providing a musculature base for Kegel exercises to build upon in reducing the vaginal laxness created by tissue stretching during childbirth. Also, there should be good bowel control and sphincter tone in the event the external anal sphincter was severed. Good functional results also include not creating functional problems during the process of repair, for example, not creating fistulas due to misplacement of stitches providing a channel between orifices, or not creating sexual problems by placing stitches in the hymenal ring, or by not approximating tissue anatomically, or by reuniting the bulbocavernosus muscle too tightly — all of which can cause dyspareunia.

The artistry relates to the cosmetic results. Cosmetic results are important because an episiotomy and lacerations do constitute an assault on the woman's body which, like any type of surgery or injury elsewhere on the body, affects the woman's self-image and body concept. Further, the perineum has become a much more visible portion of the woman's body both to herself and to her sexual partner. It should not be a disfigured portion of her body because of careless repair of episiotomies or lacerations. The perfection to strive for is a repair that results in a scar the breadth of a hair and with all aspects of the perineum in precise anatomical alignment without wrinkles, puckers, or overlapping skin edges. This may not always be possible or within the individual clinician's ability to achieve but does constitute a goal for which to aim. It has been observed that clinicians who do needlework (e.g., sewing, embroidery, needlepoint) generally have an advantage in doing the fine needlework in episiotomy and laceration repair.

Adequate anesthesia is an essential prerequisite to episiotomy or laceration repair. The area of repair is sensitive both physically and psychologically. This should be recognized and respected as evidenced by concern that the woman not feel pain during the repair. Pudendal block or local infiltration for repair will provide adequate anesthesia and are described earlier in this part of the book. The woman should be prepared to differentiate between pressure and pain since she may still feel pressure even though not feeling pain.

The aids to wound healing listed earlier that are pertinent during the actual repair are as follows with further elaboration:

1. Strict adherence to aseptic technique. This includes changing gloves and redraping if necessary; using an extra sterile glove over the sterile glove you already have on your examining hand for checking the rectum and discarding the extra glove immediately after use; and positioning a sterile drape (hand towel) across the rectal area and below, to beneath the level of the table, in order to provide a noncontaminated field in the event suture drops to that level and brushes against whatever is there.

2. Prevention of unnecessary further trauma to the incisional tissues. Examples of unnecessary further trauma include the following:

    a. use of an eyed needle pulling a double strand of suture through the tissue when eyeless or swaged-on needles pulling a single strand of suture through the tissue are available.

    b. using suture with suture gauge and needle size larger than needed. The following is generally used for episiotomy and laceration repairs:

        (1) 4-0 chromic catgut is used for (a) repair of the anterior wall of the rectum in fourth degree lacerations, (b) repair of clitoral lacerations, or (c) repair of any other place when very fine sutures are desired.

        (2) 3-0 chromic catgut is used for (a) repair of the vaginal mucosa, (b) the subcutaneous stitches, (c) the subcuticular stitches, and (d) repair of periurethral lacerations.

        (3) 2-0 chromic catgut is used for (a) repair of the external anal sphincter, (b) repair of cervical lacerations, (c) repair of lateral vaginal wall lac-

erations, and (d) deep interrupted stitches of pelvic muscles (these may also be repaired with 3-0 chromic catgut if the cut or laceration is not too extensive).

It helps when selecting suture gauge to remember that muscle requires a stronger suture. The smaller the gauge number the finer the suture (e.g., 4-0, 6-0, 8-0) and the larger the gauge number the heavier the suture and the stronger the tensile strength of the suture (e.g., 2-0, 1, 4).

The size and type of needle usually used is the atraumatic, swaged-on General Closure needle. An atraumatic swaged-on G-I needle may be used in doing very fine, tiny stitches as might be indicated in repairing a clitoral laceration.

    c. inappropriate use of a traumatic cutting needle rather than an atraumatic round needle. A cutting needle is triangular-shaped with each edge a cutting edge. Many clinicians feel that a cutting needle is not needed for the repair work under discussion. They prefer the round needle which has a tapered point and will go through soft tissues easily with less trauma than a cutting needle. There is also less chance of nicking or lacerating a blood vessel with a round needle than with a cutting needle. Other clinicians feel that since the cutting needle is designed for the tougher, less vascular tissues it is valid to use a cutting needle for placing stitches in these areas. The subcutaneous and subcuticular tissues would be examples of this type of tissue.

    d. unnecessary, excessive number of needle punctures as a result of:

        (1) misplacement of stitches, requiring removal and replacement.

        (2) too many stitches, too close together. Too many stitches also means exces-

sive suture in the wound, which slows the healing process as a result of the inflammatory reaction they cause as foreign material. Stitches should be carefully planned before the woman is stuck. Good visualization facilitates proper placement of stitches.

e. tissue strangulation because stitches are too tight. Tissue strangulation devitalizes the tissue and, if the stitches are so tight that circulation is inadequate, may even cause the tissue to slough.

f. unnecessary repeated sponging and probing of the wound. This can cause further trauma and disrupt clotting, especially if the sponge is used to rub rather than blot. Constant probing and sponging usually are due to anxiety secondary to insecurity in performance. This is common in the learner, who should make a conscious effort not to sponge and probe repeatedly.

g. use of instruments that crush tissue. This refers specifically to the use of pickup forceps. Learn to use them so you can hold tissue securely with them without crushing the tissue. Forceps with teeth should be avoided.

3. Removal of blood clots and debris prior to closure. If blood clots and debris are stitched over they can become foci for bacterial growth, inflammatory reaction, and tissue and repair breakdown.

4. Visible hemostasis prior to closure. This avoids the formation of hematomas that can totally disrupt a repair with infection and tissue and repair breakdown. All significant bleeders, whether pumping or oozing, should be tied off before the repair is begun.

5. Precise approximation of tissues, the closure of which obliterates all dead space. Dead space, by not approximating the tissue in that area, weakens both its healing ability and its function when healed. It also provides a non-pressure-producing spot conducive to hematoma formation and nonconducive to hemostasis. As such, it may also be a focus for bacterial growth and infection. It is also important that dead space not be created by allowing knots to slip while being tied. They should be snug to assure approximation but not tight, which might cause tissue necrosis.

The suture used in repair of episiotomies and lacerations is chromic catgut. Catgut is an absorbable suture as it is made from animal tissue (sheep intestine) and is composed primarily of collagen. As such it is a foreign protein in the human body and is dissolved by digestive enzyme action (proteolysis). Chromic catgut is catgut that has been treated with chrome salts. The function of the chrome salts is to delay the process of proteolysis by which catgut is absorbed, thereby extending the length of time the suture holds the tissue together during the healing process. Plain catgut will absorb in approximately one week and will begin to lose its strength in about 3 days. Chromic catgut delays absorption for 10 to 40 days, depending on the amount of chrome salts used, but generally will retain its strength for 2 to 3 weeks. This gives support to the wound for a longer period of time while it is healing. Absorbable suture is used, however, because artificial support is not needed indefinitely. Catgut has the disadvantage of causing marked tissue inflammatory reaction. This, in turn, can produce edema, which places tension on the sutures and may cause tissue necrosis. The result of this is excessive scarring, which means a weaker functional repair. This inflammatory reaction can be minimized by using only sufficient suture to assure hemostasis, closure of dead space, and approximation of the tissues — and not one stitch more. Artistry does *not* mean excessive decorative stitchery.

Hemostasis is one of the purposes for doing episiotomy and laceration repair. It is accomplished not only by tying off both pumping and oozing bleeders, by closure that eliminates dead space, and by avoiding a cutting needle, as mentioned before, but also by the following:

1. Probing the depth of the wound before stitching in order to identify the true depth that needs repair beneath the mucosal layer
2. Starting any line of suture at least 1 centimeter beyond the apex of the wound in order to include any retracted blood vessels
3. Using types of suture stitches that facilitate hemostasis in the most vascular areas, such as the blanket (continuous locked) suture stitch

In doing episiotomy and laceration repair it is imperative that you have good visualization of the field. This includes proper positioning of light to illumine the field; proper exposure of the field (which may mean asking someone to scrub in to hold retractors and instruments, such as for cervical lacerations or high vaginal lacerations); use of a tamponade to provide a field that is clean and dry, that is, without a continual uterine blood flow obscuring the field; and proper positioning of yourself for maximum efficiency in visualization and manipulation of tissues, materials, and equipment.

Finally, a happy balance has to be struck between the learner's need for time, without feeling rushed, in performing an episiotomy or laceration repair and the woman's need to be in stirrups no longer than absolutely necessary. Being in stirrups over time can fatigue and become uncomfortable for the woman. Being in stirrups also impairs circulation, which if continued for a long time may be a causative factor in postpartal thrombophlebitis. A total of 1½ hours in stirrups should be considered the maximum amount of time. One effective way of handling this situation is for the learner to have a set amount of time for doing the repair, after which any work not yet done will be completed by an experienced

clinician. The learner can then pace him- or herself in accord with his or her learning needs. It is also possible to do episiotomy or minor repairs with the woman in the dorsal position.

REPAIR OF A MIDLINE EPISIOTOMY

Following are the steps, listed in sequence, to take in repairing a midline episiotomy. As in other skills, this is only one way of doing it; there are other methods. This method is sound and will yield satisfactory functional and cosmetic results. Be open to other methods and individual variations, seeking always the underlying rationale, and formulating your own basic methodology and individual variations. The method presented here will give you a valid base from which to develop, experiment, and decide to continue or change this methodology.

1. Insert a tamponade to provide a field free of uterine bleeding. The most common tampon is a tailed, rolled, vaginal gauze sponge. It should be inserted in such a way that both of the following goals are met:
   a. the woman's discomfort during insertion is minimized as much as possible. To do this the tampon should not scrape along the tender and recently traumatized vaginal walls. This is accomplished by:
   (1) lightly moistening the outside of the tampon to reduce friction and the scratchiness of dry gauze.
   (2) inserting three fingers along the posterior vaginal wall with the fingertips extending into the posterior vaginal fornix and exerting strong downward pressure (this braces the wound and creates space for insertion of the tampon).
   (3) inserting the tampon by (a) hold-

ing it between the palmar surface of the index and middle fingers and the thumb of your inserting hand with the tail tucked into your palm; (b) inserting your index and middle fingers so that the back of them protects the anterior structures and vaginal wall from the gauze tampon; (c) pushing the tampon with your thumb the length of the vagina between the protective splinting and space provided by your two hands; and (d) clamping the tail of the tampon onto the abdominal drape, as a safeguard reminder to remove it when no longer needed.

b. the tampon should be inserted far enough to be well beyond the apex of the wound to allow for good visualization and room for the first stitch.

2. Identify the following structures and their anatomical juxtaposition both with the episiotomy open and with it gently pushed together with your fingers:
a. depth of the cut or laceration.
b. vaginal apex of the cut or laceration.
c. hymenal ring.
d. mucocutaneous junction.
e. tissue layers.
f. muscles.
g. rectal sphincter.
h. perineal apex of the cut or laceration.

3. Repair the vaginal mucosa with a 3-0 chromic catgut suture using an atraumatic (swaged-on) needle.
a. place your anchoring stitch approximately 1 centimeter above (beyond) the vaginal apex of the cut to catch any retracted blood vessels and provide hemostasis.
b. tie a knot after taking the anchoring stitch. Cut off the short end close to the knot.
c. plan ahead the number of stitches you will need between the anchoring stitch

and a stitch placed right behind the hymenal ring.
d. close the vaginal mucosa with the other end of the suture using the blanket (locked continuous) suture stitches (see this procedure earlier in this section).
e. if the incision is deep, do not completely close the vaginal mucosa at this time, as to do so will make it too difficult to get into the area for the deep interrupted stitches.
f. Close the vaginal mucosa to the mucocutaneous junction (the junction of the vaginal mucosa with the perineal skin).
g. a stitch should not be placed in the hymenal ring as this may cause dyspareunia. To avoid this yet carry on the closure of the vaginal mucosa:
(1) lock the stitch immediately behind (inside) the hymenal ring by inserting the needle on the same side of the incision as you just exited for that stitch.
(2) swing the needle through the tissue underneath the hymenal ring.
(3) exit on the same side only now in front of the hymenal ring.
(4) continue closure of the vaginal mucosa as before.
h. the first stitch or two of the blanket suture should consist of bites large enough to close the cut in the area completely. This can be checked by feeling the tip of the needle at the apex of the cut in the midline with the tip of your palpating finger before taking the other half of your stitch. Thereafter, the stitches include only the vaginal mucosa, with the apex of the cut and area beneath the vaginal mucosa being closed next with the deep interrupted stitches.
i. clamp the needle of the suture remaining after completion of closure of the vaginal mucosa onto the abdominal

drape to be used later for the subcutaneous and subcuticular closure.

4. Repair the bulbocavernosus muscle with a crown stitch (see procedure earlier in this section). Use a 2-0 chromic catgut suture with an atraumatic (swaged-on) needle.

5. If the cut is quite deep, you may prefer to put in a layer of deep stitches first, then finish closure of the vaginal mucosa, then repair the bulbocavernosus muscle with the crown stitch, and then put in a second layer of deep stitches. In a cut or laceration this deep, the first layer of deep stitches would close the deep transverse perineal muscle and the second layer of deep stitches would close the superficial transverse perineal muscles.

6. Repair the superficial transverse perineal muscles with deep interrupted stitches (see procedure earlier in this section). Use 2-0 chromic catgut suture with an atraumatic (swaged-on) needle. Again, plan before taking any stitches, the number of deep interrupted stitches that will be needed to effect hemostasis, close dead space, and approximate the tissue. Also check in the midline with the tip of your palpating finger to feel the tip of the needle just beyond the apex of the cut after taking half the stitch, to assure closure of the area without dead space.

7. After placing the deep interrupted stitches, especially if the cut was deep and two layers of deep interrupted stitches made, put another glove on top of the glove already on your examining hand. Do a rectal examination to determine whether or not any of the stitches accidentally entered the rectum. Discard the cover glove after completion of the examination, as it is grossly contaminated.

If a stitch is in the rectum the episiotomy repair must be taken apart to the extent of identifying which stitch it is and removing it. Such a stitch is removed because of its being a path for contamination and bacteria from the rectum, thereby being the potential cause of infection and development of a sinus tract or fistula. Discovery now entails much less in the way of taking apart and redoing the episiotomy repair with its additional trauma to the tissues than would discovery later. Stitches in the rectum can be avoided if care is taken to direct the bite of the needle laterally and straight back, *not* down.

8. Repair the perineal subcutaneous fascia. Use the same suture for this repair as you used for repair of the vaginal mucosa, unclamping the needle from where you attached it to the abdominal drape in Step 3 i. above.

   a. start the suture line of continuous stitches at the upper end of the perineal body by:
      (1) locking the stitch at the mucocutaneous junction by inserting the needle on the same side of the incision as the exit of the last stitch.
      (2) swinging the needle through the vaginal mucosa on that same side.
      (3) exiting in the perineal subcutaneous fascia on the same side.

   b. close the subcutaneous fascia using the continuous suture stitches (see procedure earlier in this section).

   c. again, plan, before taking any stitches, the number of stitches you will need before the last one, which is placed differently (see e. below).

   d. care must be taken to leave sufficient and equilateral room on both sides for the final layer of subcuticular stitches.

   e. the last stitch is placed differently since its exit point becomes the start of the layer of the subcuticular suture stitches. Therefore, from the entry point, instead of going straight across as with the preceding stitches, come through the subcutaneous tissue on the same side, going a little beneath the perineal apex to include any retracted blood vessels, and exit one cell layer underneath the skin precisely at the perineal apex.

9. Close the skin edges of the episiotomy or laceration with a layer of subcuticular suture stitches. Use the remainder of the same 3-0 chromic catgut for this repair as was used for repair of the vaginal mucosa and the subcutaneous fascia. Subcuticular closure is done using the mattress suture stitch (see procedure earlier in this section). Start the suture line on the side of the incision opposite the side on which the last subcutaneous continuous stitch was taken.

10. Tie off the suture as follows:
    a. when the mucocutaneous junction is reached and the skin edges are completely closed, take a stitch through the perineal subcutaneous fascia and swing the needle on up through the vaginal mucosa, exiting just in front of the hymenal ring.
    b. take a final stitch in front of the hymenal ring for the purpose of creating ties with which to knot the suture. Try to place this stitch so that the cut ends of the knot will not be sticking the woman. The entry point of this stitch should be on the same side as, and close to the exit point of, the preceding stitch, and the exit point should be straight across on the opposite side.
    c. do *not* draw the suture all the way through the tissue with this stitch. Instead, leave a length of suture, actually a loop, to tie with.
    d. cut the needle off the other end if you desire.
    e. tie your knot slightly loose to allow for some edema resulting from inflammatory reaction to the suture.
    f. cut the ends short.

11. Remove the tampon gently and quickly. Protect the vaginal suture line with the fingers of one hand while removing the tampon with your other hand.

12. Do a vaginal examination to:
    a. inspect the vaginal suture line.
    b. make sure all foreign objects (e.g., sponges) have been removed.
    c. remove any blood clots in the vaginal fornices.
    d. help contract the uterus.
    e. check for hematomas.

13. Do a rectovaginal examination to feel the rectovaginal wall and perineal body muscle support after repair.

14. Do a rectal examination to assure that there are no rectal stitches and to check for hematomas. Discard this glove.

REPAIR OF A MEDIOLATERAL EPISIOTOMY

The repair of a mediolateral episiotomy, irrespective of which side it is on, is essentially the same as the repair of a midline episiotomy insofar as the type of suture stitches used and their sequence is concerned. There is, however, one important difference. The mediolateral episiotomy was cut on a slant in relation to the perpendicular midline of the perineum. This affects repair in two ways:

1. In a mediolateral episiotomy the medial aspect of the incision tends to retract more than the lateral aspect. Therefore, be careful when taking the medial half of the stitches to secure the tissue involved without entering the rectum.

2. Stitching from side to side of the incision must be done in accord with the angle of the incision (on a slant) and *not* done straight across as though at right angles to a perpendicular midline. This is facilitated by holding the needleholder parallel to the edges of the incision. In a mediolateral episiotomy there will be more tissue on the lateral side than on the medial side of

the incision; therefore, care must be taken in properly aligning and approximating the tissues. This is done by including more tissue in the lateral bite and half of the stitch than in the medial bite and half of the stitch and recognizing that the interval between the stitches on the medial aspect of a row of suture stitches will be closer together than will be the interval between the stitches on the lateral aspect of a row of suture stitches.

Keeping this important difference of angle in mind, repair the mediolateral episiotomy in the same sequence of suture stitches and steps as repair of a midline episiotomy (see procedure earlier in this section):

1. Insert a tamponade.
2. Identify the pertinent structures.
3. Repair the vaginal mucosa.
4. Repair the bulbocavernosus muscle.
5. Repair the pubococcygeus and deep transverse perineal muscles with one layer of deep interrupted stitches.
6. Repair the superficial transverse perineal muscle with another layer of deep interrupted stitches.
7. Do a rectal examination to check for sutures in the rectum.
8. Repair the perineal subcutaneous fascia.
9. Close the skin edges.
10. Tie off the suture.
11. Remove the tampon.
12. Do a vaginal examination.
13. Do a rectovaginal examination.
14. Do a rectal examination.

REPAIR OF FIRST AND SECOND DEGREE LACERATIONS AND SULCUS TEARS

First degree (1°) lacerations are those that involve the vaginal mucosa, posterior fourchette, and perineal skin. Second degree (2°) lacerations are those that involve the vaginal mucosa, posterior fourchette, perineal skin, and perineal muscles. Muscle involvement depends on the depth and direction of the tear, therefore possibly involving any or all of the following: bulbocavernosus, superificial transverse perineal, deep transverse perineal, and pubococcygeus of the levator ani.

Sulcus tears are a type of second degree laceration in which the vaginal mucosa and underlying tissue lacerates along one (unilateral) or both (bilateral) sides of the posterior column of the vagina instead of up the middle. The posterior column of the vagina is a longitudinal ridge of the inner surface of the lining extending the length of the vagina. The lateral edges of the column as they meld into the lateral vaginal walls create a slight groove (sulcus) from which a laceration extending any distance up this groove derives its name.

Repair of first degree lacerations depends on their extent. Some vaginal nicks or skid marks barely lacerate the vaginal mucosa and will heal by themselves without stitches since the edges approximate and stay together once the woman's legs are together again. More extensive first degree lacerations can be repaired using the blanket suture stitch for the vaginal mucosa, the continuous suture stitch for the perineal fascia, and the continuous mattress suture stitch for subcuticular closure of the skin edges.

Repair of second degree lacerations uses the same sequence of suture stitches and steps (1 to 14) as does repair of episiotomies. However, lacerations often are jagged wounds with ragged edges, making approximation of tissue more difficult. Care must also be taken to place all stitches in accord with the angle of the wound, recognizing that the angle may change in a jagged tear.

Repair of sulcus tears differs only in the repair of the vaginal mucosa if it is a bilateral sulcus tear. In this event there are two apexes and two suture lines of blanket stitches to close the separate tears in the vaginal mucosa. At their common base one line of suture stitches is tied off with a final stitch and a square knot while the other continues to draw the larger base opening together. Sulcus tears usually are deep lacerations and often necessitate two layers of deep interrupted stitches. Because of this, you may want to repair the vaginal mucosa just a stitch or two into the common base of the bilateral tear for approximation of the tissues, then put in your deep interrupted stitches, and then return to complete your repair of the vaginal mucosa.

REPAIR OF THIRD DEGREE LACERATIONS

Third degree (3°) lacerations are those that involve the vaginal mucosa, posterior fourchette, perineal skin, perineal muscles (which ones depending on the depth of the tear); and external anal sphincter. Some authorities refer to this as a partial third degree laceration, with a complete third degree laceration involving also the anterior rectal wall. Other authorities refer to this latter as a fourth degree laceration; this is the designation given it in this book. Sometimes the equivalent of a third degree laceration is cut deliberately (sphincterotomy). Third degree lacerations may occur in deliveries in which no episiotomy has been cut; however, frequently they are a lacerated extension of a midline episiotomy.

The first step in repair of a third degree laceration is to identify it. This is done as follows:

1. Observation. Observe for the ends of the torn external anal sphincter in the open wound. As the torn ends retract, these are found flush with, or as dimples in, the lateral walls at the bottom of the perineal aspect of the wound near the surface. The muscle fibers of the sphincter are obviously different from the surrounding fascia and look rough and stringy.
2. Palpation. The experienced clinician can often tell by palpating in the open wound

whether or not the rectal sphincter is intact. However, if you are not sure, put another glove over the glove already on your examining hand and put a finger in the woman's rectum. You should be able to palpate the sphincter between your finger inside the rectum and your thumb outside the rectum or to feel its absence anteriorly in the area of the perineal laceration. Be sure to discard the cover glove as soon as you finish with your rectal palpation because it is grossly contaminated.

3. Ask the woman to tighten her rectal sphincter if she is able. You can observe the constriction of the sphincter and also feel it close around your palpating rectal finger if it is intact. It is not possible for her to tighten her sphincter if she has had any type of spinal anesthesia or is under the effects of a pudendal block.
4. The final proof is when you grasp each torn end with an Allis clamp and pull them towards each other, causing them to meet by crossing the Allis clamps and thereby demonstrating the drawing up of perineal tissue on both sides.

Repair of the lacerated external anal sphincter is with interrupted stitches approximating the torn ends grasped by the Allis clamps. Inclusion of the anterior and posterior fascial layers will strengthen the repair. Use 2-0 chromic catgut suture. The remainder of the repair is the same as for repair of an episiotomy or a second degree laceration. Some clinicians prefer to first anchor a 3-0 chromic catgut suture within the inferior apex of the skin extension of the laceration and take a few subcuticular stitches, then laying it aside until the end. They do this in order to avoid later difficulty, which sometimes arises, from being unable to visualize this apex after repair of the sphincter.

After repairing the sphincter and before continuing with the remainder of the repair, do a rectal examination to make sure that you have not placed any suture through the rectal mucosa. If you have, that suture will have to be removed so that it does not become a pathway for infection or cause the development of a fistula. Either put on a cover glove which you remove and discard after the examination, or use the glove you have on and change gloves after the examination.

REPAIR OF FOURTH DEGREE LACERATIONS

Fourth degree (4°) lacerations are those that involve the vaginal mucosa, posterior fourchette, perineal skin, perineal muscles (which ones depending on the depth of the tear); external anal sphincter, and anterior rectal wall. After identification of the tear in the anterior rectal wall and the torn ends of the anal sphincter, repair is begun with repair of the anterior rectal wall. This is repaired in two layers with 4-0 chromic catgut on a swaged-on atraumatic needle:

1. The first layer starts at the apex and consists of a row of interrupted stitches placed in the rectal submucosa to approximate the rectal mucosa without placing stitches in the lumen of the bowel. This suturing requires painstaking care.
2. The second layer covers the first layer and consists of either a row of interrupted stitches or a continuous suture line approximating the overlaying layers of fascia. This layer reinforces the line of repair.

After checking for suture in the rectal lumen, repair the external anal sphincter as described for repair of a third degree laceration, and the remainder of the laceration as described for repair of an episiotomy or a second degree laceration. Special care must be taken in rebuilding the muscle layers of the perineal body which have been totally rent.

REPAIR OF PERIURETHRAL LACERATIONS

Periurethral lacerations derive their name from the fact that they occur near the urethra. Usually they are longitudinal lacerations which follow, for a variable distance, the general contour of the vestibule of the perineum. They vary in depth as well as in length, with the longest extending into the clitoris. At other times they may be transverse lacerations extending into the labia minora. Their repair depends on their depth or, if superficial, whether or not they are bleeding (either actively or oozing), or the need for repair on a cosmetic basis. Repair of any periurethral laceration close to the urethra should be preceded by insertion of a urinary catheter to prevent accidental closure of the urethra.

Small superficial periurethral lacerations will heal spontaneously without stitches, as the edges of the tear will be approximated when the woman's legs are together again. If you are unsure that a laceration fits this category, you may take a single interrupted stitch in the middle of the laceration to facilitate this approximation. Any laceration that is oozing must be repaired. Larger periurethral lacerations can be repaired with interrupted sutures. However, it is more cosmetic to use a mattress or, if deep enough, a layer of continuous suture covered with a subcuticular closure using mattress suture stitches.

All periurethral lacerations should be repaired with 3-0 chromic catgut on a swaged-on needle, except clitoral lacerations, for which 4-0 chromic catgut is used. Such repairs challenge the ingenuity and artistry of the clinician for a cosmetic result since they often involve jagged skin edges. Because of this, there is no precise pattern or sequence of stitches as enumerated for repair of the other lacerations and for episiotomies. Instead you have an arsenal of skills in various suture stitches, a knowledge of the pertinent anatomy, a gentle approach, and a caring philosophy.

REPAIR OF CERVICAL LACERATIONS

The keys to quick and easy repair of cervical lacerations are two:

1. Good visualization. This means proper placement of the light source, retraction of the vaginal wall, effective use of the ring forceps on the cervix to bring the cervix and its laceration into full view, and a well contracted uterus so obscuring bleeding is minimal.
2. An extra pair of hands. An assistant is invaluable in this situation to hold the retractors that will enable good visualization.

Cervical lacerations more than approximately 1 centimeter in length should be repaired in order to prevent possible future problems that might occur if left unrepaired — erosions, chronic ascending infections, and so forth. Repair is with 2-0 chromic catgut on a swaged-on needle. Cervical lacerations that extend into the lower uterine segment require repair by the physician.

Approximation of the two sides of the tear is facilitated by the placement of a ring forceps on each side of the laceration. These should be close enough to the edges to be of use but far enough away from the edges that the bites of the stitches can be taken without sewing through the ring of the forceps and thereby including it in a stitch. On longer lacerations forceps impingement can be avoided for a while by clamping the ring forceps only on the lower portion of the laceration, which means they will be out of the way during repair of the upper reaches of the laceration.

Cervical lacerations are repaired with either interrupted stitches, or a continuous suture, or a blanket (continuous locked) suture. The first stitch should be placed approximately 1 centimeter above (beyond) the apex of the laceration to catch any retracted blood vessels. Care should be taken in the placement of each stitch approximating the two sides of the tear that only one side of the cervix is included in the stitch, thereby maintaining the patency of the cervical canal.

REFERENCE

1. Zikria, B. *Manual of Surgical Knots.* Somerville, N. J.: Ethicon, 1981.

61

Gestational Age Assessment

Mead Johnson and Company has developed and mass produced the "Unified System for Gestational Age Evaluation and Classification of the Newborn." This system includes forms for estimation of gestational age based on a rating of neuromuscular and physical maturity. These forms are reproduced here as Figure 61-1, Tables 61-1 and 61-2, and in the following description of the procedure to be used in classifying babies by estimated gestational age (1).

The assessment should be unhurried, systematic, and complete. It should be done when the infant is assumed stable and in the *quiet alert* state. See Figure 61-1 for the scoring form and proceed as follows:

1. Fill in information from the infant's record, concerning:
   a. Gestation by history (EDC) in weeks
   b. Birth date and hour
   c. APGAR score at 1 minute and 5 minutes
2. Perform assessment of Neuromuscular Maturity as instructed in Table 61-1. Mark the appropriate square on Figure 61-1 for each of the six areas evaluated (X for first exam and O for second exam).

3. Perform assessment of Physical Maturity in accord with Table 61-2. Mark the appropriate square on Figure 61-1 for each of the six areas evaluated (X for first exam and O for second exam).
4. Add up the values given for the six areas of the Neuromuscular Maturity assessment plus the score for the six areas of the Physical Maturity assessment.
5. Using the Maturity Rating Chart in Figure 61-1, determine the Estimated Gestational Age in weeks, using the total score obtained in Step 4.
6. Record the date, time, and age at examination, and place signature in designated area.

REFERENCE

1. "Unified System for Gestational Age Evaluation and Classification of the Newborn." Evansville, Indiana: Mead Johnson and Company, 1977.

TABLE 61-1.   Assessment of Neuromuscular Maturity*

Procedure	Scoring	
Posture: with the infant supine and quiet, score as indicated at right	Arms and legs extended	= 0
	Slight or moderate flexion of hips and knees	= 1
	Moderate to strong flexion of hips and knees	= 2
	Legs flexed and abducted, arms slightly flexed	= 3
	Full flexion of arms and legs	= 4
Square window: flex the hand at the wrist; exert pressure sufficient to get as much flexion as possible	The angle between the hypothenar eminence and the anterior aspect of the forearm is measured and scored (see Fig. 61-1); *do not rotate the wrist*	
Arm recoil: with the infant supine, fully flex the forearm for 5 seconds, then fully extend by pulling the hands and release	Score arm reaction according to:	
	Extended or random movements — 180°	= 0
	Incomplete or partial flexion — 100–180°	= 2
	Increased flexion — 90–100°	= 3
	Brisk return to full flexion — < 90°	= 4
Popliteal angle: with the infant supine and the pelvis flat on the examining surface, the leg is flexed on the thigh and the thigh fully flexed with the use of one hand; with the other hand, the leg is then extended	The angle attained is scored as indicated in Figure 61-1	
Scarf sign: with the infant supine, take the infant's hand and draw it across the neck and as far across the opposite shoulder as possible; assistance to the elbow is permissible by lifting it across the body	Score according to the location of the elbow:	
	Elbow reaches the opposite anterior axillary line	= 0
	Elbow between opposite anterior axillary line and midline of thorax	= 2
	Elbow at midline of thorax	= 3
	Elbow does not reach midline of thorax	= 4
Heel-to-ear maneuver: with the infant supine, hold the infant's foot with one hand and move it as near to the head as possible *without forcing it*; keep the pelvis flat on the examining surface	Score according to Figure 61-1	

*Reproduced by permission of Mead Johnson and Company, Evansville, Indiana 47721.

ESTIMATION OF GESTATIONAL AGE BY MATURITY RATING

Symbols: X - 1st Exam   O - 2nd Exam

NEUROMUSCULAR MATURITY

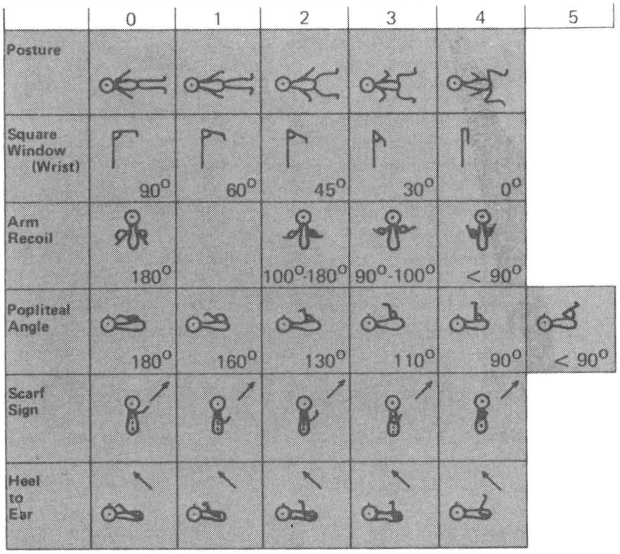

Scoring system: Ballard JL, *et al*: A Simplified Assessment of Gestational Age, Pediatr Res 11:374, 1977. Figures adapted from "Classification of the Low-Birth-Weight Infant" by AY Sweet in Care of the High-Risk Infant by MH Klaus and AA Fanaroff, WB Saunders Co, Philadelphia, 1977, p. 47.

	0	1	2	3	4	5
Posture						
Square Window (Wrist)	90°	60°	45°	30°	0°	
Arm Recoil	180°		100°-180°	90°-100°	< 90°	
Popliteal Angle	180°	160°	130°	110°	90°	< 90°
Scarf Sign						
Heel to Ear						

Gestation by Dates _____ wks

Birth Date _____ Hour _____ am pm

APGAR _____ 1 min _____ 5 min

MATURITY RATING

Score	Wks
5	26
10	28
15	30
20	32
25	34
30	36
35	38
40	40
45	42
50	44

PHYSICAL MATURITY

	0	1	2	3	4	5
SKIN	gelatinous red, transparent	smooth pink, visible veins	superficial peeling &/or rash, few veins	cracking pale area, rare veins	parchment, deep cracking, no vessels	leathery, cracked, wrinkled
LANUGO	none	abundant	thinning	bald areas	mostly bald	
PLANTAR CREASES	no crease	faint red marks	anterior transverse crease only	creases ant. 2/3	creases cover entire sole	
BREAST	barely percept.	flat areola, no bud	stippled areola, 1–2 mm bud	raised areola, 3–4 mm bud	full areola, 5–10 mm bud	
EAR	pinna flat, stays folded	sl. curved pinna, soft with slow recoil	well-curv. pinna, soft but ready recoil	formed & firm with instant recoil	thick cartilage, ear stiff	
GENITALS Male	scrotum empty, no rugae		testes descending, few rugae	testes down, good rugae	testes pendulous, deep rugae	
GENITALS Female	prominent clitoris & labia minora		majora & minora equally prominent	majora large, minora small	clitoris & minora completely covered	

SCORING SECTION

	1st Exam=X	2nd Exam=O
Estimating Gest. Age by Maturity Rating	_____ Weeks	_____ Weeks
Time of Exam	Date _____ am Hour _____ pm	Date _____ am Hour _____ pm
Age at Exam	_____ Hours	_____ Hours
Signature of Examiner	_____ M.D.	_____ M.D.

FIGURE 61-1.   (Reprinted by permission of Mead Johnson and Company, Evansville, Indiana 47721.)

TABLE 61-2.   Scoring System for Physical Maturity*

External Sign	0	1	2	3	4
Skin:					
Texture	Very thin, gelatinous	Thin and smooth	Smooth; medium thickness. Rash or superficial peeling	Slight thickening. Superficial cracking and peeling, especially of hands and feet	Thick and parchmentlike; superficial or deep cracking
Color	Dark red	Uniformly pink	Pale pink; variable over body	Pale; only pink over ears, lips, palms, or soles	
Opacity (trunk)	Numerous veins and venules clearly seen, especially over abdomen	Veins and tributaries seen	A few large vessels clearly seen over abdomen	A few large vessels seen indistinctly over abdomen	No blood vessels seen
Lanugo (over back)	No lanugo	Abundant; long and thick over whole back	Hair thinning, especially over lower back	Small amount of lanugo and bald areas	At least half of back devoid of lanugo
Plantar creases	No skin creases	Faint red marks over anterior half of sole	Definite red marks over > anterior half; indentations over < anterior third	Indentations over > anterior third	Definite deep indentations over > anterior third

Breast:					
Areola	Nipple barely visible; no areola	Nipple well defined; areola smooth and flat, diameter < 0.75 cm.	Areola stippled, edge not raised, diameter < 0.75 cm.	Areola stippled, edge raised, diameter > 0.75 cm.	Full areola
Bud	No breast bud palpable	Breast bud on one or both sides, < 0.5 mm. diameter	Breast bud both sides; one or both 1–2 mm.	Breast bud both sides; one or both 3–4 mm.	Breast bud both sides; one or both 5–10 mm.
Ear:					
Form	Pinna flat and shapeless, little or no incurving of edge	Incurving of part of edge of pinna	Partial incurving whole of upper pinna	Well-defined incurving whole of upper pinna	Thick ear cartilage
Firmness	Pinna soft, easily folded, no recoil	Pinna soft, easily folded, slow recoil	Cartilage to edge of pinna, but soft in places, ready recoil	Pinna firm, cartilage to edge; instant recoil	Ear stiff
Genitals:					
Male	Neither testis in scrotum; no rugae		At least one testis high in scrotum; few rugae	At least one testis down; good rugae	Testes pendulous; deep rugae
Female (with hips ½ abducted)	Labia majora widely separated, labia minora protruding; prominent clitoris		Labia majora and minora equally prominent	Labia majora almost covers labia minora	Clitoris and labia minora completely covered

*Reproduced by permission of Mead Johnson and Company, Evansville, Indian 47721.

BIBLIOGRAPHY FOR PART VII

Anderson, M. *Principles of Wound Healing in the Repair of the Episiotomy.* Hawthorne, N. Y.: Margaret Anderson, 1975.

Bates, B. *A Guide to Physical Examination.* Philadelphia: Lippincott, 1974.

Bonica, J. J. *Principles and Practice of Obstetric Analgesia & Anesthesia.* Philadelphia: F. A. Davis, 1967.

Caldeyro-Barcia, R. The influence of maternal position during the second stage of labor. *ICEA Conference Proceedings,* 1978.

Cavanagh, D. et al. *Obstetric Emergencies, 3rd.* Philadelphia: Harper & Row, 1982.

College of Medicine and Dentistry of New Jersey, New Jersey Medical School, Nurse-Midwifery Education Program. Curriculum Modules: Base Skills, Physical Assessment, and Pelvic Gynecological Screening, 1975.

Department of Health, Education and Welfare, Public Health Service, Health Services and Mental Health Administration, Center for Disease Control, State and Community Services Division, Venereal Disease Branch. *Criteria and Techniques for the Diagnosis of Gonorrhea.* (pamphlet) Atlanta, Georgia, 1972.

Garrey, M. M. et al. *Obstetrics Illustrated, 3rd.* New York: Churchill Livingstone, 1980.

Goss, C. M. (Ed.). *Gray's Anatomy of the Human Body,* (29th.) Philadelphia: Lea & Febiger, 1973.

Greenhill, J. P., and Friedman, E. A. *Biological Principles and Modern Practice of Obstetrics.* Philadelphia: Saunders, 1974.

Haagensen, C. D. *Diseases of the Breast,* (2nd.) Philadelphia: Saunders, 1971.

Hibbard, L., Ulene, A., and Christensen, W. Submodule 1: Anatomy and physiology of the breast. *OMNI Module: Breast Examination.* N. J.: Ortho Pharmaceutical, 1974.

Jeffcoate, T. N. A. *Principles of Gynaecology, 4th.* New York: Butterworth, 1975.

Judge, R., and Zuidema, G. D. (Eds.). *Physical Diagnosis: A Physiologic Approach to the Clinical Examination, 2nd.* Boston: Little, Brown, 1968.

Klink, E. W. Perineal nerve block. *Obstet. Gynecol.* 1:136, 1953.

Liston, J., and Liston E. H., Jr. The mirror pelvic examination: Assessment in a clinic setting. *J. Obstet. Gynecol. Neonat. Nurs.,* p. 47. (March/April) 1978.

Manual of Operative Procedure and Surgical Knots. Somerville, N. J.: Ethicon, 1970.

Medical University of South Carolina, College of Nursing, Nurse-Midwifery Education Program. Curriculum Modules: Base Skills, Physical Assessment, Pelvic/Gynecology, and Antepartal, 1975.

Myers, M. B. Sutures and wound healing. *Am. J. Nurs.* 71:1725, 1971.

Myles, M. F. *A Textbook for Midwives, 6th and 8th.* London: Livingstone, 1968 and 1975.

Netter, F. H. *The Ciba Collection of Medical Illustrations, Volume II: Reproductive System.* Summit, N. J.: Ciba Pharmaceutical Company, 1965.

Noble, E. Rationale for prenatal and postpartum exercises, *International Childbirth Education Association Proceedings,* 1978.

OMNI. *Module: Breast Examination.* Raritan, N. J. Ortho Pharmaceutical, 1974.

Oxorn, H., and Foote, W. R. *Human Labor and Birth, 4th.* New York: Appleton-Century-Crofts, 1980.

Prior, J. A., and Silberstein, J. S. *Physical Diagnosis.* St. Louis: Mosby, 1969.

Pritchard, J. A., MacDonald, P. C., and Gant N. F. *Williams Obstetrics, 17th.* Norwalk Conn.: Appleton-Century-Crofts, 1985.

Reid, D. E., Ryan, K. J., and Benirschke, K. *Principles and Management of Human Reproduction.* Philadelphia: Saunders, 1972.

State University of New York, Downstate Medical Center, College of Health Related Professions, Nurse-Midwifery Education Program. Curriculum Modules: Physical Assessment, Pelvic, and Antepartal, 1974.

Steer, C. M. *Maloy's Evaluation of the Pelvis in Obstetrics, 3rd.* New York: Plenum, 1975.

Taub, H. and Walker, L. *Student Manual for Fundamental Skills in the Clinical Laboratory, Unit 1: Specimen Processing — Drawing Capillary Blood.* Los Angeles: Allied Health Professions Project, University of California, 1971.

Taub, H., and Walker L. *Student Manual for Fundamental Skills in the Clinical Laboratory, Unit 1: Specimen Processing — Drawing Venous Blood.* Los Angeles: Allied Health Professions Project, University of California, 1972.

Taylor, E. S. *Beck's Obstetrical Practice, 9th.* Baltimore: Williams & Wilkins, 1971.

Thoms, H. *Pelvimetry.* New York: Hoeber-Harper, 1956.

Thorek, P. *Anatomy in Surgery.* Philadelphia: Lippincott, 1962.

University of Mississippi Medical Center, Nurse-Midwifery Education Program. Curriculum Modules: Base Skills, Physical Assessment, Pelvic/Gynecology, and Antepartal, 1973–1975, and Intrapartum, 1973 and 1976.

Warwick, R., and Williams, P. L. (Eds.). *Gray's Anatomy, 35th.* Philadelphia: Saunders, 1973.

Wiedenbach, E. *Family-Centered Maternity Nursing, 2nd.* New York: G. P. Putnam's Sons, 1967.

Wilds, P. L. Transvaginal pudendal-nerve block: An improved anatomical approach. *Obstet. Gynecol.* 8:385, 1956.

Ziegel, E., and VanBlarcom, C. C. *Obstetric Nursing, 6th.* New York: Macmillan, 1972.

Zikria, B. A. *Manual of Surgical Knots.* Somerville, N. J.: Ethicon, 1981.

Index

Index